Vascular and Interventional Imaging

CASE REVIEW

Series Editor

David M. Yousem, MD, MBA
Professor of Radiology
Director of Neuroradiology
Russell H. Morgan Department of Radiology and Radiological Science
The Johns Hopkins Medical Institutions
Baltimore, Maryland

Series Foreword

I have been very gratified by the popularity and positive feedback that the authors of the Case Review series have received on the publication of their volumes. Reviews in journals and online sites as well as word-of-mouth comments have been uniformly favorable. The authors have done an outstanding job in filling the niche of an affordable, easy-to-access, case-based learning tool that supplements the material in The Requisites series. I have been told by residents, fellows, and practicing radiologists that the Case Review series books are the ideal means for studying for rotations and clinical practice.

Although some students learn best in a non-interactive study book mode, others need the anxiety or excitement of being quizzed. The selected format for the Case Review series (which consists of showing a few images needed to construct a differential diagnosis and then asking a few clinical and imaging questions) was designed to simulate the board examination experience. The only difference is that the Case Review books provide the correct answer and immediate feedback. The limit and range of the reader's knowledge are tested through scaled cases ranging from relatively easy to very hard. The Case Review series also offers feedback on the answers, a brief discussion of each case, a link back to the pertinent The Requisites volume, and up-to-date references from the literature. In addition, we have recently included labeled figures, figure legends, and supplemental figures in a new section at the end of the book, which provide the reader more information about the case and diagnosis.

Because of the popularity of online learning, we have been rolling out new editions on the web. The Case Reviews are now hosted online at https://expertconsult.inkling.com. The interactive test-taking format allows users to get real-time feedback, "pinch-and-zoom" figures for easier viewing, and links to supplemental figures and online references. Personally, I am very excited about the future. Join us.

David M. Yousem

Vascular and Interventional Imaging

CASE REVIEW

Third Edition

Wael E. Saad, MBBCh, FSIR
Professor of Radiology
Director, Vascular & Interventional Radiology
Director, Neurointerventional Radiology
Department of Radiology
University of Michigan Medical Center
Ann Arbor, Michigan

Minhaj S. Khaja, MD, MBA
Assistant Professor of Radiology
Vascular & Interventional Radiology
Department of Radiology
University of Michigan Medical Center
Ann Arbor, Michigan

Suresh Vedantham, MD
Professor of Radiology & Surgery
Mallinckrodt Institute of Radiology
Washington University School of Medicine
St. Louis, Missouri

ELSEVIER

ELSEVIER

1600 John F. Kennedy Blvd.
Ste 1800
Philadelphia, PA 19103-2899

VASCULAR AND INTERVENTIONAL IMAGING, CASE REVIEW   ISBN: 978-1-4557-7630-6

Notices

Knowledge and best practice in this field are constantly changing. As new research and experience broaden our understanding, changes in research methods, professional practices, or medical treatment may become necessary.

Practitioners and researchers must always rely on their own experience and knowledge in evaluating and using any information, methods, compounds, or experiments described herein. In using such information or methods they should be mindful of their own safety and the safety of others, including parties for whom they have a professional responsibility.

With respect to any drug or pharmaceutical products identified, readers are advised to check the most current information provided (i) on procedures featured or (ii) by the manufacturer of each product to be administered, to verify the recommended dose or formula, the method and duration of administration, and contraindications. It is the responsibility of practitioners, relying on their own experience and knowledge of their patients, to make diagnoses, to determine dosages and the best treatment for each individual patient, and to take all appropriate safety precautions.

To the fullest extent of the law, neither the Publisher nor the authors, contributors, or editors, assume any liability for any injury and/or damage to persons or property as a matter of products liability, negligence or otherwise, or from any use or operation of any methods, products, instructions, or ideas contained in the material herein.

Library of Congress Cataloging-in-Publication Data
Saad, Wael E., author.
  Vascular and interventional imaging / Wael E. Saad, Minhaj S. Khaja, Suresh Vedantham. – Third edition.
      p. ; cm. – (Case review series)
  Preceded by Vascular and interventional imaging / Nael E.A. Saad, Suresh Vedantham, Jennifer Gould. 2nd ed. c2010.
  Includes bibliographical references and indexes.
  ISBN 978-1-4557-7630-6 (pbk. : alk. paper)
  I. Khaja, Minhaj S., authr. II. Vedantham, Suresh, author. III. Saad, Nael E. A. Vascular and interventional imaging. Preceded by (work): IV. Title. V. Series: Case review series.
  [DNLM: 1. Vascular Diseases–radiography–Case Reports.   2. Vascular Diseases–radiography–Problems and Exercises.   3. Radiography, Interventional–methods–Case Reports.   4. Radiography, Interventional–methods–Problems and Exercises. WG 18.2]
  RC683.5.R3
  616.1'307572–dc23
                                                                                2015029183

Content Strategist: Robin Carter
Content Development Specialist: Jillian Crull
Publishing Services Manager: Patricia Tannian
Project Manager: Ted Rodgers
Designer: Amy Buxton
Cover photos: Courtesy of Dr. Curtis L. Anderson

Printed in the United States of America

Last digit is the print number: 9   8   7   6   5   4   3

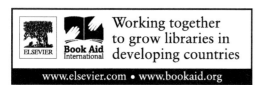

Sarah Allgeier, MD, PhD
University of Michigan Health System
Ann Arbor, Michigan

Jared H. Bailey, MD
University of Michigan Health System
Ann Arbor, Michigan

Alok Bhatt, MD
University of Southern California
Los Angeles, California

Lucia Flors Blasco, MD, PhD
University of Virginia Health System
Charlottesville, Virginia

Adam Bracha, MD, DABR
University of Michigan Health System
Ann Arbor, Michigan

Jordan Castle, MD
The Ohio State University Wexner Medical Center
Columbus, Ohio

Michael Cline, MD
University of Michigan Health System
Ann Arbor, Michigan

Kyle J. Cooper, MD
Miami Cardiac & Vascular Institute
Miami, Florida

Steven Doukides, MD
The Ohio State University Wexner Medical Center
Columbus, Ohio

Jeremy S. Feldman, MD
University of Michigan Health System
Ann Arbor, Michigan

Andrew Ferdinand, MD
University of Virginia Health System
Charlottesville, Virginia

James Frencher, MD, PhD
Mount Sinai School of Medicine
New York, New York

Christopher M. Graham, MD
The Ohio State University Wexner Medical Center
Columbus, Ohio

Jason Grove, MS, PA
University of Michigan Health System
Ann Arbor, Michigan

Klaus D. Hagspiel, MD
University of Virginia Health System
Charlottesville, Virginia

Kevin Hannawa, MD
University of Michigan Health System
Ann Arbor, Michigan

Nicholas J. Hendricks, MD
University of Virginia Health System
Charlottesville, Virginia

Matthew Hermann, MD
University of Michigan Health System
Ann Arbor, Michigan

Alexandria Jo, MD
University of Michigan Health System
Ann Arbor, Michigan

Abrar Khan, MS, DO
Michigan State University Health System
Pontiac, Michigan

Mamdouh Khayat, MD
The Ohio State University Wexner Medical Center
Columbus, Ohio

Bill S. Majdalany, MD
University of Michigan Health System
Ann Arbor, Michigan

David M. Mauro, MD
University of Virginia Health System
Charlottesville, Virginia

Douglas Murrey, MD, MS
The Ohio State University Wexner Medical Center
Columbus, Ohio

David Nicholson, RT (R) (CV)
University of Virginia Health System
Charlottesville, Virginia

Andrew Niekamp, MD
University of Texas Medical School at Houston
Houston, Texas

Brandon Olivieri, MD
Mount Sinai Medical Center
Miami Beach, Florida

Kushal Parikh, MD, MBA
University of Michigan Health System
Ann Arbor, Michigan

Nishant Patel, MD, MBA
University of Michigan Health System
Ann Arbor, Michigan

Feraz Rahman, MD, MS
Emory University
Atlanta, Georgia

W. Tania Rahman, MD, BA
University of Michigan Health System
Ann Arbor, Michigan

Arnold Saha, MD
University of Michigan Health System
Ann Arbor, Michigan

William Sherk, MD
University of Michigan Health System
  Ann Arbor, Michigan

Vikram Sood, MD
University of Michigan Health System
  Ann Arbor, Michigan

Andre Uflacker, MD
University of Virginia Health System
  Charlottesville, Virginia

Marco A. Ugas, MD
University of Virginia Health System
  Charlottesville, Virginia

Candace L. White, MA, MD
Mount Sinai Medical Center
  Miami Beach, Florida

Zachary Wilseck, MD
University of Michigan Health System
  Ann Arbor, Michigan

I am happy to present the third edition of *Vascular and Interventional Imaging* of the Case Review Series featuring Drs. Wael E. Saad, Minhaj S. Khaja, and Suresh Vedantham for your reading pleasure. The authors have updated the vascular and non-vascular cases with the latest knowledge and procedures being performed in 2015 and reformatted the material for online education. The material will prepare residents and fellows for general radiology and interventional radiology-based patient care. The emphasis on physics, clinical evaluation, and treatment follows the new emphasis of medicine as espoused by The Joint Commission as well as the Accreditation Council for Graduate Medical Education. However, for those who have specialized in this field, the book will also serve as a challenging review of the subspecialty.

Vascular and Interventional Imaging is one of the most popular works in the Case Review Series. I am sure that this edition will continue that strong favorable history. Congratulations to the authors and to the readers, who will benefit from their wisdom.

David M. Yousem, MD, MBA

The Case Review Series provides an interactive case review format, which challenges the reader to demonstrate both interpretive accuracy and an understanding of the clinical relevance of imaging findings. As such, it could not be better suited to address the unique and dynamic challenges associated with learning interventional radiology.

In the third edition, we showcase numerous diagnostic and therapeutic procedures, which are performed by the modern interventional radiologist. The image of interventional radiology held by typical radiology trainees often reflects only those few case types to which they have been exposed. However, the reader of this book will discover cases involving a broad range of arterial, venous, oncology, portal hypertension, and non-vascular procedures, and will observe their impact upon many disease processes. Included throughout the book, but specifically within the Fair Game and Challenge sections, are cases involving several very new procedures, which define the outer edge of interventional radiology knowledge in 2015. Our sincere hope is that the "impressive" display of this broad spectrum will stimulate trainees to explore the possibilities of subspecializing in this exciting field.

Additionally, the reader will notice that a significant amount of presented material pertains to the proper *clinical evaluation* and *treatment* of patients. In our view, this material is critical in enabling the reader to develop and convey (to referring physicians or colleagues) a fundamentally mature procedure-related clinical judgment level, which every radiologist should possess. The speed with which interventionalists are adopting the practice patterns and responsibilities of our clinical colleagues in other disciplines is accelerating, and only a superb grounding in clinical and therapeutic principles will enable the modern trainee to keep pace.

In the third edition, we have added several procedures that have developed and gained favor in the field of modern Interventional Radiology. We also have strived to add multiple imaging modalities to as many cases as possible in order to direct the reader's eye to the findings across different types of studies. Finally, we have updated references and existing case discussions to reflect the current data in the literature.

We certainly hope that *Vascular and Interventional Imaging* will prove to be a valuable resource for all current practitioners and trainees in Vascular and Interventional Radiology.

Wael E. Saad, MBBCh, FSIR
Minhaj S. Khaja, MD, MBA
Suresh Vedantham, MD

We sincerely thank and acknowledge the many contributions of our interventional radiology colleagues. Specifically, we are indebted to Drs. Alan Matsumoto, David Williams, Daniel Brown, Thomas Vesely, Narasimham Dasika, J. Fritz Angle, Klaus Hagspiel, Bill Majdalany, James Duncan, David Hovsepian, Michael Darcy, Sailendra Naidu, and Daniel Picus for being exceedingly generous in sharing the clinical gems hidden in their personal teaching files. We appreciate the help of Zainab Ashraf in preparing the individual case templates. Many thanks also go to our publishing team at Elsevier: Katy Meert, Jillian Crull, and Robin Carter. We also acknowledge Series editor Dr. David Yousem for his vision, guidance, and encouragement, and for the wonderful opportunity he has given us.

CONTENTS

Opening Round

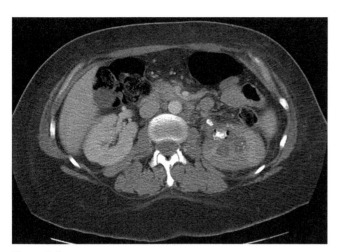

Figure 1-1

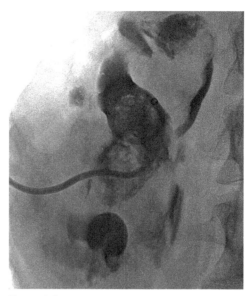

Figure 1-2

HISTORY: A 24-year-old female presenting with fever and dysuria.

1. Which of the following would be included in the differential diagnosis for the imaging findings presented? (Choose all that apply.)
   A. Urothelial carcinoma
   B. Renal artery stenosis
   C. Hydronephrosis
   D. Pyonephrosis

2. What is the ideal puncture site into the kidney for percutaneous nephrostomy tube placement?
   A. Anterior calyx
   B. Posterior calyx
   C. Upper pole calyx
   D. Lower pole calyx

3. What is the most common pathogen associated with pyonephrosis?
   A. *Bacteroides fragilis*
   B. *Staphylococcus aureus*
   C. *Escherichia coli*
   D. *Klebsiella pneumoniae*

4. Two days following the placement of a percutaneous nephrostomy tube and the initiation of intravenous antibiotics, the patient remains febrile and tachycardiac. What is the most likely diagnosis?
   A. Extrarenal catheter placement
   B. Pulmonary embolus
   C. Perinephric hematoma
   D. Perinephric abscess

See Supplemental Figures section for additional figures and legends for this case.

CASE 1

Pyonephrosis

1. **C and D.** The computed tomography (CT) image demonstrates an obstructed left renal collecting system with multiple calculi, gas, and a heterogeneous delayed left nephrogram. These findings are consistent with pyonephrosis.

2. **B.** The optimal location for access into the renal collecting is via a posterior calyx. This is the best location for two main reasons. First, this approach may traverse Brodel's avascular plane, which can reduce the incidence of bleeding complications. Second, posterior calyceal access results in a straighter percutaneous tract into the renal collecting system. This results in easier subsequent catheter placement, dilation, and manipulation.

3. **C.** *E. coli* is the most common pathogen implicated in pyonephrosis (as in this case). *K. pneumoniae* is also a common urinary tract pathogen, although not as common as *E. coli*.

4. **D.** Given the contrast extravasation noted during the percutaneous nephrostomy catheter placement (Figure S1-2) and the patient's persistent sepsis, a perinephric abscess should be suspected. Subsequent imaging (Figure S1-3) confirmed the presence of a perinephric abscess which required drain placement. A perinephric hematoma is also possible, but not as likely based on the imaging and clinical findings.

Comment

Patient Presentation

The CT examination demonstrates left hydronephrosis and collecting system gas (Figure S1-1). Although percutaneous nephrostomy tubes can be inserted electively for relief of urinary obstruction, clinical signs of infection are concerning for pyonephrosis: infected urine within the obstructed urinary collecting system. Such patients are at risk for sepsis, and percutaneous nephrostomy should be performed urgently.

In the patient who already exhibits signs of sepsis, percutaneous nephrostomy can be life-saving and must be performed emergently.

Procedural Technique

Percutaneous nephrostomy tubes can be placed using a variety of imaging guidance techniques. If contrast material is already present from an existing study or if an existing ureteral stent or radiopaque renal calculus is present, then fluoroscopic guidance alone may be sufficient. Otherwise, ultrasound-guided or CT-guided puncture of a posterior calyx can be performed (one-pass method). Alternatively, if a dilated posterior calyx is not clearly visible, then the renal pelvis can be punctured with a 22-gauge needle. A small amount of contrast and air are injected to opacify a posterior calyx, which is then definitively punctured using an 18-gauge needle under fluoroscopic guidance (two-pass method) (Figure S1-2).

Etiology

Although any cause of urinary tract obstruction can lead to hydronephrosis or pyonephrosis, more than 50% of cases result from urinary tract calculi. Another common cause is ureteral compression by a pelvic mass lesion. Definitive removal of the obstructing agent should be deferred to a time when the patient's infection has resolved, because excessive manipulation can precipitate sepsis. Complications include perinephric abscess formation (Figures S1-3 and S1-4).

References

Li A, Regalado S. Emergent percutaneous nephrostomy for the diagnosis and management of pyonephrosis. *Semin Intervent Radiol.* 2012;29:218–225.

Watson RA, Esposito M, Richter F. Percutaneous nephrostomy as adjunct management in advanced upper urinary tract infection. *Urology.* 1999;54:234–239.

Cross-reference

Vascular and Interventional Radiology: The Requisites, 2nd ed, 488–495.

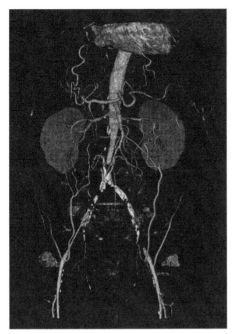

Figure 2-1. *Courtesy of Dr. Klaus D. Hagspiel.*

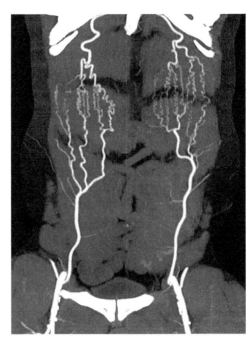

Figure 2-2. *Courtesy of Dr. Klaus D. Hagspiel.*

HISTORY: A 47-year-old male with intermittent claudication.

1. Which of the following is the most likely diagnosis for the imaging findings presented?
   A. Aortic dissection
   B. Aortitis
   C. Aortic occlusion
   D. Midaortic syndrome

2. Which of the following is the collateral pathway from the aorta to the lower extremities shown in this case?
   A. Superior to inferior epigastric artery pathway
   B. Superior mesenteric artery (SMA) to inferior mesenteric artery (IMA) via superior hemorrhoidal arteries
   C. Intercostal/lumbar arteries to circumflex arteries
   D. Intercostal/lumbar arteries to superior gluteal arteries

3. Which symptom is NOT classically seen in Leriche's syndrome?
   A. Hip and buttock claudication
   B. Hypertension
   C. Impotence
   D. Absent femoral pulses

4. What is the treatment of choice for this condition?
   A. Thrombolysis
   B. Endarterectomy
   C. Endovascular aortic repair
   D. Aortobifemoral bypass graft

See Supplemental Figures section for additional figures and legends for this case.

CASE 2

Abdominal Aortic Occlusion

1. **C.** Imaging shows aortoiliac occlusion, which is a result of severe atherosclerotic disease and thrombosis of the abdominal aorta. Mid aortic syndrome, however, is progressive abdominal aortic narrowing, commonly seen in children and young adults.

2. **A.** All of the answer choices represent possible collateral pathways.
   - Subclavian→internal mammary→superior epigastric→inferior epigastric→external iliac artery is the collateral pathway shown in the case, also known as the pathway of Winslow
   - SMA→marginal artery of Drummond/arc of Riolan→IMA→superior hemorrhoidal→middle/inferior hemorrhoidal→external iliac artery
   - Intercostal/lumbar→circumflex→external iliac
   - Intercostal/lumbar→superior gluteal/iliolumbar→internal iliac→external iliac

3. **B.** Leriche's syndrome (aortoiliac occlusive disease) classically includes hip and buttock claudication, absent femoral pulses, and impotence.

4. **D.** Chronic aortoiliac occlusion must be corrected by surgical bypass. In patients who are not surgical candidates, endoluminal recanalization and stenting of the occluded aorta and iliac arteries may be performed. Additionally, given the chronic nature of the disease, thrombolysis will not be effective in relieving the patient of the clot burden.

Comment

Clinical Presentation

Occlusion of the abdominal aorta can result from a variety of causes including trauma, thromboembolism, or iatrogenic dissection. In this case, thrombosis is superimposed on chronic atherosclerotic stenosis, a condition known as Leriche's syndrome (Figure S2-1). In these patients, symptoms of ischemia might not appear until occlusion is imminent, and some patients present after the vessel has occluded. The classic symptoms of Leriche's syndrome are seen in men and include hip and buttock claudication, absent femoral pulses, impotence (due to limitation of blood flow into the internal iliac artery territories), and cool lower extremities.

Treatment Methods

The slow progression of the atherosclerotic occlusion allows the development of large intercostal, lumbar, and epigastric collaterals that provide flow to the iliac arteries and lower-extremity vessels (Figure S2-2). The treatment of choice for Leriche's syndrome is surgical bypass graft placement; in this case, an aortobifemoral bypass graft would be appropriate. Endovascular aortic repair is not the first-line therapy due to the complexity of the recanalization and possible suprarenal aortic dissection or injury.

References

Bosch JL, Huninck MC. Meta-analysis of the results of percutaneous transluminal angioplasty and stent placement for aorto-iliac occlusive disease. *Radiology.* 1997;204:87–96.

Hardman RL, Lopera JE, Cardan RA, Trimmer CK, Josephs SC. Common and rare collateral pathways in aortoiliac occlusive disease: a pictorial essay. *AJR Am J Roentgenol.* 2011;197:19–24.

Cross-reference

Vascular and Interventional Radiology: The Requisites, 2nd ed, 209–214.

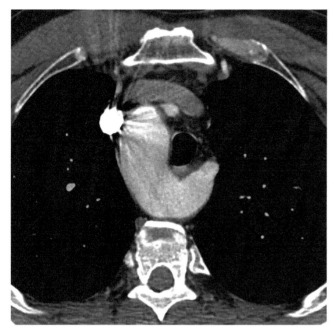

Figure 3-1

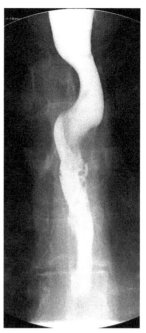

Figure 3-2

HISTORY: A 42-year-old male with difficulty swallowing.

1. Which of the following is the most likely diagnosis for the imaging findings presented?
   A. Pulmonary sling
   B. Left aortic arch with aberrant right subclavian
   C. Right aortic arch with aberrant left subclavian
   D. Right aortic arch with mirror image branching

2. Which of the choices has the highest incidence of associated congenital heart disease?
   A. Right aortic arch with mirror image branching
   B. Right aortic arch with aberrant left subclavian
   C. Pulmonary sling
   D. Left aortic arch with aberrant right subclavian

3. Which of the listed congenital heart defects is most common in patients with this diagnosis?
   A. Aortic coarctation
   B. Atrial septal defect (ASD)
   C. Tetralogy of Fallot (TOF)
   D. Ventricular septal defect (VSD)

4. Dilatation of the origin of an aberrant subclavian artery is known as:
   A. Sano aneurysm
   B. Hutch diverticulum
   C. Diverticulum of Kommerell
   D. Norwood diverticulum

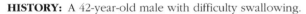

See Supplemental Figures section for additional figures and legends for this case.

CASE 3

Right-Sided Aortic Arch

1. **C.** The computed tomography demonstrates a right-sided aorta with the left subclavian artery coursing behind the trachea to reach the left upper extremity. In patients with a right arch with mirror image branching, the branch vessels course anterior to the trachea just like in a normal arch, but from the opposite side.

2. **A.** Right arch with mirror image branching is associated with congenital heart disease 98% of the time. Right arch with aberrant left subclavian is associated with congenital heart defects 10% of the time.

3. **C.** The most common congenital heart defect in these patients is TOF. TOF consists of right ventricular hypertrophy, overriding aortic arch, VSD, and pulmonary stenosis. VSD, ASD, and coarctation are less commonly seen independently.

4. **C.** Dilatation of the origin of the aberrant subclavian artery is seen in approximately 60% of patients and is known as the diverticulum of Kommerell. Hutch diverticulum is an outpouching of the bladder. Norwood and Sano are both surgeons who have their names attached to congenital heart operations.

Comment

Main Teaching Point

A right-sided aortic arch with aberrant left subclavian artery occurs in 0.05% to 0.10% of the population. The aortic arch passes over the right mainstem bronchus and descends to the right of the esophagus and trachea (Figure S3-1). The left subclavian artery arises as the last branch, often from a diverticulum of Kommerell, as in this case, and passes behind the trachea and esophagus to supply the left arm (Figure S3-2). Symptoms of respiratory and esophageal compression are seen in only 5% of cases. Esophageal compression as a result of the aberrant subclavian artery is called *dysphagia lusoria*. Only 10% of patients have associated congenital heart disease, most commonly TOF.

Description of Anatomic Variants

Right aortic arch can also be seen with mirror-image branching. In this situation, the aortic branch vessels in order are the left brachiocephalic artery, right common carotid artery, and right subclavian artery. More than 98% of these patients have cyanotic congenital heart disease, most commonly TOF.

References

Donnelly LF, Fleck RJ, Pacharn P, et al. Aberrant subclavian arteries: cross-sectional imaging findings in infants and children referred for evaluation of extrinsic airway compression. *Am J Roentgenol.* 2002;178:1269–1274.

Franquet T, Erasmus JJ, Gimenez A. The retrotracheal space: normal anatomic and pathologic appearances. *Radiographies.* 2002;22: S231–S246.

Cross-reference

Vascular and Interventional Radiology: The Requisites, 2nd ed, 177–179.

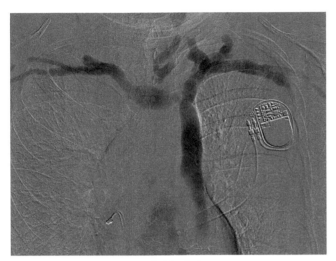

Figure 4-1. *Courtesy of Dr. Minhaj S. Khaja.*

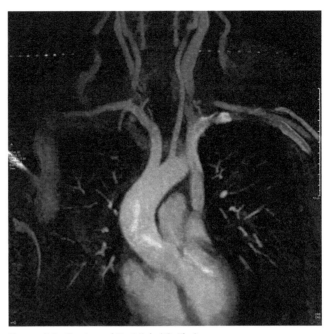

Figure 4-2. *Courtesy of Dr. Minhaj S. Khaja.*

HISTORY: A 55-year-old male with arrhythmia presents for venogram prior to pacemaker upgrade.

1. Which of the following is the most likely diagnosis for the imaging findings presented?
   A. Anomalous pulmonary venous return
   B. Left superior vena cava (SVC)
   C. Left superior intercostal vein
   D. Collateral vessels

2. Where does the aforementioned structure most commonly drain?
   A. Right atrium
   B. Left atrium
   C. Coronary sinus
   D. Pulmonary vein

3. Which of the following is most commonly associated with this anomaly?
   A. Congenital heart disease
   B. Duplicated inferior vena cava
   C. Anomalous pulmonary venous return
   D. Absence of the left brachiocephalic vein

4. Which of the following patients is most likely symptomatic from their variant vascular anatomy?
   A. Left-sided SVC that drains into the coronary sinus
   B. Left-sided SVC that drains into the left atrium
   C. Presence of a left superior intercostal vein
   D. Left aortic arch with an aberrant right subclavian artery

See Supplemental Figures section for additional figures and legends for this case.

CASE 4

Variant Anatomy: Left Superior Vena Cava

1. **B.** This is a persistent left SVC, which results from the failure of regression of left anterior cardinal vein. The left superior intercostal vein is a normal structure and serves as an important collateral pathway in cases of SVC obstruction.

2. **C.** The left SVC most commonly drains into the coronary sinus and into the right atrium. More rarely, it drains into the left atrium. In these cases, there often is associated congenital heart disease.

3. **D.** In most cases, the presence of a persistent left SVC is associated with absence of the left brachiocephalic vein. The venous tributaries, which normally enter the left brachiocephalic vein, drain via the left SVC. A left SVC may be associated with congenital disease.

4. **B.** Patients with a left SVC that drains into the left atrium very commonly have congenital heart disease. A left SVC that drains into the coronary sinus is benign and not symptomatic. The left superior intercostal vein is a normal structure.

Comment

Main Teaching Point

A left SVC results from persistence of the left anterior cardinal vein. This usually occurs in association with congenital heart disease, although it occurs rarely as an isolated abnormality associated with situs inversus. Typically, the left SVC drains to the right atrium via the coronary sinus, but occasionally it drains directly into the left atrium (Figures S4-1 and S4-2).

Other Variant Anatomy

Duplication of the SVC is more common and is even more often associated with congenital heart disease. It can be associated with anomalous pulmonary venous return. Similar to the isolated left SVC, the left moiety typically drains into the coronary sinus.

References

Minniti S, Visentini S, Procacci C. Congenital anomalies of the venae cavae: embryological origin, imaging features and report of three new variants. *Eur Radiol.* 2002;12:2040–2055.

Povoski S, Khabiri H. Persistent left superior vena cava: review of the literature, clinical implications, and relevance of alterations in thoracic central venous anatomy as pertaining to the general principles of central venous access device placement and venography in cancer patients. *World J Surg Oncol.* 2011;9:173.

Cross-reference

Vascular and Interventional Radiology: The Requisites, 2nd ed, 137–138.

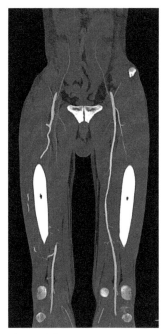

Figure 5-1

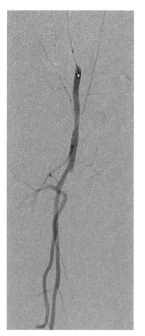

Figure 5-2

HISTORY: A 54-year-old male with chronic right calf claudication.

1. Which of the following is the most likely diagnosis for the imaging findings presented?
   A. External iliac artery occlusion
   B. Superficial femoral artery (SFA) occlusion
   C. Deep vein thrombosis of the femoral vein
   D. Arterial entrapment in Hunter's canal

2. How would you categorize this lesion based on the TransAtlantic InterSociety Consensus (TASC) classification system, based on the fact that this is a 12 cm lesion?
   A. TASC A
   B. TASC B
   C. TASC C
   D. TASC D

3. Under what ankle-brachial index (ABI) would you expect a patient to experience tissue loss?
   A. Less than 1
   B. Less than 0.8
   C. Less than 0.6
   D. Less than 0.4

4. What anatomic structure marks the transition of the SFA to the popliteal artery on a digital subtraction angiogram?
   A. Intercondylar notch
   B. Articulating surface of the femoral condyle
   C. Origin on the geniculate arteries
   D. Medial cortex of the femur

See Supplemental Figures section for additional figures and legends for this case.

CASE 5

Occluded Superficial Femoral Artery

1. **B.** The computed tomography angiogram and initial angiogram image demonstrate occlusion at the origin of the SFA. Additionally noted is a large profunda femoris artery on the angiogram without extensive collateralization.

2. **B.** Given that this is an occlusion of the SFA that is greater than 5 cm, but less than 15 cm, this would be TASC B.

3. **D.** An ABI between 0.9 and 0.41 indicates mild to moderate peripheral arterial disease. An ABI below 0.4 suggests severe peripheral arterial disease called critical limb ischemia. Tissue loss is seen in Rutherford category 5 and 6 disease.

4. **D.** As the SFA crosses the medial femoral cortex, it becomes the popliteal artery.

Comment

Clinical Presentation

The SFA represents an extremely common site of atherosclerotic disease. Stenotic lesions in this vessel are most commonly observed at the level of the adductor (Hunter's) canal. These lesions are a common cause of calf claudication and can contribute (in the presence of other lesions) to rest pain and limb-threatening ischemia. Progressive SFA stenosis often leads to complete SFA occlusion as seen in Figures S5-1 and S5-2.

Imaging Interpretation

When describing a lesion in the SFA, several observations are important to make: (1) The status of the ipsilateral common femoral artery is important because this vessel nearly always represents the source vessel for a therapeutic bypass graft. (2) The point at which the distal circulation reconstitutes, as well as its continuity with pedal flow, determines the distal anastomotic site of the bypass graft. (3) The status of the ipsilateral profunda femoral artery often determines the clinical status of the limb, because this vessel provides the source for the collaterals that reconstitute the distal circulation.

Treatment Methods

The standard treatment of isolated SFA occlusion with popliteal reconstitution is femoropopliteal bypass graft placement. This procedure has a 5-year patency of 50% to 80%, depending on whether the distal anastomosis is placed above or below the knee and depending on the number and quality of patent runoff vessels. Catheter-directed thrombolysis with subsequent angioplasty (Figure S5-3) and stenting can be used to recanalize native SFA occlusions, but patency rates following this procedure are less than those of surgical therapy.

The Rutherford classification system is frequently used to categorize claudicants:

Category 0: Asymptomatic
Category 1: Mild claudication
Category 2: Moderate claudication
Category 3: Severe claudication
Category 4: Rest pain
Category 5: Minor tissue loss
Category 6: Major tissue loss and gangrene

References

Gibbs JM, Peña CS, Benenati JF. Treating the diseased superficial femoral artery. *Tech Vasc Interv Radiol.* 2010;13:37–42.

Hunink M, Wong J, Donaldson M, et al. Revascularization for femoropopliteal disease: a decision and cost-effectiveness analysis. *JAMA.* 1995;274:165–171.

Cross-reference

Vascular and Interventional Radiology: The Requisites, 2nd ed, 343–351.

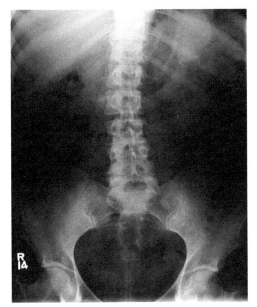

Figure 6-1

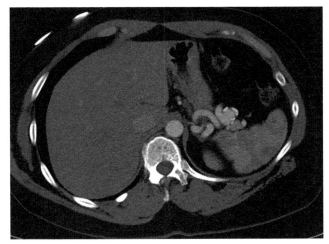

Figure 6-2

HISTORY: A 49-year-old atraumatic female with back pain; incidental finding on plain film with subsequent computed tomography (CT). Normal white count and erythrocyte sedimentation rate.

1. Which of the following is the most likely diagnosis for the imaging findings presented?
   A. Splenic artery pseudoaneurysm
   B. Vasculitis
   C. Splenic artery aneurysm
   D. Fibromuscular dysplasia

2. What is the most common location of a visceral artery aneurysm?
   A. Hepatic artery
   B. Splenic artery
   C. Gastroduodenal artery
   D. Superior mesenteric artery

3. What is the first line of treatment for this lesion?
   A. 1-year follow-up CT
   B. Open surgical ligation
   C. Covered stent placement
   D. Coil embolization

4. What is the most common cause of splenic artery pseudoaneurysm?
   A. Trauma
   B. Pancreatitis
   C. Infection
   D. Iatrogenic

See Supplemental Figures section for additional figures and legends for this case.

CASE 6

Splenic Artery Aneurysm

1. **C.** True splenic aneurysms are overall more common than pseudoaneurysms. True aneurysms have a female predilection, whereas pseudoaneurysms are more common in men. There are no adjacent imaging findings to suggest infection or fibromuscular dysplasia.

2. **B.** Splenic artery aneurysms account for 60% of all visceral aneurysms. The hepatic artery is the second most common location at 20%.

3. **D.** Coil embolization or covered stent exclusion is the treatment of choice for splenic artery aneurysms. In this case, due to the tortuosity of the vessel, coil embolization would be preferred.

4. **B.** While all of the answer choices are possible causes of pseudoaneurysm formation, pancreatitis is the most common.

Comment

Etiology

The splenic artery is the most common site of visceral artery aneurysms (approximately 60%), followed by the hepatic artery (approximately 20%). Splenic artery aneurysms are four times more common in women than men. The most common etiology is medial degeneration with superimposed atherosclerosis. There appears to be some relationship to pregnancy because the majority of women who have splenic artery aneurysms have had at least two pregnancies, and pregnancy is associated with an increased risk of rupture. Other causes of visceral aneurysms include trauma, pancreatitis, infection, congenital portal hypertension, collagen vascular disease, hypersplenism, fibromuscular dysplasia, and vasculitis.

Disease Progression

Many aneurysms are discovered incidentally on cross-sectional imaging or radiograph (Figures S6-1, S6-2, and S6-3). The main risk is aneurysm rupture, which carries a high mortality. These patients typically present with abdominal pain and/or hypotension. Nevertheless, less than 10% of aneurysms rupture, and the majority of ruptures are associated with pregnancy. Therefore, treatment is not recommended for all unruptured aneurysms. Treatment is typically recommended for aneurysms greater than 20 mm, pseudoaneurysms, aneurysms in patients who may become pregnant, and aneurysms in patients who may undergo a liver transplant.

Treatment Methods

Treatment is directed at eliminating flow into the aneurysm sac. Transcatheter embolization is the preferred treatment, and coils are the most commonly used agents (Figures S6-4 and S6-5). It is important to embolize from distal to proximal across the aneurysm neck to prevent retrograde flow into the aneurysm from collateral vessels filling the distal splenic artery. Splenic infarction or abscess formation is rare owing to collateral flow to the spleen. Splenic artery aneurysms can be treated surgically by removing the spleen and aneurysm or by ligating the artery proximal and distal to the aneurysm.

References

Berceli S. Hepatic and splenic artery aneurysms. *Semin Vasc Surg.* 2005;18(4):196–201.

Stanley C. Mesenteric arterial occlusive and aneurysmal disease. *Cardiol Clin.* 2002;20:611–622.

Yasumoto T, Osuga K, Yamamoto H, et al. Long-term outcomes of coil packing for visceral aneurysms: correlation between packing density and incidence of coil compaction or recanalization. *J Vasc Interv Radiol.* 2013;24:1798–1807.

Cross-reference

Vascular and Interventional Radiology: The Requisites, 2nd ed, 256–258.

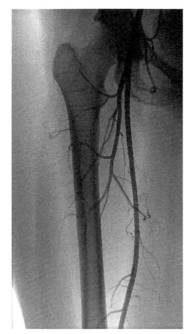

Figure 7-1. *Courtesy of Dr. Alan H. Matsumoto.*

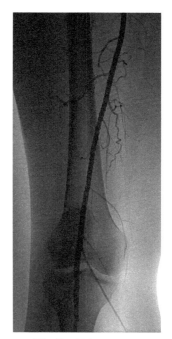

Figure 7-2. *Courtesy of Dr. Alan H. Matsumoto.*

HISTORY: A 30-year-old female with known right calf/ankle venous malformation presenting with increasing leg swelling.

1. Which of the following would be included in the differential diagnosis for the imaging findings presented? (Choose all that apply.)
   A. Fibomuscular dysplasia (FMD)
   B. Standing waves
   C. Popliteal entrapment
   D. Raynaud's phenomenon

2. Which of the following noninvasive techniques can eliminate this finding on further angiography? (Choose all that apply.)
   A. Vasodilators
   B. Decrease of contrast injection rate
   C. Increase of filming rate
   D. Larger volume of contrast

3. What vascular beds most commonly demonstrate this finding? (Choose all that apply.)
   A. Extremity arteries
   B. Mesenteric vessels
   C. Carotid arteries
   D. Internal iliac arteries

4. What is the likely explanation of this finding?
   A. Fibrous bands squeezing the vessels
   B. Motion artifact
   C. Vasculitis
   D. Flow and pressure changes during contrast injection into a high-resistance vascular bed

See Supplemental Figures section for additional figures and legends for this case.

CASE 7

Standing Waves

1. **B.** Standing waves are a regular corrugated appearance of the arteries. FMD is an underlying dysplastic process in the media of the vessel wall. Popliteal entrapment is compression of the popliteal artery by adjacent muscular structures.

2. **A and B.** Standing waves can be reduced by either injecting a vasodilator or injecting a slower rate of contrast. Increasing the frame rate will not decrease the appearance of standing waves.

3. **A and B.** Standing waves are most commonly seen in the extremities and mesenteric vessels. The superficial femoral artery is the most commonly visualized location.

4. **D.** It is noted that flow and pressure changes during contrast injection into a high-resistance vascular bed can cause pressure on the arterial wall.

Comment

Imaging Interpretation

Standing waves are a benign phenomenon of uncertain etiology. As seen in Figures S7-1, S7-2, and S7-3, standing waves have a regular, corrugated appearance of the vessels. The proposed mechanisms for this phenomenon are usually based on vasospasm, particularly given case reports of resolution of standing waves after administration of vasodilators. However, there also have been reports of resolution of standing waves seen on immediate repeat angiography without administration of vasodilators. Other mechanisms for standing waves have been proposed, including a physiological response of the vasculature to rapid injection of contrast or artifact from flow-related disruption of contrast medium layering in vessels. Although standing waves have been reported predominantly during conventional arteriography, they also have been reported in magnetic resonance angiography. In contrast to FMD, a fixed irregular filling defect, standing waves are regular and transient and therefore may not be reproduced on repeat contrast injections.

References

Norton PT, Hagspiel KD. Stationary waves in magnetic resonance angiography. *J Vasc Interv Radiol.* 2005;16:423–424.

Reuter SR, Redman HC, Cho KJ. Vascular diseases. In: *Gastrointestinal Angiography.* 3rd ed. Philadelphia: Saunders; 1986:120–121.

Cross-reference

Vascular and Interventional Radiology: The Requisites, 2nd ed, 15–17.

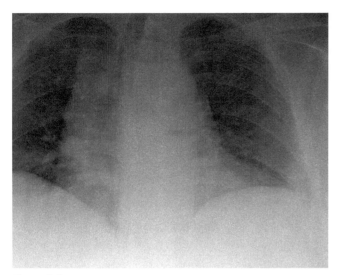

Figure 8-1

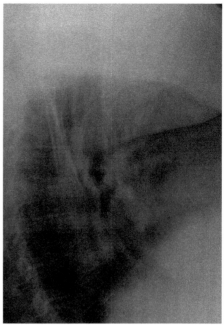

Figure 8-2

HISTORY: A 57-year-old male presents with suspected pneumonia. Recent bedside left peripherally inserted central venous catheter (PICC) placement.

1. Which of the following is the most likely diagnosis for the imaging findings presented?
   A. Central venous catheter tip within the internal jugular (IJ) vein
   B. Central venous catheter tip within the superior vena cava (SVC)
   C. Central venous catheter tip within the azygous vein
   D. Central venous catheter tip within the right atrium

2. What is the major complication associated with a central venous catheter tip in the right atrium?
   A. Arrhythmias
   B. Rapid fibrin sheath formation
   C. Poor flow through the catheter
   D. Spontaneous repositioning of the catheter tip

3. What is the major complication associated with a central venous catheter tip in the upper SVC?
   A. Arrhythmias
   B. Rapid fibrin sheath formation
   C. Poor flow through the catheter
   D. Spontaneous repositioning of the catheter tip

4. A 45-year-old male with chronic renal failure presents for emergent dialysis catheter placement. Which of the following access locations is preferred in this patient?
   A. Subclavian access
   B. Translumbar inferior vena cava (IVC) access
   C. IJ access
   D. Femoral vein access

See Supplemental Figures section for additional figures and legends for this case.

CASE 8

Central Venous Catheter Malposition

1. **C.** The images demonstrate a left PICC with tip curved posteriorly into the azygous vein. The catheter should be repositioned to avoid complications.

2. **A.** A central venous catheter tip within the right atrium is associated with arrhythmias. Spontaneous repositioning of the tip is associated with a tip in the SVC as described in the following question. A fibrin sheath theoretically could form along a catheter in any location but is less common in higher flow areas.

3. **D.** A central venous catheter tip within the SVC is associated with spontaneous repositioning (i.e., into the IJ or contralateral brachiocephalic veins).

4. **B.** The IJ vein is generally the preferred approach for placing long-term catheters and ports. In this specific case, the subclavian vein should be avoided, as the patient may need an upper extremity arteriovenous fistula or graft for hemodialysis in the future. Femoral access is less desirable as femoral catheters limit patient mobility and have higher rates of infection. Translumbar IVC access should only be used if other, more peripheral veins are non-accessible.

Comment

Main Teaching Point

Radiologists can place the entire gamut of central venous catheters: (1) PICC lines: these small-caliber catheters are used for short-term (2 to 6 weeks) venous access and are inserted via an arm vein (Figures S8-1 through S8-4); (2) nontunneled or tunneled (for long-term access) catheters for administering blood transfusions, antibiotics, other parenteral medications, and/or total parenteral nutrition; (3) nontunneled or tunneled pheresis catheters; (4) nontunneled or tunneled hemodialysis catheters; and (5) implantable ports for intermittent access.

Endovascular Management

In general, the IJ vein is the preferred approach for placing tunneled (long-term) catheters and ports. The IJ approach is associated with a lower incidence of catheter migration, pinch-off syndrome, and symptomatic venous occlusion. Furthermore, IJ access spares the subclavian veins; this is extremely important in patients with chronic renal failure for whom upper extremity dialysis access might eventually be needed. For nontunneled catheters, the subclavian vein is generally preferred because chest wall exit sites are associated with a lower infection rate than neck or groin exit sites. However, notable exceptions to this rule include the aforementioned patients with chronic renal failure and those with impaired coagulation, because the subclavian vein is located in a less-compressible location than the IJ. Although most organizational guidelines recommend placing the catheter tip in the distal SVC, a significant number of physicians are placing hemodialysis and pheresis catheters in the proximal right atrium in order to achieve better flow rates.

References

Engstrom B, Horvath J, Steward J, et al. Tunneled internal jugular hemodialysis catheters: impact of laterality and tip position on catheter dysfunction and infection rates. *J Vasc Interv Radiol.* 2013;24:1295–1302.

Schutz J, Patel A, Clark T, et al. Relationship between chest port catheter tip position and port malfunction after interventional radiologic placement. *J Vasc Interv Radiol.* 2004;15:581–587.

Vesely T. Central venous catheter tip position: a continuing controversy. *J Vasc Interv Radiol.* 2003;14:527–534.

Cross-reference

Vascular and Interventional Radiology: The Requisites, 2nd ed, 145–150.

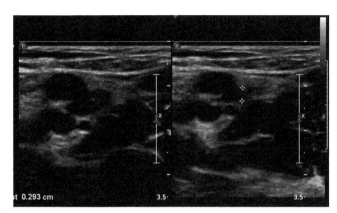

Figure 9-1. *Courtesy of Dr. Minhaj S. Khaja.*

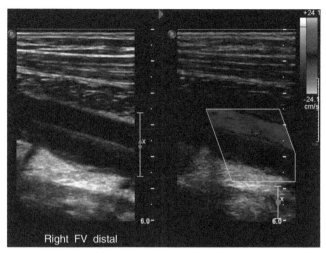

Figure 9-2. *Courtesy of Dr. Minhaj S. Khaja.*

HISTORY: A 35-year-old male with acute onset of lower-extremity swelling.

1. Which of the following would be included in the differential diagnosis for the imaging findings presented? (Choose all that apply.)
   A. Chronic deep venous thrombosis (DVT)
   B. Femoral artery embolism
   C. Acute DVT
   D. Phlebitis

2. Which of the following studies is the first-line modality used in diagnosing this entity?
   A. Magnetic resonance (MR) venography
   B. Doppler and compressional ultrasonography
   C. Nuclear studies
   D. Conventional venography

3. Which of the following clinical manifestations of acute DVT describes the *phlegmasia cerulea dolens* phenomenon?
   A. Edema, pain, swelling, and erythema within the extremity
   B. Pale, painful, extremity with weak pulses; usually transient
   C. Cyanotic, extremely painful, pulseless extremity; limb loss likely
   D. Tender, erythematous, cord-like, palpable veins within the extremity

4. What treatment options are available? (Choose all that apply.)
   A. Systemic anticoagulation
   B. Vena cava filters
   C. Surgical thrombectomy
   D. Catheter-directed thrombolysis

See Supplemental Figures section for additional figures and legends for this case.

CASE 9

Acute Deep Venous Thrombosis

1. **C.** In acute DVT, the filling defect is smooth and usually resides within an enlarged vein. In chronic DVTs, the defect is irregular and contracted, with the involved vein generally appearing smaller in size than normal. Furthermore, as in this case, the absence of collateral veins and varicosities is suggestive of an acute rather than chronic thrombus (<14 days in age). Phlebitis most commonly occurs in the superficial veins of the lower extremity.

2. **B.** Low cost, lack of radiation, and wide availability are some of the major advantages of ultrasonography. MR venography is considered extremely sensitive and specific in the detection of lower-extremity DVT. However, drawbacks of MR venography include cost, time, and relatively limited availability. Finally, while conventional venography remains the gold standard in evaluation of DVT, cost, invasiveness, and radiation have led to its use for intervention rather than diagnosis.

3. **C.** *Phlegmasia cerulea dolens* is extensive venous thrombosis, which results in arterial collapse due to the resultant soft tissue edema. Answer choice A is a description of the garden-variety DVT. Answer choice B describes the complication of phlegmasia alba dolens, which is thought to be caused by arterial spasm secondary to venous thrombosis. Answer choice D describes superficial thrombophlebitis, which is a clinical diagnosis.

4. **A, B, C, and D.** Anticoagulation is the first-line treatment option for patients with DVT. The purpose of anticoagulation is to prevent new thrombus formation while the body's endogenous processes lyse the existing thrombotic burden. Vena cava filters are the prophylaxis of choice for patients who have contraindication to, or have failed, anticoagulation. Inferior vena cava filters do not, in and of themselves, treat DVT in any way, just the potential complication of pulmonary embolism. Surgical thrombectomy is usually reserved for cases in which patients demonstrate impending or advanced *phlegmasia cerulea dolens*. Catheter-directed thrombolysis has replaced surgical thrombectomy as the interventional procedure of choice for extensive, symptomatic, acute iliofemoral DVT, although its effect on the post-thrombotic syndrome is under investigation.

Comment

Clinical Presentation

Lower-extremity DVT is a significant cause of morbidity and long-term disability. The immediate complications of DVT can include pulmonary embolism and limb-threatening phlegmasia. In the long term, a large fraction of DVT patients experience postthrombotic symptoms, which include limb heaviness and aching, ambulatory edema, venous claudication, and lower-extremity ulcerations.

Diagnostic Imaging

The diagnosis of DVT in the femoropopliteal veins can be made with high accuracy using duplex ultrasound (Figures S9-1 and S9-2). In contrast, lower-extremity venography, the gold standard for the diagnosis of DVT, is only infrequently required for diagnosis. Venography is more often used to evaluate for DVT in the iliac venous system, which is often not well visualized by ultrasound. However, MR or computed tomography venogram is increasing in popularity for the diagnosis of iliac venous DVT. Venographic findings of acute (<2 weeks) DVT typically include globular filling defects within a vein, abrupt occlusion of the vein, and/or dilation of the peripheral distal venous system (Figure S9-3).

Treatment Methods

Patients with iliofemoral DVT have a particularly high risk of developing a severe form of postthrombotic syndrome. For this reason, selected patients with acute iliofemoral DVT are treated with catheter-directed thrombolysis or surgical venous thrombectomy. The standard treatment for patients with DVT is anticoagulation using low-molecular-weight or unfractionated heparin followed by warfarin and compression for at least 3 months in most instances. However, in appropriate patients, catheter-directed thrombolysis may be an option.

References

Vedantham S, Millward SF, Cardella JF, et al. Society of Interventional Radiology: Society of Interventional Radiology position statement. Treatment of acute iliofemoral deep vein thrombosis with use of adjunctive catheter-directed intrathrombus thrombolysis. *J Vasc Interv Radiol.* 2006;17:613–616.

Wells PS, Forgie MA, Rodger MA. Treatment of venous thromboembolism. *JAMA.* 2014;311:717–728.

Cross-reference

Vascular and Interventional Radiology: The Requisites, 2nd ed, 370–375.

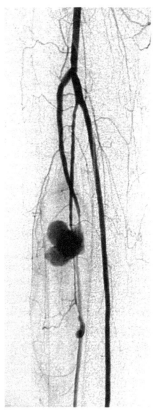

Figure 10-1

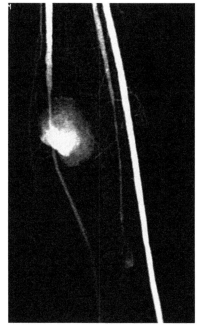

Figure 10-2

HISTORY: A 43-year-old male with right lower-extremity injury during motor vehicle collision.

1. Which of the following is the most likely diagnosis for the imaging findings presented?
   A. Vascular malformation
   B. Pseudoaneurysm
   C. True aneurysm
   D. Hematoma

2. Which of the following is the most common etiology for peripheral artery pseudoaneurysms?
   A. Postsurgical
   B. Mycotic/infectious
   C. Malignancy
   D. Atherosclerotic vascular disease

3. Which of the following therapies would be most appropriate in treating this patient?
   A. Coil embolization
   B. Ultrasound-guided thrombin injection
   C. Ultrasound-guided external compression
   D. Operative repair

4. In the case of a mycotic pseudoaneurysm, which of the following treatment options is relatively contraindicated?
   A. Ultrasonography (US)-guided compression
   B. Exclusion of the pseudoaneurysm using a stent graft
   C. US-guided thrombin injection
   D. Operative repair

See Supplemental Figures section for additional figures and legends for this case.

CASE 10

Peripheral Artery Pseudoaneurysm

1. **B.** Pseudoaneurysms are the result of disruptions in arterial walls. High arterial pressures cause blood to dissect into the surrounding tissues. The pseudoaneurysm is contained by media and adventitia, which differs from a true aneurysm.

2. **A.** Pseudoaneurysms are most commonly the result of trauma, whether it is iatrogenic or due to blunt or penetrating trauma. Atherosclerotic vascular disease will more commonly result in areas of stenosis or true aneurysm formation. Mycotic pseudoaneurysms tend to be very rare, particularly in the extremities.

3. **D.** All of the options may be used to treat pseudoaneurysms in various arterial beds. Given the peripheral location (lower extremity) of this lesion, large size, and wide neck, an operative repair is the best option for this patient. Coil embolization, while feasible, would require limb-salvaging bypass surgery.

4. **B.** Mycotic aneurysms are caused by infection or inflammation affecting the arterial wall. In the setting of infection, placing foreign material such as a stent graft is relatively contraindicated. None of the other options is contraindicated in the setting of infection.

Comment

Etiology

Peripheral pseudoaneurysms of medium-sized vessels most commonly occur in the setting of trauma. Although mycotic aneurysm is rare, the possibility should be considered when saccular or irregular aneurysms are seen in the periphery.

Diagnostic Evaluation

Although computed tomography angiography and duplex US can diagnose and localize the pseudoaneurysm, arteriography is important in planning appropriate therapy (Figures S10-1 and S10-2). It is important to determine the exact location of the entry into the pseudoaneurysm and to completely evaluate the arterial runoff to the extremity. When the injured vessel still makes a significant contribution, as in this case, to perfusion of the lower extremity, surgical repair of the vessel or ligation with distal bypass is clearly indicated. In select instances when this is not the case, arterial embolization may be undertaken.

References

Saad N, Saad W, Davies MG, et al. Pseudoaneurysms and the role of minimally invasive techniques in their management. *Radiographics*. 2005;25:173–190.

Wolford H, Peterson SL, Ray C, et al. Delayed arteriovenous fistula and pseudoaneurysm after an open tibial fracture successfully managed with selective angiographic embolization. *J Trauma*. 2001;51:781–783.

Cross-reference

Vascular and Interventional Radiology: The Requisites, 2nd ed, 354–359.

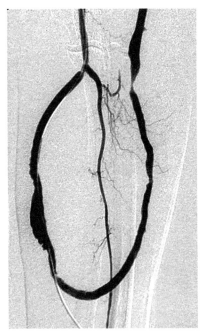

Figure 11-1. *Courtesy of Dr. Thomas Vesely.*

HISTORY: A 58-year-old male with end-stage renal disease presenting with incomplete dialysis and increased venous pressures.

1. Which of the following is the most likely diagnosis for the imaging findings presented?
   A. Pseudoaneurysm formation
   B. Patent hemodialysis arteriovenous fistula
   C. Stenosed hemodialysis arteriovenous graft
   D. Vascular steal syndrome

2. What symptoms are most likely to be present in this patient?
   A. Pain and cyanotic swelling with skin thickening or ulceration of the involved extremity
   B. Dilatation of vein walls
   C. Coolness, pallor, and pain with ischemic gangrene of the graft that worsens with dialysis
   D. High recirculation during dialysis or low flow rates

3. Which location is the most common site of stenosis in a prosthetic arteriovenous graft?
   A. At the venous anastomosis
   B. Within the graft itself
   C. At the arterial anastomosis
   D. In the parent artery

4. What is the current recommended first-line treatment of the above abnormality?
   A. Surgical repair
   B. Balloon angioplasty
   C. Balloon angioplasty with subsequent stent placement
   D. Placement of a central venous catheter, preferably in an internal jugular vein

See Supplemental Figures section for additional figures and legends for this case.

CASE 11

Dialysis Graft Stenosis

1. **C.** This image shows multiple stenoses throughout the graft, most noticeably at the venous anastomosis with the other two areas involved being within the graft itself. The imaging findings of vascular steal syndrome may be quite normal, and the diagnosis would rely heavily on the physical exam findings of pallor and diminished pulses distal to the fistula/graft with ischemic symptoms in the hand.

2. **D.** The most likely symptoms that this patient would be experiencing would be limited low flow rates and high recirculation during dialysis given the fact that the graft still shows flow across the stenosis. The other options listed would indicate more advanced disease such as frank thrombosis or aneurysmal formation.

3. **A.** The most common location for stenosis is at the venous anastomosis. This is due to the large increase in shear stress in the thin-walled outflow vein leading to fibromuscular hyperplasia and fibrosis.

4. **B.** The current first-line therapy for revision of stenosed hemodialysis-access grafts is balloon angioplasty in order to prevent graft thombosis. Stent graft placement has been shown to improve the chances of being free from subsequent interventions. Second-line therapies include surgical revision and central venous access.

Comment

Main Teaching Point

Hemodialysis can be performed from a variety of access routes: (1) A native fistula can be created between an extremity artery—usually a radial artery or brachial artery—and an adjacent vein; (2) a prosthetic graft—usually polytetrafluoroethylene—can be placed to attach a parent artery to an outflow vein; or (3) a dialysis access catheter may be placed from a suitable central vein, preferably an internal jugular vein. When a native fistula or prosthetic graft is used, suboptimal dialysis can occur due to formation of stenotic lesions somewhere in the vascular access circuit. The venous anastomosis of the graft is by far the most common site of stenosis in patients with prosthetic grafts, as in this case (Figure S11-1). However, suboptimal dialysis can also result from flow-limiting stenoses within the graft, within the outflow veins draining the graft, within the central venous system, at the arterial anastomosis, or even in the parent artery. Such lesions, in addition to causing suboptimal dialysis, ultimately lead to graft thrombosis in the majority of cases.

Treatment Methods

Improved duration of graft patency and improved dialysis quality can be achieved via successful treatment of stenotic lesions. This can be achieved surgically or via percutaneous transluminal angioplasty and/or stent graft placement. The interventional management of stenosed fistulas results in successful hemodialysis for at least 30 days in 92% of patients and 6-month patency rates of 61%.

References

Bittl JA. Catheter interventions for hemodialysis fistulas and grafts. *J Am Coll Cardiol Intv.* 2010;3:1–11.

Haskal Z, Trerotola S, Domatch B, et al. Stent graft versus balloon angioplasty for failing dialysis-access grafts. *N Engl J Med.* 2010;362: 494–503.

National Kidney Foundation. Guidelines for vascular access. *Kidney Disease Outcomes Quality Initiative Clinical Practice Guidelines.* New York: National Kidney Foundation; 2000.

Cross-reference

Vascular and Interventional Radiology: The Requisites, 151–157.

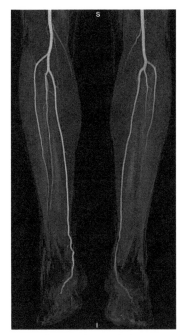

Figure 12-1. *Courtesy of Dr. Minhaj S. Khaja.*

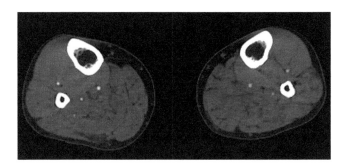

Figure 12-2. *Courtesy of Dr. Minhaj S. Khaja.*

HISTORY: A 44-year-old male with right lower-extremity pain.

1. Which of the following is the most likely diagnosis for the imaging findings presented?
   A. Peronea arteria magna (PAM)
   B. Peripheral vascular disease
   C. Normal lower-extremity arterial runoff
   D. Critical limb ischemia

2. Which of the following represents the *conventional* branching of the pattern of the popliteal artery?
   A. Trifurcation into anterior tibial (AT), posterior tibial (PT), and peroneal arteries
   B. AT artery and tibioperoneal trunk
   C. Main tibial artery and peroneal artery
   D. Superficial and deep popliteal arteries

3. Which of the following represents the proper continuation of calf artery into the foot?
   A. AT artery—dorsalis pedis; PT artery—plantar arteries
   B. PT artery—dorsalis pedis; AT artery—plantar arteries
   C. Peroneal artery—dorsalis pedis; PT artery—plantar arteries
   D. AT artery—dorsalis pedis; peroneal artery—plantar arteries

4. Which of the following arteries terminate above the ankle in a *normal* three-vessel runoff?
   A. AT artery
   B. Peroneal artery
   C. PT artery
   D. Dorsalis pedis artery

See Supplemental Figures section for additional figures and legends for this case.

CASE 12

Normal Tibial Artery Anatomy

1. **C.** Three patent calf arteries are visualized without significant atherosclerotic calcifications or flow-limiting stenosis. This is the standard branching pattern of the calf arteries. PAM is a conventional variant where the peroneal artery is the only vascular supply to the foot.

2. **B.** Normal variant anatomy can include a trifurcation of the popliteal artery, although the most common pattern includes an AT artery and tibioperoneal trunk, which bifurcates into peroneal and PT arteries.

3. **A.** D may occur in PAM with hypoplastic PT and normal AT artery.

4. **B.** The peroneal artery gives terminal branches, which anastomose with the PT and AT artery branches. A lower-extremity runoff exam should not be reported to have only two-vessel patency just because the peroneal artery is not visualized to the level of the foot.

Comment

Conventional Anatomy

The popliteal artery begins distal to the adductor canal and passes through the popliteal fossa between the heads of the gastrocnemius muscle. At its terminal aspect, it typically bifurcates into the AT artery and tibioperoneal trunk. After 2 to 3 cm, the tibioperoneal trunk in turn bifurcates into the peroneal and PT arteries (Figures S12-1 through S12-4). A true trifurcation of the popliteal artery is only present in a minority (2%) of patients. In the normal patient, the AT artery continues across the ankle as the dorsalis pedis artery; the PT artery passes behind the medial malleolus into the foot, where it divides into the lateral and medial plantar arteries. These vessels then anastomose through dorsal and plantar arches within the foot. The peroneal artery runs in the interosseous membrane and typically gives off terminal branches proximal to the ankle that anastomose with branches from the PT and AT arteries.

Variant Anatomy

Arterial variant anatomy has been described in a large (albeit, older) series. The two most commonly described variants are a high take-off of the AT artery (Figure S12-5, 4%), and PAM (Figure S12-6, 4%). The latter condition is not particularly well defined. Most plastic and vascular surgeons define PAM as single dominant peroneal artery with hypoplastic AT and PT arteries (0.2%). However, it is more common to have a dominant peroneal artery supplying the plantar arteries with a normal AT and hypoplastic PT (3.8%). The potential presence of a PAM prompts preoperative computed tomography angiogram with lower-extremity runoff prior to fibular flap reconstruction at many institutions for fear of disrupting the only arterial supply to the foot.

References

Fernandez N, McEnaney R, Marone L, et al. Predictors of failure and success of tibial interventions for critical limb ischemia. *J Vasc Surg.* 2010;52:834–842.

Kim D, Orron D, Skillman J. Surgical significance of popliteal arterial variants: a unified angiographic classification. *Ann Surg.* 1989;210:776–781.

Toussarkissian B, Mejia A, Smilanich RP. Noninvasive localization of infrainguinal arterial occlusive disease in diabetics. *Ann Vasc Surg.* 2001;13:714–721.

Cross-reference

Vascular and Interventional Radiology: The Requisites, 2nd ed, 334–337.

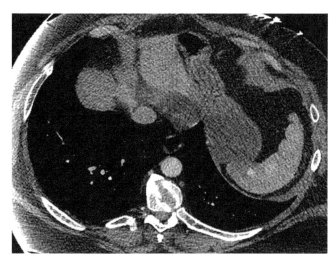

Figure 13-1. *Courtesy of Dr. Wael E. Saad.*

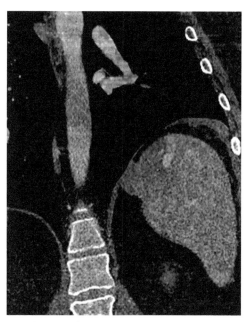

Figure 13-2. *Courtesy of Dr. Wael E. Saad.*

HISTORY: A 32-year-old male presents with left upper quadrant pain after falling off a ladder.

1. Which of the following is the most likely diagnosis for the imaging findings presented?
   A. Splenic laceration
   B. Splenic pseudoaneurysm
   C. Hepatic laceration
   D. Hemoperitoneum

2. In a hemodynamically unstable adult, what is the preferred treatment?
   A. Proximal coil embolization
   B. Subselective distal splenic embolization
   C. Observation
   D. Laparotomy

3. Where is the appropriate place to position an embolization coil when performing proximal coil embolization?
   A. Between the dorsal pancreatic and pancreatica magna arteries
   B. Proximal to the dorsal pancreatic artery
   C. Distal to the pancreatica magna artery
   D. Distal to the caudal pancreatic artery

4. What is the ideal coil size for proximal embolization?
   A. 100% larger than vessel diameter
   B. 75% larger than vessel diameter
   C. 25% larger than vessel diameter
   D. Exactly the same as vessel diameter

See Supplemental Figures section for additional figures and legends for this case.

CASE 13

Traumatic Splenic Artery Injury

1. **B.** Focal areas of hyperdensity are noted within the spleen. No linear hypodensity is seen to suggest splenic or hepatic laceration.

2. **D.** Unstable patients should proceed to laparotomy. Splenic embolization or observation is reserved for hemodynamically stable patients.

3. **A.** Coil placement between the dorsal pancreatic and pancreatica magna arteries decreases the pressure head of blood flow, while still allowing collateral supply to the spleen. Embolization proximal to the dorsal pancreatic artery, distal to the pancreatica magna artery, or distal to the caudal pancreatic artery negates collateral supply via the transverse pancreatic artery and places the spleen at risk for infarction.

4. **C.** The coil should be over-sized by approximately 25% to provide sufficient radial force to stabilize the coil. Sizes larger than this may cause the coil to not form properly. Sizes smaller than this place the coil at risk for migration.

Comment

Preprocedural Planning

When evaluating the patient with abdominal trauma, a reasonable plan for identifying the bleeding artery can only be developed after reviewing an abdominal computed tomography scan, the results of diagnostic peritoneal lavage, and surgical findings (if the patient has already been explored) (Figures S13-1 and S13-2). Because time is of the essence, the angiographer must direct his or her attention to the most likely source of bleeding. An abdominal aortogram may be performed initially. Although this only detects the grossest forms of branch vessel hemorrhage, it can help in selecting branch vessels in patients with distorted anatomy. The visceral vessels should then be evaluated with selective arteriography, and the vessels most likely to represent the source of bleeding should be studied first.

Imaging Interpretation

Angiographic findings of visceral arterial trauma can include displacement or splaying of arterial branches due to hematoma formation, pseudoaneurysms, contrast extravasation, arterial filling defects due to thrombosis or dissection, and diffuse vasoconstriction due to hypovolemic shock (Figure S13-3). In the latter instance, the extremely small caliber of the visceral vessels can occasionally render selective catheterization difficult.

Endovascular Management

Traditional treatment of trauma-induced splenic arterial injuries has been splenic artery ligation with splenectomy. In recent years, transcatheter embolization has evolved into a less morbid alternative that might allow the spleen to be conserved (Figure S13-4). However, because splenic infarcts occur with moderate frequency following embolization, patients should receive appropriate immunizations to prevent later episodes of bacteremia.

References

Kluger Y, Rabau M. Improved success in nonoperative management of blunt splenic injury: embolization of splenic artery pseudoaneurysm. *J Trauma*. 1998;45:980–981.
Schnuriger B, Inaba K, Konstantinidis A, et al. Outcomes of proximal versus distal splenic artery embolization after trauma: a systematic review and meta-analysis. *J Trauma*. 2011;70:252–260.

Cross-reference

Vascular and Interventional Radiology: The Requisites, 2nd ed, 255–256.

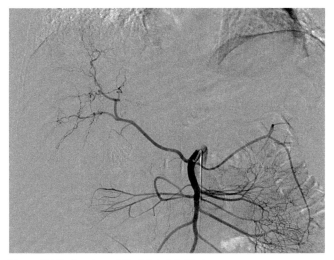

Figure 14-1. *Courtesy of Dr. Minhaj S. Khaja.*

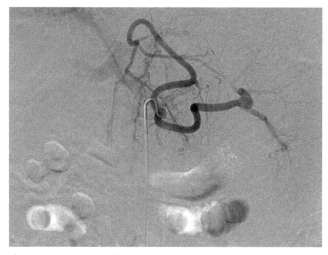

Figure 14-2. *Courtesy of Dr. Minhaj S. Khaja.*

HISTORY: A 48-year-old male with cirrhosis.

1. Which of the following is the most likely diagnosis for the imaging findings presented in the first image?
   A. Accessory right hepatic artery
   B. Gastroduodenal artery
   C. Proper hepatic artery
   D. Replaced right hepatic artery

2. With regard to variant hepatic arterial anatomy, which of the following is true of accessory arteries and replaced arteries?
   A. Replaced arteries should generally be preserved during transplant surgery as opposed to accessory arteries, which do not necessarily need to be preserved.
   B. Accessory arteries are generally larger than their associated vessel of normal origin.
   C. Replaced arteries are generally redundant and are typically of little clinical significance.
   D. Patients with replaced arteries typically also have accessory arteries.

3. Which of the following best describes a replaced left hepatic artery?
   A. Left hepatic artery arising from the proper hepatic artery
   B. Left hepatic artery arising from the left gastric artery
   C. Left hepatic artery supplying the left hepatic lobe that branches, supplying part of the right hepatic lobe
   D. Left hepatic artery coupled with another vessel that both supply the left hepatic lobe

4. Which of the following correctly defines an accessory artery?
   A. An artery that anastomoses with another artery in the same organ
   B. An artery that takes an abnormal course
   C. An artery with an abnormal origin
   D. An artery that supplies a portion of the liver that is also supplied by a vessel of normal origin

See Supplemental Figures section for additional figures and legends for this case.

CASE 14

Variant Anatomy: Replaced Hepatic Arteries

1. **D.** The image shows a replaced right hepatic artery arising from the superior mesenteric artery.

2. **A.** Replaced arteries generally have to be preserved whereas accessory arteries do not, because in the latter, there is often flow through the additional conventional vessel.

3. **B.** By definition, a replaced vessel is one that has an abnormal origin. Therefore, a left hepatic artery arising from the left gastric artery should be characterized as replaced. Choice A represents conventional anatomy.

4. **D.** By definition, an accessory artery supplies the same region as the normal vessel of normal origin. Choice C describes a replaced artery.

Comment

Main Teaching Point

It is important to recognize the common variants in the arterial supply to the liver. Vessels can be *replaced* or *accessory*, but vessels supplying the liver are typically not redundant. A *replaced* artery exists when the vessel supplying an entire hepatic lobe arises aberrantly. An *accessory* artery exists when a portion of a hepatic lobe is supplied by a vessel of normal origin but an additional vessel of aberrant origin also supplies a portion of the lobe.

Description of Variant Anatomy

Estimates vary, but approximately 15% to 25% of people have an accessory or replaced left hepatic artery arising from the left gastric artery (Figure S14-2). When it is difficult to determine whether left hepatic branches are arising from the left gastric artery, steep left anterior oblique and lateral views can help to separate hepatic branches (which run anteriorly to the left liver lobe) and gastric fundal branches. Approximately 15% to 20% of people have an accessory or replaced right hepatic artery arising from the superior mesenteric artery (Figure S14-1). The replaced hepatic artery is almost invariably the first branch from the superior mesenteric artery in such cases. Additional rare variants have been described in which the entire hepatic arterial supply is derived from the superior mesenteric artery or aorta (Figures S14-3 and S14-4).

Reference

Covey AM, Brody LA, Maluccio MA, et al. Variant hepatic arterial anatomy revisited: digital subtraction angiography performed in 600 patients. *Radiology.* 2002;224:542–547.

Cross-reference

Vascular and Interventional Radiology: The Requisites, 2nd ed, 229–232.

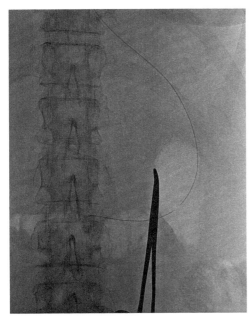

Figure 15-1

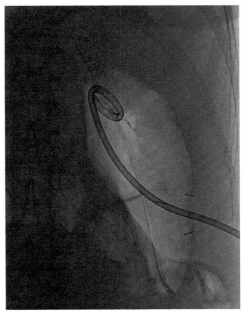

Figure 15-2

HISTORY: A 63-year-old woman with metastatic ovarian cancer and dysphagia.

1. For the procedure depicted in the image, which of the below statements is FALSE?
   A. Visualization of rugal folds after injection of contrast helps confirm appropriate intraluminal positioning.
   B. The stomach should be punctured near the pylorus.
   C. The procedure is most often performed under fluoroscopic guidance.
   D. Administration of glucagon may be helpful during this procedure.

2. Which of the below statements is CORRECT?
   A. A gastrostomy tube (G-tube) can be safely removed no sooner than 6 months after placement.
   B. The patient's nasogastric feeding tube should be removed prior to placing a G-tube.
   C. Colonic interposition may increase the difficulty of placing the G-tube.
   D. The stomach should be decompressed prior to the procedure to reduce the risk of gastric injury.

3. Which of the following is NOT a contraindication to this procedure?
   A. Massive ascites
   B. Anterior gastric wall neoplasm
   C. Bleeding diathesis
   D. Hiatal hernia

4. Which of the below statements is CORRECT?
   A. Compared with endoscopic placement, percutaneous G-tubes have higher rates of postprocedural infection.
   B. Compared with surgical placement, percutaneous G-tubes have higher rates of postprocedural hemorrhage.
   C. A gastrojejunostomy tube may be preferable in patients with gastric outlet obstruction or a documented history of aspiration.
   D. G-tubes should be left in place for no longer than 2 months.

See Supplemental Figures section for additional figures and legends for this case.

CASE 15

Percutaneous Gastrostomy Placement

1. **B.** The stomach should be punctured in the gastric body. Visualization of rugal folds after injection of contrast helps confirm appropriate intraluminal positioning of the tube. In rare cases, such as patients with severe colonic or hepatic interposition, computed tomography may be helpful to cross a narrow gastrostomy window. Otherwise, the procedure is commonly performed under fluoroscopic guidance.

2. **C.** Colonic interposition may increase the difficulty of placing the G-tube. Insufflation of the stomach helps displace the colon away from the stomach puncture site. Additionally, barium can be instilled via the rectum to delineate the colon, if needed. A G-tube can be removed after the formation of a tract, which usually occurs within 4 to 6 weeks. A nasogastric tube (NG) tube should be placed in the stomach for insufflation prior to percutaneous puncture.

3. **D.** Massive ascites may result in leaking around the tube site. Bleeding diathesis and anterior wall neoplasm may cause severe hemorrhage during the procedure. Coagulopathy should be treated prior to the procedure.

4. **C.** A gastrojejunostomy tube may be preferable in patients with gastric outlet obstruction or a documented history of aspiration. Such patients require postpyloric feeding to reduce the risk of aspiration or postprandial discomfort. Percutaneous placement of G-tubes has a lower rate of infectious and hemorrhagic complications and does not require endoscopy.

Comment

Indication

Percutaneous G-tube placement is performed for nutritional support in patients with inadequate oral intake or for gastric decompression in patients with chronic obstruction of the small bowel. Advantages of percutaneous G-tube placement over surgical placement include elimination of general anesthesia and its associated morbidity. Endoscopic placement has a higher incidence of aspiration and wound infection.

Procedural Technique

The basic method of G-tube placement involves the following steps: (1) The stomach is insufflated with air through an NG tube (Figures S15-1 and S15-3). (2) Fluoroscopic confirmation of a safe access window into the stomach is confirmed, with careful attention to avoiding transcolonic or transhepatic puncture. (3) Percutaneous gastropexy may be performed via insertion of two to four metallic T-fasteners, which bring the anterior gastric wall up to the anterior abdominal wall. This is done routinely in some centers and selectively in others. Selected patients include those with ascites and patients who have diminished ability to form a secure transperitoneal tract around the catheter (e.g., patients receiving steroids). (4) A needle is placed in the gastric body, and contrast is injected to confirm intragastric positioning (Figure S15-3). (5) Over a guidewire, the tract is enlarged using sequential dilators. (6) The gastrostomy catheter is positioned in the stomach, and contrast is injected to confirm adequate positioning (Figures S15-2 and S15-4).

Complications

Complications of percutaneous G-tube placement can include peritonitis, aspiration, hemorrhage, and tube migration. Contraindications include uncorrectable bleeding diatheses, lack of a safe access window into the stomach, massive ascites, anterior gastric wall neoplasm, and the presence of a ventriculoperitoneal shunt.

References

Laasch HU, Wilbraham L, Bullen K. Gastrostomy insertion: comparing the options-PEG, RIG or PIG? *Clin Radiol.* 2003;58:398–405.

Lyon SM, Pascoe DM. Percutaneous gastrostomy and gastrojejunostomy. *Semin Intervent Radiol.* 2004;21:181–189.

Cross-reference

Vascular and Interventional Radiology: The Requisites, 2nd ed, 425–432.

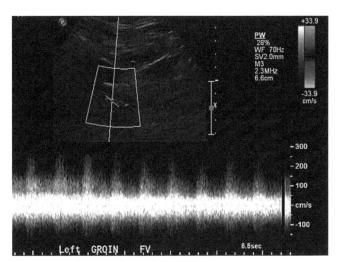

Figure 16-1. *Courtesy of Dr. Luke R. Wilkins.*

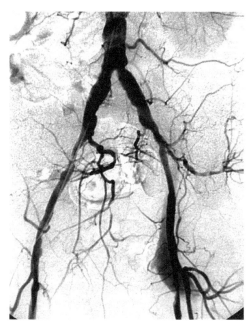

Figure 16-2.

HISTORY: A 46-year-old male who recently underwent cardiac catheterization.

1. Which of the following is the correct diagnosis for the imaging findings presented?
   A. Neoplasm
   B. Venous thromboembolism
   C. Femoral arteriovenous fistula (AVF)
   D. Superficial femoral artery aneurysm

2. What are risk factors for development of such a lesion? (Choose all that apply.)
   A. Low groin punture
   B. Tachycardia
   C. Male gender
   D. Anticoagulation

3. Which of these is a clinical problem associated with this lesion?
   A. Infection
   B. High-output cardiac failure
   C. Hemorrhage
   D. Thrombosis

4. What is the standard treatment for this lesion?
   A. Ultrasound-guided compression
   B. Surgical repair
   C. Endovascular placement of a covered vascular stent
   D. Coil embolization

See Supplemental Figures section for additional figures and legends for this case.

CASE 16

Femoral Arteriovenous Fistula

1. **C.** There is early filling of the left iliofemoral venous system during the early arterial phase of the angiogram as well as arterialized flow within the femoral vein on ultrasonography, consistent with a left femoral AVF. A neoplasm would appear as a mass neovascularity and parenchymal blush. A true aneurysm would demonstrate uniform contrast filling of a dilated vessel and a pseudoaneurysm would appear as a focal outpouching of contrast within the vessel.

2. **A and D.** Low groin puncture and anticoagulation such as high heparin dosages or warfarin therapy predispose patients to AVF formation as do arterial hypertension and female gender. Tachycardia is not a known risk factor of AVF formation.

3. **B.** The increased venous return from an AVF that causes arterial to venous shunting can lead to high-output heart failure. Infection and thrombosis are uncommon complications. Hemorrhage is a risk factor to the development of an AVF or a complication of surgical repair of the AVF.

4. **B.** The gold standard for treatment of an AVF is surgical repair with fistula tract identification, resection, and primary or patch closure repair. Other options include ultrasound-guided compression or endovascular techniques; however, they are less successful than surgical repair in most cases. Endovascular treatment may be precluded by location of the AVF, especially if it is in close proximity to the common femoral artery (CFA) bifurcation or has ischemic complications related to coil deployment or stent malfunction.

Comment

Diagnostic Imaging

Duplex ultrasonography, computed tomography angiography, and angiography may be used in the diagnosis of AVF (Figures S16-1 through S16-4). Duplex ultrasonography is noninvasive and requires no radiation and is, therefore, the appropriate initial exam. In some cases, however, angiography may be performed prior to planned treatment. The proper evaluation of an angiogram starts with several important observations: (1) The type of examination should be stated. (2) The catheter position and vascular approach should be noted, and the reader should specify whether nonselective or selective catheter placement has been performed. (3) The reader should be sure to observe whether the image viewed was obtained in the early arterial, late arterial, parenchymal, or venous phases of the dynamic angiographic run.

Etiology

Complications of arteriography include groin infection, groin hematomas, contrast-related renal dysfunction or allergy, and arterial injuries. Injury to the femoral artery at the puncture site can result in formation of a pseudoaneurysm (which occurs in 1% of angiograms) with or without an AVF. The optimal site of femoral artery puncture is at the femoral head level; at this level, the CFA and vein lie side by side. However, abnormally low punctures of the femoral artery can result in traversal of the femoral vein, with formation of an AVF upon removal of the catheter. AVF may also be the result of blunt or penetrating trauma (Figure S16-4).

Symptoms

AVFs are usually asymptomatic, but they occasionally enlarge and cause arterial steal or high-output cardiac failure. Surgical ligation or covered stent placement of femoral AVFs may be performed in patients who have symptomatic AVFs that fail to spontaneously close.

References

Perings SM, Kelm M, Jax T. A prospective study on incidence and risk factors of arteriovenous fistulae following transfemoral cardiac catheterization. *Int J Cardiol.* 2003;88:223–228.
Porter J, Al-Jarrah Q, Richarson S. A case of femoral arteriovenous fistula causing high-output cardiac failure, originally misdiagnosed as chronic fatigue syndrome. *Case Rep Vasc Med.* 2014;2014:510429.

Cross-reference

Vascular and Interventional Radiology: The Requisites, 2nd ed, 40–43.

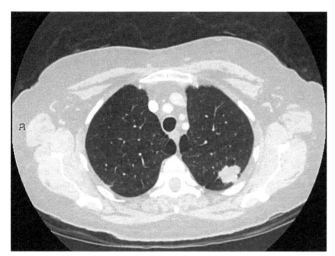

Figure 17-1

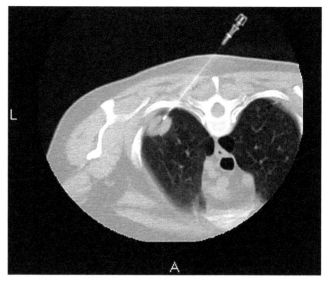

Figure 17-2

HISTORY: A 63-year-old male with a cough, history of lung mass detected on recent chest computed tomography (CT).

1. Which of the following would be included in the differential diagnosis for the imaging findings presented? (Choose all that apply.)
   A. Primary bronchogenic carcinoma
   B. Granuloma
   C. Pulmonary arteriovenous malformation (AVM)
   D. Cystic adenomatoid malformation

2. The referring physician has requested a biopsy of the mass, with fine needle aspiration and core biopsy. Which of the following is most correct?
   A. Perform the biopsy under ultrasound as it would visualize both types of needles.
   B. Perform the biopsy under CT guidance, making passes with the fine needle first, then removing the needle, and placing a new access for the core needle.
   C. Perform the biopsy under CT guidance, using a coaxial trocar needle technique, for both the fine needle aspiration and the core needle.
   D. Avoid performing the biopsy because of the risk of tract seeding.

3. Which of the following is true regarding image-guided biopsy of the lung?
   A. Traversing a fissure with a needle results in no increased risk of pneumothorax.
   B. Local hemorrhage and hemoptysis are serious complications of biopsy.
   C. Lung zones below the hili are the most affected by respiratory motion.
   D. The middle lobe is the area most sensitive to cardiac motion.

4. If a 17-gauge needle is left without a stylet within a small pulmonary vein, the patient is at increased risk for which of the following? (Choose all that apply.)
   A. Air embolism
   B. Hemorrhage
   C. Pneumothorax
   D. Failed biopsy

See Supplemental Figures section for additional figures and legends for this case.

CASE 17

CT-Guided Lung Biopsy

1. **A and B.** Primary bronchogenic carcinoma appears as a spiculated solid mass. While unusual for granulomatous disease, these could also have a similar appearance but commonly have associated calcifications. Pulmonary AVM's commonly have a visible draining vein, while cystic adenomatoid malformations should have very low attenuations (well below soft tissue).

2. **C.** Today most lung biopsies are performed with a coaxial trocar needle, which allows only a single puncture of the pleura and can accommodate both the fine needle and the core biopsy needle, thus minimizing passes through the pleura and risk of complication.

3. **C.** The lung bases are the most susceptible to respiratory motion and most difficult to biopsy under CT guidance. Traversing a fissure increases the risk of pneumothorax, and the lingula is the area most sensitive to cardiac motion. Local hemorrhage during the procedure is almost always found, and hemoptysis is expected after the procedure, and these should not be considered serious complications unless the patient requires additional intervention.

4. **A, B, and D.** Air embolism can occur if a large needle is left open to air within a pulmonary vein. A needle that transverses a pulmonary vein can cause hemorrhage, which will not be significant in most cases, but can cause obscuration of the field, leading to a failed biopsy.

Comment

Preprocedural Planning

Percutaneous lung biopsy is a safe procedure when performed by radiologists who are capable of managing its potential complications. For spiculated masses for which primary lung cancer is suspected, multiple fine needle aspiration specimens often suffice to make the diagnosis. For more complex lesions and when lymphoma is a diagnostic possibility, core biopsy is needed. Preprocedure planning should include careful evaluation of the CT scan and a review of the patient's overall cardiopulmonary status. As seen in this case, CT is helpful in both planning and performing the procedure itself (Figures S17-1 and S17-2).

Complications

It is common (25%) for patients to experience a small amount of hemoptysis following the procedure, but massive hemoptysis and significant hemothorax are rare. Pneumothorax occurs in 15% to 30% of patients undergoing lung biopsy, but it only requires chest tube placement in 2% to 5%. Patients with chronic obstructive pulmonary disease, however, have a significantly higher risk of postbiopsy pneumothorax, with a more significant fraction requiring chest tube placement. In general, when chest tube placement is required, a small-bore tube (10 to 12 F) may be used and the tube can usually be removed within 1 to 3 days. The incidence of pneumothorax may be reduced by the use of the coaxial technique; by minimizing the number of pleural surfaces crossed by the needle, minimizing needle path length, and avoiding oblique passes across pleural surfaces. A cytopathologist should be present to verify that sufficient tissue is obtained for confident diagnosis with a minimum number of needle passes.

References

Ohno Y, Hatabu H, Takenaka D, et al. CT-guided transthoracic needle aspiration biopsy of small solitary pulmonary nodules. *AJR Am J Roentgenol.* 2003;180:1665–1669.

Tsai I, Tsai W, Chen M, et al. CT-guided core biopsy of lung lesion: a primer. *AJR Am J Roentgenol.* 2009;193:1228–1235.

Cross-reference

Vascular and Interventional Radiology: The Requisites, 2nd ed, 395–399.

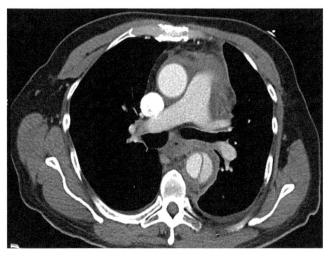

Figure 18-1. *Courtesy of Dr. David M. Williams.*

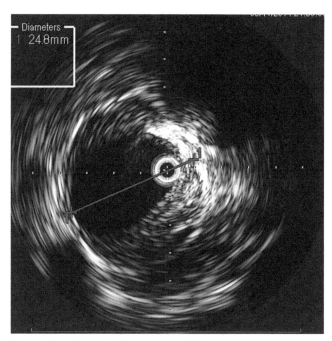

Figure 18-2. *Courtesy of Dr. David M. Williams.*

HISTORY: A 71-year-old male presents with crushing chest pain.

1. Which of the following would be included in the differential diagnosis for the imaging findings presented? (Choose all that apply.)
   A. Aortic rupture
   B. Aortic dissection
   C. Aortic aneurysm
   D. Penetrating atherosclerotic ulcer

2. What is/are the most widely used classification system(s) for aortic dissection?
   A. Stanford and DeBakey
   B. European Society of Cardiology
   C. DISSECT
   D. None of the above

3. Which is NOT a risk factor for aortic dissection?
   A. Prior cardiac surgery
   B. Hypertension
   C. Marfan syndrome
   D. Female gender

4. Which is an indication for surgical or endovascular treatment of Stanford B dissection? (Choose all that apply.)
   A. Malperfusion
   B. Intractable pain
   C. Acute expansion of the false lumen
   D. Contained rupture

See Supplemental Figures section for additional figures and legends for this case.

CASE 18

Aortic Dissection

1. **A and B.** An intimal flap is present, consistent with aortic dissection. There is also mediastinal hemorrhage, which is suspicious for aortic rupture. The aorta is not aneurysmal and there is no penetrating atherosclerotic ulcer.

2. **A.** The most widely used systems are Stanford and DeBakey. Stanford type A dissection involves the ascending aorta, while type B dissections involve the aorta beyond the left subclavian artery. Developed in 2001, the European Society of Cardiology classification is less widely used. The DISSECT classification is a mnemonic-based system published by the DEFINE project investigators in 2013.

3. **D.** Male gender is a risk factor for dissection, not female gender. Prior cardiac surgery (especially of the aortic valve), hypertension, and Marfan syndrome are all risk factors for dissection.

4. **A, B, C, and D.** Limb and visceral malperfusion, intractable pain despite antihypertensive medication, acute expansion of the false lumen, and contained rupture are all indications for procedural treatment of Stanford type B dissection.

Comment

Diagnostic Evaluation

Acute aortic dissection is a life-threatening disease with a mortality of about 1% per hour during the first 48 hours. The definitive diagnosis of aortic dissection is made using helical computed tomography, magnetic resonance imaging, intravascular ultrasound, or multiplanar transesophageal echocardiography (Figures S18-1 and S18-2). Angiography is used when branch vessels must be assessed before surgical aortic repair or endovascular therapy (Figures S18-4 and S18-5).

Classification Schema

Stanford type A dissections involve the ascending aorta with (DeBakey type I) or without (DeBakey type II) concomitant involvement of the descending aorta. Stanford type B dissections (DeBakey type III) involve only the aorta distal to the left subclavian artery. Patients with Stanford type A dissections undergo emergent surgical ascending aortic replacement to prevent the complications of coronary artery occlusion, aortic valvular insufficiency, and rupture into the pericardial sac. Patients with uncomplicated Stanford type B dissections are treated with pharmacologic therapy to reduce the systemic blood pressure and cardiac impulse force.

Treatment Methods

Treatment options for Stanford type B dissections complicated by branch vessel ischemia include surgical aortic replacement and endovascular therapy. Endovascular interventions include balloon fenestration of the dissection flap, stenting of compromised branch vessels, and placement of aortic stents or stent grafts (Figure S18-3).

References

Dake MD, Thompson M, van Sambeek M, Vermassen F, Morales JP, DEFINE Investigators. DISSECT: a new mnemonic-based approach to the categorization of aortic dissection. *Eur J Vasc Endovasc Surg.* 2013;46:175–190.

Erbel R, Alfonso F, Boileau C, et al. Task force on aortic dissection diagnosis and management of aortic dissection. *Eur Heart J.* 2001;22:1642–1681.

Vedantham S, Picus D, Sanchez LA, et al. Percutaneous management of ischemic complications in patients with type-B aortic dissection. *J Vasc Interv Radiol.* 2003;14:181–193.

Williams DM, Lee DY, Hamilton BH, et al. The dissected aorta: percutaneous treatments of ischemic complications—principles and results. *J Vasc Interv Radiol.* 1997;8:605–625.

Cross-reference

Vascular and Interventional Radiology: The Requisites, 2nd ed, 188–192.

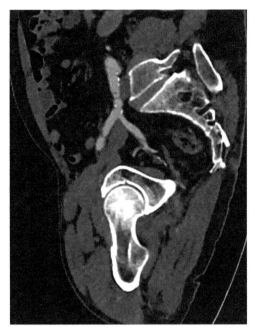

Figure 19-1. *Courtesy of Dr. Saher S. Sabri.*

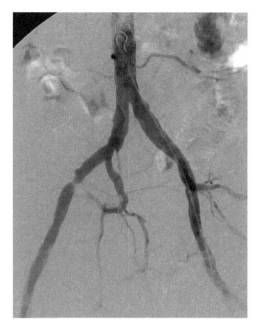

Figure 19-2. *Courtesy of Dr. Saher S. Sabri.*

HISTORY: A 69-year-old male with right lower-extremity claudication.

1. Which of the following is the most likely diagnosis for the imaging findings presented?
   A. Right common iliac artery occlusion
   B. Right external iliac artery stenosis
   C. Right external iliac artery dissection
   D. Right common femoral artery stenosis

2. What is the most likely etiology of the condition presented?
   A. Penetrating ulcer
   B. Fibromuscular dysplasia
   C. Atherosclerotic disease
   D. Embolic disease

3. What is the best fluoroscopic projection to demonstrate the right common iliac artery, right external iliac artery, and right internal iliac artery in profile?
   A. Posterior-anterior
   B. Right posterior oblique (RPO)
   C. Left posterior oblique (LPO)
   D. Right anterior oblique (RAO)

4. What would be considered a normal Ankle Brachial Index (ABI)?
   A. Greater than or equal to 1.3
   B. 0.9 to 1.1
   C. 0.6 to 0.8
   D. Less than or equal to 0.5

See Supplemental Figures section for additional figures and legends for this case.

CASE 19

Iliac Artery Stenosis

1. **B.** Key angiographic references for demarcating iliofemoral arterial segments include the bifurcation of the external and internal iliac arteries, the origin of the inferior epigastric artery, and bifurcation of the superficial femoral and profunda femoral arteries. No dissection flap is seen in the external iliac artery segment.

2. **C.** Atherosclerotic disease is the most likely cause for the stenosis in this case given the patient's age and overall angiographic appearance. Fibromuscular dysplasia can affect the iliac arteries, but typically has a beaded angiographic appearance and occurs in younger patients. This is not the typical appearance for a penetrating ulcer, and embolic disease usually presents with acute symptoms and angiographic stenosis/occlusion at bifurcation points.

3. **B.** RPO will show the right common iliac, right external iliac, and right internal iliac arteries in profile. LPO and RAO would give the same projection and would be useful for visualizing the left iliac arteries in profile, and posterioranterior would result in overlap of the external and internal iliac arteries.

4. **B.** An ABI greater than or equal to 1.3 indicates noncompressible vessels, which are heavily calcified. An ABI less than or equal to 0.8 indicates ischemia, which is critical below 0.4.

Comment

Diagnostic Imaging

Computed tomography angiography is increasingly more commonly employed in the diagnosis of claudication as it can assist in diagnosis and treatment planning (Figure S19-1). Magnetic resonance angiography may also be used in patients with poor renal function and contraindication for iodinated contrast dyes.

Treatment Methods

Percutaneous transluminal angioplasty and endoluminal stenting are well-accepted procedures for treating aortoiliac occlusive disease. Treatment is appropriate in patients with claudication that limits lifestyle and in patients with limb-threatening ischemia. Concentric, noncalcified stenoses less than 3 cm in length have the best long-term patency after treatment and often respond well to angioplasty alone.

Endovascular Intervention

Stent insertion following angioplasty is appropriate for greater than 30% residual stenoses, a residual systolic pressure gradient of greater than 10 mm Hg at rest or greater than 20 mm Hg after administration of a vasodilator, development of a hemodynamically significant dissection, or late restenosis at the angioplasty site. Primary stenting is useful when there is a higher risk of dissection or distal embolization with angioplasty alone—generally for eccentric, calcified plaques or those with small amounts of associated fresh thrombus. This case is an example of primary stenting in a patient with residual stenosis postangioplasty (Figures S19-2 through S19-4). Generally, the secondary patencies of iliac artery angioplasty and stenting are comparable to those of surgical reconstruction but with lower morbidity and mortality rates.

References

Bosch JL, Tetteroo E, Mall WP, et al. Iliac arterial occlusive disease: cost-effectiveness analysis of stent placement versus percutaneous transluminal angioplasty. *Radiology.* 1998;208:641–648.

Sabri SS, Choudhri A, Orgera G, et al. Outcomes of covered kissing stent placement compared with bare metal stent placement in the treatment of atherosclerotic occlusive disease at the aortic bifurcation. *J Vasc Interv Radiol.* 2010;21:995–1003.

Cross-reference

Vascular and Interventional Radiology: The Requisites, 2nd ed, 209–214.

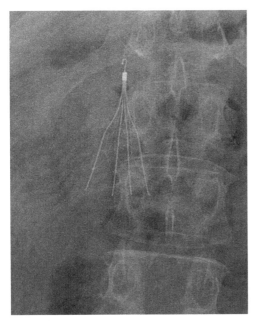

Figure 20-1

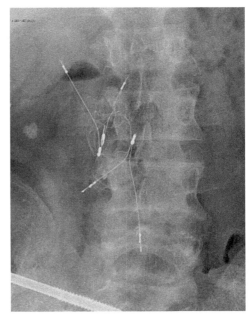

Figure 20-2

HISTORY: A 52-year-old female with history of pulmonary embolism (PE), previously failed anticoagulation.

1. Which of the devices shown would be suitable for a vena cava with a diameter more than 30 mm?
   A. Denali
   B. Greenfield
   C. Bird's Nest
   D. Gunther Tulip

2. Which of the following is the desired location for successful inferior vena cava (IVC) filter placement?
   A. T11
   B. Immediately below the lowermost renal vein entry point
   C. Immediately above the most superior renal vein entry point
   D. Immediately at the confluence of the common iliac veins to form the IVC

3. Which of the following is considered a failure of anticoagulation?
   A. A 28-year-old female with a past medical history (PMH) of deep vein thrombosis (DVT) successfully treated with warfarin for 6 months develops a second acute DVT while on a cross-country road trip 2 months after cessation of therapy.

B. A 56-year-old male with a PMH of osteoarthritis was recently discharged from the hospital after an arthroscopic knee surgery with a 5-day course of prophylactic enoxaparin develops an acute DVT on treatment day 3 of 5.
C. A 66-year-old newly vegetarian female develops an acute PE after being on chronic warfarin therapy for 13 years for a past DVT.
D. A 73-year-old female with a history of atrial fibrillation on chronic warfarin therapy (INR 2.5) and metastatic breast cancer develops an acute DVT.

4. Which of the following devices is a "retrievable" filter?
   A. Bird's Nest
   B. Greenfield
   C. Gunther Tulip
   D. Venatech LP

See Supplemental Figures section for additional figures and legends for this case.

CASE 20

Inferior Vena Cava Filters

1. **C.** The only IVC filter Food and Drug Administration–approved for a vena cava greater than 30 mm is the Bird's Nest filter. A cava of this size would be considered a megacava, which is a vena cava greater than 28 mm.

2. **B.** The commonly preferred location for placement of an IVC filter is immediately below the ostium of the lowermost renal vein. This location minimizes the effects of thrombosis due to continuous inflow of blood near the filter.

3. **D.** This patient has failed anticoagulation therapy due to the fact that she has been chronically anticoagulated on a therapeutic dose of warfarin and still developed an acute DVT. The 56-year-old male was not on a therapeutic dose of enoxaparin, the 28-year-old female's new DVT was a provoked DVT (car ride), and the 66-year-old newly vegetarian patient most likely has a subtherapeutic INR due to her large increase in consumption of leafy green vegetables, which can inhibit the effect of warfarin.

4. **D.** Out of all the options listed, the Gunther Tulip IVC filter is the only one designed specifically for retrieval, although there are now several other retrievable IVC filters including the Denali, Optease, Crux, and Option Elite, among others.

Comment

Main Teaching Point

Different IVC filters vary in terms of their physical characteristics, cost, and deployment method, but all serve to prevent PE in patients with documented lower-extremity DVT and as prophylaxis in selected patients who are at high risk for developing lower-extremity DVT. An inferior vena cavogram is performed to obtain four specific pieces of information that guide filter selection and placement: (1) presence of IVC thrombus—this can interfere with proper seating of the filter and might mandate placement at a higher level in the IVC; (2) location of the lowermost renal vein on each side, because the preferred location of IVC filters is immediately below the renal vein entry; (3) presence of caval or renal vein anomalies; and (4) IVC diameter.

Endovascular Management

Any filter (Greenfield, Boston Scientific; Venatech, Braun; Simon-Nitinol, Bard; Gunther Tulip, Cook Medical; Crux Vena Cava Filter, Volcano Corporation; Option, Argon Medical; Optease, Cordis; Denali, Bard) can be inserted into an IVC that measures 18 to 28 mm. However, between 1% and 3% of patients have a megacava, in which the IVC diameter is greater than 28 mm. The TrapEase filter (Cordis) can be inserted into an IVC measuring 18 to 30 mm, and the Bird's Nest filter (Cook) can be inserted into an IVC measuring up to 40 mm. In the rare situation where the IVC diameter is greater than 40 mm, two filters can be inserted, one into each common iliac vein (Figures S20-1 through S20-6).

References

Grassi CJ, Swan TL, Cardella JF, et al. Quality improvement guidelines for percutaneous permanent inferior vena cava filter placement for the prevention of pulmonary embolism. *J Vasc Interv Radiol.* 2001;12:137–141.

Kim HS, Young MJ, Narayan AK. A comparison of clinical outcomes with retrievable and permanent inferior vena cava filters. *J Vasc Interv Radiol.* 2008;19:393–399.

Cross-reference

Vascular and Interventional Radiology: The Requisites, 2nd ed, 296–301.

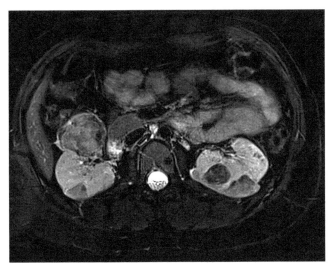

Figure 21-1. *Courtesy of Dr. J. Fritz Angle.*

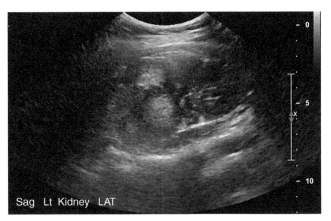

Figure 21-2. *Courtesy of Dr. J. Fritz Angle.*

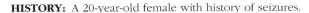

HISTORY: A 20-year-old female with history of seizures.

1. Which of the following is the most likely diagnosis for the imaging findings presented?
   A. Renal cell carcinoma (RCC)
   B. Simple cyst
   C. Angiomyolipoma (AML)
   D. Oncocytoma

2. Given the constellation of findings, what disorder does this patient likely have?
   A. Von Hippel-Lindau
   B. Polyarteritis nodosa
   C. Churg-Strauss
   D. Tuberous sclerosis

3. What is the complication of this renal mass that warrants endovascular treatment?
   A. Ectopic hormone secretion
   B. Hemorrhage
   C. Infarction
   D. Infection

4. At what size is prophylactic treatment of this lesion generally recommended?
   A. 0.5 cm
   B. 1 cm
   C. 4 cm
   D. 10 cm

See Supplemental Figures section for additional figures and legends for this case.

CASE 21

Renal Angiomyolipoma

1. **C.** There are multiple fat-containing masses seen on the ultrasound and the fat-suppressed enhanced magnetic resonance imaging (MRI) most consistent with AML. Although rarely RCC lesions can engulf fat, this would be extremely rare in a young patient with multiple lesions.

2. **D.** Tuberous sclerosis is associated with multiple renal AMLs, cystic lung lesions (lymphangioleiomyomatosis), facial angiofibromas, cardiac rhabdomyomas, and cortical tubers and subependymal nodules in the brain. Patients often present with seizures due to the CNS lesions.

3. **B.** AMLs are very hypervascular lesions that have a propensity to bleed spontaneously, sometimes to a life-threatening degree. Other symptoms of renal AML include flank pain and hematuria.

4. **C.** Prophylactic treatment is generally recommended for lesions greater than 4 cm. Any AML, however, that is symptomatic should be treated.

Comment

Etiology

AMLs are hamartomatous lesions containing fat, smooth muscle, and blood vessels. Approximately 80% of patients with tuberous sclerosis have AMLs, which are often multiple and bilateral in these patients.

Imaging Interpretation

AMLs are often diagnosed on cross-sectional imaging owing to the presence of fat within a renal lesion, which nearly always indicates AML (Figures S21-1 and S21-2). AMLs are usually hypervascular, and this property gives them a characteristic appearance on angiography as well as strong contrast enhancement on MRI and computed tomography (Figures S21-1 and S21-3). Angiographic features include hypervascularity with large, tortuous feeding arteries arranged circumferentially, occasional small arterial aneurysms, and a sunburst appearance in the parenchymal phase. Arteriovenous shunting does not commonly occur in these lesions. Angiographic differentiation from RCC is usually not definitive.

AMLs are generally treated if they are large (>4 cm) or symptomatic or if they bleed spontaneously. Treatment may include surgical resection or percutaneous catheter-based embolization with particulate or liquid embolic agents.

References

Hocquelet A, Cornelis F, Le Bras Y, et al. Long-term results of preventive embolization of renal angiomyolipomas: evaluation of predictive factors of volume decrease. *Eur Radiol.* 2014;24:1785–1793.

Siegel C. Renal angiomyolipoma: relationships between tumor size, aneurysm formation, and rupture. *J Urol.* 2003;169:1598–1599.

Cross-reference

Vascular and Interventional Radiology: The Requisites, 2nd ed, 278–279.

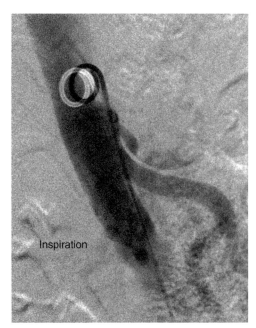

Figure 22-1. *Courtesy of Dr. Minhaj S. Khaja.*

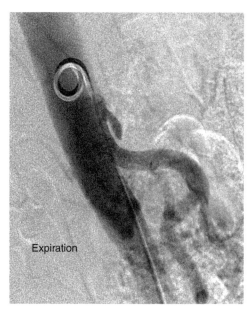

Figure 22-2. *Courtesy of Dr. Minhaj S. Khaja.*

HISTORY: A 30-year-old female presents with crampy abdominal pain and concern for malabsorption.

1. Which of the following is the most likely diagnosis for the imaging findings presented?
   A. Median arcuate ligament compression
   B. Celiac artery atherosclerotic stenosis
   C. Mesenteric ischemia
   D. Fibromuscular dysplasia

2. With what patient maneuver does compression worsen?
   A. Inspiration
   B. Expiration
   C. Leaning forward
   D. Leaning backward

3. What is the correct treatment for this entity?
   A. Endovascular stenting
   B. Surgical release
   C. Gaining weight
   D. Losing weight

4. What imaging tests can be used to make the diagnosis? (Choose all that apply.)
   A. Ultrasound with Doppler
   B. Catheter angiography
   C. Computed tomography angiography
   D. Magnetic resonance (MR) angiography

See Supplemental Figures section for additional figures and legends for this case.

CASE 22

Median Arcuate Ligament Syndrome

1. **A.** Compression of the celiac artery is most pronounced during expiration. The syndrome is present when the imaging findings are accompanied by crampy abdominal pain and malabsorption (weight loss). Celiac stenosis due to atherosclerotic disease does not change with provocative maneuvers, and there is no evidence of luminal narrowing due to plaque. Mesenteric ischemia can result from occlusion of the mesenteric vessels; however, this patient has clear retrograde filling of the celiac vessels from the superior mesenteric artery.

2. **B.** During expiration the diaphragm rises and the celiac artery gets impinged by the diaphragmatic crura, whereas during inspiration the diaphragmatic crura move away from the celiac trunk. Weight loss has little impact on celiac artery compression but can impact superior mesenteric artery compression.

3. **B.** Surgical release is the correct and definitive treatment for median arcuate ligament syndrome (MALS). The problem with a stenting approach is that the long-term patency in an area of repeated pressure may be low and fracture may result. Gaining and losing weight may affect splenic artery compression but not celiac artery compression.

4. **A, B, C, and D.** All of these imaging modalities can aid in the diagnosis of MALS. Ultrasound and MR have the benefit of not requiring radiation. All four modalities allow imaging in both inspiration and expiration, which should prove exacerbation of the celiac stenosis during expiration, although angiography is the gold standard.

Comment

Etiology

MALS, or celiac artery compression syndrome, is the most common visceral arterial compression syndrome. Patients with this syndrome have extrinsic compression of the celiac artery by the median crus of the diaphragm and/or the celiac neural plexuses and connective tissues. The majority of patients with this diagnosis are young, thin women who are asymptomatic, despite stenoses of more than 50% diameter. However, some patients develop crampy abdominal pain and malabsorption that has been attributed to celiac artery compression.

Imaging Findings

The arterial compression usually varies with respiration and worsens with expiration (Figures S22-1 and S22-2). Also commonly seen is poststenotic dilation of the celiac artery (Figures S22-1 through S22-3). As in this case, the compression can be severe enough that injection of the superior mesenteric artery produces celiac artery opacification in retrograde fashion via the gastroduodenal and pancreaticoduodenal arteries (Figure S22-4).

Treatment Methods

Surgery to enlarge the diaphragmatic hiatus or resect the celiac ganglion is the preferred therapy because this compression does not respond to angioplasty. Stents are contraindicated due to possible device fatigue.

References

Douard R, Ettore GM, Chevalier JM, et al. Celiac trunk compression by arcuate ligament and living-related liver transplantation: a two-step strategy for flow-induced enlargement of donor hepatic artery. *Surg Radiol Anat.* 2002;24:327–331.

Sultan S, Hynes N, Elsafty N, Tawfick W. Eight years experience in the management of median arcuate ligament syndrome by decompression, celiac ganglion sympathectomy, and selective revascularization. *Vasc Endovascular Surg.* 2013;47:614–619.

Cross-reference

Vascular and Interventional Radiology: The Requisites, 2nd ed, 238–239.

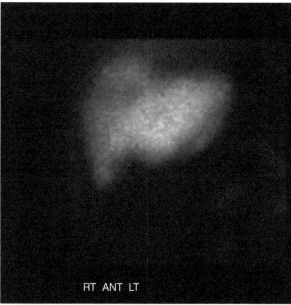

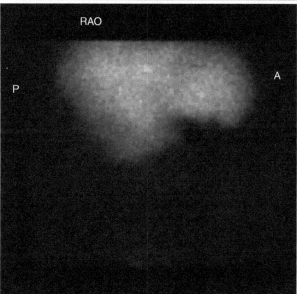

RT ANT LT

RAO

P   A

Figure 23-2. *Courtesy of Dr. Minhaj S. Khaja.*

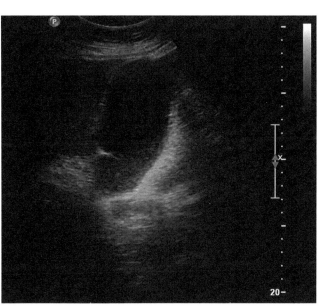

20—

Figure 23-1. *Courtesy of Dr. Minhaj S. Khaja.*

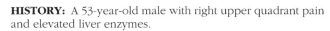

HISTORY: A 53-year-old male with right upper quadrant pain and elevated liver enzymes.

1. Which of the following is the most likely diagnosis for the imaging findings presented?
   A. Emphysematous cholecystitis
   B. Acute pyogenic cholecystitis
   C. Cholangiocarcinoma
   D. Gallbladder adenocarcinoma

2. If the patient is currently a poor surgical candidate, which of the following is the most appropriate intervention?
   A. Percutaneous biliary drainage
   B. Peritoneal drainage catheter placement
   C. Percutaneous cholecystostomy
   D. Fluoroscopic-guided biopsy

3. Which of the following is a relevant contraindication to the intervention?
   A. Acute pancreatitis
   B. Liver malignancy
   C. History of human immunodeficiency virus
   D. Uncontrolled bleeding diathesis

4. Which of the following is one of the major complications of the intervention?
   A. Bile peritonitis
   B. Pancreatitis
   C. Bowel obstruction
   D. Cirrhosis

See Supplemental Figures section for additional figures and legends for this case.

CASE 23

Percutaneous Cholecystostomy

1. **B.** The ultrasound image demonstrates a distended gallbladder with sludge. However, no definite cholelithiasis was seen. Hepatobiliary iminodiacetic acid confirms obstruction of the cystic duct. In a patient presenting with right upper quadrant pain and fever, the findings may be concerning for acute cholecystitis. There is no evidence for a mass or intramural gas to suggest an alternative diagnosis.

2. **C.** The appropriate intervention would be decompression of the gallbladder until the patient was a surgical candidate. Cholecystectomy remains the definitive treatment for patients with acute cholecystitis. Drainage of the biliary tree may be helpful in a patient with choledocholithiasis and ascending cholangitis. Biopsy may be helpful in cases where neoplasm was suspected.

3. **D.** The absolute contraindications to percutaneous cholecystostomy are few and mostly include untreated or severe bleeding diathesis. Interposition of bowel may be a concern; however, this can be avoided via a transhepatic approach. Some of the other relative contraindications include perforated gallbladder, gallbladder cancer, and a stone-filled gallbladder, which may not accommodate a catheter.

4. **A.** The most common acute complications include hemorrhage, sepsis, vasovagal reactions, catheter migration (most common), bile leak, bowel perforation, and pneumothorax. The most common complication via the transhepatic access route is bleeding, whereas bile peritonitis occurs more commonly via the transperitoneal approach.

Comment

Clinical Indication

The current indications for percutaneous gallbladder drainage include acute calculous or acalculous cholecystitis, access for percutaneous stone dissolution or removal, diagnostic cholangiography, and drainage of the biliary system when the common bile duct is obstructed. For many of these patients, the diagnosis of cholecystitis is difficult because the patients are unable to provide history because of mechanical ventilation or depressed mental status. Diagnosis with imaging may include ultrasound, magnetic resonance imaging, nuclear medicine hepatobiliary scan, or computed tomography (Figures S23-1 and S23-2).

Percutaneous Management

There are two different potential routes to percutaneously drain the gallbladder, each with advantages and disadvantages. Transhepatic access is favored by many because there is a reduced incidence of bile leakage into the peritoneum due to the fixation of the gallbladder to the liver surface (Figures S23-3 through S23-6). However, disadvantages include the potential for liver laceration and bleeding. Therefore, some favor the transperitoneal route, although this route is more commonly associated with bile peritonitis. The aspirated bile should be cultured, although negative cultures are found in as many as 40% of patients despite obvious cholecystitis.

Clinical Follow-up

To reduce the risk of sepsis, the tube should not be manipulated until the patient improves clinically. Subsequently, cholangiography via the tube is performed to establish cystic and common bile duct patency and to establish the presence or absence of stones that will require further treatment. No drainage catheter should be removed until the underlying problem has resolved and a complete fibrous tract has developed around the catheter from the gallbladder to the skin surface to prevent bile peritonitis. Cholecystectomy remains the definitive treatment for these patients; therefore, these patients should also be followed by general surgery for a potential definitive operation.

References

Little MW, Briggs JH, Tapping CR, et al. Percutaneous cholecystostomy: the radiologist's role in treating acute cholecystitis. *Clin Radiol.* 2013;68:654–660.

Menu Y, Vuillerme MP. Non-traumatic abdominal emergencies: imaging and intervention in acute biliary conditions. *Eur Radiol.* 2002;12:2397–2406.

Cross-reference

Vascular and Interventional Radiology: The Requisites, 2nd ed, 474–480.

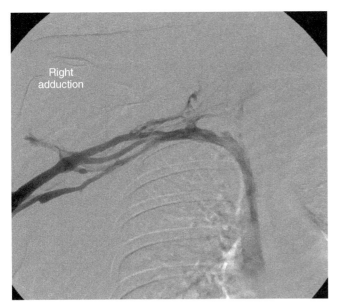

Figure 24-1

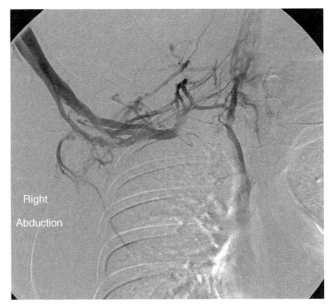

Figure 24-2

HISTORY: An 18-year-old female with a history of right upper extremity pain and swelling.

1. Which of the following is the most likely diagnosis for the imaging findings presented?
   A. Subclavian steal syndrome
   B. Superior vena cava (SVC) occlusion
   C. Subclavian vein occlusion
   D. Arteriovenous fistula

2. Which of the following would NOT be considered an appropriate therapy in treatment of this condition?
   A. Venous thrombolysis
   B. First rib resection
   C. Primary stenting with a balloon-expandable stent
   D. Anticoagulation

3. What are potential complications of this condition? (Choose all that apply.)
   A. Ischemic digits
   B. Pulmonary embolus
   C. Muscle wasting
   D. Postthrombotic syndrome

4. Which of the following structures are commonly implicated in this condition?
   A. Subclavius muscle
   B. Sternocleidomastoid muscle
   C. Aneurysmal subclavian artery
   D. Posterior scalene muscle

_____

See Supplemental Figures section for additional figures and legends for this case.

CASE 24

Subclavian Vein Occlusion

1. **C.** Subclavian vein occlusion is shown, in this case secondary to venous thoracic outlet syndrome, which is most common in younger patients who are involved in athletics or other strenuous activity. The SVC is not occluded on the images provided and no arterial images are shown, making the other answer choices incorrect.

2. **C.** Primary stenting with a balloon-expandable stent would not be an appropriate therapy given high mechanical shear forces from an external compression within the area of placement, which could result in stent crushing/fracture. The other choices are typically used in combination to treat axillo-subclavian vein occlusion secondary to venous thoracic outlet syndrome.

3. **B and D.** Pulmonary embolus and postthrombotic syndrome are complications of venous thrombosis, especially if reocclusion occurs. The other answer choices would be more characteristic of arterial and neurogenic thoracic outlet syndrome.

4. **A.** A hypertrophied subclavius muscle or anterior scalene, in addition to the clavicle or first rib, causes external shearing-type compression of the subclavian vein most prominent during upper extremity abduction. This is why it is crucial to perform adduction and abduction venography if venous thoracic outlet syndrome is suspected.

Comment

Clinical Presentation

Primary axillo-subclavian vein occlusion is caused by mechanical compression of the vein at its point of entry into the thorax. This disorder most commonly is seen in young patients, particularly those with well-developed musculature. The compression induces an intimal reaction in the vein as well as perivascular fibrosis, which produce symptoms of upper extremity swelling and/or pain. If the occlusion is left undiagnosed, thrombosis often occurs.

Diagnostic Evaluation

The diagnosis of subclavian vein stenosis or thrombosis is usually made by venography. When evaluating a patient for primary axillo-subclavian vein occlusion, it is important to perform venographic runs with the arm abducted and during arm abduction with pectoralis flexion (Figures S24-1 and S24-2). These maneuvers often demonstrate pronounced compression or occlusion of the vein. The disorder is commonly bilateral, so it is important to also evaluate the contralateral upper extremity.

Treatment Methods

The treatment of primary axillo-subclavian occlusion centers on early removal of thrombus via catheter-directed thrombolysis, followed by surgical thoracic outlet decompression (Figure S24-3). Angioplasty of the underlying subclavian vein stenosis is typically avoided initially to avoid further trauma to the vein; however, it may be used for persistent stenoses following surgical decompression (Figure S24-4). Stent placement is contraindicated as initial therapy because of the risk of stent fracture resulting from mechanical compression in this area.

References

Meissner MH. Axillary-subclavian venous thrombosis. *Rev Cardiovasc Med.* 2002;3:S76–S83.

Thompson JF, Winterborn RJ, Bays S, et al. Venous thoracic outlet compression and the Paget-Schroetter syndrome: a review and recommendations for management. *Cardiovasc Intervent Radiol.* 2011;34:903–910.

Cross-reference

Vascular and Interventional Radiology: The Requisites, 2nd ed, 140–144.

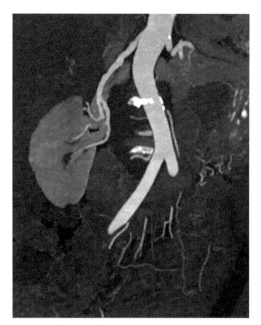

Figure 25-1. *Courtesy of Dr. Alan H. Matsumoto.*

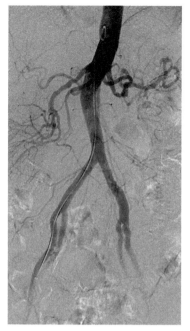

Figure 25-2. *Courtesy of Dr. Alan H. Matsumoto.*

HISTORY: A 60-year-old woman with refractory hypertension, currently on four antihypertensive medications.

1. Which of the following would be included in the differential diagnosis for the imaging findings presented? (Choose all that apply.)
   A. Atherosclerotic renal artery stenosis (ARAS)
   B. Fibromuscular dysplasia (FMD)
   C. Polyarteritis nodosa
   D. Segmental arterial mediolysis

2. Which of the following is the standard first-line treatment for hemodynamically significant FMD of the renal arteries?
   A. Stenting
   B. Balloon angioplasty
   C. Embolization
   D. Surgical bypass

3. Which site is the LEAST likely to be affected by FMD?
   A. Iliac artery
   B. Renal artery
   C. Carotid artery
   D. Brachial artery

4. On Doppler ultrasonography, which of the following are suggestive of renal artery stenosis? (Choose all that apply.)
   A. Tardus parvus waveform
   B. Increased resistive indices
   C. Decreased renal-aortic ratio
   D. Increased peak systolic velocity

See Supplemental Figures section for additional figures and legends for this case.

CASE 25

Fibromuscular Dysplasia with Renal Artery Stenosis

1. **A and B.** This case represents a typical patient with FMD as the lesion is in the middle portion of the main renal artery. However, ARAS should also be considered, although those lesions are most commonly ostial in location.

2. **B.** Balloon angioplasty alone is the standard first-line treatment for FMD; approximately 80% of patients have resolution or improvement of hypertension. Stenting is reserved for complications of angioplasty.

3. **D.** Although the brachial arteries may be affected by FMD, the renal, carotid, iliac, and vertebral arteries are more commonly affected.

4. **A, B, and D.** All of the choices except C are seen in renal artery stenosis. In fact, patients with renal artery stenosis have increased renal-aortic ratios, with a ratio greater than 3.5 representing stenosis.

Comment

Patient Presentation

FMD is a disorder of unknown cause that most commonly affects the renal arteries. It is the second most common cause of renovascular hypertension (behind ARAS). The mid and distal portions of the main renal artery are most commonly affected, but the entire artery can be involved (Figures S25-1 and S25-2). Rarely, only the proximal portion is affected. When FMD is unilateral, the right renal artery is more commonly affected. The disease involves renal artery branch vessels in nearly 20% of cases. In less than 5% of cases, only the branch vessels are diseased.

Subtypes of FMD

The most common angiographic finding is the string-of-beads appearance seen in the medial fibroplasia variant. Five additional variants have been described. In decreasing order of frequency, these are perimedial fibroplasia, medial hyperplasia, medial dissection, intimal fibroplasia, and adventitial fibroplasia.

Treatment Methods

In this case, the preferred treatment modality is percutaneous transluminal angioplasty (Figures S25-3 and S25-4). The expected technical success is similar to angioplasty of atherosclerotic stenoses, but the expected clinical success is better. About 40% of patients are cured of their hypertension, and an additional 40% demonstrate significantly improved blood pressure control following angioplasty. The 5-year patency rates following angioplasty for renal artery FMD are about 90%. Stents are reserved for cases in which iatrogenic dissection occurs following angioplasty.

References

Gowda MS, Loeb AL, Crouse L. Complementary roles of color-flow duplex imaging and intravascular ultrasound in the diagnosis of renal artery fibromuscular dysplasia (FMD): should renal arteriography serve as the "gold standard"? *J Am Coll Cardiol.* 2003;41:1305–1311.

Olin JW, Sealove BA. Diagnosis, management, and future developments of fibromuscular dysplasia. *J Vasc Surg.* 2011;53:826–836.

Cross-reference

Vascular and Interventional Radiology: The Requisites, 2nd ed, 268–275.

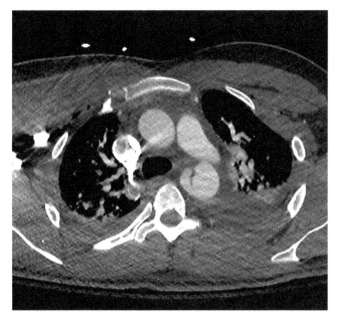

Figure 26-1. *Courtesy of Dr. David M. Williams.*

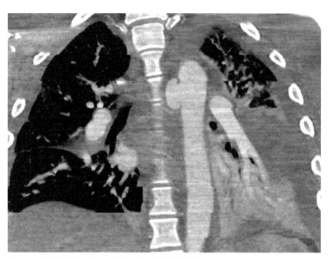

Figure 26-2. *Courtesy of Dr. David M. Williams.*

HISTORY: A 26-year-old male presents after a motorcycle accident.

1. Which of the following is the most likely diagnosis for the imaging findings presented?
   A. Dissection
   B. Pseudoaneurysm
   C. Aneurysm
   D. Ductus bump

2. What is the initial management of patients with contained aortic transection?
   A. Aortic interposition tube graft
   B. Endovascular stent graft
   C. Blood pressure and rate control
   D. Lumbar drain

3. What is the most common location of thoracic aortic injury seen on angiography due to blunt trauma?
   A. Ascending thoracic aorta
   B. Great vessel origin
   C. Mid or distal descending thoracic aorta
   D. Proximal descending thoracic aorta

4. Which of the following is the most common cause of late failure in thoracic stent grafts?
   A. Incomplete graft apposition
   B. Device infolding
   C. Component separation
   D. Branch occlusion

See Supplemental Figures section for additional figures and legends for this case.

CASE 26

Acute Traumatic Aortic Injury

1. **B.** A focal outpouching of the aorta with sharp margins at the aortic isthmus and periaortic fluid are seen on cross-sectional imaging. Although a ductus bump or ductus arteriosus remnant is included in the differential diagnosis for pathological condition at the aortic isthmus, focal outpouching with adjacent fluid and a history of high-speed trauma are indicative of pseudoaneurysm.

2. **C.** Blood pressure and rate control are the initial steps taken to prevent or minimize exsanguination. Endovascular stent graft or surgical tube graft placement are potential next steps in management. A lumbar drain placement is an adjunct procedure to open or endovascular repair used to help maintain spinal perfusion and minimize ischemia.

3. **D.** The proximal descending thoracic aorta, just distal to the origin of the left subclavian artery, is the most common site seen angiographically. Patients with ascending aortic injury commonly expire before imaging can be performed. The other sites are less commonly seen.

4. **A.** Component separation (or Type III endoleak) is a known late failure of modular endograft systems. Separation is most likely to occur at junctions near a curve and within the main aneurysmal segment. Treatment involves placement of a bridging endograft between the separating components. The remainder of the complications occur at initial stent graft placement.

Comment

Clinical Presentation

Acute traumatic aortic injury (ATAI) is associated with significant mortality. Aortic rupture is the cause of death in approximately 16% of motor vehicle crashes involving sudden deceleration. Only 15% of patients with ATAI live long enough to survive transfer to the hospital, and the mortality when ATAI is undiagnosed is 30% at 6 hours, 50% at 24 hours, and 90% within 4 months.

Imaging Interpretation

Sudden deceleration causes stress at points of maximal fixation in the aorta. The most common traumatic aortic injury seen on angiography (>80%) is a laceration just distal to the left subclavian artery at the aortic isthmus, resulting in development of a pseudoaneurysm. The pseudoaneurysm typically appears as a bulge of the aortic contour that can involve the entire circumference of the aorta or only a portion of it (Figures S26-2 and S26-3). As in the case shown, a linear lucency representing a flap of involved intima and media may be identified (Figure S26-1). Less common sites of injury seen on angiography include the ascending aorta (most patients with this injury expire before angiography can be obtained) and the descending thoracic aorta at the diaphragm level.

Endovascular Management

The treatment of choice for ATAI was previously an operative repair; however, advances in technology and user experience have led to significantly increased use of stent grafts and improved outcomes in patients with ATAI (Figures S26-4 and S26-5).

References

Demetriades D, Velmahos G, Scalea T, et al. Operative repair or endovascular stent graft in blunt traumatic thoracic aortic injuries: results of an American Association for the Surgery of Trauma Multicenter Study. *J Trauma.* 2008;64:561–570.

Fattori R, Napoli G, Lovato L, et al. Indications for, timing of, and results of catheter-based treatment of traumatic injury to the aorta. *AJR Am J Roentgenol.* 2002;179:603–609.

Lee WA. Failure modes of thoracic endografts: prevention and management. *J Vasc Surg.* 2009;49:792–799.

Cross-reference

Vascular and Interventional Radiology: The Requisites, 2nd ed, 193–195.

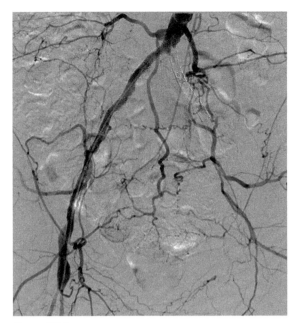

Figure 27-1

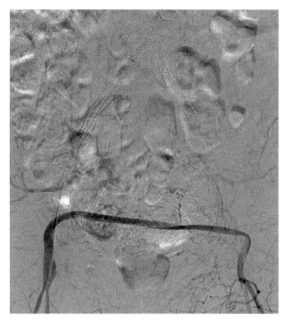

Figure 27-2

HISTORY: A 75-year-old male presenting with lower-extremity pain.

1. Which of the following is the most likely diagnosis for the imaging findings presented?
   A. Femoral arteriovenous loop graft
   B. Iliofemoral arterial bypass graft
   C. Femorofemoral arterial bypass graft
   D. Femorofemoral vein bypass (Palma procedure)

2. What was the probable indication for selecting this procedure?
   A. Iliac vein occlusion
   B. Right common femoral artery total occlusion
   C. Left iliac artery total occlusion
   D. Hemodialysis access

3. What factors are associated with higher patency rates of the imaged structure?
   A. Preoperative angioplasty of stenosis in the donor iliac system
   B. Systemic anticoagulation with warfarin
   C. Postoperative hypertension
   D. Infrainguinal venous patency

4. What would have been another possible treatment option for this patient?
   A. Aortofemoral bypass
   B. Venous thrombolysis
   C. Right common femoral artery angioplasty
   D. Left iliac artery embolectomy

See Supplemental Figures section for additional figures and legends for this case.

CASE 27

Patent Femorofemoral Bypass Graft

1. **C.** The images demonstrate a left iliac artery occlusion treated with a crossover femorofemoral arterial bypass. No venous component is seen to suggest a venous bypass or shunt.

2. **C.** The left iliac artery is occluded. Previously placed bilateral iliac artery stents are also noted.

3. **A.** Success of any bypass is highly dependent on hemodynamically adequate inflow from the donor artery and outflow into at least one healthy recipient artery.

4. **A.** While femorofemoral bypass is often used because of its less invasive tunneled nature, aortofemoral, crossover iliofemoral, or axillofemoral bypasses (extra-anatomic bypasses) could potentially have been used in this patient. Although challenging, endovascular approaches can also be feasible in some patients with unilateral iliac arterial occlusion.

Comment

Indication

A femorofemoral bypass graft is an extra-anatomic vascular bypass usually used to treat unilateral iliac artery occlusion. Extra-anatomic bypass grafts are preferred in patients with unilateral iliac disease, patients who are poor candidates for surgery, patients with severe scarring from prior vascular procedures, patients with current abdominal or groin infections, or patients in whom one limb of an aortobifemoral bypass graft is occluded.

Disease Progression

The degree of disease in the native donor and recipient arteries typically determines the long-term patency of the graft. Disease in the donor iliac artery can result in significant flow reduction to both limbs, and in severe cases it can lead to flow reversal in the graft. The presence of superficial femoral artery occlusion reduces the duration of graft patency as well as the likelihood of achieving symptomatic relief. Complications of femorofemoral bypass placement can include graft thrombosis, femoral steal phenomenon, anastomotic pseudoaneurysms, and anastomotic stenoses.

Endovascular Evaluation

Arteriography is typically performed by catheterizing the donor femoral artery, but other approaches include the axillary artery, the translumbar aorta, and direct graft puncture (Figures S27-1 through S27-3). Due to the tendency for complications to occur at the anastomoses, it is important to obtain images in different projections to optimally profile these regions. If a stenosis is present, angioplasty can be performed as indicated. Computed tomography angiography and duplex ultrasonography can also be performed to evaluate the bypass graft in a noninvasive manner (Figure S27-4).

References

AbuRahma AF, Robinson PA, Cook CC, Hopkins ES. Selecting patients for combined femorofemoral bypass grafting and iliac balloon angioplasty and stenting for bilateral iliac disease. *J Vasc Surg.* 2001;33:S93–S99.

Bismuth J, Duran C. Bypass surgery in limb salvage: inflow procedures. *Methodist Debakey Cardiovasc J.* 2013;9:66–68.

Huded CP, Goodney PP, Powell RJ, et al. The impact of adjunctive iliac stenting on femoral-femoral bypass in contemporary practice. *J Vasc Surg.* 2012;55:739–745.

Nazzal MM, Hoballah JJ, Jacobovicz C, et al. A comparative evaluation of femorofemoral crossover bypass and iliofemoral bypass for unilateral iliac artery occlusive disease. *Angiology.* 1998;49:259–265.

Cross-reference

Vascular and Interventional Radiology: The Requisites, 2nd ed, 209–214.

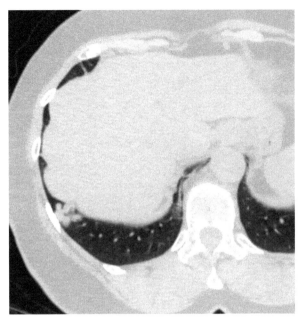

Figure 28-1. *Courtesy of Dr. Bill S. Majdalany.*

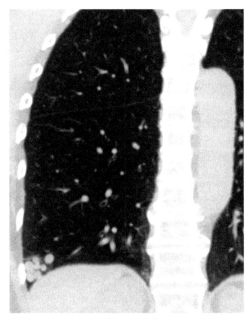

Figure 28-2. *Courtesy of Dr. Bill S. Majdalany.*

HISTORY: A 48-year-old male with history of recurrent nose-bleeds presenting with acute mental status changes.

1. Which of the following would be included in the differential diagnosis for the imaging findings presented? (Choose all that apply.)
   A. Pulmonary artery pseudoaneurysm
   B. Bronchogenic carcinoma
   C. Pulmonary arteriovenous malformation (pAVM)
   D. Pulmonary varix

2. With which of the following hereditary syndromes is this entity most commonly associated?
   A. Sturge-Weber syndrome
   B. Churg-Strauss syndrome
   C. Klippel-Trénaunay-Weber syndrome
   D. Osler-Weber-Rendu syndrome

3. All of the following are indications for endovascular treatment EXCEPT:
   A. Progressive enlargement of the lesion(s)
   B. Orthodeoxia
   C. Paradoxic embolization
   D. Feeding vessels 3 mm or larger

4. Which of the following are possible complications of endovascular treatment of this entity? (Choose all that apply.)
   A. Pulmonary hypertension
   B. Air embolus
   C. Recanalization
   D. Coil migration

See Supplemental Figures section for additional figures and legends for this case.

CASE 28

Pulmonary Arteriovenous Malformation

1. **A and C.** The computed tomography (CT) images demonstrate a well-defined serpiginous mass within the right lung base. Pulmonary artery pseudoaneurysms and pAVMs can demonstrate similar characteristics on cross-sectional imaging and angiography. A feeding artery and draining vein confirm the diagnosis of arteriovenous malformation (AVM).

2. **D.** The imaging findings are consistent with a diagnosis of pAVM. The wide majority of pAVMs (~85%) occur as part of the autosomal dominant disorder known as hereditary hemorrhagic telangiectasia (HHT), also known as Osler-Weber-Rendu syndrome. This syndrome demonstrates a classic triad on presentation of epistaxis, multiple mucocutaneous telangiectasias, and positive first degree family members/automsomal dominant inheritance pattern.

3. **B.** Orthodeoxia (desaturation with upright positioning) is a phenomenon seen in the setting of pAVMs whereby upright positioning forces greater perfusion to the lung bases, exacerbating the degree of shunting through the pAVM. This causes the characteristic desaturation as higher levels of unoxygenated blood is returned to the left heart for systemic circulation. While this is a fairly common symptom seen in patients with pAVMs, it is not considered an indication for invasive intervention.

4. **A, B, C, and D.** The most feared complication of pAVM coil embolization is migration of coil material into the systemic circulation. Meticulous attention must also be paid during the procedure to prevent the formation of air emboli. Even so, air emboli are not uncommon occurrences (encountered in <5% cases). In terms of pulmonary artery pressures, most patients with pAVMs have normal to low PA pressures, owing to the shunting mechanism. However, it has been found that significant numbers of patients who undergo embolization for treatment of pAVMs subsequently develop pulmonary hypertension. Finally, recanalization/recurrence is a rare possible complication, likely due to aneurysmal wall fragility.

Comment
Clinical Presentation

HHT has a reported prevalence of 2 to 3 per 100,000, but it is probably more common because in many patients with mild symptoms it can go undiagnosed. The disorder has a classic triad of mucocutaneous telangiectasias, epistaxis, and autosomal dominant inheritance. About 15% of patients with HHT have pAVMs, but the risk is higher when there is a family member with a pulmonary AVM. Although most patients present with the central nervous system manifestations (stroke and brain abscess), the most common clinical manifestations are dyspnea, fatigue, cyanosis, clubbing, and polycythemia. Diagnosis can be confirmed with cross-sectional imaging such as CT or angiography (Figures S28-1 through S28-3).

Treatment Methods

Treatment options include surgical resection of the involved lung and embolotherapy with coils or other devices (Figures S28-4 and S28-5). Because the overwhelming majority of pulmonary AVMs have a single feeding artery and a single draining vein, with an intervening thin-walled aneurysm, the goal of therapy is to eliminate arterial inflow. This is in contrast to peripheral (nonpulmonary) AVMs, in which the goal of therapy is to eliminate the nidus when possible. Family members of patients with HHT should undergo screening.

References

Haitjema T, Disch F, Overtoom TT, et al. Screening family members of patients with hereditary hemorrhagic telangiectasia. *Am J Med.* 1995;99:519–524.

Meek M, Meek J, Beheshti M. Management of pulmonary arteriovenous malformations. *Semin Intervent Radiol.* 2011;28:24–31.

Zylak C, Eyler W, Spizamy D, et al. Developmental lung anomalies in the adult: radiologic–pathologic correlation. *Radiographics.* 2002;22:S25–S43.

Cross-reference

Vascular and Interventional Radiology: The Requisites, 2nd ed, 169–171.

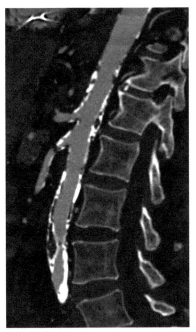

Figure 29-1. *Courtesy of Dr. Alan H. Matsumoto.*

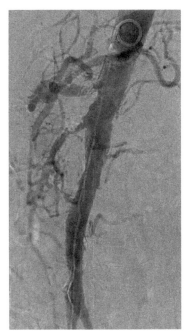

Figure 29-2. *Courtesy of Dr. Alan H. Matsumoto.*

HISTORY: A 65-year-old female with hyperlipidemia presents with 6-month history of worsening postprandial abdominal pain and weight loss.

1. Which of the following is the most likely diagnosis for the imaging findings presented?
   A. Penetrating aortic ulcer
   B. Celiac artery compression syndrome
   C. Mesenteric ischemia
   D. Aortic dissection with involvement of the mesenteric artery origins

2. Risk factors for chronic mesenteric ischemia include which of the following? (Choose all that apply.)
   A. Hypertension
   B. Diabetes mellitus
   C. Hyperlipidemia
   D. Smoking

3. What is the classic clinical presentation of patients with chronic mesenteric ischemia?
   A. Hypotension
   B. Metabolic acidosis
   C. Altered mental status
   D. Chronic postprandial abdominal pain and food avoidance

4. Patients with chronic mesenteric ischemia often have robust collateral formation. What are the collateral pathways between the superior mesenteric artery (SMA) and inferior mesenteric artery (IMA) circulations? (Choose all that apply.)
   A. Pancreaticoduodenal arcade
   B. Gastroduodenal artery
   C. Marginal artery of Drummond
   D. Arc of Riolan

See Supplemental Figures section for additional figures and legends for this case.

CASE 29

Chronic Mesenteric Ischemia

1. **C.** Median arcuate compression and involvement by aortic dissection would be considerations in the differential of chronic mesenteric ischemia, although the findings in the images are suggestive of atherosclerosis as the cause.

2. **A, B, C, and D.** All of the answer choices listed are risk factors for the development of chronic mesenteric ischemia.

3. **D.** The classic clinical findings in chronic mesenteric ischemia are postprandial abdominal pain, food avoidance, and weight loss. The other answer choices listed would suggest a more acute presentation of mesenteric ischemia.

4. **C and D.** The marginal artery of Drummond and the arc of Riolan are the names of collateral pathways between the SMA and IMA. The pancreaticoduodenal arcades and gastroduodenal arteries are the collateral pathways between the celiac axis and the SMA.

Comment

Etiology

Chronic mesenteric ischemia is less common than acute mesenteric ischemia. The primary cause is atherosclerosis, usually due to aortic plaques that involve the mesenteric artery ostia. These stenoses are typically circumferential and can exhibit poststenotic dilation. The stenosis can progress to thrombotic occlusion. Most patients are elderly women with risk factors for atherosclerosis. In addition to the classic symptoms listed above, some patients develop nausea, vomiting, and/or diarrhea due to malabsorption. Physical examination is typically unremarkable, although an epigastric bruit may be heard.

Diagnostic Evaluation

It is generally agreed that the diagnosis requires that at least two of the three mesenteric arteries have significant stenoses or occlusions because the splanchnic system has efficient collateral channels. However, milder degrees of stenosis can become symptomatic when cardiac output is reduced. Imaging evaluation of patients with suspected mesenteric ischemia may include computed tomography angiography, magnetic resonance angiography, ultrasonography, or angiography (Figures S29-1 and S29-2). Typically, enlarged collaterals are identified at arteriography because the disease is chronic. The main collaterals between the celiac and SMA circulations are the gastroduodenal and pancreaticoduodenal arteries. The primary collaterals between the SMA and IMA circulations are the marginal artery of Drummond and the arc of Riolan. The IMA can receive flow from the internal iliac arteries via the hemorrhoidal arterial system as well.

Treatment Methods

These patients are managed similarly to patients with coronary or peripheral vascular disease, which includes smoking cessation, aspirin, statin medications, and exercise. For those patients requiring invasive treatments, surgical bypass or endarterectomy may be performed. Endovascular angioplasty and stenting are increasing in favor among those who treat this disease process given their results and lower immediate postprocedural morbidity and mortality (Figures S29-2 through S29-6).

References

Matsumoto AH, Angle JF, Spinosa DJ. Percutaneous transluminal angioplasty and stenting in the treatment of chronic mesenteric ischemia: results and long-term follow-up. *J Am Coll Surg*. 2002; 194:S22–S31.

Park WM, Cherry KJ, Chua HK. Current results of open revascularization for chronic mesenteric ischemia: a standard for comparison. *J Vasc Surg*. 2002;35:853–859.

Turba UC, Saad WE, Arslan B, et al. Chronic mesenteric ischaemia: 28-year experience of endovascular treatment. *Eur Radiol*. 2012; 22:1372–1384.

Cross-reference

Vascular and Interventional Radiology: The Requisites, 2nd ed, 238–239.

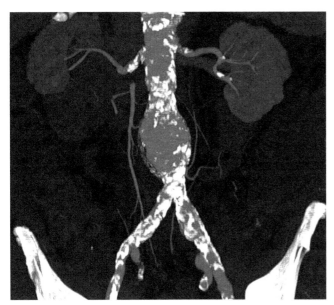

Figure 30-1. *Courtesy of Dr. Klaus D. Hagspiel.*

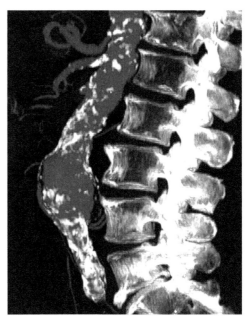

Figure 30-2. *Courtesy of Dr. Klaus D. Hagspiel.*

HISTORY: A 65-year-old Caucasian male with past medical history significant for long-standing hypertension, hyperlipidemia, and 30-pack/year smoking history presents for computed tomography angiography (CTA) to further evaluate an incidental finding on an abdominal ultrasound.

1. Which of the following is the most likely diagnosis for the imaging findings presented?
   A. Aortic aneurysm
   B. Aortic dissection
   C. Aortitis
   D. Leriche syndrome

2. What is the most common location for abdominal aortic aneurysm (AAA)?
   A. Suprarenal
   B. Juxtarenal
   C. Infrarenal
   D. Pararenal

3. What is the most common age/gender combination that this condition affects?
   A. Women over 60
   B. Men over 60
   C. Women from 40 to 60
   D. Men from 40 to 60

4. Appropriate anatomic considerations for endovascular aneurysm repair (EVAR) include which of the following? (Choose all that apply.)
   A. Adequate infrarenal neck length for proximal graft seal
   B. Adequate distal iliac artery seal zone
   C. Appropriate caliber access vessels
   D. Appropriate course of access vessels (absence of excessive tortuosity)

See Supplemental Figures section for additional figures and legends for this case.

CASE 30

Abdominal Aortic Aneurysm

1. **A.** There is a 5.2 cm infrarenal fusiform aneurysm of the abdominal aorta. There is no dissection flap or enhancement and thickening of the aortic wall to suggest dissection or aortitis, respectively. Leriche syndrome is an atherosclerotic occlusive disease involving the abdominal aorta and bifurcation.

2. **C.** The most common location for AAA is in the infrarenal position that is greater than 1 cm below the level of the renal arteries. A juxtarenal aneurysm would occur within 1 cm of the renal artery origin. A suprarenal aneurysm extends above the level of the renal arteries.

3. **B.** AAA most commonly affects men over the age of 60. Other risk factors include hypertension, hyperlipidemia, smoking history, and family history of AAA.

4. **A, B, C, and D.** All of the listed choices are appropriate anatomic considerations when planning EVAR. An adequate, normal minimally calcified aortic wall should be available for appropriate graft approximation and thereby aneurysm exclusion with minimal risk for endoleak.

Comment

Etiology

AAAs usually results from atherosclerotic disease. The most important complications of AAAs are aneurysm rupture and distal embolization. Rupture carries a high mortality rate, and rupture risk increases with larger aneurysm size. AAA treatment is indicated for aneurysms greater than 5 cm in diameter or those that cause distal embolization; a lower size threshold is used in women and in patients with connective tissue disorders.

Diagnostic Evaluation

Imaging diagnosis of AAA is commonly made by ultrasonography or computed tomography, both of which are highly sensitive for AAA. These modalities enable precise diameter measurements of the aneurysm and adjacent normal aortic segments to be obtained. In contrast, when thrombus is present within an aneurysm sac, arteriography can be insensitive for the diagnosis of AAA and often underestimates aneurysm diameter. CTA is invaluable in obtaining measurements needed for planning stent-graft repair of AAAs (Figures S30-1 and S30-2). Arteriography is primarily used intraprocedurally to evaluate visceral branch vessel relationships to the aneurysm, to evaluate the suitability of the iliac arteries as access vessels for stent-graft placement, and to enable proper stent-graft device selection and sizing.

Treatment Methods

The traditional standard treatment of AAA is operative repair with bypass graft placement. In recent years, endovascular stent-graft placement has been employed in patients with suitable anatomy and is clearly indicated in high-risk patients with medical contraindications to aortic surgery. Compared with operative repair, stent grafts have demonstrated diminished periprocedural morbidity and hospital stays. CTA is commonly employed following intervention to monitor aneurysm exclusion and complications such as endoleak or graft migration (Figure S30-3).

References

Golzarian J. Imaging after endovascular repair of abdominal aortic aneurysm. *Abdom Imaging*. 2003;28:236–243.

Walker TG, Kalva SP, Yeddula K, et al. Clinical practice guidelines for endovascular abdominal aortic aneurysm repair: written by the Standards of Practice Committee for the Society of Interventional Radiology and endorsed by the Cardiovascular and Interventional Radiological Society of Europe and the Canadian Interventional Radiology Association. *J Vasc Interv Radiol*. 2010;21:1632–1655.

Cross-reference

Vascular and Interventional Radiology: The Requisites, 2nd ed, 203–209.

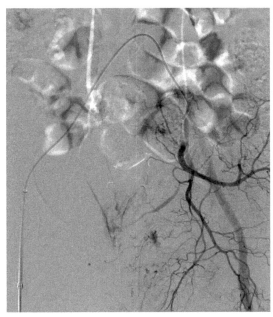

Figure 31-2

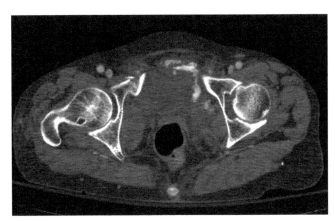

Figure 31-1

HISTORY: Middle-aged male status post motor vehicle collision.

1. Which of the following best describes the findings in the images shown?
   A. Pelvic fractures with active extravasation
   B. Pelvic fractures with a pudendal blush
   C. Pelvic fractures with extraperitoneal bladder rupture
   D. Pelvic fractures with intraperitoneal bladder rupture

2. Which of the following is NOT considered a permanent embolic agent?
   A. Gelfoam
   B. Particles
   C. Liquid embolics
   D. Beads

3. Which of the following places the risk level at increased risk of significant hemorrhage in the setting of traumatic pelvic fractures?
   A. Persistent sciatic artery
   B. Aberrant obturator artery arising from the external iliac artery
   C. Deep circumflex artery
   D. Iliopsoas artery

4. Which of the following hemodynamic parameters warrants emergent intervention for hemorrhagic shock?
   A. Normal pulmonary capillary wedge pressure (PCWP), increased cardiac output, decreased systemic vascular resistance
   B. Increased PCWP, decreased cardiac output, increased systemic vascular resistance
   C. Decreased PCWP, increased cardiac output, decreased systemic vascular resistance
   D. Decreased PCWP, increased cardiac output, increased systemic vascular resistance

See Supplemental Figures section for additional figures and legends for this case.

CASE 31

Pelvic Trauma with Active Extravasation

1. **A.** Pelvic fractures with active extravasation as manifested by the hyperattenuating foci adjacent to multiple pelvic fractures. The bladder is not well seen in the given images but care should be taken to exclude bladder rupture in the setting of significant pelvic trauma. The "pudendal blush" refers to the distal branches of the internal pudendal artery that can mimic a bleed when there is none.

2. **A.** Gelfoam is the only one of the provided embolic agents that is not considered permanent. Recanalization may occur as early as 2 to 3 weeks after the procedure. It is often the ideal embolic agent to use in the traumatic setting as it temporarily occludes an injured vessel, giving it the opportunity to heal. Side effects, such as sexual dysfunction, may improve with time as well.

3. **B.** The aberrant obturator artery arising from the external iliac artery is a normal variant and is seen in up to 10% to 30% of patients. It courses adjacent to the superior pubic ramus, rendering it prone to injury in the setting of pelvic fractures. This anatomic variant is known as the corona mortis, or "crown of death." The sciatic artery is a continuation of the internal iliac artery, which supplies the lower extremity during fetal development. It typically involutes by birth but may persist.

4. **D.** During hemorrhagic shock, there is decreased preload (decreased PCWP), increased cardiac output, and increased afterload (increased systemic vascular resistance). Choice B is seen in cases of distributive shock and choice C is seen in the setting of sepsis.

Comment

Clinical Presentation

Blunt pelvic trauma usually results from motor vehicle collisions, falls from a height, and crush injuries. Approximately 10% of patients with pelvic fractures have pelvic bleeding that requires therapy. These patients are often hypotensive and have multiple organ injuries. Prompt treatment of active hemorrhage is necessary because mortality is primarily related to hemorrhage and sepsis. Commonly injured vessels are the superior gluteal and internal pudendal arteries, and injury results from adjacent pelvic fractures.

Endovascular Evaluation

The focus of extravasation may be evident on contrast-enhanced computed tomography and/or nonselective angiography of the abdominal aorta (Figure S31-1). However, it is necessary to select both internal iliac arteries to exclude a vascular injury, and the entire pelvis, including the femoral regions should be studied because there may be multiple sites of bleeding. Arteriographic findings can include contrast extravasation, pseudoaneurysm, vasospasm, vascular occlusion, and hematoma (displacement, compression, and/or stretching of arterial branches), and/or arteriovenous fistula (Figures S31-2 and S31-4).

Endovascular Management

Transcatheter embolization with coils or Gelfoam is the preferred treatment (Figure S31-3). Both internal iliac artery branches should be treated if the bleeding site is midline so as to prevent continued hemorrhage from collateral flow. Selective embolization is preferred if possible, but in the unstable patient, embolization of the proximal internal iliac artery may be necessary and is usually well tolerated.

References

Kertesz J, Anderson S, Murakami A, et al. Detection of vascular injuries in patients with blunt pelvic trauma by using 64-channel multidetector CT. *Radiographics*. 2009;29:151–164.

Lopera J. Embolization in trauma: principles and techniques. *Semin Intervent Radiol*. 2010;27:14–28.

Velmahos GC, Toutozas KJ, Vassiliu P, et al. A prospective study on the safety and efficacy of angiographic embolization for pelvic and visceral injuries. *J Trauma*. 2002;53:303–308.

Cross-reference

Vascular and Interventional Radiology: The Requisites, 2nd ed, 220–222.

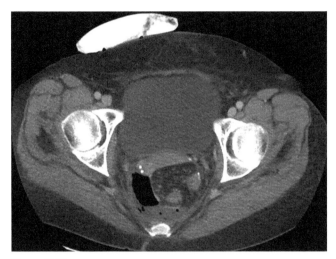

Figure 32-1

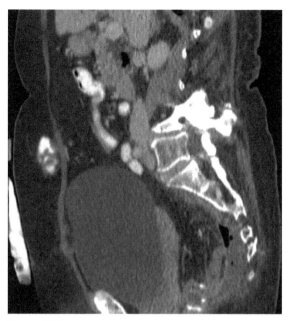

Figure 32-2

HISTORY: A 68-year-old female with recently diagnosed rectal cancer status post low anterior resection presents with worsening rectal pain.

1. Which of the following would be included in the differential diagnosis for the imaging findings presented? (Choose all that apply.)
   A. Fistula
   B. Abscess
   C. Perforation
   D. Bowel obstruction

2. Which complication is especially concerning given these imaging findings?
   A. Necrotizing fasciitis
   B. Bowel necrosis
   C. Osteomyelitis
   D. Pneumaturia

3. What is the preferred treatment for this condition?
   A. Image-guided drain placement
   B. Antibiotics
   C. Image-guided drain placement plus antibiotics
   D. Surgical drainage

4. Which of the following findings suggests a fistulous connection with a drained fluid collection?
   A. Persistent fevers
   B. Pneumaturia
   C. Persistent pain
   D. Persistent copious drainage

See Supplemental Figures section for additional figures and legends for this case.

CASE 32

Percutaneous Abscess Drainage

1. **A and B.** This is a gas-filled fluid collection that could represent perirectal abscess with or without fistula. Such a contained perforation would be unlikely, and no dilated loops of bowel were seen to suggest obstruction.

2. **C.** Sacral osteomyelitis is a real concern given the proximity of this collection to the sacrum. Pneumaturia can be seen in vesicocolic or vesicovaginal fistulae. Necrotizing fasciitis cannot occur within the abdominopelvic cavity, by definition, due to lack of fascia. Abdominal wall necrotizing fasciitis is possible, although unrelated to these imaging findings.

3. **C.** Patients with abscesses that are not drained have mortality rates ranging from 45% to 100% per the literature. Antibiotics are also required for treatment. Surgery is reserved for extremely complex cases or fistulae after acute infection is under control.

4. **D.** Persistent copious drainage is a sign suggesting a fistulous connection with a nearby entity. Persistent fevers and pain may be a sign of persistent abscess, due to drain malfunction.

Comment

Treatment Methods

Percutaneous catheter drainage of an infected fluid collection is a common procedure performed by the interventional radiologist. Percutaneous drainage has nearly replaced surgical drainage as the treatment of choice for abscesses or other fluid collections because it is less invasive and has lower morbidity and expense. Overall, radiologic drainage is effective in greater than 80% of cases.

Percutaneous Management

A safe route to the fluid collection is required for percutaneous drainage, and typically fluoroscopy, ultrasound, or computed tomography can be used to guide safe passage of the needle so that vital structures are not transgressed (Figures S32-1 through S32-4). The best candidate for fluid collections are those that are unilocular, well-defined, and free flowing. More-complex collections (e.g., multilocular or debris laden) can be drained percutaneously, but complete drainage may be slow or impossible.

Clinical Management

Because drainage of infected collections can cause transient bacteremia, all patients should receive antibiotics before and after the procedure. A sample of the fluid should be acquired for culture, so that the antibiotics can be tailored to treat the organisms involved. The clinical condition of most patients improves significantly within 24 to 48 hours of effective drainage. Follow-up imaging is necessary to establish satisfactory drainage and exclude the presence of undrained components or fistulae, particularly when the clinical condition does not improve or there is continued daily output that does not taper in volume (Figure S32-5).

References

Lee MJ. Non-traumatic abdominal emergencies: imaging and intervention in sepsis. *Eur Radiol.* 2002;12:2172–2179.

Robert B, Yzet T, Regimbeau JM. Radiologic drainage of post-operative collections and abscesses. *J Visc Surg.* 2013;150S:S11–S18.

Cross-reference

Vascular and Interventional Radiology: The Requisites, 2nd ed, 401–418.

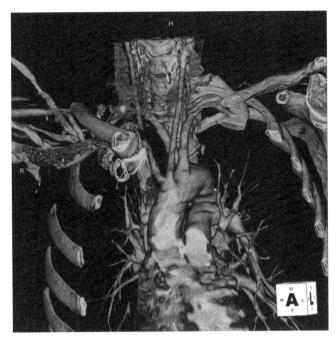

Figure 33-1. *Courtesy of Dr. Klaus D. Hagspiel.*

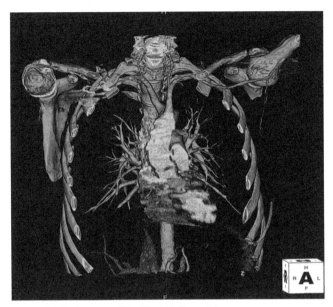

Figure 33-2. *Courtesy of Dr. Klaus D. Hagspiel.*

HISTORY: Computed tomography angiography of the chest following motor vehicle collision.

1. Which of the following would be included in the differential diagnosis for the imaging findings presented in Figure 33-1? (Choose all that apply.)
   A. Normal branching pattern of the aortic arch
   B. Common origin of bilateral common carotid arteries
   C. Aberrant right subclavian artery
   D. Common origin of the brachiocephalic trunk and left common carotid artery

2. Which of the following would be included in the differential diagnosis for the imaging findings presented in Figure 33-2?
   A. Normal branching pattern of the aortic arch
   B. Common origin of the brachiocephalic trunk and left common carotid artery
   C. Aberrant right subclavian artery
   D. Aberrant left subclavian artery

3. What is the normal order of branching of the aortic arch from proximal to distal?
   A. Brachiocephalic trunk-left common carotid-left vertebral artery
   B. Right vertebral artery-right common carotid-brachiocephalic trunk
   C. Brachiocephalic trunk-left common carotid-left subclavian artery
   D. Right subclavian-right common carotid-left subclavian

4. What is the most common normal variant of aortic arch branching?
   A. Aberrant right subclavian artery
   B. Common origin of the brachiocephalic trunk and left common carotid artery
   C. Left brachiocephalic trunk
   D. Left vertebral artery arises from aortic arch

See Supplemental Figures section for additional figures and legends for this case.

CASE 33

Variant Anatomy: Aortic Arch

1. **B and C.** The patient in Figure S33-1 has an aberrant right subclavian artery, which passes posterior to the esophagus causing posterior compression (not shown). This patient also has common origins of the common carotid arteries. This configuration is considerably rarer than that in the patient in Figure S33-2.

2. **C.** Figure S33-2 demonstrates an aberrant right subclavian artery passing posteriorly in the mediastinum.

3. **C.** The normal branching pattern of the aortic arch is present in only 70% of the population and is the brachiocephalic trunk, left common carotid, and left subclavian artery in that order.

4. **B.** The most common normal variant of aortic arch branching is the so-called bovine arch configuration, also known as common origin of the brachiocephalic trunk and left common carotid artery. This configuration, in reality, has little resemblance to bovine anatomy.

Comment

Main Teaching Point

Normally there are three branch vessels arising from the aortic arch. In order, these are the brachiocephalic artery, the left common carotid artery, and the left subclavian artery. Although this is the typical configuration, it is seen in only about 70% of patients. Multiple anatomic variants comprise the remainder. The most common of these is a common origin of the right brachiocephalic and left common carotid arteries. Following this in decreasing order of frequency include direct origin of the left vertebral artery from the aortic arch, common origin of the common carotid arteries (Figure S33-1), presence of two brachiocephalic arteries, and separate origin of each of the four great vessels from the aortic arch. The aberrant origin of the right subclavian artery (Figure S33-2) has been found to cause compression of the esophagus resulting in dysphagia, termed *dysphagia lusoria*.

Reference

Morgan-Hughes G, Roobottom C, Ring N. Anomalous aortic arch anatomy: three-dimensional visualization with multislice computed tomography. *Postgrad Med J.* 2003;79(929):167.

Cross-reference

Vascular and Interventional Radiology: The Requisites, 2nd ed, 177–183.

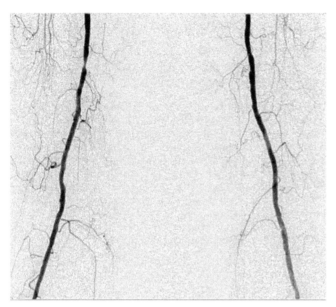

Figure 34-1

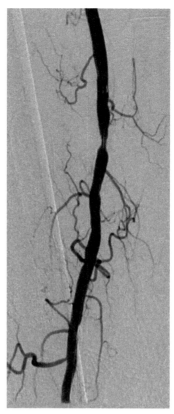

Figure 34-2

HISTORY: A 75-year-old female presenting with lifestyle-limiting calf pain after ambulating three blocks. Her symptoms are persistent despite adhering to an exercise regimen and medical therapy.

1. Which of the following is the most likely diagnosis for the imaging findings presented?
   A. Superficial femoral vein DVT (deep vein thrombosis)
   B. Common femoral artery dissection
   C. Profunda femoris stenosis
   D. Superficial femoral artery (SFA) stenosis

2. Based upon these images, if no other vascular lesions were present, what would the patient's ankle-brachial index (ABI) likely be?
   A. Below 0.4
   B. 0.5 to 0.9
   C. 1.0 to 1.2
   D. Above 1.2

3. In general, what is the first step in treatment when a patient is initially diagnosed with peripheral arterial disease?
   A. Angioplasty and stent placement
   B. Angioplasty
   C. Optimal medical therapy
   D. Femoropopliteal bypass

4. How would you treat the patient given the clinical presentation above?
   A. Endarterectomy
   B. Percutaneous revascularization
   C. Femoropopliteal bypass
   D. Aortofemoral bypass

See Supplemental Figures section for additional figures and legends for this case.

CASE 34

Superficial Femoral Artery Stenosis

1. **D.** These images depict a focal high-grade right SFA stenosis. No dissection or DVT is seen on these images.

2. **B.** 0.5 to 0.9. Since this patient has only one level of vascular disease, is experiencing intermittent claudication, and has no history of rest pain or tissue loss, the ABI is likely 0.5 to 0.9. An ABI of greater than 1.2 suggests vessel wall calcification and incompressibility and less than 0.4 usually correlates with rest pain and critical limb ischemia.

3. **C.** A therapeutic trial with optimal medical therapy should be attempted prior to intervention. Optimal medical therapy not only focuses on treatment aimed at symptomatic relief, it also includes cardiovascular risk factor modification, including smoking cessation, a supervised exercise regimen, statin therapy, blood pressure and diabetes control, antiplatelet therapy, and a trial of cilostazol, if appropriate.

4. **B.** Based on the clinical history of lifestyle-limiting symptoms refractory to optimal medical therapy, intervention should be considered in this patient. Percutaneous revascularization is the least invasive method with percutaneous angioplasty (PTA) alone being an acceptable option given the short lesion length. Femoropopliteal bypass could be considered, although endovascular options, which carry much lower rates of morbidity, should be considered first in this elderly patient.

Comment

Clinical Presentation

In general, patients with a single vascular level of disease are likely to experience intermittent claudication without rest pain and are likely to have an ABI of 0.5 to 0.9. Patients with rest pain nearly always have more than one level of vascular disease (for example, iliac artery disease and femoral artery disease), and they typically have an ABI under 0.4. The major indications for invasive treatment of lower-extremity atherosclerotic disease are limb-threatening rest pain or ulceration, lifestyle-limiting intermittent claudication, and the presence of a lesion that is suspected of being a source of distal embolization.

Endovascular Treatment

Traditionally the endovascular treatment of SFA stenosis consisted of PTA with stenting reserved for technical complications such as dissection (also known as provisional PTA with bailout stenting) (Figures S34-1 through S34-3). However, a wealth of new technological advances has recently changed the way that SFA disease is treated. While an in-depth discussion on the subject is beyond the scope of this text, there have been many randomized controlled trials evaluating the various therapies available.

Treatment Outcomes

The expected 5-year patency of a femoropopliteal bypass graft is 50% to 80%, depending upon the level of the distal anastomosis and the quality of the runoff vessels. In contrast, the expected 2-year patency of a SFA plain balloon angioplasty procedure is 50% to 70%, with 5-year patency well under 50%. However, the morbidity of endovascular treatment is significantly lower than that of surgical bypass grafting, and bypass can potentially be performed following failure of endovascular therapy or disease recurrence. The BASIL trial demonstrated equivalent rates of amputation-free survival between those randomized to open surgery versus percutaneous revascularization, with decreased morbidity and decreased costs within the first year in the endovascular arm. For these reasons, patients with peripheral arterial disease are often treated with an endovascular-first strategy.

References

Adam DJ, Beard JD, Cleveland T, et al. on behalf of the BASIL trial participants. Bypass versus angioplasty in severe ischaemia of the leg (BASIL): multicentre, randomised controlled trial. *Lancet.* 2005;366:1925–1934.

Chowdhury MM, McLain AD, Twine CP. Angioplasty versus bare metal stenting for superficial femoral artery lesions. *Cochrane Database Syst Rev.* 2014;24(6):CD006767.

Dick P, Wallner H, Sabeti S, et al. Balloon angioplasty versus stenting with nitinol stents in intermediate length superficial femoral artery lesions. *Catheter Cardiovasc Interv.* 2009;74:1090–1095.

Schillinger M, Sabeti S, Dick P, et al. Sustained benefit at 2 years of primary femoropopliteal stenting compared with balloon angioplasty with optional stenting. *Circulation.* 2007;115:2745–2749.

Cross-reference

Vascular and Interventional Radiology: The Requisites, 2nd ed, 343–350.

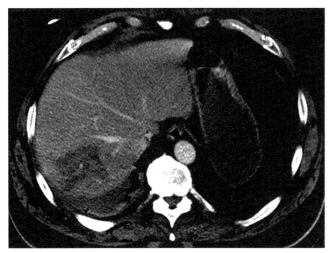

Figure 35-1

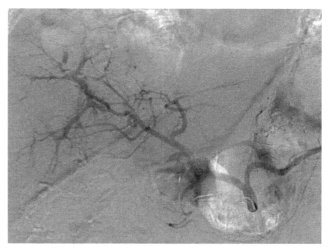

Figure 35-2

HISTORY: A 62-year-old male status post motor vehicle collision.

1. Which of the following is the most likely diagnosis for the imaging findings presented?
   A. Traumatic portal thrombosis
   B. Traumatic hepatic infarct
   C. Liver laceration without evidence of active bleeding
   D. Liver laceration with active extravasation

2. What is the embolic agent of choice for traumatic hepatic injuries?
   A. Gelfoam and coils
   B. Gelfoam and particles
   C. Coils and particles
   D. Gelfoam and glue

3. What concomitant condition increases the risk for hepatic infarction following embolization?
   A. Peripheral location
   B. Multicentric extravasation
   C. Portal thrombus
   D. Hemobilia

4. What is a common location of non-targeted embolization?
   A. Gallbladder
   B. Spleen
   C. Small bowel
   D. Stomach

See Supplemental Figures section for additional figures and legends for this case.

CASE 35

Traumatic Hepatic Laceration

1. **D.** The arterial phase image shows a small focus of arterial blush that dissipates on the portal venous phase, imaging consistent with active extravasation within a hepatic dome laceration.

2. **A.** Gelfoam and coils are the embolic agents of choice. Gelfoam is a temporary embolic agent that can be used nonselectively for embolization rather than selecting and coil embolizing each branch.

3. **C.** There is a dual blood supply to the liver with roughly 70% derived from the portal vein. Patients with portal vein thrombosis and portal hypertension are at increased risk of hepatic ischemia following hepatic artery embolization.

4. **A.** The cystic artery should be identified prior to embolization. Nontarget embolization of the cystic artery can lead to gallbladder necrosis.

Comment

Imaging Interpretation

Patients with blunt abdominal trauma are initially evaluated with contrast-enhanced computed tomography (CT) imaging (Figure S35-1). Hepatic injuries are typically categorized on CT into five categories, and in many institutions patients with CT evidence of contrast extravasation and most patients with grade 3 to 5 injuries (grade 3 = laceration 3 to 10 cm in length or hematoma 3 to 10 cm in thickness) typically undergo arteriography to search for arterial bleeding (Figure S35-2). When bleeding is seen, embolization can be performed with a high likelihood of success.

Treatment Methods

Hepatic ischemia following embolization is uncommon because approximately 70% of hepatic blood supply is derived from the portal venous system. For these reasons, when a laceration involves a large part of the hepatic parenchyma and multiple bleeding arteries are present, Gelfoam can be used to embolize an entire hepatic lobe rather than attempting to coil embolize each individual branch. However, patients with portal venous thrombosis and those with portal hypertension are at increased risk for hepatic ischemia, and embolization in these patients should be performed judiciously (portal hypertension patients) or not at all (portal vein thrombosis patients). This patient was treated with a combination of coils and Gelfoam (Figures S35-3 and S35-4).

References

Hagiwara A, Murata A, Matsuda T, et al. The efficacy and limitations of transarterial embolization for severe hepatic injury. *J Trauma.* 2002;52:1091–1096.

Hardy AH, Phan H, Khanna P, Nolan T, Dong P. Transcatheter treatment of liver lacerations from blunt trauma. *Semin Intervent Radiol.* 2012;29:197–200.

Romano L, Giovine S, Guidi G, Tortora G, Cinque T, Romano S. Hepatic trauma: CT findings and considerations based on our experience in emergency diagnostic imaging. *Eur J Radiol.* 2004;50:59–66.

Cross-reference

Vascular and Interventional Radiology: The Requisites, 2nd ed, 255–256.

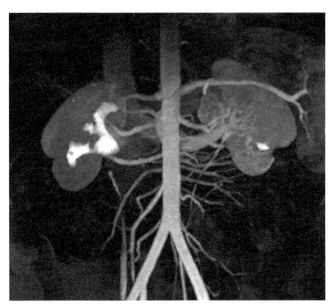

Figure 36-1. *Courtesy of Dr. J. Fritz Angle.*

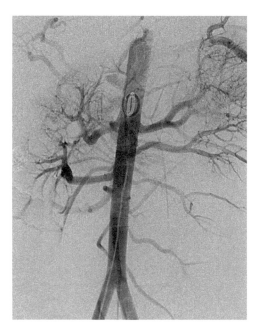

Figure 36-2. *Courtesy of Dr. J. Fritz Angle.*

HISTORY: A 23-year-old male undergoing evaluation as a renal transplant donor.

1. Which of the following is the most likely diagnosis for the imaging findings presented?
   A. Duplicate renal veins
   B. Duplicate renal arteries
   C. Circumaortic renal vein
   D. Early branching of the segmental renal arteries

2. Which kidney is generally preferred by surgeons for renal transplantation?
   A. Right kidney
   B. Left kidney
   C. The one with a single renal artery
   D. No preference

3. What findings in a renal artery angiogram completely rule out harvest for transplantation?
   A. Unilateral atherosclerotic renal ostial disease
   B. Parenchymal scarring
   C. Three renal arteries, one of which is a superior pole artery measuring 1.5 mm
   D. Bilateral string of beads appearance of the renal arteries

4. Which branch vessels least commonly arise from the renal arteries?
   A. Ureteral arteries
   B. Inferior phrenic arteries
   C. Adrenal arteries
   D. Capsular arteries

See Supplemental Figures section for additional figures and legends for this case.

CASE 36

Variant Anatomy: Multiple Renal Arteries

1. **B.** There is bilateral duplication of the renal arteries as can be seen on both the coronal maximum intensity projection magnetic resonance angiography (MRA) and the aortogram, which is confirmed on selective renal arteriograms. Early renal artery bifurcation is present when the bifurcation occurs less than 1 cm from the aortic origin, not present in this case. The renal veins appear normal on limited evaluation. Retroaortic and circumaortic renal veins are avoided in renal harvest because of increased venous injury risk.

2. **B.** The left kidney has a longer renal vein and is therefore preferred for healthy donor transplant nephrectomy. Kidneys with a single renal artery are preferred over those with multiple renal arteries, but the longer renal vein in a left kidney with two renal arteries is preferred over a right kidney with a single renal artery. Kidneys with accessory lower pole renal arteries are less desirable because of injury risk to the collecting system.

3. **D.** The string of beads appearance is seen in patients with fibromuscular dysplasia (FMD). Bilateral FMD precludes harvest for transplantation. The other characteristics described are relative contraindications. With the acceptance of older donors, atherosclerotic disease is more prevalent and can be dealt with by endarterectomy at time of harvest if unilateral. Small parenchymal scars do not rule out transplantation.

4. **B.** Inferior phrenic arteries most commonly arise directly from the aorta or celiac axis but can rarely arise from the renal arteries.

Comment

Main Teaching Point

Patients being considered as donors for renal transplantation may undergo preoperative imaging and angiographic evaluation directed at determining several specific pieces of information. (1) The size and number of renal arteries on each side and the presence of any anatomic variants: Generally, kidneys with a single renal artery of significant size are preferred. (2) The presence of early bifurcation of the renal artery: This is important because there must be sufficient room to place a clamp (which measures approximately 1 cm in width) across the donor main renal artery before its division. (3) The presence of stenosis or any evidence of FMD: Patients with these disorders are not generally considered candidates for transplantation. (4) The presence of parenchymal or ureteral anomalies that are not detected on other imaging examinations: In recent years, many institutions rely instead upon noninvasive modalities such as MRA or computed tomography angiography to evaluate renal donors (Figure S36-1).

Anatomy

Renal arteries are of three types: hilar, polar, and capsular. Multiple renal arteries occur in 30% of patients, and they represent the most common anomaly of the renal arteries. Accessory hilar renal arteries most commonly arise from the aorta inferior to the main renal artery, but they can arise anywhere in the abdominal aorta or from the iliac arteries. If the flush aortogram does not clearly demonstrate what parenchymal distribution is supplied by a particular artery suspected of providing renal supply, then selective arteriography can be performed to clarify this (Figures S36-2 through S36-6).

References

Liem YS, Kock MC, Ijzermans JN, et al. Living renal donors: optimizing the imaging strategy-decision and cost-effectiveness analysis. *Radiology.* 2003;226:53–62.

Sebastià C, Peri L, Salvador R, et al. Multidetector CT of living renal donors: lessons learned from surgeons. *Radiographics.* 2010;30:1875–1890.

Shetty A, Adiyat KT. Comparison between helical computed tomography angiography and intraoperative findings. *Urol Ann.* 2014;6:192–197.

Cross-reference

Vascular and Interventional Radiology: The Requisites, 2nd ed, 265–268.

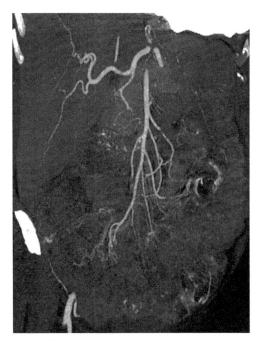

Figure 37-1

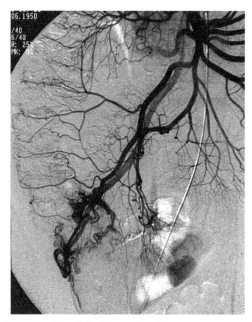

Figure 37-2. *Courtesy of Dr. Thomas Vesely.*

HISTORY: A 73-year-old female presents with hematochezia and acute decrease in hemoglobin.

1. Which of the following is the most likely diagnosis for the imaging findings presented?
   A. Metastatic endometrial cancer
   B. Bleeding diverticulum
   C. Angiodysplasia
   D. Post-radiation changes

2. What is the preferred treatment for this condition in the *acute* phase?
   A. Embolization
   B. Hormonal therapy
   C. Surgical resection
   D. Endoscopic treatment

3. What is the typical location for this condition?
   A. Small bowel
   B. Descending and sigmoid colon
   C. Cecum and ascending colon
   D. Stomach

4. What percentage of gastrointestinal (GI) bleeding is attributed to this condition?
   A. Less than 1%
   B. 3% to 5%
   C. 10% to 15%
   D. 25% to 30%

See Supplemental Figures section for additional figures and legends for this case.

CASE 37

Angiodysplasia

1. **C.** There is no mass and no active bleeding. Radiation changes tend to cause vascular stenosis rather than a tangle of vessels with early draining vein as noted in this case.

2. **D.** Endoscopic management is the preferred method of treatment in the acute phase, if possible. There is a high rate of rebleeding with embolization. Hormonal therapy is used in the chronic phase. Surgical resection can also be performed, but generally this is reserved for dire situations or after angiographic localization of the acute site of bleed.

3. **C.** Greater than 70% of angiodysplasia occurs in the cecum or ascending colon; it is the second most common cause of GI bleeding in patients greater than 60. Diverticulosis more commonly occurs on the left side and is the most common cause of lower GI bleeding in the adult population. Up to 15% occur in the jejunum or ileum, making it the second most common location for angiodysplasia.

4. **B.** Diverticulosis is responsible for approximately 60% of lower GI bleeding in adults. Angiodysplasia is estimated to occur in 3% to 5% of patients, although some estimates place it as high as 7%.

Comment

Patient Presentation

Angiodysplasia is a vascular abnormality that may be the cause of chronic intermittent GI bleeding or, rarely, acute massive bleeding in up to 50% of persons older than 55 years. However, because it has been identified incidentally in 15% of nonbleeding patients at mesenteric angiography, the presence of angiodysplasia does not confirm that it is the source of bleeding. Active contrast extravasation is only identified in 10% of cases. Therefore, in the evaluation of GI bleeding, one should diligently search for an alternate cause of bleeding if angiodysplasia without active extravasation is identified.

Diagnostic Imaging

Although these lesions can be located anywhere along the GI tract, they are typically located within the right colon and particularly within the cecum (Figure S37-1). They range in size from very tiny to very large, as in this case. The imaging characteristics include a vascular tuft or tangle of vessels with early, intense filling of the draining vein that then slowly empties (Figures S37-2 and S37-3). In order to make the diagnosis, one needs to see simultaneous opacification of the artery and vein that, because they run in parallel, typically creates a tram-track appearance. This lesion can be missed at colonoscopy, so angiography is very useful in diagnosis.

Treatment Methods

Because of the abnormal vessels, bleeding from angiodysplasia is typically not responsive to vasopressin infusion. Surgical resection is curative. Endoscopic therapy is usually the first-line treatment, but with a rebleeding rate of up to 36%. Embolization has been attempted with variable success but carries a fairly high rate of rebleeding and complications such as bowel ischemia; it has a role in the management of acute life-threatening hemorrhage. Interventional radiology catheter localization with dye injection of angiodysplasia prior to surgical resection has been reported, but widespread use of this technique has yet to surface. Use of somatostatin has been proposed for use in the subacute or chronic phase.

References

Jackson C, Gerson L. Management of gastrointestinal angiodysplastic lesions (GIADs): a systematic review and meta-analysis. *Am J Gastroenterol.* 2014;109:474–483.

Junquera F, Quiroga S, Saperas E, et al. Accuracy of helical computed tomographic angiography for the diagnosis of colonic angiodysplasia. *Gastroenterology.* 2000;119:293–299.

Cross-reference

Vascular and Interventional Radiology: The Requisites, 2nd ed, 259–260.

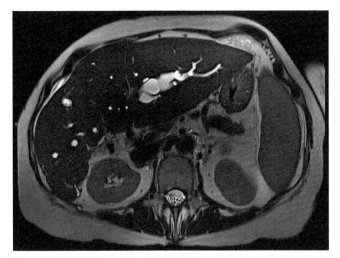

Figure 38-1. *Courtesy of Dr. J. Fritz Angle.*

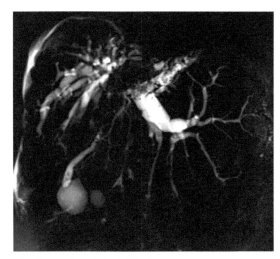

Figure 38-2. *Courtesy of Dr. J. Fritz Angle.*

HISTORY: A 58-year-old woman presents with pruritus and abdominal pain.

1. Which of the following would be included in the differential diagnosis for the imaging findings presented? (Choose all that apply.)
   A. Caroli's disease
   B. Cholangiocarcinoma
   C. Primary biliary cirrhosis
   D. Primary sclerosing cholangitis

2. Prior to performing a hepatobiliary intervention, which of the following antibiotics could be administered to decrease risk of sepsis?
   A. Trimethoprim-sulfamethoxazole
   B. Levofloxacin
   C. Vancomycin
   D. Ampicillin

3. Stents can be used to treat both malignant and benign biliary strictures. Which of the following should NOT be used to treat a benign biliary stricture?
   A. Metallic stent
   B. Plastic stent
   C. Surgical revision of the stricture
   D. Internal-external biliary drain

4. Which of the following is NOT a risk factor for cholangiocarcinoma?
   A. Ulcerative colitis
   B. Primary sclerosing cholangitis
   C. Hepatolithiasis
   D. Cholelithiasis

See Supplemental Figures section for additional figures and legends for this case.

CASE 38

Cholangiocarcinoma (Klatskin Tumor)

1. **A, B, and D.** The images are most representative of a Klatskin tumor, which is a cholangiocarcinoma at the confluence of the right and left hepatic ducts causing significant dilatation of the intrahepatic biliary tree. Caroli's disease, a genetic disorder that results in segmental or lobar dilatation of the intrahepatic bile ducts, can also have this appearance. It is also a risk factor for cholangiocarcinoma. Primary sclerosing cholangitis (choice D) typically manifests as multiple focal biliary strictures, which are commonly associated with biliary ductal dilatation.

2. **B.** Hepatobiliary interventions place patients at risk for bacterial translocation into the bloodstream and subsequent sepsis. The risk is higher if the patient already has cholangitis. Broad-spectrum antibiotic coverage is warranted, which cover common pathogens infecting the biliary tree. These pathogens include intestinal flora such as anaerobes, *Escherichia coli*, *Klebsiella*, or *Enterococcus*. Levofloxacin, a fluoroquinolone, provides excellent biliary bioavailability and provides appropriate coverage. Vancomycin only covers gram-positive cocci. Ampicillin is inappropriate monotherapy but may be administered with an aminoglycoside. Ceftriaxone is another antibiotic that is commonly administered.

3. **A.** Biliary stent placement can be performed both endoscopically and transhepatically. Despite what method is used, metallic stents are most commonly used if the patient's expected life span is less than 6 months because they generally cannot be retrieved and are prone to occlusion and failure. Therefore, they should not be used to treat benign biliary strictures where the prognosis is better with other appropriate therapies. All of the other options can be used to treat benign biliary strictures. Plastic stents are often used and exchanged at regularly scheduled intervals.

4. **D.** Cholelithiasis is not a risk factor for cholangiocarcinoma, whereas all the other choices are known risk factors.

Comment

Indication

Percutaneous transhepatic cholangiography (PTC) has largely been replaced by endoscopic retrograde cholangiopancreatography (ERCP) for the treatment of obstructive biliary disease. However, the primary indications for PTC are evaluation and treatment of biliary obstructive disease in symptomatic patients who are not amenable to or who fail ERCP. Diagnostic imaging may also guide clinicians in decision making as to whether ERCP or PTC and drainage should be attempted (Figures S38-1 and S38-2).

Percutaneous Management

Bacterial overgrowth is common in patients with biliary obstruction. Therefore, all patients should receive preprocedural antibiotics to cover gram-negative species, even in the absence of overt signs and symptoms of cholangitis. A bile duct sample should be sent for culture. A fluid sample can be sent for cytologic analysis when neoplasm is suspected. Material can also be acquired using a brush biopsy device or fine needle aspiration. Larger specimens can be obtained using biopsy forceps or atherectomy devices.

Procedural Technique

If it is necessary to drain the liver percutaneously, a peripheral biliary radical should be selected from the cholangiogram images for needle and subsequent catheter insertion, if the initial needle entry site is unfavorable (Figures S38-3 and S38-4). Manipulation should be minimized in patients with signs and symptoms of suppurative cholangitis, and in these patients, temporary external drainage is preferred. Definitive internal drainage via internal-external biliary drains or internal stents may be delayed several days to allow resolution of cholangitis (Figure S38-5). Contraindications to PTC include uncorrectable coagulopathy and massive ascites due to danger of hemorrhage and leak of ascites around the catheter insertion site, respectively.

References

Szklaruk J, Tamm E, Charnsangevej C. Preoperative imaging of biliary tract cancers. *Surg Oncol Clin N Am.* 2002;11:865–876.

Venkatesan A, Kundu S, Sacks D, et al. Practice guideline for adult antibiotic prophylaxis during vascular and interventional radiology procedures. *J Vasc Interv Radiol.* 2010;21:1611–1630.

Cross-reference

Vascular and Interventional Radiology: The Requisites, 2nd ed, 451–473.

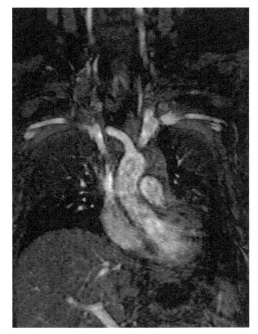

Figure 39-1. *Courtesy of Dr. David M. Williams.*

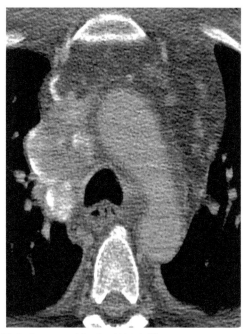

Figure 39-2. *Courtesy of Dr. David M. Williams.*

HISTORY: A 67-year-old female with a history of colon cancer who presents with syncope, swelling, and congestion of the upper half of her body.

1. Which of the following is the most likely diagnosis for the imaging findings presented?
   A. Aortic dissection
   B. Superior vena cava obstruction (SVCO)
   C. Subclavian steal syndrome
   D. Pulmonary arteriovenous malformation (AVM)

2. What is the most common underlying etiology of the diagnosis?
   A. Prior radiation therapy
   B. Presence of a pacemaker
   C. Cardiac catheterization
   D. Intrathoracic malignancy

3. Which of the following indications is NOT an emergent treatment of a patient with this diagnosis?
   A. Cerebral edema
   B. Pulmonary edema
   C. Laryngeal edema
   D. Hemodynamic compromise

4. What endovascular treatment modality is safe and effective in treating this diagnosis?
   A. Chemoembolization
   B. Coil embolization
   C. Endovascular stent placement
   D. Radiofrequency ablation

See Supplemental Figures section for additional figures and legends for this case.

CASE 39

Superior Vena Cava Obstruction

1. **B.** The images demonstrate an area of stenosis at the superior vena cava (SVC), consistent with the diagnosis of SVCO, which is most commonly due to extraluminal compression from an intrathoracic malignancy. Limited images do not demonstrate aortic dissection and the pulmonary vasculature is not visualized on these images, making pulmonary AVM unlikely.

2. **D.** Malignancy is the most common cause of SVCO, specifically lung carcinoma and lymphoma. Other neoplastic conditions associated with SVCO include metastatic mediastinal nodes, germ cell tumors, and malignant thymomas. Radiation therapy, pacemaker use, and central venous catheter placement are risk factors for the development of SVCO but are not as commonly the cause as malignancy. Cardiac catheterization is not a known risk factor for SVCO.

3. **B.** Cerebral edema, laryngeal edema, and hemodynamic compromise are all reasons for emergent endovascular treatment of SVCO. Pulmonary edema is not a common sequela of SVCO.

4. **C.** Endovascular stent placement with or without balloon angioplasty provides safe and rapid symptom relief to patients with SVCO. It also allows for future histological assessment of the malignancy responsible for SVC compression. Oftentimes, stent placement is utilized for malignant SVCO and primary angioplasty for benign causes with stenting reserved for recurrent or nonresponsive stenoses. Chemoembolization, coil embolization, and radiofrequency ablation are not as rapid or effective at treating malignant SVCO and its symptoms.

Comment

Clinical Presentation

Patients with SVCO commonly experience pronounced facial and arm swelling, headaches, hoarseness, dysphagia, and dyspnea. In severe cases, SVCO can cause syncope, visual and cognitive disturbances, seizures, and even coma. The most common cause of SVCO is intrathoracic malignancy, commonly bronchogenic carcinoma or lymphoma (Figures S39-1 and S39-2). Other risk factors for the development of SVCO include the use of central venous catheters, pacemakers, and prior radiation therapy.

Treatment Methods

Patients with malignant SVCO are typically treated with external-beam irradiation with or without adjunctive chemotherapy depending upon tumor histology and stage. This approach produces symptomatic improvement in 60% to 75% of patients within 2 to 4 weeks. Patients with benign causes of SVCO are usually treated with anticoagulation, and selected patients are offered surgical venous bypass.

Endovascular Management

Endovascular methods have been used to treat SVCO with good success. When SVCO is caused by SVC stenosis without thrombus formation, endovascular stents can be placed (Figures S39-3 through S39-5). When SVC thrombosis is present, catheter-directed thrombolysis can first be used to remove the thrombus before the stent is placed. Response to endovascular therapy occurs in 95% of patients within a few days.

References

Katabathina VS, Restrepo CS, Betancourt Cuellar SL, et al. Imaging of oncologic emergencies: what every radiologist should know. *Radiographics*. 2013;33:1533–1553.

Nicholson AA, Ettles DF, Arnold A, et al. Treatment of malignant superior vena cava obstruction: metal stents or radiation therapy. *J Vasc Intervent Radiol*. 1997;8:781–788.

Rachapalli V, Boucher L. Superior vena cava syndrome: role of the interventionalist. *Can Assoc Radiol J*. 2014;65:168–176.

Vedantham S. Endovascular strategies for superior vena cava obstruction. *Tech Vasc Intervent Radiol*. 2000;3:29–39.

Cross-reference

Vascular and Interventional Radiology: The Requisites, 2nd ed, 144–145.

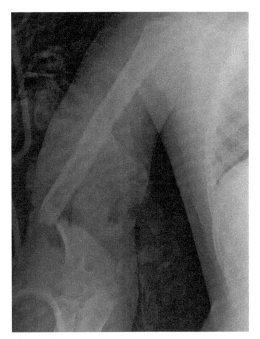

Figure 40-1

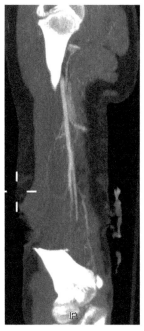

Figure 40-2

HISTORY: A 10-year-old male presenting with an acutely pulseless right upper extremity.

1. Which of the following would be included in the differential diagnosis for the imaging findings presented? (Choose all that apply.)
   A. Acute traumatic injury to the brachial artery
   B. Non-accidental trauma
   C. Early branching of the right radial artery at the mid-humerus
   D. Pathologic fracture due to infection

2. Regarding the differential diagnosis for brachial artery trauma, which of the following is TRUE?
   A. Includes vasospasm, transection, and pseudoaneurysm
   B. Includes vasospasm, intramural hematoma, and transection
   C. Includes dissection, true aneurysm, and occlusion
   D. Includes wall thickening, friability, and penetrating ulcer

3. The most appropriate management of an acute traumatic brachial artery transection with ischemia of the ipsilateral limb includes which one of the following?
   A. Balloon angioplasty and stenting
   B. Catheter-directed thrombolytic therapy
   C. Open surgical repair
   D. Expectant management, with distal perfusion via collaterals

4. Which of the following statements regarding brachial artery trauma is TRUE?
   A. Prognosis for limb salvage is more favorable with injury proximal to the profunda brachii
   B. Vascular, instead of nerve injury, is the most important prognostic factor for long-term extremity function
   C. The ulnar nerve courses along the entire length of the brachial artery
   D. Brachial artery injury is associated with nerve injury, particularly the median nerve

See Supplemental Figures section for additional figures and legends for this case.

CASE 40

Traumatic Brachial Artery Occlusion

1. **A and C.** The finding is secondary to acute injury to the brachial artery in the setting of a displaced, comminuted spiral fracture of the right humerus in a pediatric victim of a motor vehicle accident. Incidental note is also made of an early branching right radial artery, which is a common anatomic variant. While option B could be true, it is much less likely.

2. **A.** The findings associated with trauma most commonly include vasospasm, transection, dissection, pseudoaneurysm, occlusion, and frank extravasation. The other findings are possible, but much less likely to be present in a case of acute trauma.

3. **C.** Open surgical management is the mainstay of therapy for traumatic brachial artery transection. Angiography is used to guide surgical repair, with select cases of brachial artery trauma amenable to percutaneous therapy.

4. **D.** The median nerve courses along the length of the brachial artery, predisposing victims to a high association of nerve injury in cases of brachial artery injury. Nerve injury is the most important prognostic factor for restoration of limb function, and limb salvage is reduced when injury occurs proximal to the profunda brachii.

Comment

Clinical Indications

When hard clinical signs of upper-extremity arterial injury are present, angiography should be performed promptly to guide surgical repair. When hard clinical signs are absent, indications for angiography include a shotgun blast etiology, a bullet following the course of a major artery over a long segment, history of peripheral vascular disease in the involved limb, thoracic outlet injury location, or the presence of extensive injury to bone or soft tissue (Figures S40-1 and S40-2). Angiography can be performed electively in proximity injuries.

Endovascular Evaluation

Catheter angiography is the gold standard for evaluating injuries to upper-extremity arteries. However, upper-extremity computed tomography angiography is now being employed more commonly (Figure S40-2). Guidewire and catheter manipulation within the area suspected of being injured should be avoided whenever possible in order to avoid inducing vasospasm that could be mistaken for an injury. Angiography provides information about the presence and location of arterial injury as well as the extent of injury. The presence of unsuspected injuries and the etiology of any pulse deficits might also be indicated by angiography. Common pitfalls in diagnosis include mistaking lacerated intima for thrombus or embolus, mistaking vasospasm for occlusion, and missing an intimal injury because of dense contrast or overlying bone. Two projections should be used for a complete study.

References

Bozlar U, Ogur T, Norton PT, et al. CT angiography of the upper extremity arterial system – part 1: anatomy, technique and use in trauma patients. *AJR*. 2013;201:745–752.

Soto JA, Munera F, Morales C. Focal arterial injuries of the proximal extremities: helical CT arteriography as the initial method of diagnosis. *Radiology*. 2001;218:188–194.

Cross-reference

Vascular and Interventional Radiology: The Requisites, 2nd ed, 131–134.

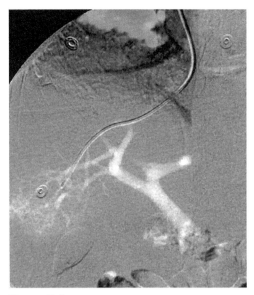

Figure 41-1

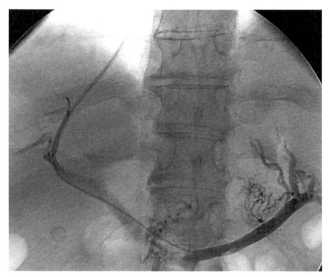

Figure 41-2

HISTORY: A 61-year-old man presents with recurrent ascites and right pleural effusion.

1. What contrast agent was used to acquire the first image?
   A. Full-strength iodinated contrast
   B. Gadavist
   C. ¼-strength iodinated contrast
   D. Carbon dioxide

2. What portosystemic gradient is associated with an increased risk for variceal hemorrhage?
   A. 4 mm Hg
   B. 8 mm Hg
   C. 11 mm Hg
   D. 16 mm Hg

3. Which of the following combinations is a long-term complication of a transjugular intrahepatic portosystemic shunt (TIPS)?
   A. Progressive liver failure and encephalopathy
   B. Progressive coagulopathy and pulmonary hypertension
   C. Spontaneous bacterial peritonitis and progressive encephalopathy
   D. TIPS stenosis and stroke

4. Wedged venography from a catheter in the right hepatic vein opacifies which vessel first?
   A. Left portal vein
   B. Right portal vein
   C. Main portal vein
   D. Left and right portal veins simultaneously

See Supplemental Figures section for additional figures and legends for this case.

CASE 41

TIPS: Portography and Wallstent

1. **D.** This wedged portogram was obtained using carbon dioxide as the portal system appears white on digital subtraction imaging.

2. **D.** A portosystemic gradient of 12 mm Hg or higher is associated with increased risk of variceal hemorrhage. Hence, the goal of a TIPS is to decrease this gradient to less than 12 mm Hg.

3. **A.** Progressive liver failure, encephalopathy, TIPS stenosis/thrombosis, and pulmonary hypertension are all long-term complications seen following TIPS.

4. **B.** The right portal vein will be opacified first as the hepatic sinusoids from the right portal system drain to the right hepatic vein.

Comment

Main Teaching Point

Portography is typically performed prior to accessing the portal system for safer targeting, compared to anatomic landmarks alone. Intra-procedural, pre-TIPS portography is not essential to the TIPS procedure. There are options both in apparatus and contrast for performing portography. The catheter or sheath may be wedged within the hepatic parenchyma or a balloon may be used for occlusion. Wedged portograms are faster to perform but do carry an increased risk of hepatic injury secondary to pressure induced on the hepatic parenchyma from contrast injection. Alternatively, portography may be performed using a balloon occlusion catheter. The pressure from contrast injected is dispersed over a larger surface area (greater vicinity of liver parenchyma and greater number of sinusoids), decreasing risk of pressure induced hepatic injury. The disadvantage of balloon occlusion is the risk of a poor contrast portogram due to outflow from hepatic venous collaterals. Regardless of apparatus, the contrast reaches the portal system due to high pressures in the hepatic sinusoids pushing contrast from the hepatic veins to the portal system. In other words: carbon dioxide (a compressible and highly soluble gas) is force-squeezed retrograde from the wedged hepatic venule through the sinusoids and retrograde into the afferent portal venules and then the greater portal vein branches. Both iodinated contrast and carbon dioxide may be used as the contrast agent (carbon dioxide is considerably safer). Iodinated contrast typically provides higher quality imaging. However, it also bears an increased risk of hepatic injury given the high viscosity. Carbon dioxide carries a lower risk or hepatic injury and does not add to the overall contrast load of the case.

Procedural Technique

A portogram allows the radiologist to determine in which hepatic vein the catheter or sheath is placed. An injection from the right hepatic vein will opacify the right portal vein first and then subsequently fill the left and main (Figure S41-1). A left hepatic vein injection will opacify to the left portal vein first and then the right and main. An injection from the middle portal vein will simultaneously opacify the left and right portal veins. After the portal vein is identified, the remainder of the procedure is performed as described in a subsequent case (Figures S41-2 through S41-4).

References

Gaba R, Khiatani V, Knuttinen G, et al. Comprehensive review of TIPS technical complications and how to avoid them. *AJR Am J Roentgenol.* 2011;196:675–685.

Maleux G, Nevens F, Heye S, et al. The use of carbon dioxide wedged hepatic venography to identify the portal vein: comparison with direct catheter portography with iodinated contrast medium and analysis of predictive factors influencing level of opacification. *J Vasc Interv Radiol.* 2006;17:1771–1779.

Cross-reference

Vascular and Interventional Radiology: The Requisites, 2nd ed, 311–325.

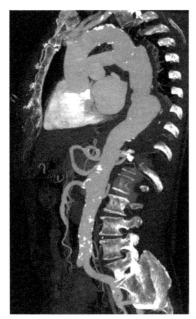

Figure 42-1. *Courtesy of Dr. Narasimham L. Dasika.*

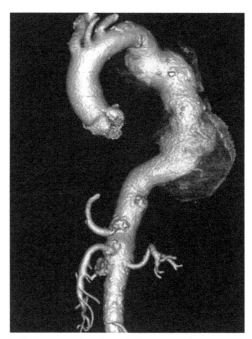

Figure 42-2. *Courtesy of Dr. Narasimham L. Dasika.*

HISTORY: A 55-year-old male with history of atherosclerosis.

1. Which of the following would be included in the differential diagnosis for the imaging findings presented? (Choose all that apply.)
   A. Syphilis
   B. Marfan syndrome
   C. Atherosclerosis
   D. Traumatic aortic injury

2. What is the definition of an aneurysmal thoracic aorta? (Choose all that apply.)
   A. Ascending aorta greater than 3 cm
   B. Descending aorta greater than 2 cm
   C. Ascending aorta greater than 4.5 cm
   D. Descending aorta greater than 4 cm

3. What method of treatment is preferred for a rapidly expanding (>10 mm per year) ascending aortic aneurysm?
   A. Regular follow-up
   B. Medical management
   C. Endovascular treatment
   D. Open surgical repair

4. What is a common complication of endovascular AND surgical thoracic aortic repair?
   A. Spinal cord ischemia
   B. Endoleak
   C. Hypertension
   D. Pulmonary embolism

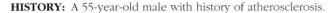

See Supplemental Figures section for additional figures and legends for this case.

CASE 42

Thoracic Aortic Aneurysm

1. **A, B, C, and D.** All of these choices can cause aortic aneurysms. Atherosclerosis and trauma are far more common than Marfan syndrome and syphilis.

2. **C and D.** These are the diameters generally agreed upon to represent aneurysmal thoracic aortic disease. However, parameters regarding when to repair the aneurysm have not yet been universally agreed upon. Generally, rapid expansion of an aneurysm (>10 mm per year), aneurysms of ascending aorta greater than 5 to 6 cm, and aneurysms of descending aorta greater than 6 to 7 cm are treated.

3. **D.** Surgical repair is performed for ascending aortic aneurysms—endovascular repair is not performed in these cases at this time.

4. **A.** Spinal cord ischemia is a risk of both open and endovascular surgical repair with similar percentage occurrence in each case. Endoleaks only occur with endovascular repair.

Comment

Etiology

Thoracic aortic aneurysms (TAAs) are commonly the result of atherosclerotic disease, although they can also result from trauma, connective tissue disorders, syphilis, infection, and other conditions. The main complication of TAAs is that of rupture, which occurs in 30% of aneurysms greater than 6 cm in diameter. For these reasons, TAAs 5.5 to 6.0 cm in diameter are generally repaired surgically. In female patients and those with connective tissue disorders, TAAs tend to rupture at smaller diameters, and these patients are therefore usually referred earlier for surgical repair.

Diagnostic Evaluation

The diagnosis of TAA is generally made using computed tomography (CT) or magnetic resonance imaging (MRI) (Figures S42-1 and S42-2). Angiography is rarely used for the diagnosis of TAA, and it does not provide accurate aneurysm diameter measurements in comparison with CT and MRI. However, angiography provides fairly accurate measurements of the length of the aorta and the degree of angulation in the proximal neck of the aneurysm, and it accurately depicts the aneurysm's relationship to the origins of the great vessels, as does intravascular ultrasound. These findings can be extremely important in surgical planning and in selecting a device and access route for endovascular stent-graft repair.

Treatment Methods

The most important drawbacks of surgical TAA repair are significant rates of perioperative mortality (6% to 12%), paraplegia (3% to 16%), and cardiopulmonary complications (5% to 30%). Early results suggest that significant improvements in perioperative mortality and morbidity are likely to be achieved with endovascular repair, although the durability of these procedures is not fully established (Figure S42-3). More recent studies suggest that endovascular repair of chronic type B aortic dissections undergoing aneurysmal enlargement is a technically feasible option with comparable morbidity and mortality to open repair. Follow-up imaging is performed after endovascular repair in order to monitor change in aneurysm sac size or other complications such as endoleak (Figures S42-4 and S42-5).

References

Mitchell RS. Stent grafts for the thoracic aorta: a new paradigm? *Ann Thorac Surg*. 2002;74:S1818–S1820.

Scali S, Feezor R, Chang C, et al. Efficacy of thoracic endovascular stent repair for chronic type B aortic dissection with aneurysmal degeneration. *J Vasc Surg*. 2013;58:10–17.

Cross-reference

Vascular and Interventional Radiology: The Requisites, 2nd ed, 183–188.

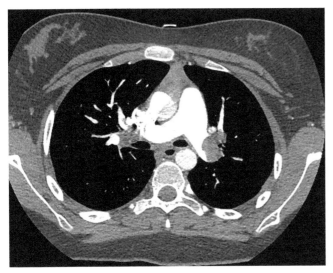

Figure 43-1. *Courtesy of Dr. Wael E. Saad.*

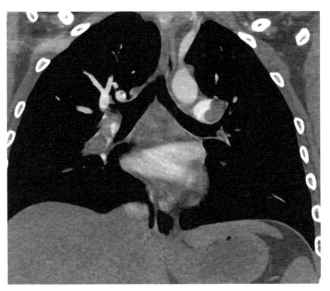

Figure 43-2. *Courtesy of Dr. Wael E. Saad.*

HISTORY: A 22-year-old female with chest pain, family history of Factor V Leiden mutation.

1. Which of the following would be included in the differential diagnosis for the imaging findings presented? (Choose all that apply.)
   A. Pulmonary artery sarcoma
   B. Acute pulmonary embolism
   C. Transient interruption of contrast
   D. Chronic pulmonary embolism

2. Which of the following modalities is LEAST beneficial in the workup of this entity?
   A. Magnetic resonance (MR) angiography
   B. Unenhanced chest computed tomography (CT)
   C. Xenon/^{Tc99m}MAA (technetium macro aggregated albumin) ventilation-perfusion scan (V/Q scan)
   D. Chest radiograph

3. Where is the most common location for this entity to occur in the acute setting?
   A. Subsegmental pulmonary arteries
   B. Pulmonary artery branching points
   C. Bronchial arteries
   D. Segmental pulmonary arteries

4. Which of the following is a treatment option for this entity?
   A. Surgical thrombectomy
   B. Anticoagulation
   C. Catheter-directed thrombolysis
   D. All of the above

See Supplemental Figures section for additional figures and legends for this case.

CASE 43

Acute Pulmonary Embolism

1. **A, B, C, and D.** Figures 43-1 and 43-2 demonstrate large filling defects in bilateral pulmonary artery branches. This can be seen in the setting of a pulmonary artery sarcoma, which can demonstrate similar CT and angiographic findings. Both acute and chronic pulmonary emboli (PE) manifest as intraluminal filling defects. Key factors aiding in the differentiation of these two entities include thrombus location within the vessel (peripheral vs. central), presence or absence of intraluminal webs, and presence or absence of smooth/nodular wall thickening, with the latter set of factors favoring an acute etiology.

2. **B.** The fundamental criteria for diagnosing pulmonary embolism on cross-sectional imaging revolves around the presence of an intraluminal filling defect within an involved pulmonary artery. Thus, an unenhanced CT would be the least beneficial study for this purpose. MR angiography would demonstrate a filling defect and can be an alternative modality used in patients who have a CT contrast dye allergy. The V/Q scan is a nuclear medicine study that is also commonly used in the evaluation of PE. A chest radiograph is considered a beneficial adjunct to the cross-sectional and nuclear medicine studies discussed above, as it can be used to reliably and efficiently rule-out other pathologies that can elicit similar symptoms of chest pain and/or shortness of breath in the patient, such as pneumonia, pulmonary edema, or atelectasis.

3. **B.** Since the overwhelming majority of pulmonary artery filling defects are caused by embolic phenomenon, rather than in situ thrombus formation, pulmonary artery branch points serve as an ideal location where the caliber of artery abruptly narrows and the site of branching inherently contributes to local turbulence of blood flow. These are factors that are amenable to lodging of traveling emboli.

4. **D.** Anticoagulation is the first-line treatment option for patients with deep vein thrombosis and/or PE. The purpose of anticoagulation is to prevent new thrombus formation while the body's endogenous processes lyse the existing thromboembolic burden. In the need for acute (usually life-saving) relief from hypoxia and right heart strain, aggressive treatment options include surgical thrombectomy/thromboendarterectomy and catheter-directed (pharmacological or mechanical) thrombolysis. Factors indicating which of the two interventions is favored are numerous, but include the time frame within which the intervention must be performed as well as the degree and extent of the patient's comorbidities.

Comment

Diagnostic Imaging

With the advent of spiral CT angiography, pulmonary arteriography is being performed much less often in the diagnosis of pulmonary embolism. Pulmonary arteriography has a negative predictive value of nearly 100% for vascular thromboembolism within 3 months. However, CT pulmonary angiography can be rapidly performed and is available in most medical centers and is quickly becoming the new gold standard (Figures S43-1 and S43-2).

Imaging Interpretation

The range of angiographic findings in acute pulmonary embolism includes abrupt vessel cutoff, intraluminal filling defects manifested by the tram-track sign, wedge-shaped parenchymal oligemia, absence of a draining vein from the affected segment, arterial collaterals, and hypervascularity of an infarcted segment (Figure S43-3). PEs are typically multiple and bilateral, and they tend to lodge in the lower lobe vessels.

Endovascular Intervention

The accuracy of pulmonary arteriography can be optimized with attention to several facts. Emboli lyse rapidly, so arteriography should be performed within 24 to 48 hours of symptoms. Multiple projections of both lungs should be obtained. V/Q scans and CT can be used to focus the examination to suspicious areas. Careful attention to small vessels, particularly in the lower lobes, is critical because many patients only have subsegmental emboli. Emboli can be missed because of overlapping vessels, small size of the emboli, or respiratory or patient motion, so additional imaging, including oblique or magnification views or selective vessel injection, may be necessary. Catheter-directed thrombolysis has been found to be effective in reducing right heart dysfunction in patients with acute PE (Figures S43-4 and S43-5).

References

Gaba R, Gundavaram M, Parvinian A, et al. Efficacy and safety of flow-directed pulmonary catheter thrombolysis for treatment of submassive pulmonary embolism. *AJR Am J Roentgenol.* 2014;202:1355–1360.

Harvey RB, Gester WB, Hrung JM, et al. Accuracy of CT angiography versus pulmonary angiography in the diagnosis of acute pulmonary embolism: evaluation of the literature with summary ROC curve analysis. *Acad Radiol.* 2000;7:786–797.

Kucher N, Boekstegers P, Muller O, et al. Randomized, controlled trial of ultrasound-assisted catheter-directed thrombolysis for acute intermediate-risk pulmonary embolism. *Circulation.* 2014;1 (29):479–486.

Cross-reference

Vascular and Interventional Radiology: The Requisites, 2nd ed, 159–168.

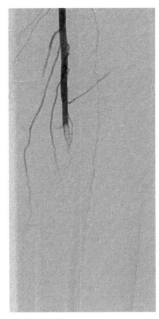

Figure 44-2

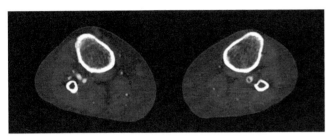

Figure 44-1

HISTORY: A 51-year-old female with atrial fibrillation presents with acute left lower-extremity pain.

1. Which of the following is the most likely diagnosis for the imaging findings presented?
   A. Giant cell arteritis
   B. Acute occlusive arterial thromboembolic disease
   C. Acute traumatic occlusion
   D. Arteriovenous fistula

2. Regarding thrombolytic therapy for acute limb ischemia, which of the following is TRUE?
   A. It is less effective in clearance of the affected microcirculation than open thrombectomy.
   B. It has an overall reduced risk of hemorrhage compared with surgery.
   C. Intravenous thrombolysis is the route of choice for delivery of thrombolytic agents.
   D. Thrombolytic therapy has become the intervention of choice in the past two decades.

3. An acutely ischemic limb, given category II-b according to the Society for Vascular Surgery Clinical Categories of Acute Limb Ischemia, would most likely have which prognosis?
   A. Major permanent tissue loss
   B. Not immediately threatened
   C. Salvageable with prompt treatment
   D. Salvageable with immediate treatment

4. A patient with atrial fibrillation on chronic warfarin therapy and an international normalized ratio of 1.8 presents with clinical findings of acute thromboembolic limb ischemia. He has no history of myocardial infarction. What anatomic site would be the most likely culprit for an acute arterial thrombus?
   A. Left atrial appendage
   B. Left ventricular true aneurysm
   C. Left common femoral vein deep venous thrombus via an atrial septal defect
   D. Infectious mitral valve vegetation

See Supplemental Figures section for additional figures and legends for this case.

CASE 44

Embolic Lower Extremity Arterial Occlusion

1. **B.** All of the other choices are not reasonable differential diagnoses for the appearance of an acute thrombus in the lumen of an artery with a meniscus sign. Other differential diagnostic considerations for this appearance would include septic thromboemboli, tumor thrombus, or in situ thrombosis, although a meniscus makes these less likely.

2. **D.** Catheter-directed thrombolysis has become the intervention of choice in most cases of acute limb ischemia secondary to acute thromboembolism or thrombosis. Thrombolysis is more effective than open surgery in clearing the microcirculation, carries a higher risk of hemorrhagic complications, and is no longer commonly performed via the venous route.

3. **D.** A Rutherford acute limb ischemia category II-b limb is immediately threatened, and is identified by rest pain, sensory loss at a distribution greater than the toes, and mild to moderate muscle weakness on clinical exam. A limb with the above findings merits emergent intervention.

4. **A.** The most common source of thrombus in a patient with atrial fibrillation who is subtherapeutic on warfarin is the left atrial appendage. The other choices are plausible but less likely. A left ventricular aneurysm would be rare in the absence of chronic infarction.

Comment

Clinical Presentation

Patients with acute limb ischemia typically present with a cold painful leg with pallor, cyanosis, and/or paresthesias. A careful pulse examination often suggests the level of obstruction. Profound sensory loss, muscle weakness, or paralysis are concerning for irreversible ischemia. Most macroemboli lodge near branch points in the femoral or popliteal arteries (Figure S44-1).

Endovascular Evaluation

The role of angiography in the evaluation of acute limb ischemia is fourfold (Figure S44-2): (1) determine the level of arterial obstruction and reconstitution; (2) determine whether the occlusion is embolic or thrombotic; (3) assist in finding the source of embolus. The most common source of emboli by far is the left heart, due to left atrial or ventricular dilation, dysrhythmia, valvular heart disease, left ventricular aneurysm, or rarely, left heart tumor; for this reason, echocardiography is often indicated. Angiography can sometimes localize the source of noncardiac emboli, which can originate from aneurysms or ulcerated plaque in the aortoiliac vessels; (4) in selected cases, reopen the artery.

Treatment Methods

Treatment is chosen based upon the presumed cause, the severity of the symptoms, and the patient's clinical condition. Acute embolization is treated with surgical embolectomy or bypass grafting if the limb appears severely threatened. Thrombolytic therapy can reduce the thrombus burden, but it can be ineffective in lysing the embolic nidus itself, which is composed of organized thrombus or plaque material. Ultimately, the embolic source must be treated to prevent recurrence.

References

Ebben H, Nederhoed J, Lely R, et al. Low-dose thrombolysis for thromboembolic lower extremity arterial occlusions is effective without major hemorrhagic complications. *Eur J Vasc Surg.* 2014;48 (5):551–558.

Ouriel K. Current status of thrombolysis for peripheral arterial occlusive disease. *Ann Vasc Surg.* 2002;16:797–804.

Cross-reference

Vascular and Interventional Radiology: The Requisites, 2nd ed, 351–357.

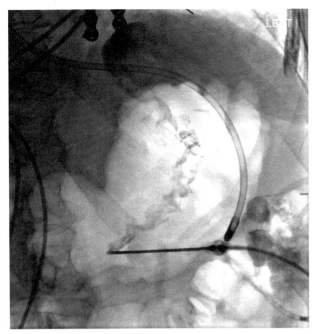

Figure 45-1

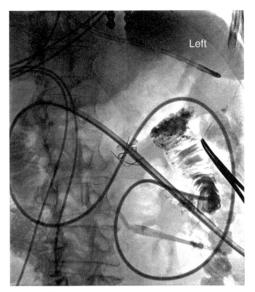

Figure 45-2

HISTORY: An 81-year-old female with a mass obstructing the duodenum.

1. Which of the following is the most likely procedure performed based on the imaging presented?
   A. Gastrostomy tube placement
   B. Gastrojejunostomy (GJ) tube placement
   C. Nephrostomy tube placement
   D. Cholecystostomy tube placement

2. Which of the following is NOT an indication for percutaneous GJ placement?
   A. Aspiration with gastric feeding
   B. Failed swallow evaluation
   C. Diabetic gastroparesis
   D. Gastric outlet obstruction

3. Which of the following is an absolute contraindication for percutaneous GJ placement?
   A. Transverse colon interposed between the stomach and anterior abdominal wall on recent computed tomography
   B. International normalized ratio 1.4
   C. Gastric varices
   D. Severe gastroparesis

4. The morning following a percutaneous gastrostomy placement, no fluid is identified within the gastrostomy drainage bag and the patient is complaining of severe abdominal pain. What is the next step in management?
   A. Begin enteral feeding through the gastrostomy tube.
   B. Wait an additional day to begin feeding through the gastrostomy tube.
   C. Inject contrast into the tube under fluoroscopy to evaluate for intraperitoneal placement.
   D. Consult gastroenterology for esophagogastroduodenoscopy.

See Supplemental Figures section for additional figures and legends for this case.

CASE 45

Percutaneous Gastrojejunostomy Placement

1. **B.** The figures demonstrate placement of a percutaneous GJ tube. The first figure was obtained after contrast injection demonstrating intragastric needle placement. The second image was obtained after tube placement and injection of the jejunal port demonstrating intrajejunal tube placement.

2. **B.** While failing a swallow evaluation is a common indication for gastrostomy tube placement, it alone is not an indication for GJ-tube placement. The indications for GJ tube placement include severe gastroparesis, gastric outlet obstruction, and aspiration with gastric feeding.

3. **C.** Due to the risk of severe bleeding, percutaneous gastrostomy/GJ should not be performed in patients with known gastric varices.

4. **C.** The absence of drained gastric fluid overnight in addition to the patient's abdominal pain is concerning for intraperitoneal tube placement. The tube should be evaluated prior to the initiation of any feeding.

Comment

Indication

The indications for placement of a percutaneous GJ tube (either de novo or via conversion of an existing gastrostomy tube to a GJ tube) include aspiration with gastric feeding, known severe gastroesophageal reflux, gastric outlet obstruction, and decreased gastric motility (e.g., patients with diabetic gastroparesis).

Procedural Technique

From a technical standpoint, three differences from percutaneous gastrostomy tube placement are present. First, because of the increased catheter manipulation required for GJ-tube placement, gastropexy with placement of two to four T-fasteners is strongly recommended (Figure S45-1). Second, catheterization of the duodenum can be challenging in patients with pyloric stenosis or unfavorable angulation of the initial gastrostomy tract. Third, extreme care must be used to avoid buckling a loop of catheter into the stomach during placement; this can result in loss of hard-earned access into the duodenum and can lengthen procedure time. The optimal positioning of the distal part of the tube is in the proximal jejunum beyond the ligament of Treitz (Figure S45-2).

References

Bell S, Carmody E, Yeung E, et al. Percutaneous gastrostomy and gastrojejunostomy: additional experience in 519 procedures. *Radiology.* 1995;194:817–820.

Lyon SM, Pascoe D. Percutaneous gastrostomy and gastrojejunostomy. *Semin Intervent Radiol.* 2004;21:181–189.

Cross-reference

Vascular and Interventional Radiology: The Requisites, 2nd ed, 432–436.

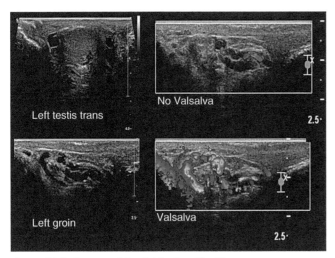

Figure 46-1. *Courtesy of Dr. C. Matthew Hawkins.*

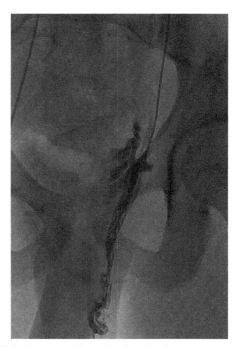

Figure 46-2. *Courtesy of Dr. C. Matthew Hawkins.*

HISTORY: An 18-year-old male presents to his physician with a painful knot of "worms" in his left scrotum.

1. Which of the following is the most likely diagnosis for the imaging findings presented?
   A. Spermatocele
   B. Testicular neoplasm
   C. Varicocele
   D. Hydrocele

2. When does this finding raise concern for malignancy?
   A. Never
   B. When it is only right sided
   C. When it is only left sided
   D. When it is bilateral

3. Which of the following is commonly associated?
   A. Orchitis
   B. Impotence
   C. Thrombophlebitis
   D. Infertility

4. Interventional management of the entity includes which of the following? (Choose all that apply.)
   A. Sclerosis
   B. Coil embolization
   C. Ablation
   D. None, management is surgical

See Supplemental Figures section for additional figures and legends for this case.

CASE 46

Male Varicocele

1. **C.** Ultrasound images demonstrate a left varicocele, which increases in size during Valsalva maneuver. Angiographic image with a catheter injecting contrast into the left gonadal vein demonstrates the varicocele.

2. **B.** Spontaneous unilateral varicoceles are much less common on the right, as the right gonadal vein drains directly into the inferior vena cava. Blood returning from the left testis has a more tortuous course through the left renal vein and is therefore more prone to obstruction and subsequent varicocele. For this reason, an isolated right varicocele is usually due to extrinsic compression, possibly from a mass, malignancy, or lymphadenopathy. Bilateral varicoceles are much more common and less ominous.

3. **B.** Infertility is the most common side effect of varicoceles, and nearly 50% of males evaluated for infertility have hydroceles. Improper temperature regulation of sperm is thought to be the culprit.

4. **A and B.** Both sclerosis with sotradecol foam or boiling hot contrast and embolization with coils or plugs have been shown to have high success rates as minimally invasive varicocele treatments. Success rates are similar to surgical procedures such as resection, but complications of hydrocele are greater in surgery.

Comment

Etiology

Varicocele is a dilation of the pampiniform plexus that affects 10% to 15% of males. Many theories have been proposed to explain primary varicocele, including abnormalities of the internal spermatic vein valves and left renal vein compression causing venous hypertension. A unilateral right varicocele or sudden onset of a varicocele in an older man should raise concern for an abdominal or pelvic mass causing venous compression and impaired venous drainage.

Patient Presentation

Most men are asymptomatic, but infertility resulting from impaired sperm motility and number, scrotal pain, and scrotal swelling and disfigurement can result. Nearly 50% of men evaluated for infertility have unilateral or bilateral varicocele. Leading theories suggest a relation to elevated scrotal temperature or reflux of metabolites from the renal and adrenal veins. Most varicoceles are detected on physical examination, but sonography, scintigraphy, venography, and magnetic resonance imaging are useful when the examination is normal or equivocal (Figures S46-1 and S46-2).

Treatment Methods

Surgical ligation and interventional sclerotherapy or embolization are the primary treatment modalities. Interventional methods involve performing a diagnostic venogram to confirm valvular incompetence followed by embolization or sclerosis of the internal spermatic vein from the level of the superior pubic ramus to the vein orifice with occlusion of collateral channels as necessary (Figures S46-2 through S46-6). Surgical and interventional radiology techniques demonstrate similar rates of technical success, improvement in sperm density and motility, subsequent pregnancy, and complications. Surgical techniques have higher association with hydroceles.

References

Fretz PC, Sandlow JI. Varicocele: current concepts in pathophysiology, diagnosis, and treatment. *Urol Clin North Am.* 2002;29:921–937.

Iaccarino V, Ventucci P. Interventional radiology of male varicocle: current status. *Cardiovasc Interv Radiol.* 2012;35:1263–1280.

Kwak N, Siegel D. Imaging and interventional therapy for varicoceles. *Curr Urol Rep.* 2014;15:399.

Cross-reference

Vascular and Interventional Radiology: The Requisites, 2nd ed, 306.

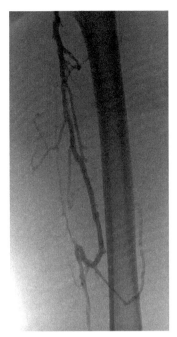

Figure 47-1. *Courtesy of Dr. Minhaj S. Khaja.*

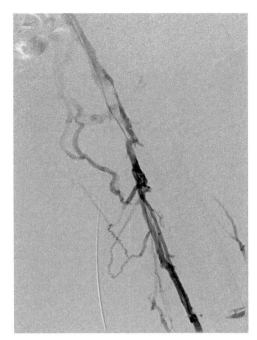

Figure 47-2. *Courtesy of Dr. Minhaj S. Khaja.*

HISTORY: A 53-year-old male with left calf swelling and discoloration.

1. Which of the following would be included in the differential diagnosis for the imaging findings presented? (Choose all that apply.)
   A. Acute deep vein thrombosis (DVT)
   B. Chronic DVT
   C. Acute superficial femoral artery thrombosis
   D. Chronic superficial femoral artery thrombosis

2. Which of the following is long-term sequela of this disorder?
   A. Calf pain, skin hyperpigmentation, ulceration, and swelling
   B. Diminished pedal pulses
   C. Increased ankle-brachial index
   D. Increased tissue oximetry values

3. What intrinsic abnormality should you consider in patients with multiple left lower extremity DVTs?
   A. *Phlegmasia alba dolens*
   B. Paget-Schroetter
   C. May-Thurner syndrome
   D. *Phlegmasia cerulea dolens*

4. Which of the following sonographic findings is NOT characteristic of this disorder?
   A. Compressible veins
   B. Noncompressible veins
   C. Wall-adherent echogenic material
   D. Synechiae

See Supplemental Figures section for additional figures and legends for this case.

CASE 47

Chronic Deep Vein Thrombosis

1. **A and B.** Venography demonstrates wall-adherent thrombus with synechiae and venous collaterals consistent with chronic DVT. Acute DVT usually causes occlusion and distension of the involved vein without extensive collateral formation but may be superimposed on chronic DVT.

2. **A.** These symptoms are all seen in postthrombotic syndrome (PTS). This syndrome is the long-term result of venous obstruction, valve reflux, and impaired venous return. The venous thrombotic event commonly damages the valves thus leading to venous reflux. Choices B, C, and D are methods used to evaluate arterial disease.

3. **C.** May-Thurner syndrome is due to the extrinsic compression of the left iliac vein by the right common iliac artery. This abnormality leads to increased incidence of DVT on the left. Paget-Schroetter disease is an upper-extremity DVT usually as a result of venous thoracic outlet syndrome. *Phlegmasia alba dolens* is a symptom of DVT characterized by pain, edema, and white (alba) appearance of the leg. *Phlegmasia cerulea dolens* results from a severe episode of DVT with occlusion of the major and collateral drainage veins of the lower extremity. This disorder results in severe pain, edema, and cyanosis (blue or cerulea) that can lead to gangrene.

4. **A.** Ultrasound findings of chronic DVT include wall-adherent echogenic thrombus, synechiae, and noncompressible veins with collateral formation. The veins can become thick walled or even appear like a fibrous cord when they fail to recanalize.

Comment
Clinical Presentation

From 25% to 50% of patients with DVT develop PTS. Patients with PTS often manifest symptoms of limb edema, aching, venous claudication, hyperpigmentation, and/or ulcerations. The symptoms are typically worse near the end of the day after the patient has been ambulatory. PTS is known to impair quality of life.

Etiology

The etiology of postthrombotic symptoms is ambulatory venous hypertension, which has two distinct components: completed valvular damage with subsequent reflux and persistent venous obstruction due to intraluminal thrombus and debris.

Image Interpretation

Venographic findings of chronic (>2 weeks) DVT often include a septated and contracted appearance of the involved vein(s) with multiple channels, relative lack of venous dilation, and the presence of large collaterals (Figures S47-1 and S47-2). Sonographic findings parallel the venographic findings and include increased echogenicity of the intraluminal material, a laminar distribution of the filling defects, and a septated appearance.

References

Nayak L, Vedantham S. Multifaceted management of the post-thrombotic syndrome. *Semin Intervent Radiol.* 2012;29:16–22.

Stain M, Schonauer V, Minar E, et al. The post-thrombotic syndrome: risk factors and impact on the course of thrombotic disease. *J Thromb Haemost.* 2005;3:2671–2676.

Cross-reference

Vascular and Interventional Radiology: The Requisites, 2nd ed, 374–375.

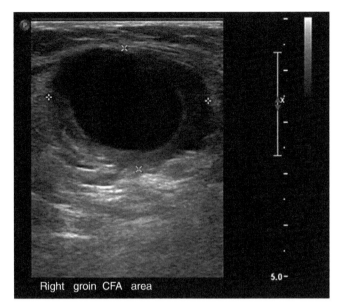

Figure 48-1. *Courtesy of Dr. Minhaj S. Khaja.*

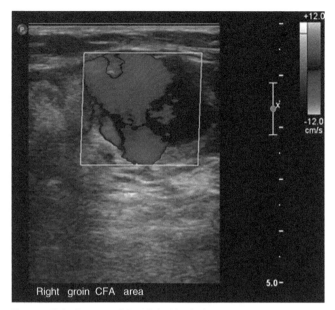

Figure 48-2. *Courtesy of Dr. Minhaj S. Khaja.*

HISTORY: A 55-year-old woman with a pulsatile right groin mass and ecchymosis, 2 days after cardiac catheterization.

1. Which of the following is the most likely diagnosis for the imaging findings presented?
   A. Pseudoaneurysm
   B. Hematoma
   C. Arteriovenous (AV) fistula
   D. Abscess

2. Which of the following is associated with decreased risk of this complication?
   A. High arterial puncture relative to the femoral head
   B. Arterial puncture in a thin patient
   C. Use of a relatively large sheath
   D. Low arterial puncture relative to the femoral head

3. Which of the following statements is correct regarding pseudoaneurysms?
   A. Color Doppler would demonstrate a "to and fro" pattern.
   B. Pseudoaneurysms contain all three histologic layers of the arterial wall.
   C. Pseudoaneurysms do not require treatment.
   D. Pseudoaneurysms are most often treated with ultrasound-guided compression of the pseudoaneurysm neck.

4. Which of the following is true regarding treatment of pseudoaneurysms with thrombin injection?
   A. 10,000 to 50,000 units of thrombin should be used.
   B. Thrombin injection has a lower success rate than ultrasound-guided pseudoaneurysm neck compression.
   C. Thrombin injection is safest in pseudoaneurysms with short necks.
   D. Thrombin injection is safest in pseudoaneurysms with narrow necks.

See Supplemental Figures section for additional figures and legends for this case.

CASE 48

Common Femoral Artery Pseudoaneurysm with Thrombin Injection

1. **A.** The images demonstrate an anechoic region adjacent to the common femoral artery with surrounding hypoechogenicity. Doppler image demonstrates to and fro motion (yin-yang sign) characteristic of pseudoaneurysm. An abscess would likely not demonstrate arterial flow. An AV fistula would show an arterial waveform within the common femoral vein.

2. **B.** Obese patients are at increased risk for pseudoaneurysm formation due to increased difficulty of compressing the artery due to overlying soft tissue. High arterial punctures can result in retroperitoneal hemorrhage. Low arterial punctures may result in AV fistula.

3. **A.** Color Doppler of the pseudoaneurysm neck shows flow directed toward and away from the transducer. Spectral Doppler demonstrates flow above and below the baseline, corresponding to flow reversal during diastole. Pseudoaneurysms are at risk of further expansion or rupture. There are a variety of methods to treat a pseudoaneurysm, including compression, thrombin injection, and surgical ligation.

4. **D.** Thrombin injection is safest in pseudoaneurysms with narrow necks. The narrow neck can be compressed with the ultrasound probe during injection, minimizing the risk of thrombin reflux out of the pseudoaneurysm sac and down the leg. Thrombin injection is reported to have a success rate of 80% to 90%.

Comment

Clinical Presentation

Pseudoaneurysm formation is an important potential complication following interventional procedures. Patients may present with a pulsatile mass, pain, and ecchymosis in the prior access site. Commonly, the diagnosis is confirmed with an ultrasound of the access site, which includes gray scale and Doppler evaluation (Figures S48-1 through S48-3); computed tomography may also be performed, although this is commonly not required (Figure S48-4). Pseudoaneurysms greater than 2 cm likely require treatment as they are unlikely to thrombose spontaneously or may become a source for emboli or infection.

Etiology

Arterial puncture at the access site weakens the normal three-layered vessel wall, allowing blood to enter and expand between the layers, forming a blood-filled pouch. As the pseudoaneurysm grows, there is an increased risk of rupture. Other risk factors for pseudoaneurysm include large sheath size, patient obesity, arterial hypertension, and inadequate post-procedure compression. Post-puncture pseudoaneurysms occur in 1% to 5% of cases.

Treatment Methods

Ultrasound-guided direct thrombin injection is the first-line treatment for most post-procedural pseudoaneurysms. A needle is placed into the pseudoaneurysm, with the tip directed away from the neck (Figure S48-5). One hundred to 500 units of thrombin is carefully injected under direct ultrasonographic visualization, typically resulting in immediate cessation of flow (Figure S48-6). This approach should be avoided in pseudoaneurysms with short, wide necks, as the thrombin may reflux out of the pseudoaneurysm and cause distal thrombosis. Other treatment methods include direct or ultrasound-guided compression or surgical ligation.

References

Hendricks NH, Saad WE. Ultrasound-guided management of vascular access pseudoaneurysms. *Ultrasound Clin.* 2012;7:299–307.

Keeling AN, Mcgrath FP, Lee MJ. Interventional radiology in the diagnosis, management, and follow-up of pseudoaneurysms. *Cardiovasc Intervent Radiol.* 2009;32:2–18.

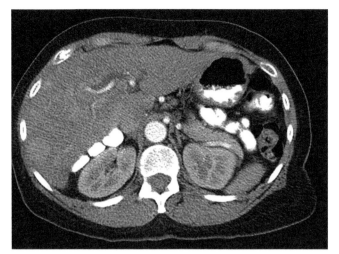

Figure 49-1. *Courtesy of Dr. Bill S. Majdalany.*

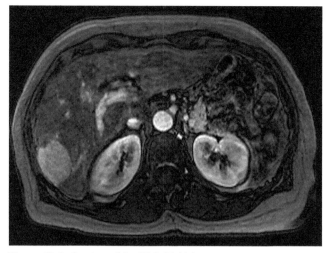

Figure 49-2. *Courtesy of Dr. Bill S. Majdalany.*

HISTORY: A 64-year-old male with history of hepatitis C cirrhosis complicated with a large hepatic mass found on screening ultrasound.

1. Which of the following would be included in the differential diagnosis for the imaging findings presented? (Choose all that apply.)
   A. Metastatic neuroendocrine tumor
   B. Hepatocellular carcinoma (HCC)
   C. Metastatic choriocarcinoma
   D. Metastatic thyroid carcinoma

2. Which of the following regarding transarterial chemoembolization (TACE) of HCC is TRUE?
   A. TACE is reserved only for patients with infection-related cirrhosis (hepatitis B and C).
   B. The vascular supply to HCCs comes primarily from the portal vein, which also supplies the majority of the hepatic parenchyma.
   C. TACE is reserved for patients with bilirubin greater than 2 mg/dL, or in cases of tumor replacing more than 50% of the liver parenchyma.
   D. TACE is based on targeted ischemia with high local chemotherapeutic drug concentrations.

3. Placement of a catheter proximal to the origin of the gastroduodenal artery during TACE in a patient with a segment 7 HCC and a replaced right hepatic artery arising from the superior mesenteric artery will most likely result in which of the following?
   A. Nontarget embolization of the left hepatic lobe, duodenum, and pancreas
   B. Nontarget embolization of the sigmoid colon
   C. Adequate embolization of the hepatic segment 7 lesion
   D. Adequate embolization of the hepatic segment 7 lesion, with tolerable nontarget embolization of uninvolved segments

4. A sample regimen of chemotherapeutic agents used in TACE includes which of the following?
   A. 5-Fluorouracil, floxuridine
   B. Cisplatin, doxorubicin, mitomycin-C
   C. Methotrexate, gemcitabine, dacarbazine
   D. Actinomycin-D, danorubicin, cladribine

See Supplemental Figures section for additional figures and legends for this case.

CASE 49

Hepatocellular Carcinoma

1. **A, B, C, and D.** All of the lesions listed would be expected to demonstrate arterial hyperenhancement on computed tomography (CT) or magnetic resonance imaging (MRI). In a cirrhotic liver, the findings are most likely consistent with HCC.

2. **D.** The other choices are false. TACE is performed in HCC due to any etiology, in patients with preferably less than 50% parenchymal replacement, and bilirubin levels under 2 mg/dL via the hepatic artery, which is the predominant supplier of blood to these tumors.

3. **A.** Injection into the proximal common hepatic artery would result in nontarget embolization of the vascular territory supplied by the gastroduodenal artery, without significant embolization reaching the segment 7 lesion, which in this case is supplied predominantly by the replaced right hepatic arising from the superior mesenteric artery.

4. **B.** The most frequently used regimen of those presented is a mixture of cisplatin, doxorubicin, and mitomycin-C. The other agents are not routinely used in combination in TACE.

Comment

Imaging Interpretation

HCC can manifest with a solitary mass, multiple masses, or diffuse hepatic involvement. Commonly found in patients with cirrhosis, it is a highly malignant neoplasm with a poor long-term prognosis. Angiographic features include enlarged feeding arteries, neovascularity, puddling, dense tumor stain, arterioportal shunting, portal vein invasion, and occasionally hepatic vein invasion (Figures S49-3 and S49-4). A central necrotic area may be present and can splay surrounding abnormal vessels. The uninvolved liver commonly shows arteriographic changes of cirrhosis, including small corkscrew-like vessels. CT and MRI with contrast are commonly employed in pre-procedural planning and follow-up and similarly may show arterially enhancing masses (Figures S49-1, S49-2, and S49-5).

Endovascular Management

Arteriography is useful for assessing tumor blood supply before surgery and for providing guidance for hepatic arterial port catheter placement or chemoembolization. It is useful to obtain portal venous images at the time of arteriography to determine the direction of portal venous flow and to detect thrombus in the portal vein. Because HCCs derive their blood supply nearly entirely from the hepatic arterial system, they are significantly more sensitive to the ischemic effects of arterial occlusion than normal hepatic parenchyma, which derives more than two thirds of its blood supply from the portal venous system. Chemoembolization, which involves intra-arterial infusion of chemotherapy immediately followed by embolization, results in two important effects that constitute the basis for this form of therapy: increased dwell time of the chemotherapeutic agents within the tumor owing to slow flow in and out of the tumor bed, and tumor ischemia.

References

Miura J, Gamblin T. Transarterial chemoembolization for primary liver malignancies and colorectal liver metastasis. *Surg Oncol Clin N Am.* 2015;24:149–166.

Sze D, Razavi M, So S, et al. Impact of multidetector CT hepatic arteriography on the planning of chemoembolization treatment of hepatocellular carcinoma. *AJR Am J Roentgenol.* 2001;177:1339–1345.

Cross-reference

Vascular and Interventional Radiology: The Requisites, 2nd ed, 247–250.

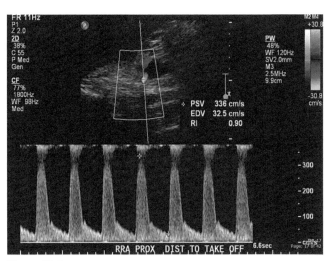

Figure 50-1

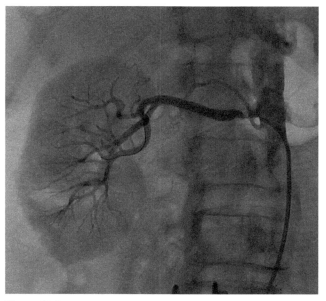

Figure 50-2

HISTORY: A 75-year-old female presenting with worsening heart failure and uncontrolled hypertension despite four antihypertensive medications.

1. Which of the following is the most likely diagnosis for the imaging findings presented?
   A. External compression of the renal artery
   B. Renal artery dissection
   C. Renal artery stenosis (RAS)
   D. Renal vein thrombosis

2. What is the most common etiology of these imaging findings?
   A. Polyarteritis nodosa
   B. Athlerosclerosis
   C. Vasculitis
   D. Dissection

3. What other disease processes should this patient be treated for?
   A. Diabetes mellitus
   B. Venous thromboembolic disease
   C. Coronary artery disease
   D. Pericarditis

4. Which of the following reasons would be an indication to treat the above imaging findings with percutaneous revascularization?
   A. 68-year-old male presents with medically controlled chronic hypertension.
   B. 75-year-old female presents with gross hematuria and right flank pain.
   C. 66-year-old male presents with recurrent episodes of flash pulmonary edema.
   D. 45-year-old female presents with severe lower extremity claudication and an aortic aneurysm.

See Supplemental Figures section for additional figures and legends for this case.

CASE 50

Atherosclerotic Renal Artery Stenosis

1. **C.** The angiographic and sonographic images demonstrate an ostial, subtotal occlusion of the right renal artery.

2. **B.** The most common causes of renal artery stenoses are atherosclerosis and fibromuscular dysplasia. Fibromuscular dysplasia is most commonly seen in younger patients.

3. **C.** Atherosclerosis is a systemic disease process, and therefore atherosclerotic RAS is considered a coronary artery disease equivalent. The patient should be treated according to current guidelines for the secondary prevention of coronary artery disease.

4. **C.** Clinical situations where percutaneous revascularization is thought to be beneficial compared to medical therapy alone are patients with RAS and recurrent flash pulmonary edema and/or refractory heart failure, failure of optimal medical therapy to control blood pressure, intolerance of optimal medical therapy, and patients with a short duration of blood pressure elevation prior to RAS diagnosis.

Comment

Etiology

Patients with RAS typically present with hypertension refractory to multiple medications or chronic renal failure resulting from ischemic nephropathy. The most common cause of RAS by far is atherosclerosis. Other causes include fibromuscular dysplasia, aortic dissection, and neurofibromatosis. Atherosclerotic lesions are most commonly located in the ostial and periostial portions of the main renal artery, as in this case, but they can also be seen distally. Because atherosclerosis is a systemic disease process, atherosclerotic RAS is considered a coronary artery disease equivalent, and the patient should therefore be treated according to current guidelines for secondary prevention of cardiovascular disease.

Treatment Methods

Once a patient has been diagnosed with RAS by diagnostic imaging (Figure S50-1), there are three potential therapeutic options: medical therapy, percutaneous angioplasty with or without stent placement, or surgical revascularization. Endovascular management with balloon angioplasty or stenting has been employed with improvement of stenosis for years (Figures S50-2 through S50-6). In multiple, recent, randomized trials, stenting of RAS did not show benefit with respect to improving kidney function, blood pressure, or major cardiovascular or renal events when compared to medical therapy alone. However, the argument has been raised that these trials were subject to selection bias, excluding subpopulations of patients with more severe RAS who would benefit from renal artery stenting. Therefore there remain situations where percutaneous revascularization of unilateral RAS is likely to have significant benefit; these include patients with unilateral RAS with recurrent flash pulmonary edema and/or refractory heart failure, unilateral RAS with failure of optimal medical therapy to control blood pressure, and patients with ischemic nephropathy with chronic kidney disease and either a solitary functioning kidney with RAS or bilateral significant RAS.

Outcomes

RAS caused by atherosclerosis has a 60% to 70% patency at 5 years when treated by percutaneous balloon angioplasty; however, angioplasty of ostial lesions is associated with substantially lower patencies (25% to 50%). A number of prospective trials have demonstrated lower rates of restenosis in patients undergoing renal artery stent placement compared with angioplasty alone, and stent placement is recommended over angioplasty alone for atherosclerotic RAS by the 2005 American College of Cardiology/American Heart Association Guidelines on peripheral arterial disease. Surgical bypass is most commonly performed in patients with lesions not amenable to percutaneous treatment.

References

Bax L, Woittiez AJ, Kouwenberg HJ, et al. Stent placement in patients with atherosclerotic renal artery stenosis and impaired renal function: a randomized trial. *Ann Intern Med.* 2009;150:840–848.

Cooper CJ, Murphy TP, Cutlip DE, et al. Stenting and medical therapy for atherosclerotic renal-artery stenosis. *N Engl J Med.* 2014;370:13–22.

Gill KS, Fowler RC. Atherosclerotic renal arterial stenosis: clinical outcomes of stent placement for hypertension and renal failure. *Radiology.* 2003;226:821–826.

Olin JW. Atherosclerotic renal artery disease. *Cardiol Clin.* 2002;20:547–562.

The ASTRAL Investigators. Revascularization versus medical therapy for renal-artery stenosis. *N Engl J Med.* 2009;361:1953–1962.

Cross-reference

Vascular and Interventional Radiology: The Requisites, 2nd ed, 28–276.

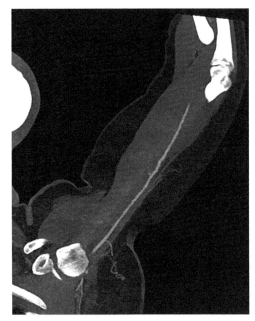

Figure 51-1. *Courtesy of Dr. Alan H. Matsumoto.*

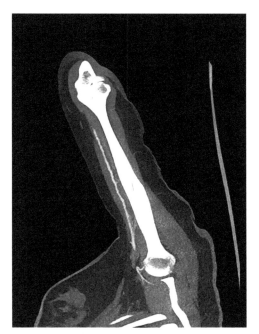

Figure 51-2. *Courtesy of Dr. Alan H. Matsumoto.*

HISTORY: A 45-year-old woman presents with left upper-extremity pain and history of hypertension.

1. Which of the following is the most likely diagnosis for the imaging findings presented?
   A. Post-ductal coarctation of the aorta
   B. Upper-extremity fibromuscular dysplasia (FMD)
   C. Brachial artery atherosclerosis
   D. Upper-extremity deep vein thrombosis

2. The patient's hypertension is likely due to disease in what location?
   A. Vertebral artery
   B. Carotid artery
   C. Coronary artery
   D. Renal artery

3. Which of the following interventions is most effective in treating this patient's hypertension?
   A. Statin and antihypertensive medications
   B. Balloon angioplasty with stent
   C. Balloon angioplasty without stent
   D. Brachial artery bypass surgery

4. Which of the following is NOT an advantage of balloon angioplasty over surgical revascularization for renal FMD?
   A. Less invasive
   B. Fewer complications
   C. Shorter recovery time
   D. Higher cure rate for hypertension

See Supplemental Figures section for additional figures and legends for this case.

CASE 51

Fibromuscular Dysplasia of the Upper Extremity

1. **B.** In young female patients with hypertension and no additional risk factors, causes of secondary hypertension should be considered (renal FMD). Computed tomography angiography demonstrates areas of beading along the brachial artery. Conventional angiography, the gold standard for diagnosing FMD shows the classic "string of beads" appearance.

2. **D.** Among patients with identified FMD, the renal arteries are most commonly involved, affecting 60% to 75% of patients. Renal artery stenosis is a common cause of secondary hypertension that is refractory to medical management. These patients can exhibit high renin and angiotensin II levels, as well as abdominal bruits.

3. **C.** Treatment of choice for hypertension caused by renal artery FMD is percutaneous transluminal angioplasty (PTA). Unlike cases where hypertension is caused by atherosclerotic renal artery stenosis, stenting is not typically performed for FMD. Less commonly, surgical revascularization of the renal arteries is performed.

4. **D.** PTA has supplanted surgical revascularization as the preferred treatment of renal artery FMD. Angioplasty can be performed with a high degree of technical and clinical success with minimal complications, is less invasive, has a markedly shorter recovery time, and is less expensive.

Comment

Pathogenesis

FMD is a rare vascular disease that is nonatherosclerotic and noninflammatory in nature and that most commonly affects the renal and cerebrovascular arterial system. Rarely the extremities are affected. Sequential thickening and thinning of segments in the affected artery give a typical "string of beads" appearance to the artery on imaging (Figures S51-1 through S51-3). FMD has been well described for the renal and cerebrovascular arteries, but other medium sized arteries can be affected. Classical pathological condition of FMD includes intimal fibroplasia, medial disease with three subclassifications (perimedial fibroplasia, medial fibroplasia, and medial hyperplasia), and periadventitial fibroplasia.

Clinical Presentation

Clinical presentation of FMD depends on location of the arteries affected. Most commonly, renal arteries are affected, causing hypertension and abdominal bruits. Diagnosis of renal artery FMD is more likely in young female hypertensive patients with no risk factors for atherosclerotic disease, as in this case. Cerebrovascular artery lesions result in headaches, neck pain, dizziness, and pulsatile ringing of the ears. Common presenting symptoms with respect to brachial involvement include signs of upper-extremity ischemia such as extremity coolness, decreased pulses, paresthesias, and pain sometimes precipitated by environmental factors.

Treatment Methods

Management of patients with FMD involves removal of the affected segment and replacement with interpositioned saphenous vein bypass or with PTA. In cases where the renal arteries are involved, angioplasty is performed without stent placement, unless a complication such as dissection arises and stenting is necessary (Figures S51-4 and S51-5).

References

Bozlar U, Ogur T, Khaja MS, et al. CT angiography of the upper extremity arterial system—part 2: clinical applications beyond trauma patients. *Am J Roentgenol.* 2013;201:753–763.

Olin JW, Sealove BA. Diagnosis, management, and future developments of fibromuscular dysplasia. *J Vasc Surg.* 2011;53:826–836.

Rice R, Armstrong P. Brachial artery fibromuscular dysplasia. *Ann Vasc Surg.* 2010;24:255, e1-4.

Cross-reference

Vascular and Interventional Radiology: The Requisites, 2nd ed, 134.

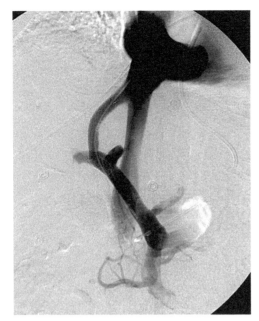

Figure 52-1. *Courtesy of Dr. Wael E. Saad.*

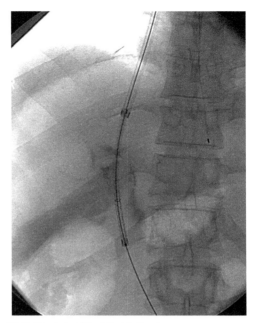

Figure 52-2. *Courtesy of Dr. Wael E. Saad.*

HISTORY: A 59-year-old male presents with intractable ascites.

1. Where is the tip of the outer sheath (10th rib level) on Figure 52-2?
   A. Hepatic vein
   B. Portal vein
   C. Inferior vena cava (IVC)
   D. Superior mesenteric vein

2. A transjugular intrahepatic portosystemic shunt (TIPS) typically directs blood flow between what two vascular structures?
   A. Portal vein to IVC
   B. Hepatic vein to portal vein
   C. Portal vein to hepatic vein
   D. Hepatic artery to hepatic vein

3. With the use of covered stents in place of bare metal stents, which TIPS complication has improved and which has remained largely unchanged?
   A. Sepsis: patency
   B. Encephalopathy: ascites
   C. Patency: encephalopathy
   D. Ascites: sepsis

4. Why is there decreased patency with bare metal stents compared to covered stents for TIPS?
   A. Early epithelialization of bare metal stents
   B. Hepatic arterial fistula causing increased turbulence within the stent
   C. Decreased comparative in-stent velocities
   D. Biliary fistula causing intrastent coagulation

See Supplemental Figures section for additional figures and legends for this case.

CASE 52

TIPS: Viatorr Deployment

1. **A.** The tip of the outer sheath is positioned within the right hepatic vein with a coaxial sheath and wire within the portal system.

2. **C.** A TIPS shunt directs blood from the portal system to the hepatic venous system, thereby surpassing the diseased hepatocytes.

3. **C.** Patency has improved with covered stents, now approximately 80% to 90% and 70% to 80% patency at 12 and 24 months. Encephalopathy as a result of shunting blood from residual active hepatocytes remains grossly unchanged.

4. **D.** Crossing biliary branches is inevitable when placing a TIPS. Bile is a coagulant and caused thrombosis of the bare metal stents as the bile leaked into the shunt. This has been overcome by covered (polytetrafluoroethylene) stents.

Comment

Procedural Technique

Multiple TIPS specific sets are commercially available. Conventionally, initial access is obtained through the right internal jugular vein. However, a left internal jugular or femoral vein approach may be employed. Serial dilation is performed to allow for a large sheath placement (e.g., 10 French). The sheath is advanced into the right atrium for acquisition of right atrial pressure measurements to evaluate for right-sided heart failure or pulmonary hypertension prior to TIPS placement. A coaxial catheter is used to select site of entry from the hepatic venous system, either the right hepatic vein or the confluence. While optional, wedged hepatic venography is typically performed to map the portal system and provide landmarks for access. Hepatic venography is depicted in further detail in Case 41. Portal access is obtained via a needle system provided in the TIPS set. Direction of needle passage is determined by anatomy and prior vein mapping. For example, a right hepatic vein to right portal vein trajectory typically requires an anterior needle pass. After each pass, the trocar needle is removed and aspiration is attempted. Successful portal access is confirmed with contrast injection. The wire and sheath are advanced into the portal system. A portal pressure is acquired directly through the sheath. The tract is dilated with balloon angioplasty. A covered stent (Viatorr, W.L. Gore and Associates, Flagstaff, AZ) (Figure S52-6) is deployed starting from the portal end (Figures S52-2 through S52-5). Repeat portal and systemic (right atrial) pressures are obtained with target gradient less than 12 mm Hg. A completion portogram is obtained to depict the new shunt (Figure S52-1). Frequently, variceal embolization is performed following TIPS placement.

References

Fidelman N, Kwan S, LaBerge J, et al. The transjugular intrahepatic portosystemic shunt: an update. *AJR Am J Roentgenol.* 2012;199:746–755.

Gaba R, Khiatani V, Knuttinen M, et al. Comprehensive review of TIPS technical complications and how to avoid them. *AJR Am J Roentgenol.* 2011;196:675–685.

Saad WE. The history and future of transjugular intrahepatic portosystemic shunt: food for thought. *Semin Intervent Radiol.* 2014;31:258–261.

Cross-reference

Vascular and Interventional Radiology: The Requisites, 2nd ed, 318–325.

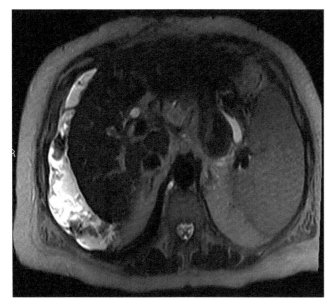

Figure 53-1

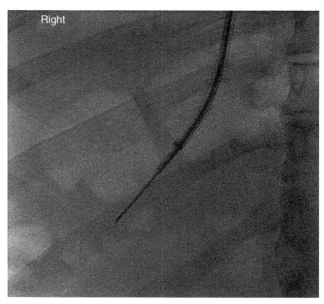

Figure 53-2

HISTORY: A 62-year-old male with history of morbid obesity, coagulopathy, and ascites referred for liver biopsy due to transaminitis and jaundice.

1. Which of the following would be included in the differential diagnosis for the imaging findings presented? (Choose all that apply.)
   A. Nonalcoholic steatohepatitis (NASH)
   B. Alcoholic cirrhosis
   C. Primary biliary cirrhosis
   D. Hepatitis C-related cirrhosis

2. Which of the following choices would be the most appropriate choice for biopsy in this patient?
   A. Transjugular liver biopsy (TJLB)
   B. Ultrasound-guided liver biopsy
   C. Computed tomography (CT)-guided liver biopsy
   D. Magnetic resonance imaging (MRI)-guided liver biopsy

3. Which structure in the liver should be transgressed during the appropriate procedure chosen in question 2?
   A. The hepatic capsule
   B. Left hepatic vein
   C. Right hepatic vein
   D. Right portal vein

4. What is the correct needle orientation for biopsy during the appropriate procedure chosen in question 2?
   A. Anterior to posterior, oriented toward the right hepatic lobe
   B. Anteriorly, from the right hepatic vein
   C. Anteriorly, from the middle hepatic vein
   D. Anteriorly, from the left hepatic vein

See Supplemental Figures section for additional figures and legends for this case.

CASE 53

Transjugular Liver Biopsy of Diffuse Liver Disease

1. **A, B, C, and D.** The etiology of cirrhosis in this patient could be attributable to any of the choices above. The incidence of NASH has been increasing in recent years.

2. **A.** The patient has several contraindications to percutaneous biopsy (ascites and coagulopathy), which would require puncture of the hepatic capsule under CT, ultrasound, and MRI guidance. The safest alternative in this case would be the transjugular approach.

3. **C.** The right hepatic vein is the most frequently used vessel for TJLB as it posteriorly located in the right hepatic lobe, allowing for more passage through liver parenchyma. The middle hepatic vein may be occasionally used, but this was not listed as a choice. Crossing the hepatic capsule in this case is incorrect, because it would mean that the operator was performing a percutaneous biopsy, which is not an appropriate option in this case.

4. **B.** During TJLB, the needle should be oriented anteriorly as the right hepatic vein is usually posterior within the right hepatic lobe. The needle should not be oriented anteriorly if using the middle hepatic vein. Answer A is incorrect because this approach requires puncturing the hepatic capsule, which is performed during percutaneous biopsy and contraindicated in this patient.

Comment

Indication

In most patients with diffuse liver lesions, tissue diagnosis may be safely obtained by transabdominal percutaneous biopsy. However, patients with impaired coagulation and those with ascites are at significant risk for intraperitoneal bleeding following needle traversal of the liver capsule (Figure S53-1). Liver biopsy from a transjugular route is associated with a lower rate of bleeding complication and represents a safer option in these situations.

Procedural Technique

To perform a TJLB, the right internal jugular vein is percutaneously accessed under ultrasound guidance. The right hepatic vein is selected and contrast venography may be used to confirm catheter position (Figure S53-3). The catheter is then exchanged for a metallic cannula. This cannula is directed anteriorly (away from the posterior liver capsule) under fluoroscopic guidance, and a specially designed long biopsy needle is used to obtain one or more core biopsy specimens from the hepatic parenchyma (Figure S53-2). If the middle hepatic vein is used instead of the right hepatic vein, then the cannula may be directed in a posterolateral direction to avoid the anterior liver capsule. The cannula is then removed and the jugular entry site is compressed for hemostasis. Hemostasis within the liver occurs quickly provided the hepatic capsule was not breached. Patients may require blood products for this procedure depending on the severity of coagulopathy.

References

Kalambokis G, Manousou P, Vibhakorn S, et al. Transjugular liver biopsy—indications, adequacy, quality of specimens, and complications—a systematic review. *J Hepatol.* 2007;47:284–294.

Wallace MJ, Narvios A, Lichtiger B, et al. Transjugular liver biopsy in patients with hematologic malignancy and severe thrombocytopenia. *J Vasc Interv Radiol.* 2003;14:323–327.

Cross-reference

Vascular and Interventional Radiology: The Requisites, 2nd ed, 332–333.

Fair Game

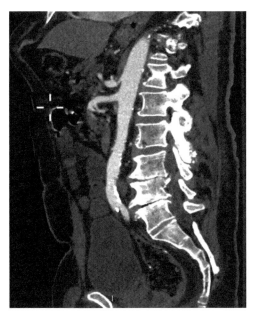

Figure 54-1

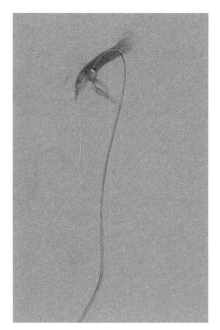

Figure 54-2

HISTORY: A 72-year-old male presents with acute onset, post-prandial abdominal pain. Patient recently stopped taking warfarin (for atrial fibrillation) due to planned orthopedic operation.

1. Which of the following is the most likely diagnosis for the imaging findings presented?
   A. Acute in situ thrombosis of the superior mesenteric artery
   B. Acute thromboembolic occlusion of the superior mesenteric artery
   C. Acute in situ thrombosis of the superior mesenteric vein
   D. Acute thromboembolic occlusion of the celiac trunk

2. After the imaging finding was communicated to the emergency room physician caring for the patient, you receive a phone call asking what Interventional Radiology can do for the patient. What is the most appropriate step in management given this imaging finding?
   A. Surgical consultation
   B. Admission to the medical intensive care unit and expectant management
   C. Colonoscopy
   D. Elective thrombolytic therapy

3. What is the most likely etiology of the imaging finding above in this case?
   A. In situ thrombus from a ruptured plaque in the setting of atherosclerotic disease
   B. Hypercoagulability in the setting of portal hypertension
   C. Thromboembolic occlusion from ruptured thoracic aortic plaque
   D. Thromboembolic occlusion from the left atrial appendage

4. If the patient above was initially taken to angiography with placement of an infusion catheter and overnight administration of papaverine, heparin and recombinant tissue plasminogen activator, and still developed worsening abdominal pain and a rising lactate, what is the most appropriate next step?
   A. Revision of the infusion dosages to a higher dose, until the lactate drops
   B. Revisit to the interventional radiology (IR) suite with exchange the infusion catheter
   C. Revisit to the IR suite with repeat angiography and possible angioplasty and stenting
   D. Exploratory laparotomy

See Supplemental Figures section for additional figures and legends for this case.

CASE 54

Superior Mesenteric Artery Embolus

1. **B.** The finding demonstrates an acutely occluded superior mesenteric artery without significant atherosclerotic disease in the proximal segment. Given the patient's history, thromboembolic phenomenon is by far the most likely scenario.

2. **A.** Acute mesenteric ischemia has traditionally been a surgical emergency. The standard therapy for acute mesenteric ischemia is open embolectomy and revascularization with resection of infarcted bowel, if present. While there is growing literature on percutaneous revascularization, the decision to perform open versus percutaneous revascularization should be made in conjunction with the surgical consultants.

3. **D.** The most likely etiology in this case is a thrombus from the left atrial appendage, as this patient recently stopped taking warfarin for his history of atrial fibrillation.

4. **D.** The patient has essentially failed percutaneous therapy. In this scenario, exploratory laparotomy and resection of infarcted bowel is mandatory. Some authors argue that if no improvement is observed within 4 hours after infusion therapy, surgery should be performed emergently.

Comment

Main Teaching Point

Acute mesenteric ischemia is associated with a mortality rate of 70%, primarily due to bowel infarction with resultant sepsis. The clinical signs of mesenteric ischemia can include abdominal pain, leukocytosis, hematochezia, and lactic acidosis. Unfortunately, the clinical signs of this disorder are insidious and are often recognized after irreversible bowel ischemia has occurred. Prompt diagnosis and therapy are absolutely imperative in avoiding mortality. Catheter-based angiography, ultrasound, magnetic resonance angiography, or catheter-based angiography are commonly employed for diagnosis (Figure S54-1 and S54-2). The etiologies of acute mesenteric ischemia include embolus (which produces ischemia within a major mesenteric vascular distribution), hypotension in patients with preexisting atherosclerotic stenoses (which can produce ischemia within a watershed distribution, usually near the splenic flexure, which represents the junction of the superior and inferior mesenteric artery territories), and acute aortic dissection.

Treatment Methods

Surgical therapy, specifically thrombectomy and/or aortomesenteric bypass with bowel resection as needed, is the treatment of choice. Endovascular methods may be used in cases where the embolus involves an extremely short segment near the origin of the superior mesenteric artery enabling the stent to be placed), but stenting has not been shown to be equivalent to surgical therapy in this clinical setting. The special subset of patients with aortic dissection complicated by mesenteric ischemia may also be treated in endovascular fashion, using stent placement and/or percutaneous balloon fenestration of the aortic flap.

References

Acosta S, Bjorck M. Modern treatment of acute mesenteric ischaemia. *Br J Surg.* 2014;101:e100–e108.

Lee R, Tung HK, Tung PH, et al. CT in acute mesenteric ischemia. *Clin Radiol.* 2003;58:279–287.

Cross-reference

Vascular and Interventional Radiology: The Requisites, 2nd ed, 236–237.

CASE 55

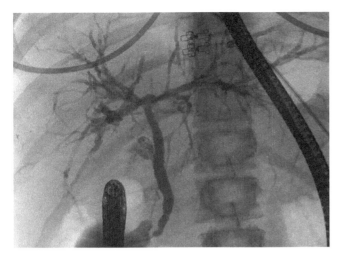

Figure 55-1

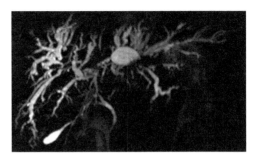

Figure 55-2

HISTORY: A 34-year-old male presents with chronic right upper quadrant pain and itching.

1. Which of the following is the most likely diagnosis for the imaging findings presented?
   A. Mirizzi syndrome
   B. Primary sclerosing cholangitis (PSC)
   C. Biloma
   D. Caroli disease

2. Which other condition is this condition most highly associated with?
   A. Ulcerative colitis
   B. Gastric carcinoma
   C. Celiac sprue
   D. Whipple's disease

3. Patients with this condition are at the most increased risk of developing which malignancy?
   A. Hepatocellular carcinoma
   B. Gallbladder carcinoma
   C. Cholangiocarcinoma
   D. Colon cancer

4. What is the only treatment modality shown to affect prognosis of PSC?
   A. Biologic medications
   B. Indwelling biliary drainage catheters
   C. Hepaticojejunostomy
   D. Liver transplant

See Supplemental Figures section for additional figures and legends for this case.

CASE 55

Sclerosing Cholangitis

1. **B.** Multifocal strictures, fibrosis, and saccular outpouchings involving the intra- and extrahepatic biliary system are characteristic of PSC. Mirizzi syndrome is obstruction of the common bile duct (CBD) due to a gallstone in the cystic duct, the CBD is relatively patent. There is no large collection seen to suggest biloma. Caroli disease is a congenital disease manifested by multifocal saccular dilation of the intrahepatic biliary tree.

2. **A.** PSC is strongly associated with inflammatory bowel disease, more so with ulcerative colitis than Crohn's disease. It is estimated that 70% of patients with PSC also have ulcerative colitis.

3. **C.** Patients with PSC are most at risk for developing cholangiocarcinoma with an estimated lifetime risk of at least 10%.

4. **D.** Liver transplant is the only treatment shown to positively impact prognosis. Percutaneous biliary drainage is used for symptomatic treatment of cholangitis and biliary obstruction.

Comment

Clinical Presentation

Sclerosing cholangitis is a progressive and chronic inflammatory and fibrotic process that affects the intra- and extrahepatic biliary ductal system. Patients often present with chronic or intermittent obstructive jaundice, abdominal pain, fatigue, and/or fever. Sclerosing cholangitis can occur as a primary idiopathic disorder or in association with other inflammatory conditions, including ulcerative colitis (most common), Crohn's disease, pancreatitis, retroperitoneal fibrosis, or mediastinal fibrosis. Long-term sequelae of this disorder include biliary cirrhosis, portal hypertension, and cholangiocarcinoma.

Imaging Interpretation

The hallmark cholangiographic findings of sclerosing cholangitis include multifocal strictures, saccular dilatation and outpouchings, and a beaded and/or pruned-tree appearance of the biliary ductal system, which may be seen on computed tomography, magnetic resonance imaging, endoscopic retrograde cholangiopancreatogram, or cholangiography (Figure S55-1 through S55-5). The CBD is almost always involved. The differential diagnosis of these findings includes sclerosing cholangiocarcinoma, primary biliary cirrhosis, autoimmune cholangitis, ascending cholangitis, and recurrent pyogenic cholangitis.

Treatment Methods

Medical management of PSC is not particularly effective. Percutaneous biliary drainage or hepaticojejunostomy can provide palliation to carefully selected patients with appropriate anatomy, but the only truly curative treatment is liver transplantation (Figure S55-5).

References

Bader T, Beavers K, Semelka R. MR imaging features of primary sclerosing cholangitis: patterns of cirrhosis in relationship to clinical severity of disease. *Radiology.* 2003;226:675–685.

Costello J, Kalb B, Chundru S, et al. MR imaging of benign and malignant biliary conditions. *Magn Reson Imaging Clin N Am.* 2014;22:467–488.

Gossardd A, Lindor K. Hepatocellular carcinoma. Low risk of HCC in patients who have PSC and cirrhosis. *Nat Rev Gastroenterol Hepatol.* 2014;115:276–277.

Cross-reference

Vascular and Interventional Radiology: The Requisites, 2nd ed, 469–471.

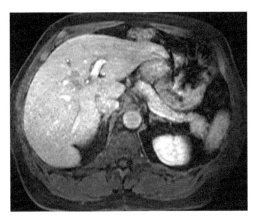

Figure 56-1

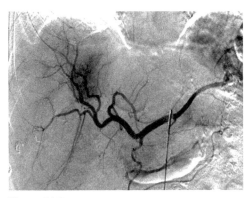

Figure 56-2

HISTORY: A 61-year-old male with hepatitis C and early cirrhosis presents for surveillance magnetic resonance imaging (MRI).

1. Which of the following would be included in the differential diagnosis for the imaging findings presented? (Choose all that apply.)
   A. Metastasis
   B. Hepatic adenoma
   C. Hepatocellular carcinoma
   D. Cholangiocarcinoma

2. Which of the following is *NOT* a risk factor for hepatocellular carcinoma?
   A. Primary sclerosing cholangitis
   B. Hepatitis C
   C. Alcoholic cirrhosis
   D. Advanced age

3. Which hepatocellular carcinoma (HCC) tumor burden can be transplanted according to Milan Criteria?
   A. 3 tumors less than 3 cm each or 1 tumor less than 5 cm
   B. 5 tumors less than 1 cm each or 2 tumors less than 6 cm
   C. Single pulmonary metastasis
   D. Right portal vein invasion

4. Which is an absolute contraindication to transarterial chemoembolization (TACE)?
   A. Left portal vein occlusion
   B. The Eastern Cooperative Oncology Group (ECOG) 4
   C. Bilobar disease
   D. Tumor greater than 8 cm

See Supplemental Figures section for additional figures and legends for this case.

CASE 56

Hepatocellular Carcinoma: DEB-TACE

1. **A, B, and C.** Metastasis, hepatic adenoma, and hepatocellular carcinoma are all in the differential diagnosis for an early arterially enhancing mass. Cholangiocarcinoma typically has delayed enhancement.

2. **A.** Primary sclerosing cholangitis is a risk factor for cholangiocarcinoma, not hepatocellular carcinoma. Hepatitis C, alcoholic cirrhosis, and advanced age are all risk factors for HCC.

3. **A.** To be within Milan Criteria, a patient's HCC burden can include up to 3 tumors less than 3 cm each or 1 tumor less than 5 cm. There must be no extrahepatic disease or vascular invasion.

4. **B.** Poor functional status is an absolute contraindication to TACE as the patient is unlikely to benefit from the procedure. ECOG classifies a "4" as a completely disabled patient who cannot perform self-care and is completely confined to a bed or chair. Portal vein occlusion is a relative contraindication. Bilobar disease and tumor burden greater than 8 cm are not contraindications and can be managed by treatment in multiple sessions.

Comment

Imaging Interpretation

Hepatocellular carcinoma can manifest with a solitary mass, multiple masses, or diffuse hepatic involvement. Commonly found in patients with cirrhosis, it is a highly malignant neoplasm with a poor long-term prognosis. The lesions are commonly diagnosed or followed by contrast-enhanced computed tomography or MRI (Figure S56-1, S56-3, and S56-4). Angiographic features include enlarged feeding arteries, neovascularity, puddling, dense tumor stain, arterioportal shunting, portal vein invasion, and occasionally hepatic vein invasion (Figure S56-2). A central necrotic area may be present and can splay surrounding abnormal vessels. The uninvolved liver commonly shows arteriographic changes of cirrhosis, including small corkscrew-like vessels. Arteriography is useful for assessing tumor blood supply before surgery and for providing guidance for hepatic arterial port catheter placement or chemoembolization. It is useful to obtain portal venous images at the time of arteriography to determine the direction of portal venous flow and to detect thrombus in the portal vein.

Endovascular Management

Because hepatocellular carcinomas derive their blood supply nearly entirely from the hepatic arterial system, they are significantly more sensitive to the ischemic effects of arterial occlusion than normal hepatic parenchyma, which derives more than two-thirds of its blood supply from the portal venous system. Chemoembolization, which involves intraarterial infusion of chemotherapy immediately followed by embolization, results in two important effects that constitute the basis for this form of therapy: increased dwell time of the chemotherapeutic agents within the tumor owing to slow flow in and out of the tumor bed, and tumor ischemia. A further refinement of this technique involves embolization with microspheres, which have been presoaked with chemotherapeutic agent (drug-eluting bead TACE). This has the theoretical advantage of more sustained, controlled drug release.

References

Malagari K, Chatzimichael K, Alexopoulou E, et al. Transarterial chemoembolization of unresectable hepatocellular carcinoma with drug eluting beads: results of an open-label study of 62 patients. *Cardiovasc Intervent Radiol.* 2008;31:269–280.

Salem R, Lewandowski RJ. Chemoembolization and radioembolization for hepatocellular carcinoma. *Clin Gastroenterol Hepatol.* 2011;11:604–611.

Sze DY, Razavi MK, So SK, et al. Impact of multidetector CT hepatic arteriography on the planning of chemoembolization treatment of hepatocellular carcinoma. *AJR Am J Roentgenol.* 2001;177:1339–1345.

Cross-reference

Vascular and Interventional Radiology: The Requisites, 2nd ed, 247–252.

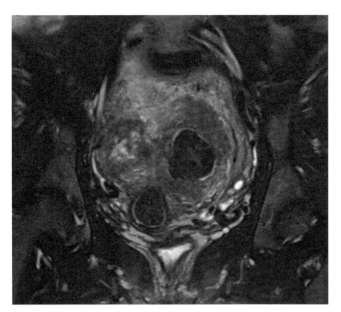

Figure 57-1. *Courtesy of Dr. Alan H. Matsumoto.*

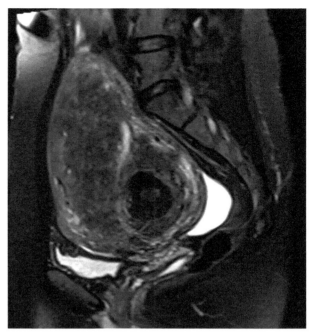

Figure 57-2. *Courtesy of Dr. Alan H. Matsumoto.*

HISTORY: A 52-year-old female presents with menorrhagia and anemia.

1. Which of the following would be included in the differential diagnosis for the imaging findings presented? (Choose all that apply.)
   A. Endometrial cancer
   B. Adenomyosis
   C. Uterine fibroids
   D. Pelvic congestion syndrome

2. What are the treatment options for uterine fibroids? (Choose all that apply.)
   A. Hysterectomy
   B. Myomectomy
   C. Uterine artery embolization (UAE)
   D. Watchful waiting

3. In addition to the uterine artery, what additional artery must be interrogated to ensure adequate therapy during an embolization procedure?
   A. Posterior division of the internal iliac artery
   B. Ovarian artery
   C. Internal pudendal artery
   D. Inferior epigastric artery

4. Which of the following complications post-UAE may present with fever, chills, and pelvic pain?
   A. Sloughed fibroids
   B. Ovarian failure
   C. Deep vein thrombosis
   D. Gluteal muscle ischemia

See Supplemental Figures section for additional figures and legends for this case.

CASE 57

Uterine Artery Embolization for Uterine Fibroids

1. **B and C.** The images shown demonstrate multiple, well-circumscribed masses that are hypointense on T2-weighted images. There is a background of thickened junctional zone, also compatible with adenomyosis. Pelvic congestion syndrome is found in the setting of enlarged pelvic venous collaterals.

2. **A, B, C, and D.** All of the options are possible treatments for uterine fibroids causing bulk symptoms or dysmenorrhea. Each therapy has benefits and risks. Interventional radiology offers fibroid embolization therapy shown here. Benefits include (a) minimally invasive, (b) outpatient, (c) no general anesthesia required, and (d) preservation of uterus.

3. **B.** The ovarian artery should be evaluated via aortic angiography during a fibroid embolization procedure to ensure that the ovarian artery has not been parasitized to supply substantial blood supply to any particular fibroid/involved myometrium. In the setting of a supplying ovarian artery, benefits of its embolization must be weighed against the risks of causing ovarian failure.

4. **A.** Sloughing of fibroids is a well-known complication of UAE for uterine fibroids, particularly when the fibroids are of the submucosal variety. When the fibroid loses its blood supply it may necrose and fall into the uterine cavity and potentially occlude the uterine entroitus, resulting in an infection.

Comment

Diagnostic Evaluation

Magnetic resonance imaging (MRI) is useful in the preembolization workup of patients with uterine fibroids for several reasons: (1) MRI is extremely accurate in diagnosing uterine fibroids and can distinguish between the diverse causes of global uterine enlargement; (2) MRI can accurately depict the local invasiveness of a mass lesion (triggering suspicion for malignancy); (3) MRI enables accurate and reproducible measurements to be obtained; (4) MRI can accurately classify fibroids as being submucosal, intramural, subserosal, and/or pedunculated. This information can affect the type of therapy employed. (5) Speculated causes of clinical failure of uterine fibroid embolization include aberrant uterine artery anatomy, untreated ovarian artery supply to fibroids, and coexistent adenomyosis, all of which can be identified by MRI (Figure S57-1 and S57-2).

Treatment Methods

Uterine fibroid tumors occur in 20% to 40% of women older than 35 years, but they cause significant symptoms only in a minority of patients. The symptoms are usually initially treated with hormonal agents, but long-term use of these agents can be associated with unfavorable side effects. Hysterectomy has long been the mainstay of therapy, but in recent years myomectomy (removal of one or more fibroids) has been used in patients desiring to preserve the uterus. Myomectomy, however, is associated with a fairly high incidence of bleeding complications when performed for multiple fibroids, and a high recurrence rate has been observed.

Endovascular Management

UAE has evolved into an excellent alternative therapy for women with symptomatic uterine fibroids who desire to preserve the uterus (Figure S57-3 through S57-6). UAE is associated with 85% to 90% success in producing significant improvement in symptoms of menorrhagia and/or pelvic pain, and it has been associated with improvements in health-related quality of life. Compared with hysterectomy, UAE is associated with less blood loss, decreased hospital stay, and decreased major complications.

References

Mohan PP, Hamblin MH, Vogelzang RL. Uterine artery embolization and its effect on fertility. *J Vasc Interv Radiol.* 2013;24:925–930.

Narayan A, Lee AS, Kuo GP, Powe N, Kim HS. Uterine artery embolization versus abdominal myomectomy: a long-term clinical outcome comparison. *J Vasc Interv Radiol.* 2010;21:1011–1017.

Scheurig-Muenkler C, Koesters C, Powerski MJ, et al. Clinical long-term outcome after uterine artery embolization: sustained symptom control and improvement of quality of life. *J Vasc Interv Radiol.* 2013;24:765–771.

Spies JB, Roth AR, Jha RC, et al. Leiomyomata treated with uterine artery embolization: factors associated with successful symptom and imaging outcome. *Radiology.* 2002;222:45–52.

Cross-reference

Vascular and Interventional Radiology: The Requisites, 2nd ed, 222–226.

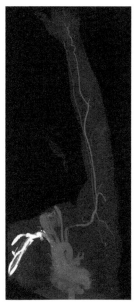

Figure 58-1. *Courtesy of Dr. Narasimham L. Dasika.*

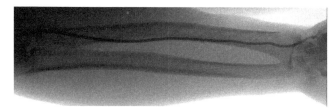

Figure 58-2. *Courtesy of Dr. Narasimham L. Dasika.*

HISTORY: A 37-year-old male with history of cerviclalia and multiple prior left shoulder dislocations presents with pain, numbness, and bluish discoloration of left index finger.

1. Which of the following is the most likely diagnosis for the imaging findings presented?
   A. Vasculitis
   B. Variant anatomy with high radial artery origin
   C. Normal anatomy
   D. Occlusion of the radial artery

2. What symptoms are commonly associated with this finding?
   A. Paresthesias and motor weakness
   B. Digital cyanosis
   C. None
   D. Shortness of breath

3. What is the recommended treatment for this finding?
   A. Anticoagulation with intravenous heparin
   B. Corticosteroids
   C. Surgical decompression
   D. No treatment recommended

4. What is the relevance of documenting this finding in the patient's medical record?
   A. This finding has no bearing or relevance with regards to the patient's medical record.
   B. This finding would be relevant to other physicians who may perform future cardiovascular interventions.
   C. This finding is a herald for future hard cardiac events and indicates a high risk of stroke.
   D. This finding is commonly associated with other autoimmune disorders (i.e., rheumatoid arthritis, inflammatory bowel disease).

See Supplemental Figures section for additional figures and legends for this case.

CASE 58

Variant Anatomy: High Radial Artery Origin

1. **B.** The reformatted computed tomographic angiography maximal intensity projection of the left upper extremity demonstrates an extremely high origin of the radial artery, which is a normal variant. This finding can be easily missed on angiography and mistaken for radial artery occlusion, if the catheter is positioned beyond the origin of the radial artery during injection. There is no evidence of vessel irregularity to suggest vasculitis.

2. **C.** High radial artery origin is an incidental finding commonly with no associated symptoms. Specifically, it does not cause nerve compression leading to paresthesias or motor weakness or contribute to cyanosis of the digits, which may be an unrelated finding.

3. **D.** This is a variant of normal anatomy. No further medical or surgical management is required.

4. **B.** Documenting this finding in the patient's medical record is especially important to a physician who may perform a future cardiovascular intervention such as a coronary intervention. Specifically, knowledge of this variant anatomy would be relevant if one were planning on performing a brachial artery puncture or radial artery puncture. There is no increased risk of stroke or hard cardiac events associated with high radial artery origin.

Comment

Main Teaching Point

Distal to the elbow joint, the brachial artery normally trifurcates into a radial artery, an ulnar artery, and an interosseous artery (Figure S58-6). Several anatomic variants of this pattern occur with enough frequency that it is important to be aware of them. For instance, in some patients the brachial artery divides proximally into two limbs that continue in parallel and then reunite distally.

Variant Anatomy

Conventionally, the radial artery arises as the first branch of the brachial artery below the elbow, and the ulnar artery divides into its named branches a few centimeters distally. However, up to 19% of persons have an early bifurcation of the brachial artery, an anomaly more commonly found on the right. Although a high radial artery origin from the brachial artery is the most common upper-extremity arterial variant (7% to 8%), the ulnar artery can also arise from the brachial artery above the elbow (Figures S58-1 through S58-5). Less commonly, the radial artery (1% to 3%) or ulnar artery (1% to 2%) can arise from the axillary artery. Physiologically, these variations are of little significance, but they can be significant when a brachial artery puncture is planned or when a patient suffers trauma to the upper extremity with associated vascular injury.

References

Kusztal M, Weyde W, Letachowicz K, et al. Anatomical vascular variations and practical implications for access creation on the upper limb. *J Vasc Access*. 2014;15:S70–S75.

Lo T, Nolan J, Fountzopoulos E, et al. Radial artery anomaly and its influence on transradial coronary procedural outcome. *Heart*. 2009;95:410–415.

Uglietta J, Kadir S. Arteriographic study of variant arterial anatomy of the upper extremities. *Cardiovasc Intervent Radiol*. 1989;12:145–148.

Cross-reference

Vascular and Interventional Radiology: The Requisites, 2nd ed.

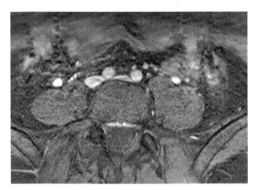

Figure 59-1. *Courtesy of Dr. David M. Williams.*

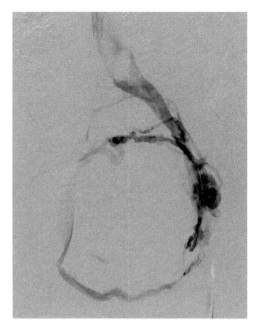

Figure 59-2. *Courtesy of Dr. David M. Williams.*

HISTORY: A 42-year-old female presents with recurrent left lower extremity deep vein thrombosis (DVT).

1. Which of the following would be included in the differential diagnosis for the imaging findings presented? (Choose all that apply.)
   A. Klippel-Trenauney-Weber syndrome
   B. Sturge-Weber syndrome
   C. May-Thurner syndrome
   D. von Hippel-Lindau syndrome

2. What is the preferred acute treatment for this condition?
   A. Antiepileptics
   B. Sclerotherapy
   C. Surgical resection
   D. Thrombolysis and stenting

3. What is the typical demographic affected by this condition?
   A. Females, 20 to 40 years
   B. Females, 5 to 15 years
   C. Males, 1 to 10 years
   D. Males, 40 to 60 years

4. Which side of the body is typically affected by this condition?
   A. Right
   B. Left
   C. Bilateral
   D. Both sides equally

See Supplemental Figures section for additional figures and legends for this case.

CASE 59

May-Thurner Syndrome

1. **C.** May-Thurner anatomy is demonstrated in these images with narrowing of the left common iliac vein by the right common iliac artery, and angiographic demonstration of stenosis, DVT, and numerous collateral vessels. Klippel-Trenauney-Weber and Sturge-Weber syndromes typically affect children and manifest with arteriovenous (AV) malformations and various other associated symptoms. Von Hippel-Lindau syndrome predisposes to certain neoplasms.

2. **D.** Endovascular treatment has been shown to work quite well for these patients, although anticoagulation is often required as well. Sclerotherapy can be used to treat AV malformations. Antiepileptics are used in Sturge-Weber syndrome, as these children are prone to seizures. Surgical resection can sometimes be used in von Hippel-Lindau syndrome for certain neoplasms.

3. **A.** Females aged 20 to 40 are typically affected by this condition. Patients may have May-Thurner anatomy without the syndrome manifesting by DVT.

4. **B.** May-Thurner syndrome is caused by compression of the left common iliac vein by the crossing right common iliac artery, resulting in inflammatory scarring and fibrosis in the vein due to arterial pulsations.

Comment

Etiology

Iliofemoral deep venous thrombosis is three to eight times more common in the left leg than in the right leg. This is thought to be due to the relative compression of the left iliac vein at the pelvic brim by the crossing right common iliac artery (Figures S59-1, S59-2, and S59-4). Iliac vein compression (May-Thurner syndrome) is a distinct entity that typically affects women in the second to fourth decades. It is differentiated from bland deep vein thrombosis of the lower extremity by the presence of a fibrous spur or adhesion in the left common iliac vein, thought to represent an inflammatory response to chronic compression of the vein and irritation of its endothelium from adjacent arterial pulsations.

Endovascular Management

Patients typically present with acute iliofemoral DVT or chronic DVT with venous insufficiency. Endovascular therapy is the treatment of choice for this disorder. Typically, catheter-directed thrombolysis is used first to remove any acute thrombus, and an endovascular stent is subsequently placed to address the venous stenosis (Figures S59-5 and S59-6). Intravascular ultrasound aids in accurate deployment of the stent at the point of compression by the right common iliac artery, although it is not always necessary (Figure S59-4). Surgical thrombectomy that does not also address the underlying left common iliac vein stenosis has a high failure rate.

References

Forauer AR, Gemmete JJ, Dasika NL, et al. Intravascular ultrasound in the diagnosis and treatment of iliac vein compression (May-Thurner) syndrome. *J Vasc Interv Radiol.* 2002;13:523–527.

Ibrahim W, Al-Safran Z, Hasan H, et al. Endovascular management of May-Thurner syndrome. *Ann Vasc Dis.* 2012;5:217–221.

Patel NH, Stookey KR, Ketcham DB, et al. Endovascular management of acute extensive iliofemoral deep venous thrombosis caused by May-Thurner syndrome. *J Vasc Interv Radiol.* 2000;11:1297–1302.

Cross-reference

Vascular and Interventional Radiology: The Requisites, 2nd ed, 370–375.

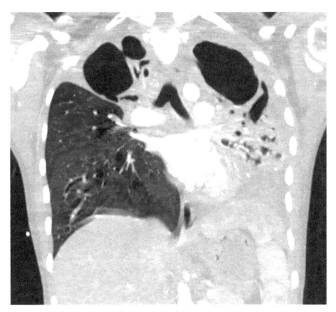

Figure 60-1. *Courtesy of Dr. Luke R. Wilkins.*

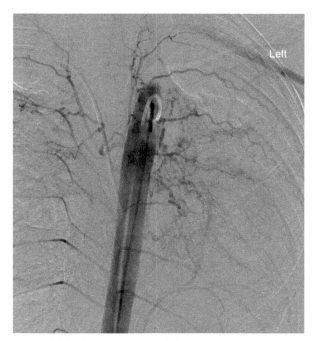

Figure 60-2. *Courtesy of Dr. Luke R. Wilkins.*

HISTORY: A 22-year-old female with a remote history of tuberculosis presenting with hemoptysis.

1. Which of the following is the most likely diagnosis for the imaging findings presented?
   A. Cystic fibrosis
   B. Pulmonary arteriovenous malformation
   C. Wegener's granulomatosis
   D. Aspergillosis

2. What is the typical threshold for performing embolization in the setting of hemoptysis?
   A. 300 mL of expectorated blood in a 24-hour period
   B. 100 mL of expectorated blood in a 24-hour period
   C. 50 mL of expectorated blood in a 24-hour period
   D. 1000 mL of expectorated blood in a 24-hour period

3. Which artery must be identified in every case of bronchial artery embolization, and what is its key characteristic?
   A. The pleural artery, which has a corkscrew appearance
   B. The esophageal artery, which has a vertical origin
   C. The medullary spinal artery, which has a hairpin loop
   D. The phrenic artery, which has a tortuous course from the aorta

4. Which of the following is the least expected finding in cases of hemoptysis?
   A. Hypervascularity
   B. Vessel hypertrophy
   C. Bronchial artery pseudoaneurysm
   D. Extravasation

See Supplemental Figures section for additional figures and legends for this case.

CASE 60

Bronchial Artery Embolization

1. **D.** While the other choices are in the differential for hemoptysis, the imaging findings and history are most consistent with a fungal infection in a cavitation.

2. **A.** Most textbooks and authors will give the 300 mL threshold for performing embolization in cases of hemoptysis. Other indications include three or more episodes of 100 mL or more within 1 week, and chronic or slowly increasing episodes.

3. **C.** The medullary spinal artery can supply the anterior spinal artery, and it must be identified in every case to prevent embolization of the thoracic spinal cord. If embolization is necessary of a branch where the medullary spinal artery is seen, it is imperative to advance the microcatheter beyond its origin and embolize cautiously.

4. **D.** The rarest finding in a bronchial angiogram is frank extravasation. The other findings are much more common.

Comment

Indication

Bronchial artery embolization has become an established procedure for treating life-threatening hemoptysis. Massive hemoptysis is usually defined by the production of 300 to 600 mL of blood per day, but the patient's clinical condition should guide therapy because smaller amounts of bleeding can be life-threatening in some instances.

Preprocedural Planning

In 90% of patients, bleeding arises from a bronchial artery. Less common sources include the pulmonary arteries, aorta, and systemic collaterals to the lungs. Localization of the bleeding site by radiography, bronchoscopy, and/or chest computed tomography before angiography and embolization is important so as to focus therapy (Figure S60-1).

Preprocedural Planning

The bronchial arteries typically originate from the descending thoracic aorta at the T5-T6 level. In about 40% of patients, there are two arteries on the left and one on the right arising from an intercostobronchial trunk. However, there is extensive variability in number, origin, and branching pattern. It is very important to identify spinal arterial branches that arise from the bronchial and intercostal arteries, because nontarget embolization of these vessels can result in spinal ischemia.

Endovascular Management

Hypertrophied and tortuous bronchial arteries, neovascularity, hypervascularity, and pulmonary arteriovenous shunting are common angiographic findings (Figures S60-2 through S60-4). Extravasation of contrast is rarely seen. In general, embolization with particles or liquid embolics is preferred. Coils are not commonly used because they produce proximal occlusion, precluding repeat embolization should hemoptysis recur. However, if pulmonary arterial fistulization is present, larger particles or coils may be necessary to shut down the fistulous connection (Figures S60-3 and S60-4).

References

Fernando HC, Stein M, Benfield JR, et al. Role of bronchial artery embolization in the management of hemoptysis. *Arch Surg.* 1998;133: 862–866.

Yoon W, Kim JK, Kim YH, et al. Bronchial and nonbronchial systemic artery embolization for life-threatening hemoptysis: a comprehensive review. *Radiographics.* 2002;22:1395–1409.

Cross-reference

Vascular and Interventional Radiology: The Requisites, 2nd ed, 174–176.

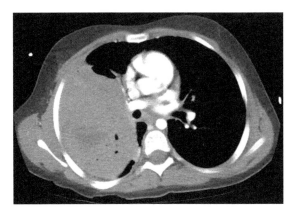

Figure 61-1

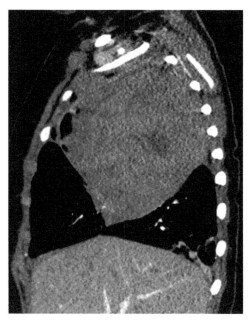

Figure 61-2

HISTORY: A 12-year-old female with hypoxia, fever, and tachycardia.

1. Which of the following is the most likely diagnosis for the imaging findings presented?
   A. Squamous cell carcinoma
   B. Infected ascites
   C. Abscess
   D. Empyema

2. Which of the following signs helps distinguish lung abscess from empyema?
   A. Split pleura sign
   B. Irregular wall
   C. Acute angles with chest wall
   D. Spherical shape

3. What is the optimal treatment for this condition?
   A. Antibiotics
   B. Percutaneous drainage
   C. A&B
   D. Surgical drainage

4. If the treatment option in Question 3 does not succeed, what additional therapy can be performed?
   A. Percutaneous drainage
   B. Fibrinolytic therapy
   C. Pleurodesis
   D. Wedge resection

See Supplemental Figures section for additional figures and legends for this case.

CASE 61

Empyema

1. **C and D.** Empyema and abscess are in the differential, and distinguishing these entities requires identification of fluid in the pleural space and pleural enhancement on both sides of the fluid collection. Abscesses are generally more aggressive, appearing to invade the lung parenchyma. Empyema generally causes mass effect. Squamous cell carcinoma is usually in the upper lobes, although it does have a somewhat similar appearance since it can be necrotic or cavitary, and is unlikely in a child. Ascites would be below the diaphragm.

2. **A.** The split pleura sign represents the contrast-enhanced computed tomography (CT) manifestation of fibrin-coating of the visceral and parietal pleura with vascular ingrowth causing enhancement. These regions coalesce at the edges of the fluid collection. The other signs are seen with lung abscesses.

3. **C.** Percutaneous drainage can be performed under image guidance (ultrasonography, fluoroscopy, CT) after CT confirmation of empyema. Needle access into the pleural space should be obtained, with the puncture site just above the rib to avoid injury of the intercostal neurovascular bundle. The patient should also be treated with antibiotics. Surgical drainage is reserved for refractory cases.

4. **B.** Injection of fibrinolytics can be performed if chest tube drainage stops but there is radiologic evidence of persistent empyema. A larger bore chest tube may also be inserted. Pleurodesis is generally performed for recurrent pleural effusions or pneumothoraces. Wedge resection generally would not be performed for empyema.

Comment

Preprocedural Planning

The images demonstrate a rim-enhancing, gas-containing complex fluid collection within the right posterior pleural space, consistent with empyema (Figures S61-1 and S61-2). Imaging-guided chest tube placement is an excellent initial therapy and can be performed under fluoroscopy, CT, or ultrasound guidance (Figures S61-3 and S61-4). Preprocedural clinical assessment should include an evaluation of whether the patient will be able to tolerate the required position on the procedure table, because many patients with empyema have significant associated pulmonary compromise. Coagulation studies and platelet level should also be obtained as bleeding is the most common but also devastating complication. Imaging is usually performed for diagnosis and planning as well (Figures S61-1, S61-2, and S61-5).

Percutaneous Management

Under imaging guidance, a needle is placed into the collection and contrast is injected to confirm proper positioning. It is important to avoid placing the needle just under a rib, because this can result in hemorrhage due to traversal of an intercostal artery. Over a guidewire, the tract is dilated and a large-bore drainage catheter is placed and attached to negative pressure. Follow-up CT scans are used to evaluate the progress of drainage. When the patient has improved clinically and the cavity is resolved, the catheter can be incrementally withdrawn to allow gradual healing of the residual cavity and tube tract.

Postprocedural Management

If drainage ceases or stabilizes before the collection completely resolves, the cavity may be loculated and intracavitary fibrinolytic agents can be given. This is successful in up to 75% of cases, but major hemorrhage is a complication reported in up to 7% of cases. However, this complication only occurred in patients who were fully anticoagulated at the time of the procedure. Another reason for failure is that the catheter might be occluded or might not be in optimal position; a repeat CT scan can be used to guide an attempt at repositioning the catheter under fluoroscopy. Alternatively, a larger catheter may be needed if the catheter is patent and in the correct position. Infrequently, the fluid may simply be too viscous for percutaneous drainage, and surgery may be required.

References

Shenoy-Bhangle A, Gervais D. Use of fibrinolytics in abdominal and pleural collections. *Semin Intervent Radiol.* 2012;29:264–269.
VanSonnenberg E, Wittich GR, Goodacre BW, et al. Percutaneous drainage of thoracic collections. *J Thorac Imaging.* 1998;13:74–82.

Cross-reference

Vascular and Interventional Radiology: The Requisites, 2nd ed, 422–423.

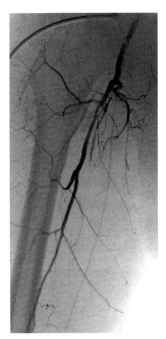

Figure 62-1. *Courtesy of Dr. Minhaj S. Khaja.*

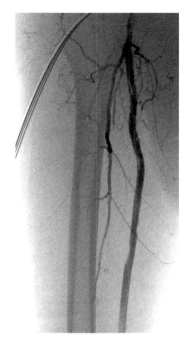

Figure 62-2. *Courtesy of Dr. Minhaj S. Khaja.*

HISTORY: A 57-year-old male with a history of diabetes and hypertension presents with a painful right lower extremity and diminished pulses.

1. Which of the following would be included in the differential diagnosis for the imaging findings presented? (Choose all that apply.)
   A. Femoral arteriovenous fistula (AVF)
   B. Occlusion of a right femoral arterial bypass graft
   C. Femoral pseudoaneurysm
   D. Acute embolic arterial occlusion

2. What are the common causes of this problem? (Choose all that apply.)
   A. Anastomotic or intragraft stenosis
   B. Mechanical compression
   C. Progression of atherosclerosis proximal or distal to the graft
   D. Hypercoagulability

3. What intervention was performed between the first two images?
   A. Endovascular stent placement
   B. Catheter-directed thrombolysis or surgical thrombectomy
   C. Amputation
   D. Balloon angioplasty

4. What are the two most feared complications of endovascular intervention in the treatment of this problem?
   A. Distant hemorrhage
   B. Distal embolization of thrombus
   C. Contrast-induced renal injury
   D. Infection

See Supplemental Figures section for additional figures and legends for this case.

CASE 62

Bypass Graft Occlusion and Thrombolysis

1. **B and D.** Based on the history and images, the diagnosis is related to acute critical limb ischemia. There is an occluded vascular structure in the images, which could be occlusion of a right femoral arterial bypass graft or acute embolic femoral arterial occlusion. The correct diagnosis is occlusion of a right common femoral arterial bypass graft. If the diagnosis were a femoral pseudoaneurysm, the images would display a contained outpouching of contrast, with a neck communicating with the vascular lumen. A femoral AVF would be suspected if there was early filling of the iliofemoral venous system during the early arterial phase of the angiogram.

2. **A, B, C, and D.** Proximal or distal anastomotic stenosis, intragraft stenosis, progression of atherosclerosis proximal or distal to the graft, hypercoagulability, and mechanical compression are all common causes of bypass graft occlusion.

3. **B.** Catheter-directed thrombolysis or surgical thrombectomy was performed and reestablished patency through the graft. There are no vascular stents present in the images. The occluded bypass graft is revascularized in subsequent images, making amputation incorrect. Balloon angioplasty alone is unlikely to clear thrombus material from the graft and reestablish patency without thrombolysis or thrombectomy.

4. **A and B.** Distant hemorrhage and distal embolization of thrombus are the most feared complications of endovascular intervention as they can lead to intracranial hemorrhage or acute embolic stroke. Acute myocardial infarction is another feared complication. Infection and contrast-induced renal injury are also potential complications of endovascular intervention. However, they are not as severe as distal embolization or hemorrhage.

Comment

Main Teaching Point

The precise role of thrombolysis in the treatment of bypass graft thrombosis is somewhat controversial. However, several published trials support its use for patients with acute (<2 weeks) graft occlusion to achieve the following benefits: (1) It avoids surgical risks in patients who often have vascular comorbidities; (2) it has potential to both declot the graft and treat an underlying stenosis using angioplasty or stent placement (Figures S62-1 through S62-6); (3) even if treatment of the underlying disorder cannot be achieved percutaneously, the diagnostic information provided by angiography after thrombolysis often guides definitive surgical therapy and enables reduction of the planned level of surgery. Endovascular therapy tends to be more successful in treating occluded synthetic grafts compared with vein grafts.

Complications

Disadvantages of thrombolysis include the longer time to reperfusion compared with surgical thrombectomy, and the risk of complications. Approximately 10% of patients require a transfusion due to bleeding, which most commonly occurs at the arterial access site. Distant bleeding occurs in 1% to 2% of patients, and intracranial bleeding occurs in 0.5% to 1.0%. Distal embolization occurs in 5% to 12% of patients, but it is usually treatable and rarely results in amputation. Compartment syndrome occurs in 2% of patients. Ischemic heart disease is a risk factor that can lead to complications such as amputation and death.

References

Koraen L, Kuoppala M, Acosta S, et al. Thrombolysis for lower extremity bypass graft occlusion. *J Vasc Surg.* 2011;54:1339–1344.

Kuoppala M, Franzén S, Lindblad B, et al. Long-term prognostic factors after thrombolysis for lower limb ischemia. *J Vasc Surg.* 2008;47:1243–1250.

Ouriel K. Current status of thrombolysis for peripheral arterial occlusive disease. *Ann Vasc Surg.* 2002;16:797–804.

Cross-reference

Vascular and Interventional Radiology: The Requisites, 2nd ed, 351–353.

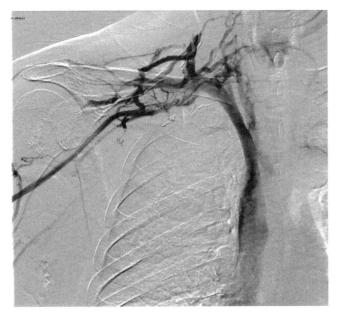

Figure 63-1

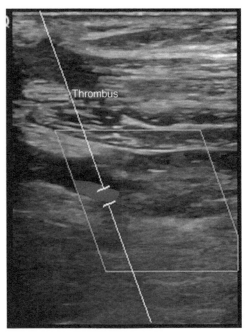

Thrombus

Figure 63-2

HISTORY: A 56-year-old male presents with right arm swelling.

1. Which of the following is the most likely diagnosis for the imaging findings presented?
   A. Lymphedema
   B. Acute venous occlusion
   C. Chronic venous occlusion
   D. Arteriovenous malformation

2. The best method of treating occlusion or stenosis in large veins is which of the following?
   A. Angioplasty
   B. Stenting
   C. Thrombolysis
   D. Thrombolysis with angioplasty

3. If the patient in this case was an athletic teenager, with no medical history other than arm swelling, the primary differential considerations would include which of the following?
   A. Pagett-Schrotter syndrome
   B. Mediastinal germ cell tumor
   C. Hodgkin's lymphoma
   D. Non-Hodgkin's lymphoma

4. The Wright's maneuver is the eponym for which one of the following?
   A. Adduction and internal rotation of the extremity while palpating the radial artery
   B. Extension of the arm and extension of the neck while rotating the head to the affected side, while palpating the radial artery
   C. Extension of the arm and internal rotation of the extremity while palpating the radial artery
   D. Abduction and external rotation of the extremity while palpating the radial artery

See Supplemental Figures section for additional figures and legends for this case.

CASE 63

Chronic Axillosubclavian Vein Occlusion

1. **C.** The imaging findings are consistent with a chronic occlusion, with abundant collaterals, and no filling defects. The other answers would not have the same venographic appearance.

2. **B.** Angioplasty of the venous system alone has poor long-term patency, with results being much better with stenting. While thrombolysis is required in acute cases (as in cases of phlegmasia) it is not necessarily indicated in chronic occlusions.

3. **A.** Acute thrombosis in the setting of venous thoracic outlet syndrome (TOS) or effort-thrombosis, is known as Pagett-Schrotter syndrome. Patients may present with an acutely edematous extremity, or with a more indolent process, in cases of venous TOS without acute thrombosis. Treatment in cases of venous TOS is aimed at restoring venous patency, relieving stenosis, and decompression of the thoracic outlet.

4. **D.** Wright's maneuver tests for occlusion of the subclavian artery and reproduction of symptoms in cases of arterial TOS by abduction of the affected extremity and external rotation. Choice B refers to Adson's maneuver, which also tests for occlusion of the subclavian artery.

Comment

Patient Presentation

Most patients with subclavian vein thrombosis experience initial upper-extremity swelling and/or pain, but these symptoms usually subside as a mature venous collateral network develops. In fact, about 80% of patients with subclavian vein thrombosis eventually become asymptomatic or minimally symptomatic with anticoagulation therapy alone.

Endovascular Management

For these reasons, endovascular interventions to restore patency in patients with subclavian vein thrombosis are reserved for carefully selected patients with primary axillosubclavian thrombosis (i.e., due to TOS), for young patients with acute secondary subclavian venous thrombosis who have good functional status, and for rare patients with special concerns such as a continuing need for central venous access where no other access sites are available. In these patients, a trial of thrombolytic therapy may be used, but most patients with chronic secondary subclavian vein thrombosis are treated with anticoagulation and removal of any central venous catheter that is present in the thrombus-containing vein.

Imaging Findings

Venographic features that strongly suggest a chronic process include the lack of significant dilation of the occluded veins, the somewhat tapered aspect of the occlusion, the lack of globular filling defects or a meniscus sign, and the presence of abundant collaterals (Figure S63-1). Duplex ultrasonography is helpful in initial screening as it may demonstrate a lack of flow and compressibility (Figure S63-2).

References

Meissner MH. Axillary-subclavian venous thrombosis. *Rev Cardiovasc Med.* 2002;3:S44–S51.

Thompson RW. Comprehensive management of subclavian vein effort thrombosis. *Semin Intervent Radiol.* 2012;29:44–51.

Cross-reference

Vascular and Interventional Radiology: The Requisites, 2nd ed, 140–144.

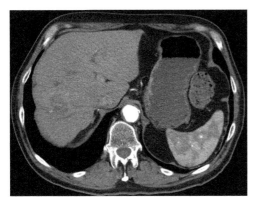

Figure 64-1

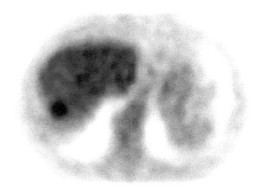

Figure 64-2

HISTORY: A 72-year-old male with a history of colon cancer presents with right upper quadrant pain.

1. Which of the following would be included in the differential diagnosis for the imaging findings presented? (Choose all that apply.)
   A. Hepatic abscess
   B. Hepatic metastasis
   C. Hepatic cyst
   D. Hepatocellular carcinoma

2. Which of the following factors may limit the therapeutic effect of radiofrequency ablation of hepatic metastasis?
   A. The presence of portal vein thrombosis
   B. A hepatic mass measuring 3 cm in size
   C. A hepatic mass in close proximity to a large vessel
   D. The presence of cirrhosis

3. In which region of the liver should radiofrequency ablation generally be avoided?
   A. At the hepatic hilum
   B. Medial left hepatic lobe
   C. Adjacent to the diaphragm
   D. Near the gallbladder fossa

4. Which of the following is the expected computed tomography (CT) appearance of a liver tumor status post successful percutaneous radiofrequency ablation?
   A. A hyperdense region with heterogeneous contrast enhancement
   B. A hypodense region with an enhancing rim, which progressively increases in size
   C. A hypodense region with an enhancing rim, which progressively decreases in size
   D. A hyperdense region without contrast enhancement

See Supplemental Figures section for additional figures and legends for this case.

CASE 64

Radiofrequency Ablation of Liver Metastasis

1. **B and D.** The differential diagnosis of a hypermetabolic, enhancing hepatic mass includes both metastatic disease and hepatocellular carcinoma. In this case, the patient had a history of colon cancer and no evidence of cirrhosis. This makes a metastatic lesion much more likely. This was confirmed by biopsy.

2. **C.** When the target lesion is adjacent to a large vessel, it may be difficult to achieve adequate ablation secondary to the heat-sink effect. Blood flow within the adjacent vessel can absorb the thermal energy from the radiofrequency probe, resulting in suboptimal ablation.

3. **A.** Radiofrequency ablation should generally be avoided for masses near the hepatic hilum. As the large bile ducts are relatively intolerant to heat, there is an increased risk of biliary strictures and/or fistulae. Techniques, such as hydrodissection, changing patient positioning, and bile aspiration can be used to avoid complications in cases where the mass abuts other important structures.

4. **C.** The expected postprocedural appearance of a liver lesion after a successful radiofrequency ablation is a hypodense region with an enhancing rim, which progressively decreases in size. The low-attenuation region is related to radiofrequency-induced necrosis. The enhancing rim is due to a peripheral inflammatory reaction. Local tumor recurrence can present as "progressive ingrowth of vascularized tissue into the necrotic area or as vascularized outgrowth away from the zone of necrosis."

Comment

Indication

Surgical resection remains the standard of care for metastatic liver lesions; however, only 5% to 15% of patients are eligible for resection. Radiofrequency ablation of nonresectable lesions can be performed in a subset of this patient population. Generally accepted selection criteria include fewer than five lesions, each less than 5 cm in diameter, and no extrahepatic disease.

Preprocedural Planning

Anatomic factors evaluated on preprocedural imaging (CT, ultrasonography (US), magnetic resonance imaging (MRI), positron emission tomography) that must be taken into consideration include the location of the tumor(s) in relation to intrahepatic structures such as the bile ducts and vessels (Figures S64-1 and S64-2). Large vessels in close proximity to the lesion can make it difficult to attain good ablation due to a heat-sink effect: Relatively high blood flow rates cause a cooling effect on the adjacent tissue. Extrahepatic structures such as the gallbladder, diaphragm, and adjacent bowel should also be evaluated for proximity to the anticipated ablation zone to prevent thermal injury to these structures.

Percutaneous Management

The mechanism of action is the transmission of radiofrequency waves to the tissues, which causes an elevation of tissue temperature leading to coagulative necrosis of the exposed tissues. Image guidance by US, CT, or even MRI is used for correct needle placement through a percutaneous approach (Figure S64-3). The procedure can be performed under moderate sedation or general anesthesia. Certain adjunctive procedures can be performed to create a safe zone between the lesion and adjacent structures to prevent thermal injury, including patient positioning and hydrodissection. Combination therapy with transarterial chemoembolization may also be performed. Follow-up imaging is commonly performed with contrast-enhanced CT or MRI (Figure S64-4).

References

Hinshaw J, Lubner M, Ziemlewicz T, et al. Percutaneous tumor ablation tools: microwave, radiofrequency, or cryoablation-what should you use and why? *Radiographics.* 2014;35:1344–1362.

Petre E, Sofocleous C, Solomon S. Ablative and catheter-directed therapies for colorectal liver and lung metastases. *Hematol Oncol Clin North Am.* 2015;29:117–133.

West J, et al. Percutaneous and intra-operative tumor ablation. *Ultrasound Clin.* 2012;7:413–420.

Cross-reference

Vascular and Interventional Radiology: The Requisites, 2nd ed, 572–579.

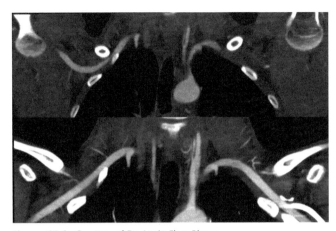

Figure 65-1. *Courtesy of Dr. Lucia Flors Blasco.*

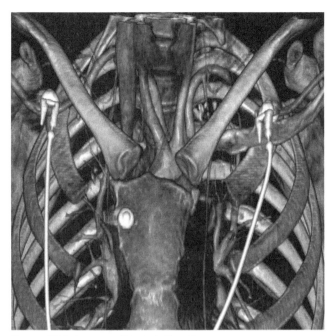

Figure 65-2. *Courtesy of Dr. Lucia Flors Blasco.*

HISTORY: A 22-year-old female with history of bilateral hand numbness, especially with extension of the arms.

1. Which of the following is the most likely diagnosis for the imaging findings presented?
   A. Arterial thoracic outlet syndrome (TOS)
   B. Occlusion of the left subclavian artery by atherosclerotic disease
   C. Arterial and venous TOS
   D. Venous TOS

2. What of the following is *NOT* a common cause of TOS?
   A. Cervical ribs
   B. Presence of a scalenus minimus muscle
   C. Pancoast tumor
   D. Healed fracture deformities of the clavicle or first rib

3. Symptoms related to TOS characteristically:
   A. Awaken the patient at night
   B. Are worse in abduction
   C. Are worse in adduction
   D. Are constant

4. Which of the following statements is *INCORRECT* regarding arterial TOS?
   A. 20% of patients with thoracic outlet compression syndrome have a cervical rib.
   B. Symptoms present in the ipsilateral hand and fingers and include pain, numbness, paresthesias, intermittent claudication, and cool skin temperature.
   C. Nearly half of patients exhibit symptoms of Raynaud's phenomenon.
   D. A systolic bruit can sometimes be heard at the site of compression.

See Supplemental Figures section for additional figures and legends for this case.

CASE 65

Arterial Thoracic Outlet Syndrome

1. **A.** Images reveal high-grade stenosis at the proximal right subclavian artery and occlusion of the left subclavian artery as they pass through the thoracic inlet when the study is performed in abduction. Patency of the bilateral subclavian arteries is seen in neutral position.

2. **C.** TOS is caused by the compression of the neurovascular bundle as it crosses the thoracic outlet, usually related by the presence of cervical ribs, a scalenus minimus muscle, wide or abnormal insertion or enlargement of the anterior scalene muscle, anomalous first rib narrowing of the costoclavicular space, healed fracture deformities of the clavicle or first rib, or muscular body habitus narrowing the pectoralis minor tunnel. Pancoast tumor is in the differential diagnosis of TOS, as patients may present with similar symptoms, but it is far less common.

3. **B.** Symptoms related to TOS often worsen with arm abduction as the extrinsic compression is at its worst.

4. **A.** Cervical ribs are present in up to 0.5% of the general population, but less than half of these patients develop symptoms of neurovascular compression. However, of patients with thoracic outlet compression syndrome, about 70% have a cervical rib.

Comment

Patient Presentation

TOS refers to the compression of the neurovascular structures as they cross through the thoracic outlet (Figure S65-1). It may be caused by arterial, venous, or neurogenic compression or as a combination. Patients with arterial TOS typically present with symptoms in the ipsilateral hand and fingers including pain, numbness, paresthesias, intermittent claudication, and cool skin temperature. Although rare, severe digital ischemia usually related to microemboli, can also occur. Nearly half exhibit symptoms of Raynaud's phenomenon. Symptoms often worsen with arm abduction. Reduction or obliteration of the radial pulse during clinical maneuvers such as passive arm hyperabduction or Adson's maneuver (deep inspiration with hyperextension of the neck while the head is rotated to the symptomatic side) are highly suggestive of the diagnosis. A systolic bruit can sometimes be heard at the site of compression.

Etiology

Cervical ribs are present in up to 0.5% of persons in the general population, but less than half of these patients develop symptoms of neurovascular compression (Figure S65-2). However, of patients with thoracic outlet compression syndrome, about 70% have a cervical rib. Other problems that can result in compression include the presence of a scalenus minimus muscle (seen in one third of normal persons), a wide or abnormal insertion or enlargement of the anterior scalene muscle, an anomalous first rib narrowing of the costoclavicular space, healed fracture deformities of the clavicle or first rib, or a muscular body habitus narrowing the pectoralis minor tunnel.

Diagnostic Imaging/Treatment

Arterial TOS is classically diagnosed by digital subtraction angiography that should be performed with selective subclavian artery injection in a neutral position and with passive abduction of the extremity. Arteriographic findings include subclavian artery compression or narrowing with or without poststenotic dilation, arterial occlusion, aneurysm, mural thrombus formation, and/or distal embolization (Figures S65-3 and S65-4). Both computed tomographic angiography and magnetic resonance angiography have been shown to be able to make the diagnosis. Treatment consists of removal of the osseous or soft-tissue abnormality, such as resection of cervical ribs or the first rib, and vascular reconstruction or thrombolysis, if necessary.

References

Bozlar U, et al. CT angiography of the upper extremity arterial system: part 1—anatomy, technique, and use in trauma patients. *AJR Am J Roentgenol.* 2013;201:745–752.

Demondion X, Bacqueville E, Paul C, et al. Thoracic outlet: assessment with MR imaging in asymptomatic and symptomatic populations. *Radiology.* 2003;227:461–468.

Cross-reference

Vascular and Interventional Radiology: The Requisites, 2nd ed, 128–129.

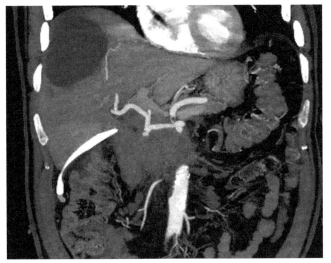

Figure 66-1. *Courtesy of Dr. Bill S. Majdalany.*

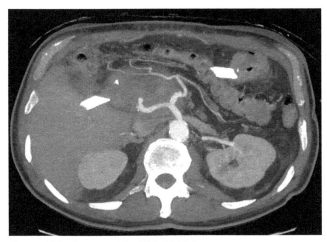

Figure 66-2. *Courtesy of Dr. Bill S. Majdalany.*

HISTORY: A 67-year-old man status post Whipple pancreaticoduodenectomy presents with increased bloody drainage from surgical drains.

1. Which of the following is the most likely diagnosis for the imaging findings presented?
   A. Hepatic artery transection
   B. Portobiliary fistula
   C. Gastroduodenal artery pseudoaneurysm
   D. Inadvertent placement of drain into portal system

2. In a hemodynamically stable patient with bleeding from a biliary drain, what is the first step in management?
   A. Gelfoam embolization through the drain
   B. Immediate angiography
   C. Exploratory laparotomy
   D. Close monitoring, frequent hemoglobin checks, and transfusion as necessary

3. Which technique for placing a transhepatic biliary drain minimizes the risk of bleeding?
   A. Insertion immediately beneath a rib
   B. Access of a central biliary duct
   C. Access of a peripheral biliary duct
   D. Insertion in a patient with ascites

4. What is the treatment of choice for this patient?
   A. Angiography and intervention
   B. Removal of biliary drain and placement of a new drain
   C. Surgical artery repair
   D. Partial hepatectomy

See Supplemental Figures section for additional figures and legends for this case.

CASE 66

Iatrogenic Arterial Pseudoaneurysm

1. **C.** There is a small, round pseudoaneurysm arising from the stump of the gastroduodenal artery. The common hepatic artery arises from the spinal muscular atrophy in this patient, a normal variant.

2. **D.** While 2% to 3% of patients undergoing biliary drain placement will experience some type of hemorrhagic complication, the majority are self-limited, particularly in stable patients. Some operators, after observation, upsize the biliary drain in order to tamponade the bleeding source.

3. **C.** Accessing a more peripheral duct minimizes risk of bleeding because the vascular branches are smaller and less crowded in the peripheral liver. The neurovascular bundle courses under the rib, so access should be above it. Ascites significantly increases the risk of bleeding.

4. **A.** In a patient with bleeding through a drain, arterial injury should be suspected. Selective arteriography can often reveal the arterial injury and intervention with coil embolization is preferred to stop the bleeding. However, covered stenting may also be possible in the appropriate situation, as seen in this case.

Comment

Main Teaching Point

Hemobilia following percutaneous biliary drainage can be a life-threatening condition, and patients should be instructed to contact the interventional radiologist immediately if they note bloody output from the drainage tube or skin site. Most bleeding, resulting from a catheter side hole within the liver parenchyma or a transient fistula between a bile duct and a portal or hepatic vein branch, is transient and resolves with conservative management. Catheter repositioning or upsizing may be necessary in some of these cases. Contrast-enhanced computed tomography may be helpful in identifying the source of bleeding in some cases (Figures S66-1 and S66-2).

Endovascular Management

Severe hemobilia is usually the result of a bile duct communication with a hepatic artery branch or a major venous branch. Arterial bleeding should be suspected when pulsatile bright red blood drains from the biliary drainage catheter; in these cases, emergent hepatic arteriography is indicated for further evaluation (Figures S66-3 and S66-5). If arteriography does not demonstrate a site of bleeding, the biliary drainage catheter should be removed over a guidewire and the angiogram should be repeated. A balloon catheter can be replaced to tamponade bleeding while the bleeding vessel is embolized. A variety of embolic agents can be used in this setting, but most interventionalists use coils for this indication. When performing coil embolization of a pseudoaneurysm, it is important to place coils distal to, across, and proximal to the pseudoaneurysm to prevent continued hemorrhage due to persistent perfusion of the pseudoaneurysm via intrahepatic collaterals (Figure S66-6). In patients with a proximal arterial pseudoaneurysm, as in this case, the site may be treated with a covered stent to exclude the bleeding source (Figure S66-4).

References

Saad WE, Davies MG, Darcy MD. Management of bleeding after percutaneous transhepatic cholangiography or transhepatic biliary drain placement. *Tech Vasc Intervent Radiol.* 2008;11:60–71.
Winick AB, Waybill PN, Venbrux AC. Complications of percutaneous transhepatic biliary interventions. *Tech Vasc Intervent Radiol.* 2001;4:200–206.

Cross-reference

Vascular and Interventional Radiology: The Requisites, 2nd ed, 462–464.

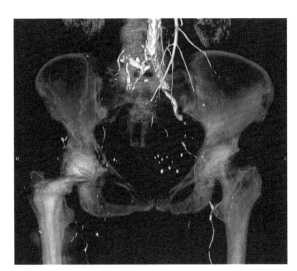

Figure 67-1. *Courtesy of Dr. Minhaj S. Khaja.*

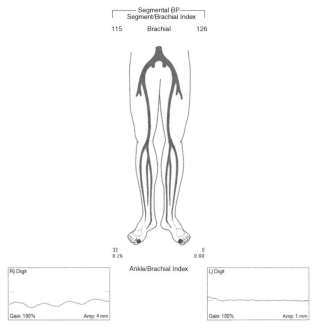

Figure 67-2. *Courtesy of Dr. Minhaj S. Khaja.*

HISTORY: A 57-year-old female with bilateral lower extremity pain, left greater than right.

1. Which of the following would be included in the differential diagnosis for the imaging findings presented? (Choose all that apply.)
   A. Bilateral internal iliac artery occlusion
   B. Bilateral external iliac artery occlusion
   C. Right common iliac artery occlusion
   D. Aortic occlusion

2. Which of the following ankle-brachial indexes (ABIs) is considered inaccurate due to incompressible vessels?
   A. 0.1 to 0.4
   B. 0.5 to 0.8
   C. 0.9 to 1
   D. Greater than 1.3

3. If the right superficial femoral artery is also occluded, which of the following may be the initial therapy attempted?
   A. Inflow surgical bypass
   B. Outflow surgical bypass
   C. Inflow endovascular revascularization
   D. Runoff revascularization

4. Which of the following is NOT an absolute contraindication for the use of thrombolysis therapy in the treatment of peripheral arterial disease (PAD)?
   A. Occult blood in the stool
   B. Central nervous system metastases
   C. Recent abdominal surgery
   D. Recent stroke

See Supplemental Figures section for additional figures and legends for this case.

CASE 67

Iliac Artery Occlusion

1. **B and C.** The CTA shows an occlusion of the right common and bilateral external iliac arteries. Additionally, the right internal iliac artery is not opacified. Numerous collaterals are seen.

2. **D.** As discussed in previous cases, ABI less than 0.4 is critical limb ischemia and present with rest pain or tissue loss. ABI greater than 1.3 is not reliable as the vessels are incompressible due to calcification.

3. **C.** Inflow revascularizatlyion, probably via an endovascular approach, would like be the initial therapy attempted. Surgical bypass is also another treatment option. Afterward, the patient should be reassessed, and if lifestyle-limiting symptoms are still present, then outflow revascularization should be performed with endovascular treatment or femoropopliteal or femoral-distal bypass could be considered.

4. **A.** Of all the options, the only one that is not an absolute indication for thrombolysis in the treatment of PAD, per the Society of Interventional Radiology, is occult blood in the stool.

Comment

Treatment Methods

Aortofemoral bypass is associated with 90% patency at 5 years. In patients who have a normal contralateral iliac artery and in whom medical comorbidities are present, femorofemoral bypass is sometimes used to revascularize the ischemic limb although endovascular techniques may be performed to recanalize the iliac artery, as seen in this case.

Endovascular Management

Endovascular recanalization of the occluded iliac artery has been performed for many years. In patients with chronic occlusions and short-segment acute occlusions, primary stent placement is considered by many to be the optimal endovascular method. In patients with acute occlusions with longer segments of thrombus, an initial course of thrombolytic therapy is favored by most physicians (Figures S67-3 through S67-5). This is done to eliminate as much thrombus as possible and thereby prevent embolization during later stent placement. Hence, in contrast to iliac artery stenoses, iliac artery occlusions are usually not treated with angioplasty alone; stents are nearly always used. In recent years, stent grafts have shown promise as a way to recanalize the occluded iliac artery with a lower potential for late restenosis. Endovascular management of iliac artery PAD is now preferred by most physicians due to the fact that procedural success and long-term outcomes are similar to surgical interventions, but with reduced morbidity and mortality. Preprocedural imaging with computed tomography or magnetic resonance may assist the physician in case planning (Figure S67-1). ABIs may also be helpful in planning and evaluation of intervention (Figures S67-2 and S67-6).

References

Klein AJ, Feldman DN, Aronow HD, et al. SCAI expert consensus statement for aorto-iliac arterial invervention and appropriate use. *Catheter Cardiovasc Interv.* 2014;84:520–528.

Lam C, Gandhi RT, Vatakencherry G, et al. Iliac artery revascularization: overview of current interventional therapies. *Interv Cardiol.* 2010;2:851–859.

Rzucidlo EM, Powell RJ, Zwolak RM, et al. Early results of stent-grafting to treat diffuse aortoiliac occlusive disease. *J Vasc Surg.* 2003;37:1175–1180.

Cross-reference

Vascular and Interventional Radiology: The Requisites, 2nd ed, 209–214.

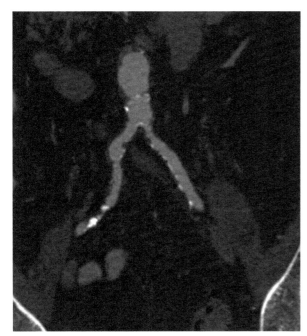

Figure 68-1. *Courtesy of Dr. Saher S. Sabri.*

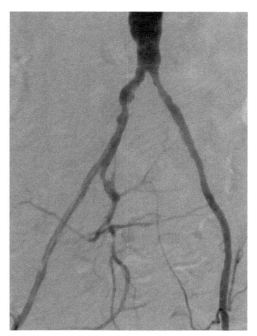

Figure 68-2. *Courtesy of Dr. Saher S. Sabri.*

HISTORY: A 78-year-old female presents with bilateral lower extremity claudication; ankle-brachial index 0.68 right and 0.61 left.

1. Which of the following is the most likely diagnosis for the imaging findings presented?
   A. Iliac stenosis
   B. Abdominal aortic aneurysm
   C. Right femoral artery aneurysm
   D. Normal aortoiliac vessels

2. A 45-year-old male smoker with a past medical history significant for diabetes and hypertension is referred to your clinic for intermittent claudication and an ankle-brachial index of 0.6. What is the most appropriate initial therapy?
   A. Referral to vascular surgery for possible revascularization
   B. Aortogram evaluation with possible endovascular intervention
   C. Cilostazol therapy
   D. Medical management of hypertension and lipids with smoking cessation encouragement

3. What TransAtlantic InterSociety Consensus (TASC) Classification would the imaging findings above be described as?
   A. TASC A
   B. TASC B
   C. TASC C
   D. TASC D

4. If the infrainguinal arteries are normal, what symptoms would this patient most likely have?
   A. Rest pain
   B. Anterior thigh claudication symptoms
   C. Hip and buttock claudication symptoms
   D. Posterior thigh claudication symptoms

See Supplemental Figures section for additional figures and legends for this case.

CASE 68

Bilateral Common Iliac Artery Stenoses (Kissing Stents)

1. **A.** There are stenoses of the bilateral common iliac arteries. There is no evidence of an abdominal aortic aneurysm or a femoral artery aneurysm on the provided images.

2. **D.** The first-line therapy of intermittent claudication symptoms is lifestyle modifications and tight control of risk factors. Even though this patient has a lower ankle-brachial index, conservative management is still the course of action. If symptoms persist or the patient worsens, further action is warranted.

3. **A.** This is a TASC A lesion as there are short stenoses of the common iliac arteries, not occlusions (which would be TASC D).

4. **C.** If the infrainguinal arteries were normal in this patient, then blood flow would be sustained to the lower extremities. Therefore the patient would be experiencing claudication symptoms proximal to those arteries, which would result in bilateral hip and buttock pain and possibly impotence for males.

Comment

Clinical Presentation

Patients with disease in the aorta or common iliac arteries typically present with hip and buttock claudication and/or impotence, because of limited flow into the internal iliac artery territories. Intermittent claudication generally occurs when ankle-brachial indices are 0.5 to 0.9. When additional levels of disease are present in the femoral and/or tibial vessels, the patient is likely to experience rest pain in the feet. Rest pain signifies limb-threatening ischemia and is associated with a high amputation rate if the vascular abnormality is not treated.

Ankle-brachial indices are generally 0.2 to 0.4 in patients with rest pain and no visible tissue loss, and they may be lower in patients with ulcers or gangrene.

Treatment Methods

Surgical aortofemoral bypass is associated with 90% patency at 5 years. The secondary patency of iliac artery angioplasty with selective stent placement is 80% to 90% at 4 years. Because endovascular therapy is associated with lower mortality and major morbidity, it is the preferred first-line treatment in patients with anatomically suitable iliac lesions.

Endovascular Management

Patients with aortoiliac junction lesions with or without actual distal aortic stenosis are often treated with kissing stents regardless of whether the contralateral iliac artery is diseased (Figures S68-1 through S68-5). This is done to effectively cover the aortic bifurcation plaque, to provide support to the other inflated balloon, and to prevent embolization down the contralateral side due to dislodged aortic bifurcation plaque. Recent studies have shown that covered stents have a higher primary patency at 2 years when compared to bare metal stents and are frequently used for kissing iliac stent interventions.

References

Abello N, Kretz B, Picquet J, et al. Long-term results of stenting the aortic bifurcation. *Ann Vasc Surg.* 2012;26:521–526.

Sabri SS, Choudhri A, Orgera G, et al. Outcomes of covered kissing stent placement compared with bare metal stent placement in the treatment of atherosclerotic occlusive disease at the aortic bifurcation. *J Vasc Interv Radiol.* 2010;21:995–1003.

Scheinert D, Schroder M, Balzer JO, et al. Stent-supported reconstruction of the aortoiliac bifurcation with the kissing balloon technique. *Circulation.* 1999;100(Suppl 19):II295–II300.

Cross-reference

Vascular and Interventional Radiology: The Requisites, 2nd ed, 209–214.

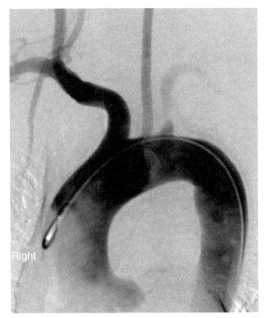

Figure 69-1. *Courtesy of Dr. Wael E. Saad.*

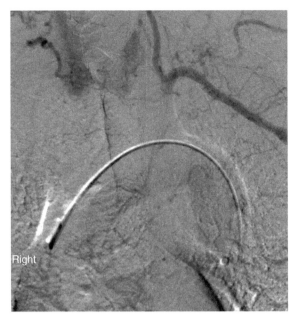

Figure 69-2. *Courtesy of Dr. Wael E. Saad.*

HISTORY: A 54-year-old female presents with dizziness and left arm claudication.

1. Which of the following is the most likely diagnosis for the imaging findings presented?
   A. Takayasu's arteritis
   B. Giant cell arteritis
   C. Subclavian stenosis with steal
   D. Fibromuscular dysplasia

2. Which of the following is Duplex ultrasonography evidence of this entity?
   A. Reversal of flow in the ipsilateral common carotid artery
   B. Reversal of flow in the ipsilateral subclavian artery
   C. Reversal of flow in the ipsilateral brachial artery
   D. Reversal of flow in the ipsilateral vertebral artery

3. Which of the following methods is *NOT* used to treat this entity?
   A. Embolization
   B. Angioplasty
   C. Stenting
   D. Surgical bypass

4. Which of the following vessels is most commonly affected in a patient with myocardial steal status post coronary artery bypass graft?
   A. Vertebral artery
   B. Lateral thoracic artery
   C. Thoracoacromial artery
   D. Internal mammary artery

See Supplemental Figures section for additional figures and legends for this case.

CASE 69

Subclavian Steal Syndrome

1. **C.** Subclavian steal syndrome occurs when a critical stenosis in the subclavian artery, proximal to the origin of the vertebral artery, results in reconstitution of the distal subclavian artery via retrograde flow through the ipsilateral vertebral artery. This results in left arm claudication with vertebrobasilar symptoms, such as syncope or dizziness. Takayasu's arteritis and giant cell arteritis commonly involve more than 1 focal vessel.

2. **D.** Duplex ultrasound reveals reversal of flow within the vertebral artery on the ipsilateral side as the proximal subclavian artery stenosis/occlusion.

3. **A.** Stenting, angioplasty, and surgical bypass of the subclavian artery lesion are all known methods to treat subclavian steal syndrome, each of which has various success rates. Embolization does not play any role in the treatment of subclavian steal syndrome.

4. **D.** Myocardial steal syndrome is similar to subclavian steal, as there is retrograde flow within an internal mammary artery bypass graft to provide flow to the left upper extremity.

Comment

Clinical Presentation

Subclavian steal syndrome can occur due to stenosis or occlusion of the proximal segment of the subclavian artery. Most commonly, this lesion causes signs of vertebrobasilar insufficiency, including syncopal or near syncopal episodes initiated by exercising the ipsilateral arm, headaches, nausea, vertigo, and other neurological symptoms. In a minority of patients, signs of brachial insufficiency are present, including upper-extremity pain, paresthesias, coolness, weakness, or fingertip necrosis.

Endovascular Management

The diagnosis is often suspected based on the clinical history and the physical finding of diminished pulse and/or diminished systolic blood pressure in the affected limb. Duplex ultrasound often demonstrates reversal of vertebral artery flow. The classic angiographic features of this diagnosis are the presence of stenosis or occlusion of the subclavian artery proximal to the vertebral artery origin, with retrograde flow down the vertebral artery seen later in the angiographic run (Figures S69-1 and S69-2). The lesion can be treated with surgical bypass, angioplasty, or stenting (Figures S69-3 and S69-4).

References

Sueoka BL. Percutaneous transluminal stent placement to treat subclavian steal syndrome. *J Vasc Interv Radiol.* 1996;7:351–356.

Taylor CL, Selman WR, Ratcheson RA. Steal affecting the central nervous system. *Neurosurgery.* 2002;50:679–688.

Cross-reference

Vascular and Interventional Radiology: The Requisites, 2nd ed, 125–126.

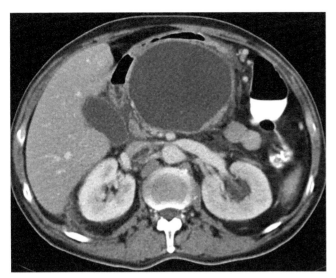

Figure 70-1

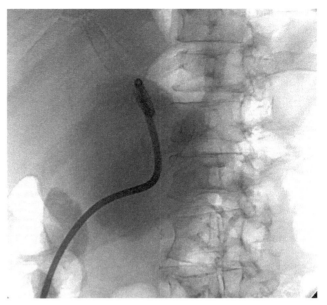

Figure 70-2

HISTORY: A 52-year-old alcoholic male with pancreatitis presents with worsening of his chronic abdominal pain.

1. Which of the following would be included in the differential diagnosis for the imaging findings presented? (Choose all that apply.)
   A. Walled-off necrosis
   B. Pancreatic pseudocyst
   C. Abscess
   D. Serous cystadenoma

2. Which of the following is *NOT* an indication for percutaneous drainage?
   A. Size greater than 6 cm
   B. Communication with the pancreatic duct
   C. Mass effect with gastric outlet obstruction
   D. Symptoms and signs of associated sepsis

3. Which of the following is true about percutaneous pseudocyst drainage?
   A. Should be performed early and aggressively
   B. Drains are usually only needed for 1 to 2 weeks
   C. Drains should be larger caliber as smaller drains can become clogged easily
   D. Drains must be placed from a retroperitoneal approach

4. After laparoscopic pancreatic necrosectomy, a patient acutely decompensates with low blood pressure. What is the next step in management?
   A. Computed tomography (CT) of the abdomen to elucidate the cause
   B. Urgent laparotomy
   C. Percutaneous drainage of the fluid collection and IV antibiotics to counteract acute sepsis
   D. Catheter-directed angiography to evaluate and treat arterial injury

See Supplemental Figures section for additional figures and legends for this case.

CASE 70

Transgastric Pancreatic Pseudocyst Drainage

1. **A, B, C, and D.** All the answer choices apply to a pancreas-associated cystic lesion seen on CT imaging. It is impossible to definitively diagnose the type of cystic lesion by CT alone. Pancreatic pseudocysts generally develop several weeks after an episode of acute pancreatitis. It is difficult to detail whether the fluid collection contents are necrotic, solid tissue, or superinfected. Magnetic resonance imaging is better at determining fluid versus solid contents. Even pancreatitis-associated pseudoaneurysms can have a similar appearance to pseudocysts on noncontrast CT.

2. **B.** Cystic lesions that communicate with the pancreatic duct are notoriously difficult to treat, and percutaneous drainage has limited benefit. All the other answer choices have been listed as reasons to attempt percutaneous drainage in addition to persistent pain beyond 6 weeks.

3. **C.** Pancreatic pseudocysts can often contain complex debris, which causes smaller tubes to clog easily and larger drains are often required for a prolonged duration. Greater than half of pseudocysts resolve with conservative therapy, and aggressive drainage should be avoided to prevent infection of a sterile space. Although a retroperitoneal approach is preferred to stay in the same space as the pancreas and prevent bowel contamination, pseudocysts can be drained from a variety of approaches including transgastric.

4. **D.** The greatest concern after pancreatic necrosectomy is injury to the splenic artery. Angiography with embolization or possibly covered stenting would be the most appropriate next step. Obtaining imaging in an unstable patient may waste critical time. Open surgical intervention is a complex procedure in a patient with postpancreatitis fluid collections and adhesions and may cause unnecessary morbidity and delay.

Comment

Pancreatic Pseudocysts

Patients with fluid collections that appear after an episode of acute pancreatitis are typically initially treated with supportive care and observation. The two primary clinical situations in which pseudocyst drainage is indicated are when there is reason to suspect that a particular fluid collection is infected and when the patient has persistent pain at least 6 weeks following the initial pancreatitis episode.

Percutaneous Management

The CT scan shown here demonstrates a large pancreatic pseudocyst immediately posterior to the stomach (Figure S70-1). A suitable window directly into this collection could not be identified, so transgastric drainage was performed. Given the large size of this pseudocyst, the procedure was performed using fluoroscopic guidance alone, using the indentation upon the gastric air pattern as a landmark for the location of the pseudocyst. Because pancreatic collections typically contain semisolid debris, a large-bore catheter was placed (Figure S70-2). Because transgastric pseudocyst drainage catheters are prone to displacement back into the stomach due to gastric peristalsis, a locking loop catheter was used.

Clinical Management

Pancreatic pseudocysts typically require several months of drainage before they can be removed. In general, the criteria for removing the catheter include minimal output (<10 mL/day for 2 days), absence of fistula to the pancreatic duct, and good clinical status (the patient is afebrile and generally improved).

References

Cruz-Santamaria DM, Taxonera C, Giner M. Update on pathogenesis and clinical management of acute pancreatitis. *World J Gastrointest Pathophysiol.* 2012;3:60–70.

Neff R. Pancreatic pseudocysts and fluid collections: percutaneous approaches. *Surg Clin North Am.* 2001;81:399–403.

Cross-reference

Vascular and Interventional Radiology: The Requisites, 2nd ed, 411–414.

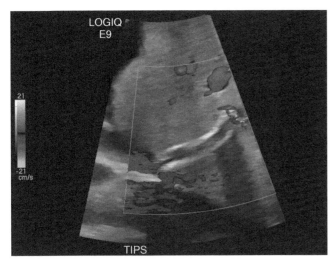

Figure 71-1. *Courtesy of Dr. Minhaj S. Khaja.*

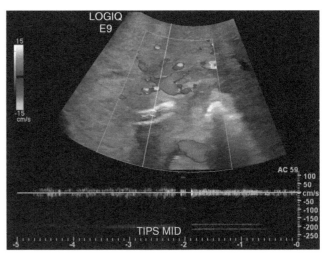

Figure 71-2. *Courtesy of Dr. Minhaj S. Khaja.*

HISTORY: A 58-year-old female status post transjugular intrahepatic portosystemic shunt (TIPS) presents with increasing ascites.

1. Which of the following is the most likely diagnosis for the imaging findings presented?
   A. TIPS in-stent stenosis
   B. Crushed TIPS
   C. Type II endoleak
   D. TIPS occlusion

2. Which of the following is a cause of early TIPS occlusion?
   A. Hypertension
   B. Fistulous connection with biliary tree
   C. Elevated international normalized ratio
   D. Refractory ascites

3. What modality is typically used for TIPS evaluation?
   A. Portography
   B. Two-phase computed tomography of abdomen
   C. Ultrasound
   D. Direct portal pressure measurement

4. Which of the following is considered within the normal velocity range for a patent TIPS?
   A. 15 to 40 cm/s
   B. 20 to 200 cm/s
   C. 90 to 190 cm/s
   D. 150 to 200 cm/s

See Supplemental Figures section for additional figures and legends for this case.

CASE 71

TIPS: Occlusion and Thrombolysis

1. **D.** The TIPS stent is thrombosed. There is no color flow seen on Doppler imaging and velocities are minimal.

2. **B.** Bile is thrombogenic and therefore biliary fistulae may result in TIPS occlusion. This has significantly decreased since the use of the covered stent.

3. **C.** There are no consensus guidelines. However, TIPS are frequently followed with ultrasound being performed after 1 month, 3 months, 6 months, then annually after placement.

4. **C.** The normal velocity range is 90 to 190 cm/s for a TIPS as evaluated by Doppler ultrasound. Both low and high velocities may indicate dysfunction.

Comment

Main Teaching Point

Currently, there are no consensus guidelines for TIPS surveillance. Doppler ultrasound is the exam of choice and is frequently performed within 1 month of placement, at 3 months, 6 months, 12 months, and then annually. Many centers only monitor TIPS if dysfunction is indicated by clinical symptoms. After TIPS placement, there is reversal of flow within the left and right portal veins towards the TIPS. Portal flow should remain directed toward the liver (and stent) in the main portal vein. There is compensatory increase in flow within the hepatic arteries. Gray-scale ultrasound images can detect anatomic defects within the stent, including kinking, luminal narrowing, and stent migration. Doppler ultrasound can further evaluate the flow dynamics (Figures S71-1 and S71-2). Normal stent velocities range between 90 and 190 cm/s. Significant velocity gradients or velocity change over time can indicate stent dysfunction. Doppler ultrasound can also demonstrate abnormal flow direction within the portal system, which may signify stenosis or occlusion.

Endovascular Management

A TIPS should not be revised based on radiographic imaging findings alone, but should be correlated with the patients clinical status. Angiographic evaluation is performed via internal jugular access. A wire and catheter are advanced into the TIPS. Both venography and pressure measurements should be employed to evaluate the shunt. If a stenosis is visualized or a pressure gradient present, a combination of angioplasty and restenting can be performed. Treatment of an occluded TIPS ranges from placement of a new TIPS to pharmacomechanical thrombolysis and angioplasty (Figures S71-3 through S71-5).

References

Brehmer WP, Saad WE. Dysfunctional transjugular intrahepatic portosystemic shunt: anatomic defects and doppler ultrasound evaluation. *Ultrasound Clin.* 2013;8:125–135.

Darcy M. Evaluation and management of transjugular intrahepatic portosystemic Shunts. *AJR Am J Roentgenol.* 2012;199:730–736.

Cross-reference

Vascular and Interventional Radiology: The Requisites, 2nd ed, 318–325.

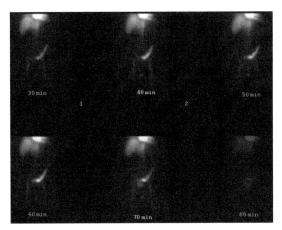

Figure 72-1

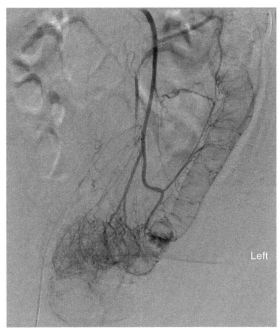

Figure 72-2

HISTORY: A 68-year-old stable male presents to the emergency department with acute hematochezia.

1. Which of the following would be included in the differential diagnosis for the imaging findings presented? (Choose all that apply.)
   A. Arteriovenous malformation
   B. Occlusive mesenteric ischemia
   C. Active bleeding
   D. Colonic neoplasm

2. What is the *MINIMAL* bleeding rate required for detection by angiography?
   A. 0.05 to 0.1 mL/min
   B. 0.1 to 0.2 mL/min
   C. 0.5 to 1.0 mL/min
   D. 2.0 to 3.0 mL/min

3. Intraarterial infusion of which pharmacologic agent can be used in the treatment of lower gastrointestinal (LGI) bleeding?
   A. Vasopressin
   B. Nitroglycerin
   C. Octreotide
   D. Cimetidine

4. Which of the following is the most common cause of LGI bleeding?
   A. Colonic cancer
   B. Colitis
   C. Angiodysplasia
   D. Diverticulosis

See Supplemental Figures section for additional figures and legends for this case.

147

CASE 72

Lower Gastrointestinal Bleed

1. **A, C, and D.** Inferior mesenteric arteriogram demonstrates active extravasation in a distal sigmoid branch, compatible with an LGI bleed. Differential consideration includes arteriovenous malformation and neoplasm. Occlusive bowel ischemia would demonstrate an intraluminal filling defect or occlusion.

2. **C.** Conventional angiography can detect active extravasation at bleeding rates of 0.5 to 1.0 mL/min. Tc-99m sulfur colloid study is the most sensitive imaging modality and can detect bleeding rates as low as 0.05 to 0.1 mL/min. In comparison, Tc-99m red cell scintigraphy requires bleeding rates of 0.1 to 0.2 mL/min for detection.

3. **A.** Vasopressin can be infused via a catheter with its tip in the vessel supplying the bleeding site, where it causes vasoconstriction. Vasopressin is not effective in the treatment of upper gastrointestinal (UGI) bleeding, and it is rarely used in that setting. Nitroglycerin is a vasodilator used to prevent vasospasm during arteriography. Intravenous octreotide infusion is an adjunct therapy for variceal UGI bleeding. Cimetidine is an H2-antagonist that may be used for prophylaxis for UGI bleeding.

4. **D.** Diverticulosis is the most common etiology of LGI bleeding (43%). The majority of diverticula occur in the left colon, though right colonic diverticula are more prone to bleeding. Though diverticular bleeding often resolves spontaneously, persistent severe bleeding warrants intervention. Colonic angiodysplasia is the second most common cause (20%).

Comment

Diagnostic Evaluation

Once patients present with signs of lower GI bleeding, the clinician must begin resuscitative efforts with acquisition of large-bore intravenous access and the administration of fluids and blood products, as necessary. The next step in management commonly includes evaluation with colonoscopy, capsule endoscopy, or diagnostic imaging. Imaging modalities include Tc99m labeled red blood cell scintigraphy, computed tomography angiography, or catheter angiography (Figures S72-1, S72-2, and S72-4).

Endovascular Management

Catheter-directed vasopressin infusion has traditionally been the first-line treatment for LGI bleeding. This is based on findings in older literature in which infarction often complicated LGI embolization. Vasopressin is a natural hormone that reduces pulse pressure and blood flow via constriction of smooth muscle in splanchnic blood vessels and bowel wall, allowing clot to form. After a bleeding site is identified, a catheter is secured with its tip in a central vessel supplying the bleeding site. Vasopressin infusion is started at 0.2 U/min. Follow-up arteriography is performed in 20 to 30 minutes to assess response. If vasopressin infusion does result in cessation of bleeding, the infusion is continued for 12 to 24 hours and the patient is closely monitored in an intensive care unit. If active extravasation is still present, the infusion is increased to 0.4 U/min, and arteriography is again repeated in 20 to 30 minutes. If active extravasation is still observed, alternative therapies (such as embolization) should be pursued. Mild abdominal discomfort at the initiation of infusion is common, but persistent pain might indicate ischemia, signaling the need to reduce the infusion rate. If continued cessation of bleeding is observed clinically, then the vasopressin infusion is tapered over the next 12 to 24 hours. Initial success rates for vasopressin infusion therapy in controlling LGI bleeding range from 60% to 90%, but rebleeding occurs in approximately 40%. Vasopressin is not effective in the treatment of UGI bleeding, and it is rarely used in that setting.

Endovascular Embolization

With modern embolization techniques, clinically significant bowel ischemia has become an uncommon complication. Although the efficacies of vasopressin and embolization are fairly comparable, embolotherapy has advantages in terms of quicker completion of therapy and decreased likelihood of systemic complications (Figures S72-3, S72-5, and S72-6). Although vasopressin is still probably preferable for diffuse lesions and cases in which super-selective catheterization is not technically possible, embolization should be considered a primary option for treating LGI bleeding.

References

Darcy M. Treatment of lower gastrointestinal (LGI) bleeding: vasopressin infusion versus embolization. *J Vasc Intervent Radiol.* 2003;14:535–543.

Hastings G. Angiographic localization and transcatheter treatment of gastrointestinal bleeding. *Radiographics.* 2000;20:1160–1168.

Navuluri R, Kang L, Patel J, et al. Acute lower gastrointestinal bleeding. *Semin Intervent Radiol.* 2012;29:178–186.

Cross-reference

Vascular and Interventional Radiology: The Requisites, 2nd ed, 239–243.

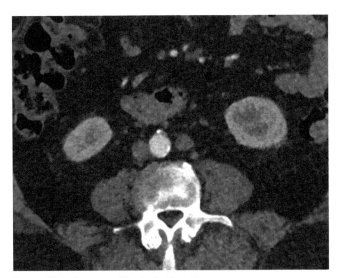

Figure 73-1 *Courtesy of Dr. Lucia Flors Blasco.*

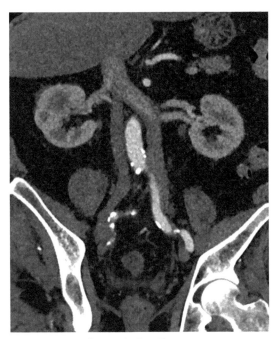

Figure 73-2 *Courtesy of Dr. Lucia Flors Blasco.*

HISTORY: A 60-year-old man with history of poorly controlled hypertension, evaluation for renal artery stenosis.

1. Which of the following is the most likely diagnosis for the imaging findings presented?
   A. Duplicated inferior vena cava (IVC)
   B. Congenitally absent IVC
   C. Left-sided IVC
   D. Retroaortic left renal vein

2. A left IVC typically drains into:
   A. The right atrium
   B. The right IVC at the level of the left renal vein
   C. The right IVC at the level of the hepatic veins
   D. The hemiazygous vein

3. Which of the following IVC congenital anomalies is most commonly seen?
   A. Left-sided IVC
   B. Duplicated IVC
   C. Retrocaval ureter
   D. Absence of the infrarenal IVC

4. In patients with duplicated IVC, which of the following is *NOT* an appropriate option for adequate protection against potential pulmonary emboli?
   A. Place two filters (one in each IVC)
   B. Suprarenal IVC filter
   C. Right IVC filter
   D. Coil embolization of the smaller IVC coupled with filter placement in the contralateral IVC

See Supplemental Figures section for additional figures and legends for this case.

CASE 73

Variant Anatomy: Duplicated IVC

1. **A.** Abdominal computed tomography shows right and left infrarenal IVCs. After drainage of the left renal vein, the left IVC crosses anterior to the aorta to form a single right-sided suprarenal IVC. No retroaortic left renal vein is seen.

2. **B.** The left-sided IVC accepts drainage from the left renal and adrenal veins and subsequently drains into the right-sided IVC.

3. **B.** Duplicated IVC has a prevalence of 1% to 3%, whereas a solitary left-sided IVC is less common, occurring in 0.2% of persons. Retrocaval ureter has a prevalence of 0.07%. Complete absence of the infrarenal IVC with preservation of the suprarenal segment is an extremely rare anomaly.

4. **C.** Potential emboli originating in both limbs should be prevented; therefore placement of a single filter within the right-sided IVC is not an adequate option to achieve sufficient protection. All of the other choices provide adequate filtration to avoid pulmonary embolism.

Comment

Clinical Importance

Normally a single IVC drains the lower extremities and iliac veins. However, several congenital anomalies of venous development exist and can affect IVC filter placement. Therefore, an inferior vena cavogram should always be performed before deploying a filter.

Duplicated Variants

Double (right and left) IVC has a prevalence of 1% to 3% and arises from the persistence of both supracardinal veins. In patients with duplication of the IVC, the left-sided IVC accepts drainage from the left renal and adrenal veins and subsequently drains into the right-sided IVC at the Ll-l2 level (Figures S73-1, tS73-3h, S73-3). Therefore, to achieve adequate protection against potential pulmonary emboli originating in both limbs, it is necessary either to place two filters (one in each IVC) or to place a single (suprarenal) filter above the confluence of the two IVCs. Coil embolization of the smaller IVC coupled with filter placement in the contralateral IVC is an alternative.

Solitary/Absent Variants

A solitary left-sided IVC is less common, occurring in 0.2% of persons. It arises from a persistent left supracardinal vein with regression of the right supracardinal vein. Similar to the duplicated IVC, this vessel drains to the right at the level of the renal veins. Congenital absence of the IVC is seen in 0.6% of patients with congenital heart disease but is more common with cyanotic heart disease. Typically, the hepatic segment of the IVC is interrupted and lower-extremity venous drainage occurs via the azygous and hemiazygous systems. The hepatic veins drain directly to the right atrium.

References

Hicks ME, Malden ES, Vesely TM, et al. Prospective anatomic study of the inferior vena cava and renal veins: comparison of selective renal venography with cavography and relevance in filter placement. *J Vasc Interv Radiol.* 1995;6:721–729.

Kandpal H, et al. Imaging the inferior vena cava: a road less traveled. *RadioGraphics.* 2008;28:669–689.

Sheth S, Fishman EK. Imaging of the inferior vena cava with MDCT. *AJR Am J Roentgenol.* 2007;189:1243–1251.

Cross-reference

Vascular and Interventional Radiology: The Requisites, 2nd ed, 287–292.

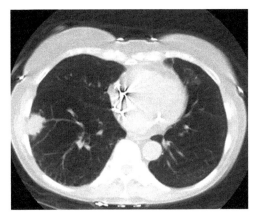

Figure 74-1. *Courtesy of Dr. Bill S. Majdalany.*

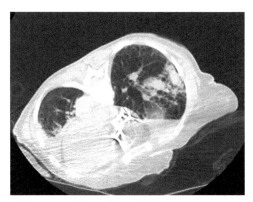

Figure 74-2. *Courtesy of Dr. Bill S. Majdalany.*

HISTORY: An 81-year-old female with chronic lung disease and a new lung nodule.

1. Which of the following would be included in the differential diagnosis for the imaging findings presented? (Choose all that apply.)
   A. Lung metastases
   B. Rounded atelectasis
   C. Pneumonia
   D. Primary lung cancer

2. Assuming that the lesion is an isolated pulmonary metastasis, what is the standard of care for this patient?
   A. Surgical resection of the lesion
   B. Chemotherapy
   C. Chemotherapy with radiation
   D. Percutaneous ablation

3. Are there any computed tomography (CT) findings that might change the management strategy for this patient? If so, what are they?
   A. No additional finding to change management
   B. Osseous metastases
   C. Atherosclerosis
   D. Emphysema

4. What is a suggested advantage of using cryoablation versus other percutaneous therapies?
   A. It is technically easier.
   B. There is a larger "ablation zone."
   C. There is better visualization of the "ablation-zone" during the procedure.
   D. Cryoablation can be done under ultrasound guidance.

See Supplemental Figures section for additional figures and legends for this case.

CASE 74

Lung Metastases: Ablation

1. **A, B, C, and D.** All of the options should be included in the differential diagnosis of a lung mass.

2. **A.** Surgical resection is the standard of care for solitary metastatic lung nodules. Adjunctivant chemotherapy and radiation can be considered on a case-by-case basis but are not considered standard of care for all solitary pulmonary metastases.

3. **D.** This patient has significant underlying emphysema and heart disease, both of which make this patient a poor operative candidate.

4. **C.** Radiologic-pathologic studies have shown that the ice-ball visualized on CT during the procedure correlates well with the pathologic zone of ablation. Note, the leading edge of the ice-ball is usually a 0°C isotherm and does not denote the active "kill-zone," which is demarcated by −20°C isotherm.

Comment

Treatment Methods

The standard of care for metastatic lung nodules with no extrapulmonary involvement is surgical resection: wedge resection, lobectomy, or even pneumonectomy. Many patients with metastatic lung disease are not candidates for surgery owing to poor pulmonary reserve or general health condition. Less-invasive therapies such as cryoablation, radiofrequency ablation, or external beam radiation can be offered to these patients. Local ablative therapies have a further advantage over external beam radiation in that they can be repeated as needed for lesions that develop further along in the course of the disease, as is typically seen in patients with metastatic disease.

Percutaneous Management

Cryoablation involves freezing and rapid thawing of tissue that leads to cell membrane disruption, resulting in cell death. The application of cryoablation includes tumors in many locations including lung, kidney, liver, bone, soft tissues, and others. Image guidance with CT or ultrasound is used for placement of the cryoprobes, and the freezing and thawing is monitored by CT imaging (Figures S74-1 through S74-4). Lung consolidation is clearly seen in the area exposed to freezing in the second image.

Complications

Hemoptysis occurs commonly; however, this is minimal in the majority of patients and requires no further intervention aside from patient reassurance. Owing to the relatively large size of the cryoprobes, pneumothorax is a common procedural complication, with rates reported at 50% to 62%. Chest tube placement is only needed in 12% of these patients.

References

Goldberg SN, Charboneau JW, Dodd III GD, et al. International working group on image-guided tumor ablation: image-guided tumor ablation: proposal for standardization of terms and reporting criteria. *Radiology.* 2003;228:335–345.

Kawamura M, Izumi Y, Tsukada N, et al. Percutaneous cryoablation of small pulmonary malignant tumors under computed tomographic guidance with local anesthesia for nonsurgical candidates. *J Thorac Cardiovasc Surg.* 2006;131:1007–1013.

Sonntag PD, Hinshaw JL, Lubner MG, et al. Thermal ablation of lung tumors. *Surg Oncol Clin N Am.* 2011;20:369–387.

Wang H, Littrup PJ, Duan Y, et al. Thoracic masses treated with percutaneous cryotherapy: initial experience with more than 200 procedures. *Radiology.* 2005;235:289–298.

Cross-reference

Vascular and Interventional Radiology: The Requisites, 2nd ed, 562–570.

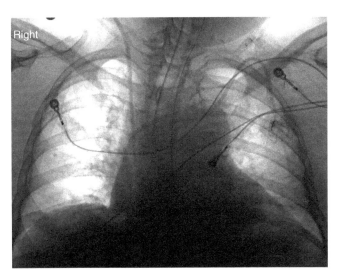

Figure 75-1

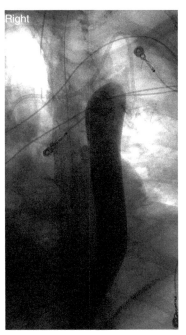

Figure 75-2

HISTORY: A 65-year-old male with esophageal cancer presents with hematemesis.

1. Which of the following would be included in the differential diagnosis for the imaging findings presented? (Choose all that apply.)
   A. Aortocaval fistula
   B. Infected (mycotic) aortic aneurysm
   C. Aortoenteric fistula
   D. Atherosclerotic abdominal aortic aneurysm

2. What location in the gastrointestinal (GI) system is the most common site for the abnormality presented in the images above?
   A. First and second parts of the duodenum
   B. Midjejunum
   C. Gastric antrum
   D. Third and fourth parts of the duodenum

3. What procedure is most likely to lead to the abnormality shown above?
   A. Push enteroscopy
   B. Repair of a perforated ulcer
   C. Biopsy of GI endothelium for suspected celiac disease
   D. Repair of an abdominal aortic aneurysm

4. Which of the following is *NOT* an indirect sign of an aortoenteric fistula?
   A. Bowel wall thickening adjacent to an aneurysm
   B. Retroperitoneal hematoma
   C. Ectopic gas adjacent to or within the aorta
   D. Disruption of the aortic fat plane

See Supplemental Figures section for additional figures and legends for this case.

CASE 75

Aortoenteric Fistula

1. **B and C.** The thoracic aortogram shows a pseudoaneurysm near the cephalad portion of an esophageal stent. The pseudoaneurysm could be due to a mycotic etiology or otherwise part of an aortoenteric fistula.

2. **C.** The third and fourth parts of the duodenum are most typically involved in an aortoenteric fistula given their anatomic position relative to the aorta, as well as their relatively fixed position. While the other options listed can become involved in an aortoenteric fistula, they are not as closely involved anatomically with the aorta.

3. **D.** The procedures that are most commonly associated with the formation of an aortoenteric fistula are reconstructions of abdominal aortic aneurysms. Most frequently, the area of communication is the suture line of the graft and the native aorta with the duodenum. This is due to the high pressures of the aorta combined with the inflammatory response of the surgical intervention.

4. **C.** Ectopic gas adjacent to or within the aorta is a direct sign that an aortoenteric fistula is present. The other answer choices are indirect signs of aortoenteric fistula.

Comment

Clinical Presentation

Formation of an aortoenteric fistula is much more common as an infrequent (0.4% to 2.4%) complication of aortic vascular procedures (termed secondary) than as a complication of aneurysm rupture (termed primary). In either situation, this disorder carries a significant risk of death or limb loss despite treatment. Patients with a direct communication between the anastomotic suture line of the aortic graft and the adjacent bowel lumen (graft-enteric fistula) often present with intermittent hematemesis or melena days to weeks after the procedure. Patients with erosion remote from the suture line with exposure of a portion of the graft prosthesis (graft-enteric erosion) commonly present with chronic GI bleeding. Patients with lesser degrees of bleeding can present with septicemia resulting from graft infection.

Endovascular Management

Most cases occur two or more years after the aortic surgery. For this reason, although aortography is not routinely performed in the angiographic evaluation of all GI bleeding patients, those with a suitable history should be studied with aortography (Figures S75-1 through S75-3). Most cases involve the third or fourth portions of the duodenum owing to the proximity of the graft anastomosis to this fairly fixated portion of bowel, but in 10% to 20% the more distal small bowel or colon is involved. Rarely, the esophagus may be involved. Endoscopy is the preferred first step in evaluation because it can diagnose many other more common causes of GI bleeding, and rarely, it can provide a definitive diagnosis by visualizing a focus of exposed graft (Figure S75-4).

References

Raman SP, Kamaya A, Federle M, et al. Aortoenteric fistulas: spectrum of CT findings. *Abdom Imaging.* 2013;38:367–375.

Ranasinghe W, Loa J, Allaf N, et al. Primary aortoenteric fistulae: the challenges in diagnosis and review of treatment. *Ann Vasc Surg.* 2011;25(386):e1–e5.

Cross-reference

Vascular and Interventional Radiology: The Requisites, 2nd ed, 206–207.

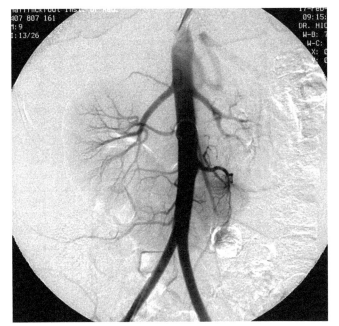

Figure 76-1

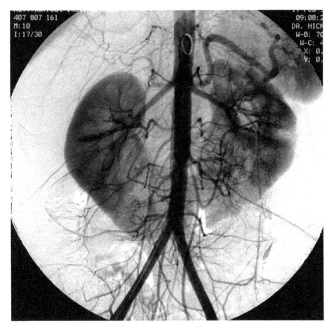

Figure 76-2

HISTORY: A 53-year-old male with hypertension.

1. What is the angiographic finding seen?
   A. Situs inversus
   B. Horseshoe kidney
   C. Crossed-fused renal ectopia
   D. Absent left kidney

2. From where can renal arteries arise in patients with a horseshoe kidney? (Choose all that apply.)
   A. Aorta
   B. Common iliac artery
   C. Hypogastric artery (internal iliac artery)
   D. Inferior mesenteric artery

3. Within what population are horseshoe kidneys most commonly seen?
   A. Male
   B. Female
   C. African-American
   D. Caucasian

4. Patient's with horseshoe kidneys are at higher risk for which of the following? (Choose all that apply.)
   A. Renal trauma
   B. Renal calculi
   C. Ureteral duplication
   D. Hydronephrosis

See Supplemental Figures section for additional figures and legends for this case.

CASE 76

Horseshoe Kidney

1. **B.** Angiogram reveals a horseshoe kidney with fused lower poles. Crossed-fused renal ectopia is another rare variant where the kidney is on the opposite of its ureteral insertion on the bladder and is fused with the contralateral kidney.

2. **A, B, C, and D.** A horseshoe kidney typically has more than two renal arteries. There is a wide array of variation within the arterial supply including origination from the aorta, common iliac artery, hypogastric artery, and inferior mesenteric artery. Most commonly, there are more than two arteries that arise from the aorta or there are more than two arteries and the isthmus is supplied from the common iliac artery/arteries. Location of the renal arteries is important for surgical planning.

3. **A.** There is a two-to-one predominance within males. There is no ethnic predominance known.

4. **A, B, C, and D.** All of the above are associated with the presence of a horseshoe kidney, in addition to other genitourinary abnormalities and anomalies of the cardiovascular, skeletal, central nervous, and gastrointestinal systems.

Comment

Variant Anatomy

In a horseshoe kidney, the two kidneys are joined at either the lower pole (90%) or upper pole (10%) by a parenchymal-fibrous isthmus (Figures S76-3 and S76-4). Typically, the long axis of each kidney is oriented somewhat more medially than normal, and the renal pelves and ureters exit their respective kidneys anteriorly. The vascular supply is often aberrant and often there are multiple renal arteries (six or more renal arteries are possible). In the case presented here, at least three renal arteries supply the right kidney, one left renal artery is present, and one more artery can be seen to supply at least part of the isthmus that joins the lower poles of the kidneys (Figures S76-1 and S76-2).

Anatomic Complications

A primary complication of horseshoe kidney is the development of renal calculi. Other associations include genitourinary abnormalities such as caudal ectopia, vesicoureteral reflux, hydronephrosis, ureteral duplication, hypospadias, undescended testis, and anomalies of the cardiovascular, skeletal, central nervous, and gastrointestinal systems.

References

Natsis K, Piagkou M, Skotsimara A, Protogerou V, Tsitouridis I, Skandalakis P. Horseshoe kidney: a review of anatomy and pathology. *Surg Radiol Anat.* 2014;36:517–526.

Raj GV, Auge BK, Weizer AZ. Percutaneous management of calculi within horseshoe kidneys. *J Urol.* 2003;170:48–51.

Cross-reference

Vascular and Interventional Radiology: The Requisites, 2nd ed, 265–268.

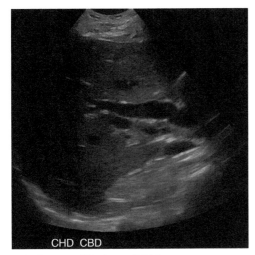

Figure 77-1. *Courtesy of Dr. James Shields.*

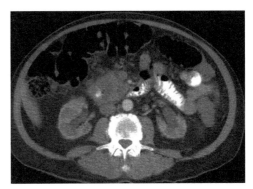

Figure 77-2. *Courtesy of Dr. James Shields.*

HISTORY: A 74-year-old male presents with 1-month history of worsening diffuse abdominal pain, weight loss, early satiety, nausea, and jaundice.

1. Which of the following is the most likely diagnosis for the imaging findings presented?
   A. Choledocholithiasis
   B. Pancreatitis
   C. Panreatic adenocarcinoma
   D. Hilar cholangiocarcinoma

2. What would be the next best test/procedure to establish a definitive diagnosis in this patient?
   A. Renal protocol computed tomography (CT)
   B. Endoscopy with brush biopsy
   C. Amylase and lipase levels
   D. CT of the chest

3. What is *NOT* an indication for plastic stent placement?
   A. Pancreatitis
   B. Choledocholithiasis
   C. Malignant obstruction
   D. Trauma

4. What is an indication for metal stent placement?
   A. Pancreatitis
   B. Choledocholithiasis
   C. Malignant obstruction
   D. Trauma

See Supplemental Figures section for additional figures and legends for this case.

CASE 77

Metallic Biliary Stent Placement

1. **C.** Given the CT of the abdomen demonstrating a mass-like density in the region of the head of the pancreas and associated upstream biliary duct dilatation as seen on the ultrasound, the most likely diagnosis given the choices above is pancreatic adenocarcinoma. Choledocholithiasis is not likely given that no stones were visualized. Pancreatitis could cause biliary duct obstruction; however, it would be unlikely to present as a mass-like density in the head of the pancreas. Cholangiocarcinoma can also present with biliary duct obstruction; however, it would be unlikely for it to present as a mass at the level of the pancreatic head and would most likely be present at the level of the hilum of the common bile duct.

2. **B.** The presence of a pancreatic head mass causing biliary duct obstruction on the abdominal CT and cholangiogram images are highly concerning for a pancreatic malignancy. Tissue sampling with endoscopy and brush biopsy is the next best test/procedure in this case in order to establish a diagnosis to further direct work-up and management.

3. **C.** Plastic biliary stents are most commonly placed for benign stricturing of the common bile duct.

4. **C.** Placement of metallic stents is generally reserved for palliation of a patient's symptoms in the setting of malignant biliary duct obstruction. This patient is a nonoperative candidate with a short life expectancy who will be undergoing chemo/radiation therapy.

Comment

Etiology

There are a wide variety of causes of biliary ductal obstruction or stricture. Benign causes include operative trauma, biliary ductal stones, scarring from prior passage of biliary stones, chronic pancreatitis, external compression, and nonoperative trauma. Malignant causes include cholangiocarcinoma, gallbladder cancer, pancreatic head carcinoma, ampullary neoplasms, and metastatic porta hepatis lymphadenopathy, which may be seen on ultrasonogram, CT, magnetic resonance imaging, or endoscopic retrograde cholangiopancreatography (Figures S77-1 and S77-2).

Percutaneous Management

Completely internalized biliary stents are often preferred to external or internal-external drainage catheters (Figures S77-3 and S77-4). However, because of the viscous nature of biliary secretions, all biliary stents must be changed regularly to prevent occlusion of the stent and/or formation of calculi. For this reason, the vast majority of internal stents and all stents placed for benign causes are made of catheter-type materials such as silicone rubber (Silastic). Permanent metallic stents should only be inserted for palliation of malignant obstructions in patients with short anticipated life expectancy. The imaging in this case demonstrates placement of an uncovered metallic stent in the common bile duct to relieve the obstruction of the distal common bile duct (Figure S77-5). Placement of a covered metallic stent is also possible to prevent tumor ingrowth; however, these have been shown to have a less superior patency rate compared to uncovered metallic stents.

References

Lee SJ, Kim MD, Lee MS, et al. Comparison of the efficacy of covered versus uncovered metallic stents in treating inoperable malignant common bile duct obstruction: a randomized trial. *J Vasc Interv Radiol.* 2014;25:1912–1920.

Schmassmann A, Von Gunten E, Knuchel J, et al. Wallstents versus plastic stents in malignant biliary obstruction: effects of stent patency of the first and second stent upon patient compliance and survival. *Am J Gastroenterol.* 1996;91:654–659.

Cross-reference

Vascular and Interventional Radiology: The Requisites, 2nd ed, 457–465.

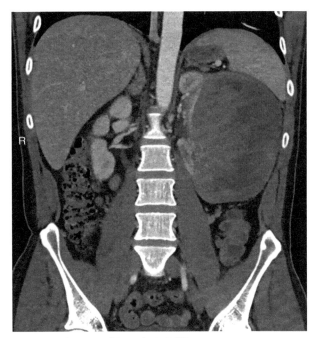

Figure 78-1. *Courtesy of Dr. Luke R. Wilkins.*

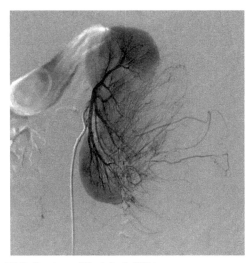

Figure 78-2. *Courtesy of Dr. Luke R. Wilkins.*

HISTORY: A 50-year-old male presents with flank pain and hematuria.

1. Which of the following would be included in the differential diagnosis for the imaging findings presented? (Choose all that apply.)
   A. Renal infarct
   B. Renal laceration
   C. Horseshoe kidney
   D. Renal cell carcinoma (RCC)

2. What lesion may have a similar angiographic appearance?
   A. Renal cyst
   B. Angiomyolipoma (AML)
   C. Polyarteritis nodosa
   D. Renal artery aneurysm

3. Which of the following treatments would *NOT* be used for this lesion?
   A. Cryoablation
   B. Direct injection of absolute alcohol
   C. Nephrectomy/partial nephrectomy
   D. Embolization

4. What disease is associated with bilateral multiple RCC?
   A. Von Hippel-Lindau
   B. Tuberous sclerosis
   C. Marchiafava-Bignami
   D. Autosomal recessive polycystic kidney disease

See Supplemental Figures section for additional figures and legends for this case.

CASE 78

Renal Cell Carcinoma Angiography

1. **D.** RCC is shown with numerous small parasitic arteries supplying the mass, which is distorting surrounding normal renal parenchyma. Renal infarct would show up as an area of hypoperfusion, no extravasation is present to indicate laceration, and no aneurysm is identified.

2. **B.** AML is a benign hypervascular hamartomatous renal mass, which often contains macroscopic fat. A renal cyst should not show increased vascularity; polyarteritis nodosa causes multiple microaneurysms; and a renal artery aneurysm is not visualized.

3. **B.** Cryoablation, nephrectomy/partial nephrectomy, and embolization may all be used to treat RCC. Cryoablation uses supercooled gas to freeze and destroy neoplastic tissue; nephrectomy/partial nephrectomy removes the entire kidney/part of the kidney with the mass. Embolization may be performed to decrease the risk of bleeding at the time of nephrectomy or treat complications such as mass rupture. Injection of absolute alcohol would be used for renal cyst sclerosis.

4. **A.** Von Hippel-Lindau is an autosomal dominant disorder with multiple manifestations including multiple bilateral RCCs, whereas tuberous sclerosis is associated with bilateral multiple AMLs. Marchiafava-Bignami is corpus callosum involvement in encephalopathy associated with alcohol use, and autosomal recessive polycystic kidney disease results in nonfunctioning kidneys requiring renal replacement.

Comment

Etiology

Risk factors for RCC include tobacco use, long-term phenacetin use, von Hippel-Lindau disease (which can cause bilateral tumors), and chronic hemodialysis. Clinically, the disorder commonly manifests with gross hematuria, flank pain, and/or weight loss; less commonly, the disorder is suspected based upon the presence of a palpable mass or a paraneoplastic syndrome (hypertension, erythrocytosis, or hypercalcemia).

Imaging Interpretation

Imaging findings of RCC include a solid mass lesion on cross-sectional imaging, which can be calcified, necrotic, and/or hemorrhagic (Figures S78-1 and S78-3). The tumor might extend into the renal vein and/or inferior vena cava. Angiographically, 95% of tumors are hypervascular, and arteriovenous shunting and venous lakes are common (Figures S78-2 and S78-4). Preoperative angiographic embolization is often performed to diminish tumor vascularity and thereby reduce perioperative blood loss (Figure S78-5).

References

Davis C, Boyett T, Caridi J. Renal artery embolization: application and success in patients with renal cell carcinoma and angiomyolipoma. *Semin Intervent Radiol.* 2007;24:111–116.

Zielinski H, Szmigielski S, Petrovich Z. Comparison of preoperative embolization followed by radical nephrectomy with radical nephrectomy alone for renal cell carcinoma. *Am J Clin Oncol.* 2000;23:6–12.

Cross-reference

Vascular and Interventional Radiology: The Requisites, 2nd ed, 278–281.

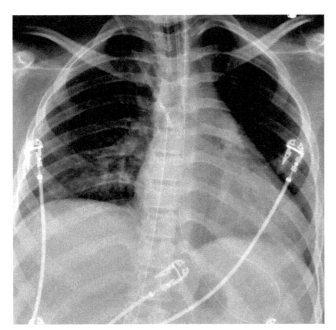

Figure 79-1

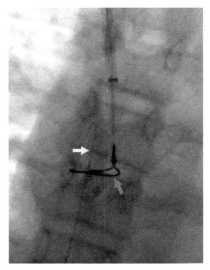

Figure 79-2

HISTORY: A 12-year-old female presents with acute renal failure.

1. Which of the following is the most likely diagnosis for the imaging findings presented?
   A. Foreign body retained in the aorta
   B. Foreign body retained in the vena cava
   C. Foreign body retained in the left ventricle
   D. Foreign body retained in the left atrium

2. Which retrieval technique is being utilized in the images presented for this case?
   A. Loop-snare technique
   B. Distal wire-grab technique
   C. Dormia basket
   D. Coaxial snare technique

3. In which scenario may it be acceptable to *NOT* retrieve a foreign body?
   A. A foreign body has lodged itself in a vein that has led to thrombosis
   B. A foreign body has become incorporated into the vessel wall
   C. A foreign body is actively causing an arrhythmia
   D. A foreign body is releasing septic emboli

4. Which of the following characteristics of nitinol-based loop snares contributes to its common use during these procedures?
   A. Cost
   B. Thermal shape stability
   C. Aluminum core
   D. Rigidity

See Supplemental Figures section for additional figures and legends for this case.

CASE 79

Foreign Body Retrieval

1. **B.** These images show a guidewire that has been retained in the patient over the right side of the body. Out of all the options listed, the vena cava is the only right-sided structure and therefore the best answer.

2. **A.** The technique used in this image sequence to retrieve the foreign body is a loop-snare technique in which the foreign body is directly grasped and removed by the snare. A Dormia basket has a distinct shape for retrieval and the distal wire grab and coaxial techniques both involve snares combined with guidewires to retrieve foreign bodies.

3. **B.** If an object is incorporated into the wall of the vessel, the risks of retrieving the object may outweigh the benefits. In such cases, it may be acceptable to continue to observe the patient and monitor for complications. The foreign body should be retrieved in the other scenarios.

4. **B.** Nitinol is a nickel titanium alloy, which has shape memory, thermal stability, and superelasticity making it a useful base for loop snares and many other endovascular devices. Cost, although an important factor, should not solely drive decision-making.

Comment

Main Teaching Point

A variety of intravascular foreign bodies have been described, including catheter and guidewire fragments, filters, stents, coils, and balloon and bullet fragments. Objects lodge in a location corresponding to their size, flexibility, and shape. Intravenous objects commonly lodge within the superior vena cava, right heart, or pulmonary artery. Large intravascular foreign bodies (as in this case) and small foreign bodies that have been present for a short time are typically removed to eliminate the potential complications of arrhythmia, thrombosis, bacteremia, and vascular or cardiac perforation (Figures S79-1 and S79-3). Small objects that have been present for prolonged periods can become incorporated into the vessel wall or endocardium, and they are often left alone unless they are causing complications.

Endovascular Management

Transcatheter retrieval is the preferred treatment. The site of percutaneous entry is selected based upon the location and orientation of the foreign body. A sheath should be inserted to minimize trauma to the access vessel when the object is removed. Typically, a guiding catheter and snare device are used. Preferably, the foreign body is snared near its tip, the snare loop is snugged around the fragment, and the object is withdrawn into the sheath and out of the vessel in a single motion (Figures S79-1 through S79-5). On occasion, a cutdown may be necessary to remove large objects or objects with sharp edges.

References

Gabelmann A, Kramer S, Gorich J. Percutaneous retrieval of lost or misplaced intravascular objects. *Am J Roentgenol.* 2001;176:1509–1513.

Woodhouse JB, Uberoi R. Techniques for intravascular foreign body retrieval. *Cardiovasc Intervent Radiol.* 2013;36:888–897.

Cross-reference

Vascular and Interventional Radiology: The Requisites, 2nd ed, 95–97.

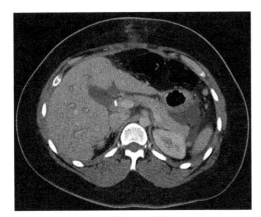

Figure 80-1. *Courtesy of Dr. Bill S. Majdalany.*

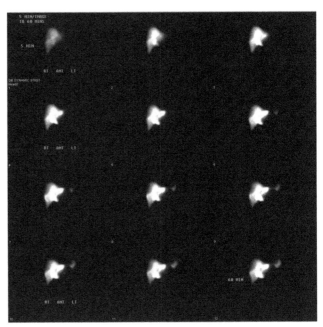

Figure 80-2. *Courtesy of Dr. Bill S. Majdalany.*

HISTORY: A 25-year-old man status post laparoscopic chole-cystectomy presents with fevers, abdominal pain, persistent drain output, and abnormal labs.

1. Which of the following would be included in the differential diagnosis for the imaging findings presented? (Choose all that apply.)
   A. Accessory hepatic duct transection
   B. Right hepatic duct laceration
   C. Common hepatic duct transection
   D. Common hepatic duct occlusion

2. Which imaging study is *LEAST* likely to add additional diagnostic information to guide the treatment of this patient?
   A. Ultrasound
   B. Endoscopic retrograde cholangiopancreatography

   C. Magnetic resonance cholangiopancreatography (MRCP)
   D. Percutaneous transhepatic cholangiogram (PTC)

3. How common are bile duct injuries during cholecystectomy?
   A. Less than 1% of cases
   B. 5% to 10% of cases
   C. 20% to 30% of cases
   D. Greater than 50% of cases

4. What is the most likely next step in management?
   A. Conservative management
   B. PTC with drain placement
   C. Laparoscopic repair
   D. Open surgical repair

_____

See Supplemental Figures section for additional figures and legends for this case.

CASE 80

Common Hepatic Duct Transection

1. **A, B, and C.** Fluid collection in the gallbladder fossa and extrahepatic accumulation of radiotracer on hepatobiliary iminodiacetic acid (HIDA) are both highly suggestive of major biliary duct injury. An occluded duct would cause biliary dilation but is less likely to manifest as a bile leak.

2. **A.** While ultrasound may confirm the presence of the gallbladder fossa fluid collection and biliary dilation, it is the least likely to reveal the precise origin of the bile leak.

3. **A.** Biliary injury during cholecystectomy, whether laparoscopic or open, is actually quite rare (approximately 0.5% and 0.2%, respectively).

4. **B.** PTC is often able to reveal the precise location of the duct injury, and drain placement can allow decompression and diversion, if able to cross. As the patient is febrile, one must be suspicious for cholangitis or abscess, and doing nothing is a poor choice. Surgical intervention is rarely first-line therapy unless injury is identified at the time of the cholecystectomy, although it may be definitive treatment.

Comment

Main Teaching Point

Bile duct injury is a dreaded complication of laparoscopic or open cholecystectomy, because in these situations, patients often require multiple radiologic interventions and/or complex surgical repair. This case demonstrates a fluid collection in the gallbladder fossa on computed tomography, suspicious for a bile leak (Figure S80-1). A bile leak is confirmed on HIDA and MRCP (Figures S80-2 and S80-3). The distal common bile duct is not visualized, indicating a complete ductal transection.

PTC was performed that showed communication of the left- and right-sided ducts, so a single right-sided external biliary drain was placed for decompression given concern for cholangitis, as well as for diversion purposes (Figures S80-4 and S80-5). A percutaneous biloma drain was also performed at the same time (not shown).

Percutaneous Management

The rate of technical failure of percutaneous biliary drainage is less than 5% in patients with dilated biliary ducts, but it can be as high as 25% in patients without ductal dilation. For this reason, in cases of major ductal injury, a percutaneous drainage catheter may first be placed within the easily accessible biloma to obtain initial control of the leak. After several weeks to a few months, a mature tract might form between the collapsed biloma cavity and the site of ductal injury. At this time, contrast injected into the biloma drain can opacify the biliary system, facilitating biliary drainage. In many cases, passage of a guidewire into the bowel is not possible; in these patients, a snare catheter may be used from the biloma access site to externalize the biliary wire and enable placement of a U-tube, which is more stable than an external biliary drainage catheter. The presence of a drainage catheter assists the surgeon in identifying the duct during dissection, because there may be significant inflammation within the hepatic hilum (Figure S80-6). Ultimately, definitive surgical repair with hepaticojejunostomy is often required.

References

Saad N, Darcy M. Iatrogenic bile duct injury during laparoscopic cholecystectomy. *Tech Vasc Interv Radiol.* 2008;11:102–110.

Thompson C, Saad N, Quazi R, et al. Management of iatrogenic bile duct injuries: Role of the interventional radiologist. *Radiographics.* 2013;33:117–135.

Cross-reference

Vascular and Interventional Radiology: The Requisites, 2nd ed, 467.

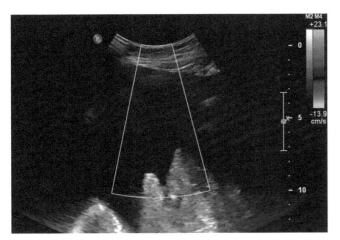

Figure 81-1

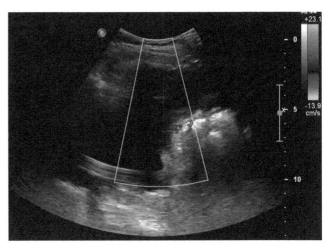

Figure 81-2

HISTORY: A 67-year-old female with history of cirrhosis and portal hypertension.

1. What is the primary abnormality seen in the image on the left?
   A. Large-volume ascites
   B. Hemoperitoneum
   C. Pneumoperitoneum
   D. Pseudomyxoma peritonei

2. What percutaneous procedure was performed on the image on the right?
   A. Percutaneous jejunostomy tube placement
   B. Transhepatic biliary drainage catheter placement
   C. Tunneled peritoneal drainage catheter placement
   D. Percutaneous nephrostomy tube placement

3. What is a serious delayed complication of this procedure?
   A. Gastrointestinal (GI) bleed
   B. Bacterial peritonitis
   C. Hemoperitoneum
   D. GI luminal perforation

4. During paracentesis of a cirrhotic patient with massive ascites, what should you consider administering during or after the procedure?
   A. ½ Normal saline
   B. Albumin
   C. Cross-matching blood
   D. Lactated Ringer's

See Supplemental Figures section for additional figures and legends for this case.

CASE 81

Massive Ascites: Tunneled Peritoneal Catheter Placement

1. **A.** A large volume of anechoic fluid consistent with ascites is visualized.

2. **C.** A percutaneous tunneled catheter is seen with ultrasonogram and by radiograph in the supplemental images.

3. **B.** Seeding of the catheter tract and subsequent bacterial peritonitis is a serious complication that can occur in patients with long-term indwelling peritoneal drains. Although luminal perforation could occur, careful attention to needle, wire, and catheter advancement will minimize this potential complication.

4. **B.** Many institutions infuse albumin to prevent massive fluid shifts following large-volume paracentesis in cirrhotic patients.

Comment

Clinical Presentation

Massive ascites can develop secondary to a variety of etiologies including portal hypertension, malignant ascites, and right-sided heart failure. The accumulation of fluid in the peritoneal cavity causes abdominal distention, which in extreme cases can result in increased pressure on the diaphragm, leading to dyspnea and easy fatigability. This can greatly affect the patient's quality of life.

Treatment Methods

Medical management with diuretics is the first-line treatment. Patients might also require therapeutic paracentesis to remove the accumulated ascites. In patients who fail to get relief of their symptoms from these measures, those who require frequent large-volume paracentesis, and those who suffer adverse effects of diuretic therapy (impaired renal function), other therapies are indicated. Transjugular intrahepatic portosystemic shunt can be performed for patients with portal hypertension; however, for patients with malignant ascites or ascites secondary to severe right-sided heart failure, placement of a tunneled peritoneal catheter is the procedure of choice.

Procedural Technique

The procedure is performed similar to tunneled central venous catheter placement with the exception that the catheter is placed within the peritoneal cavity and tunneled through the soft tissues of the anterior abdominal wall (Figures S81-1 through S81-3). The patient can then easily drain the ascitic fluid by opening the valve intermittently as needed. Bacterial peritonitis is a rare but serious potential complication.

References

Narayanan G, Pezeshkmehr A, Venkat S, et al. Safety and efficacy of the Pleurx catheter for the treatment of malignant ascites. *J Palliat Med.* 2014;17:906–912, Aug.

O'Neill M, Weissleder R, Gervais DA, et al. Tunneled peritoneal catheter placement under sonographic and fluoroscopic guidance in the palliative treatment of malignant ascites. *AJR Am J Roentgenol.* 2001;177:615–618.

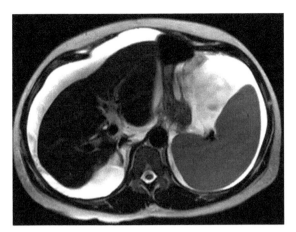

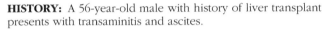

Figure 82-1

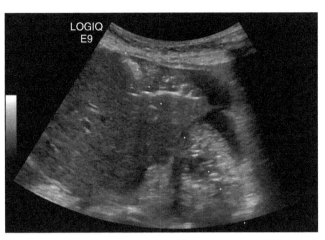

Figure 82-2

HISTORY: A 56-year-old male with history of liver transplant presents with transaminitis and ascites.

1. Which of the following is the most likely diagnosis for the imaging findings presented?
   A. Nonalcoholic steatohepatitis
   B. Secondary hemochromatosis
   C. Transplant rejection
   D. Primary sclerosing cholangitis

2. According to the Society of Interventional Radiology (SIR) guidelines, which of the following are contraindications to performing ultrasonogram (US) guided percutaneous biopsy in this patient? (Choose all that apply.)
   A. International normalized ratio (INR) greater than 1.5
   B. Cirrhosis
   C. Ascites
   D. Model for end-stage liver disease (MELD) score of 29

3. A patient on a heparin drip has been requested to undergo a percutaneous computed tomography (CT) guided liver biopsy during an admission. Which of the following is correct?
   A. The drip may be continued during the biopsy.
   B. The drip should be discontinued at least 4 hours prior to the biopsy.
   C. The drip should be discontinued at least 12 hours prior to the biopsy.
   D. The drip should be discontinued at least 24 hours prior to the biopsy.

4. A patient with history of hepatitis C infection and cirrhosis is referred to your service for a liver lesion biopsy after a multiphase magnetic resonance imaging demonstrated a 2.5 cm hepatic lesion with rapid arterial hyperenhancement and washout. Which of the following should be your response?
   A. Biopsy the lesion, if the patient has no other contraindication to the procedure.
   B. State to the requesting physician that the lesion is a LR5 lesion, and recommend treatment without biopsy.
   C. Biopsy the lesion provided that the referring physician and the patient understand the risk of track seeding.
   D. State to the requesting physician that biopsy should be performed only if repeat imaging shows interval growth in the lesion or vascular invasion.

See Supplemental Figures section for additional figures and legends for this case.

CASE 82

Percutaneous Transabdominal Liver Biopsy

1. **C.** The imaging findings are nonspecific as they demonstrate decreased T2 signal intensity within the liver with a moderate volume of ascites. In a liver transplant patient with transaminitis, rejection should be the first diagnostic consideration.

2. **A and C.** According to the SIR guidelines, the patient's INR should be 1.5 or under before undertaking an invasive procedure. While cirrhosis is not itself a contraindication to US-guided biopsy, the presence of ascites is, due to a markedly increased risk of hemorrhage secondary to disruption of the hepatic capsule. A MELD score of 29 would not necessarily be a contraindication.

3. **B.** According to the most recent guidelines, heparin should be discontinued for at least 4 hours prior to an invasive procedure.

4. **B.** This is an LR5 lesion, which according to the liver imaging reporting and data system (LI-RADS) criteria is diagnostic of hepatocellular carcinoma, and no biopsy is indicated prior to initiating treatment.

Comment

Main Teaching Point

Liver biopsy is performed from a percutaneous transabdominal route or via hepatic venous route. Fine-needle aspiration and core biopsy specimens may be obtained. Random liver biopsies are most commonly obtained in patients with diffuse liver disease while those with a focal hepatic mass have a directed biopsy.

Percutaneous Management

The potential complications of liver biopsy include severe intraperitoneal hemorrhage, hemobilia, and pneumothorax. Accordingly, preprocedure precautions should ensure that coagulation parameters and platelet level are within normal limits, particularly in patients with hepatic cirrhosis. In addition, for lesions located high within the liver parenchyma, the route of access should be carefully planned to avoid traversing the lateral sulcus of the right pleural space. For left-sided lesions, the proximity of the pericardium should be similarly kept in mind. Cross-sectional imaging is commonly performed in the patient's workup and includes ultrasound, MRI, or CT (Figure S82-1). Ultrasound or CT are used for the vast majority of image-guided biopsies (Figures S82-2 and S82-3). Ultrasound provides the advantage of real-time needle visualization and is less costly than using CT. On the other hand, many lesions are not clearly visible on ultrasound, making CT a better choice in these cases. MRI guidance is being used in some centers, primarily for hepatic dome lesions in which its multiplanar capability can be advantageous.

References

Mitchell DG, Bruix J, Sherman M, et al. LI-RADS (Liver Imaging Reporting and Data System): summary, discussion, and consensus of the LI-RADS management working group and future directions. *Hepatology.* 2014;.

Shankar S, Van Sonnenberg E, Silverman SG, et al. Interventional radiology procedures in the liver. Biopsy, drainage, and ablation. *Clin Liver Dis.* 2002;6:91–118.

Cross-reference

Vascular and Interventional Radiology: The Requisites, 2nd ed, 386–391.

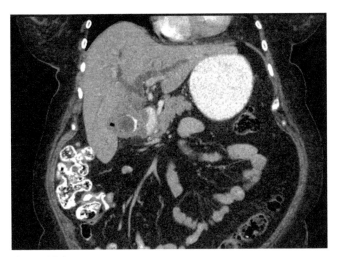

Figure 83-1

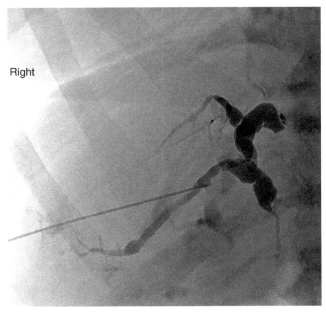

Right

Figure 83-2

HISTORY: A 63-year-old woman presents with weight loss and jaundice.

1. Which of the following is the most likely diagnosis for the imaging findings presented?
   A. Pancreatic adenocarcinoma
   B. Chronic pancreatitis
   C. Gallbladder carcinoma
   D. Iatrogenic biliary stricture

2. What is the most common cause of benign biliary strictures?
   A. Chronic pancreatitis
   B. Primary sclerosing cholangitis
   C. Iatrogenic injury
   D. Mirizzi syndrome

3. Which of the below statements is correct?
   A. Malignant biliary strictures are best treated with balloon cholangioplasty.
   B. Brush biopsy has a sensitivity of approximately 90% for diagnosis of biliary or pancreatic adenocarcinoma.

   C. Metallic biliary stents have greater long-term patency compared with plastic biliary stents.
   D. Plastic biliary stents are preferred to metal stents in patients with unresectable malignancy and short life expectancy.

4. Which of the below statements is correct?
   A. Primary sclerosing cholangitis is only associated with intrahepatic but *NOT* extrahepatic biliary strictures.
   B. Cholangiocarcinoma is the most common cause of malignant biliary strictures.
   C. External biliary drainage may be associated with electrolyte abnormalities.
   D. Percutaneous biliary drainage is most often performed under computed tomography (CT) guidance.

See Supplemental Figures section for additional figures and legends for this case.

CASE 83

Malignant Common Bile Duct Stricture

1. **C.** The elongated, rat-tail appearance of the common bile duct (CBD) is typical of a malignant entity. The presence of a mass that replaces the gallbladder and compresses the common hepatic duct (CHD) is most compatible with gallbladder carcinoma. A malignant stricture associated with pancreatic adenocarcinoma would have a very similar appearance, but the "double-duct" sign and presence of the mass centered on the gallbladder fossa favors gallbladder carcinoma.

2. **C.** Approximately 80% of biliary strictures are iatrogenic, most often from cholecystectomy or orthotopic liver transplantation. Chronic pancreatitis is the second most common cause of benign biliary strictures. The other options are rare.

3. **C.** Plastic stents have a higher rate of occlusion requiring repeat intervention. Metallic stents have a usable life of approximately 6 months. Metallic stents are preferred in these patients due to a lower need for repeat intervention. Stents improve a patient's quality of life by removing the discomfort of an external drainage apparatus. Malignant biliary strictures have poor response to balloon cholangioplasty and commonly require stenting. The sensitivity of brush biopsy is approximately 50% to 70%. A negative brush biopsy should be viewed with caution.

4. **C.** Patients are susceptible to electrolyte abnormalities due to loss of fluids and bile salts. As such, drainage volumes should be followed closely as should electrolytes so that corrective measures can be taken as needed. Primary sclerosing cholangitis is associated with both intrahepatic and extrahepatic biliary strictures. Pancreatic adenocarcinoma is the most common cause of malignant biliary strictures.

Comment

Etiology

Malignant biliary obstruction may be caused by pancreatic carcinoma, cholangiocarcinoma, gallbladder cancer, intrahepatic metastatic disease, or portal hepatic nodal disease causing extrinsic CBD or CHD compression. Although the clinical context must always be taken into account, the irregular rat-tail appearance of this CHD stricture is highly suggestive of a malignant etiology (Figure S83-2). CT or magnetic resonance diagnostic imaging is helpful in determining the etiology of the obstruction (Figure S83-1).

Percutaneous Management

The interventional radiologist might have several tasks to complete in managing the patient with malignant CBD/CHD obstruction: (1) Percutaneous transhepatic cholangiography can outline the extent of the biliary abnormality and allow selection of a duct to use for definitive biliary access; (2) biliary drainage can be performed to treat cholangitis, prevent episodes of biliary sepsis, and relieve obstructive symptoms including jaundice and pruritus (Figures S83-3 and S83-4); (3) although its diagnostic sensitivity for pancreatic or biliary adenocarcinoma is only 50% to 70%, biliary brush biopsy can sometimes provide a definitive tissue diagnosis; (4) if the malignancy is unresectable and the patient has short life expectancy, a metallic (permanent) stent can be placed to facilitate internal drainage and thereby allow removal of the externally protruding biliary drainage catheter(s).

References

Govil H, Reddy V, Kluskens L, et al. Brush cytology of the biliary tract: retrospective study of 278 cases with histopathologic correlation. *Diagn Cytopathol.* 2002;26:273–277.

Shanbhogue AK, Tirumani SH, Prasad SR, et al. Benign biliary strictures: a current comprehensive clinical and imaging review. *AJR Am J Roentgenol.* 2011;197(2):W295–W306.

Cross-reference

Vascular and Interventional Radiology: The Requisites, 2nd ed, 457–465.

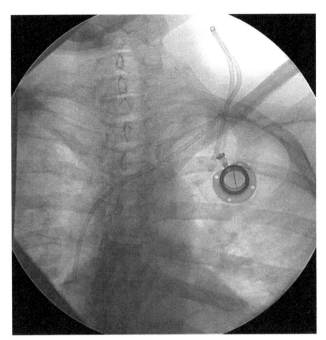

Figure 84-1

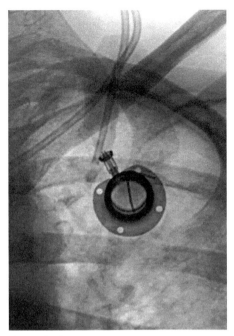

Figure 84-2

HISTORY: A 51-year-old female with breast cancer with non-functioning central venous catheter with subcutaneous reservoir.

1. Which of the following is the most likely diagnosis for the imaging findings presented?
   A. An iatrogenic pneumothorax
   B. Separation of the two attachable components of the subcutaneous infusion port
   C. Successful placement of a long-term subcutaneous infusion port
   D. An iatrogenic aortic dissection

2. In which type of patient is this device most typically used?
   A. Patient requiring immediate central venous access for large-volume resuscitation
   B. Patient requiring hemodialysis
   C. Patient requiring long-term, intermittent access
   D. Patient requiring short-term venous access

3. Which of the following abnormalities is also seen on the imaging series presented?
   A. Flipping of the port within its pocket
   B. Apical pneumothorax
   C. Kinking of the catheter
   D. Port infection

4. Which of the following scenarios is most likely to require urgent port removal?
   A. Port infection
   B. Pocket hematoma
   C. Pneumothorax
   D. Port leak

See Supplemental Figures section for additional figures and legends for this case.

CASE 84

Port Separation

1. **B.** The images presented here show the detachment of the two components of a long-term subcutaneous infusion port. Additionally noted is kinking of the catheter with apex cephalad kink.

2. **C.** The patient population in which these ports are utilized are those requiring long-term, intermittent use such as chemotherapy patients. Port catheters are not designed for large-volume resuscitation of hemodialysis flow rates.

3. **C.** This film shows no evidence of an apical pneumothorax. It does, however, show kinking of the catheter. There is a needle accessing the port, and therefore it is not flipped within the pocket. Unless subcutaneous gas were present, a port infection would likely not be seen on a radiograph.

4. **A.** If the port itself becomes infected, it almost always requires removal. Pocket hematomas may resolve by themselves or require minimal treatment, pneumothoraces can be treated with nasal cannula or chest tubes, and port leaks require replacement less than 1% of the time.

Comment

Main Teaching Point

In addition to the general complications of central venous access described earlier, a variety of device-specific complications can occur. This case demonstrates one device-specific complication of a port catheter: separation of the port and catheter components of the device (Figure S84-1). In addition, this particular catheter has been placed with an unfavorable upward curve, which may be partly extravascular (Figure S84-2).

Endovascular Devices

Several types of port catheter devices are available. In many institutions, single-piece devices are used, and in other institutions, double-piece or attachable ports are used. The attachable ports are typically assembled by the physician when the port is placed. In occasional instances, presumably related to poor initial technique in attaching the pieces and/or to local trauma, the two components can separate. This is important, because any fluid injected into the port will extravasate into the chest wall. The separation can be fixed by reopening the port incision, dissecting down to the port and catheter, and reattaching the components. Alternatively, the port can be replaced with a completely new device.

References

Funaki B, Szymski GX, Hackworth CA, et al. Radiologic placement of subcutaneous infusion chest ports for long-term central venous access. *Am J Roentgenol.* 1997;169:1431–1434.

Vesica S, Baumgartner A, Jacobs V, et al. Management of venous port systems in oncology: a review of current evidence. *Ann Oncol.* 2008;19:9–15.

Cross-reference

Vascular and Interventional Radiology: The Requisites, 2nd ed, 148–151.

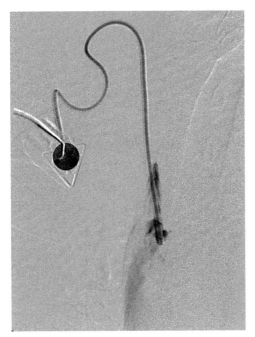

Figure 85-1

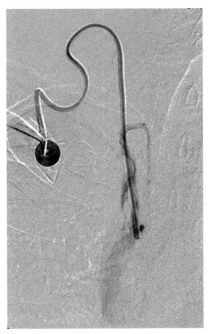

Figure 85-2

HISTORY: A 44-year-old female with colon cancer presents with a malfunctioning right chest port.

1. Which of the following is the most likely diagnosis for the imaging findings presented?
   A. Catheter occlusion
   B. Fibrin sheath
   C. Catheter kinking
   D. Inadequate port access

2. Which of the following findings can be seen with fibrin sheath formation? (Choose all that apply.)
   A. Turbulent flow jet
   B. Reflux of contrast along the catheter
   C. Contrast filling of sac at the catheter tip
   D. Extravasation of injected fluid into the soft tissues

3. Of the following, which likely results in immediate catheter dysfunction?
   A. Fibrin sheath
   B. Catheter malpositioning
   C. Venous stenosis
   D. Catheter fracture

4. Which problem is most likely to be present with use of this catheter?
   A. Difficulty injecting
   B. Difficulty aspirating
   C. Difficulty accessing
   D. None of the above

See Supplemental Figures section for additional figures and legends for this case.

CASE 85

Pericatheter Fibrin Sheath

1. **B.** The finding of contrast refluxing back along the catheter is classic for fibrin sheath formation. Contrast is clearly coursing through the catheter and being ejected from the catheter tip, therefore it is not occluded and port access is adequate.

2. **A, B, C, and D.** When fibrin surrounds the catheter tip, contrast injection produces a turbulent outflow appearance. Additionally, a thin layer of contrast can reflux between the catheter and fibrin sheath. Occasionally, a loosely adherent fibrin sac is present at the catheter tip and can fill with contrast or if the fibrin sheath is present along the entire intravascular length of the catheter, it can cause reflux of contrast back through the venotomy site and extravasation into to the subcutaneous tissues.

3. **B.** This is an early cause of catheter dysfunction caused by misplacement of the catheter tip in a nontarget vein (e.g., azygous vein), or if the catheter tip abuts a vein wall at a right angle. Fibrin sheath is a rare cause of catheter malfunction in the first 1 to 2 weeks. Fibrin sheath causes flow failure at a mean of 15 weeks after initial placement. Catheter fracture is most commonly seen with subclavian central venous catheters since they are performed from an infraclavicular approach. Over time, mechanical compression of the catheter between the clavicle and first rib can cause intermittent obstruction and, ultimately, fracture ("pinch off" syndrome).

4. **B.** The fibrin sheath acts as a one-way valve in which fluid can be injected but blood cannot be aspirated.

Comment

Etiology

Central venous catheters are prone to problems including infection, end-hole occlusion, venous thrombosis malposition, migration, kinking, vessel wall damage, and catheter fracture. One of the most common and difficult problems is the development of a fibrin sheath around the catheter tip. Shortly after placement, virtually all catheters become covered by a layer of fibrin, which eventually forms a sleeve around the catheter. When this obstructs the catheter end- and/or side-holes, the usual clinical finding is impaired ability to aspirate blood but preserved ability to inject. Dialysis catheters often demonstrate diminished flow rates in this situation. The typical venographic appearance is observed in this case: Contrast flows retrograde along the catheter within the fibrin sheath, outlining the catheter (Figures S85-1 and S85-2).

Endovascular Management

Treatment options vary. Catheter exchange over a guidewire can be performed, but it is unlikely to produce long-term improvement because the catheter is typically reinserted into the existing fibrin sheath. Alternatively, low-dose thrombolytic agents can be used, either via instillation in the catheter for 30 to 60 minutes or via infusion for several hours. Some advocate disrupting the fibrin sheath using guidewire or angioplasty balloon manipulation or stripping the fibrin sheath using a snare device inserted from another access vein. Unfortunately, most treatments lead to only temporary relief because the fibrin sheath tends to reform over time.

References

Crain MR, Horton MG, Mewissen MW. Fibrin sheaths complicating central venous catheters. *AJR Am J Roentgenol.* 1998;171:341–346.
Gray RJ, Levitin A, Buck D, et al. Percutaneous fibrin sheath stripping versus transcatheter urokinase infusion for malfunctioning well-positioned tunneled central venous dialysis catheters: a prospective, randomized trial. *J Vasc Interv Radiol.* 2000;11:1121–1129.

Cross-reference

Vascular and Interventional Radiology: The Requisites, 2nd ed, 148–151.

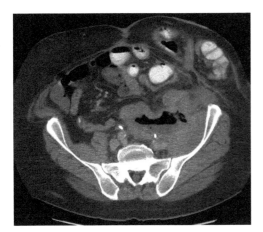

Figure 86-1

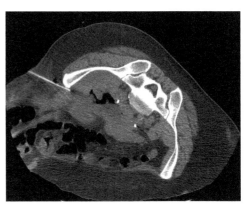

Figure 86-2

HISTORY: A 50-year-old male with a history of colon cancer status post partial colectomy presents with fever and abdominal pain.

1. Which of the following would be included in the differential diagnosis for the imaging findings presented? (Choose all that apply.)
   A. Small bowel obstruction
   B. Local metastasis
   C. Abscess
   D. Diverticulitis

2. Transgluteal catheter placement for pelvic abscesses traverses which foramen?
   A. Greater sciatic foramen
   B. Lesser sciatic foramen
   C. Obturator foramen
   D. Anterior sacral foramen

3. Which of the following approaches is preferred for transgluteal catheter placement?
   A. Inferior to the piriformis muscle
   B. Superior to the piriformis muscle
   C. Through the piriformis muscle
   D. Medial to the piriformis muscle

4. A 49-year-old female with Crohn's disease is found to have a pelvic abscess adjacent to the vagina with a sinus tract to the anterior abdominal wall. Which of the following approaches should be used for drainage catheter placement?
   A. Transgluteal catheter placement
   B. Transvaginal catheter placement
   C. Transrectal catheter placement
   D. Catheter placement through the sinus tract

See Supplemental Figures section for additional figures and legends for this case.

CASE 86

Percutaneous Drainage of Deep Pelvic Abscess

1. **B and C.** The image shows a large inflammatory soft tissue mass in the pelvis containing a collection of fluid and gas. The gas and fluid collection is consistent with an abscess, but the amount of soft tissue within the mass is also concerning for a necrotic metastatic lesion.

2. **A.** Transgluteal catheter placement traverses the greater sciatic foramen.

3. **A.** The preferred approach when placing a transgluteal catheter is infrapiriformis. This approach is at the level of the sacrospinous ligament, below the piriformis, and as close to the sacrum as possible. This approach helps avoid injury to the sciatic nerve. Depending on the location of the abscess or adjacent loops of bowel, insertion of the catheter through the piriformis may be required (transpiriformis approach).

4. **D.** When possible, placement of the drainage catheter through the existing sinus tract is preferred. Contrast can be injected into the tract to delineate the abscess cavity, and a catheter can often be inserted without the need for a needle puncture.

Comment

Percutaneous Management

The first-line management of deep pelvic abscesses is usually percutaneous imaging-guided drainage (Figures S86-2 through S86-4). Because of the presence of small bowel, bladder, and other structures within the pelvis, a simple transabdominal access route is often not available. In choosing a potential access route, the first question to ask is whether a draining sinus is present. If so, then the abscess cavity may be defined by contrast injection directly into the skin defect; in this situation a catheter can usually be advanced under fluoroscopy into the abscess without the need for needle puncture. When this option does not exist, careful examination of the computed tomography scan is critical in planning therapy (Figure S86-1).

Alternative Access Methods

When a direct transabdominal route into the collection is not present, the transvaginal and transrectal access routes are usually considered next in the absence of contraindications (e.g., a surgical bowel anastomosis in the rectal area). The advantages of the transvaginal and transrectal routes are their usual close proximity to the fluid collection and the lower risk of complications (bleeding and pain) compared with transgluteal drainage. Additionally, transgluteal drainage is occasionally technically difficult when the collection is small, because the window into the collection must be crossed with pinpoint accuracy to avoid traversing surrounding bowel and pelvic organs.

References

Harisinghani MG, Gervais DA, Maher MM, et al. Transgluteal approach for percutaneous drainage of deep pelvic abscesses: 154 cases. *Radiology.* 2003;228:701–705.

Hovsepian DM. Transrectal and transvaginal abscess drainage. *J Vasc Interv Radiol.* 1997;8:501–515.

Cross-reference

Vascular and Interventional Radiology: The Requisites, 2nd ed, 401–418.

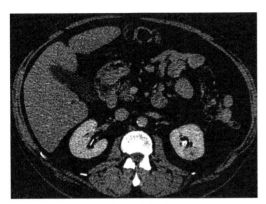

Figure 87-1. *Courtesy of Dr. Shane A. Wells.*

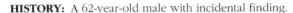

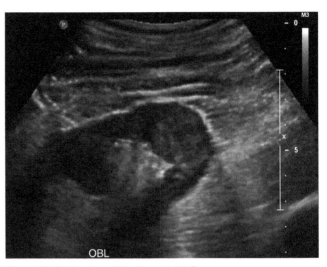

Figure 87-2. *Courtesy of Dr. Shane A. Wells.*

HISTORY: A 62-year-old male with incidental finding.

1. Which of the following would be included in the differential diagnosis for the imaging finding in the image on the left? (Choose all that apply.)
   A. Oncocytoma
   B. Renal cell carcinoma
   C. Angiomyolipoma
   D. Transitional cell carcinoma

2. Which of the following tumoral descriptions implies a higher likelihood of successful ablation? (Choose all that apply.)
   A. Size greater than 4 cm
   B. Size less than 3 cm
   C. Central location
   D. Noncentral location

3. What is the typical appearance of radiofrequency (RF) or cryoablation zones on postprocedure computed tomography (CT) and magnetic resonance imaging?
   A. CT-hypodense, T1-iso to hyperintense, T2-hypointense
   B. CT-hyperdense, T1-iso to hyperintense, T2-hypointense
   C. CT-hypodense, T1-iso to hypointense, T2-hyperintense
   D. CT-hyperdense, T1-iso to hypointense, T2-hyperintense

4. What is the appropriate treatment for a patient with low-grade fever, nausea, and vomiting following an RF ablation?
   A. Broad-spectrum antibiotics
   B. Reimaging with CT or ultrasound
   C. Acetaminophen
   D. Blood cultures and broad-spectrum antibiotics

See Supplemental Figures section for additional figures and legends for this case.

CASE 87

Renal Cell Carcinoma-Cryoablation

1. **A and B.** Solid, enhancing renal mass is seen that may be a renal cell carcinoma or oncocytoma. There is no bulk fat to suggest an angiomyolipoma. Transitional cell tends to arise from the renal pelvis.

2. **B and D.** Central location has a lower rate of complete tumoral necrosis, likely secondary to the heat sink effect of the central vessels and the risk of injury to the vascular pedicle and renal pelvis from overtreatment. Larger lesions (greater than 3 cm) also are more likely to have incomplete treatment or necessitate multiple treatments.

3. **A.** Ablation zones are low attenuation on CT and typically are T2-hypointense. Contrast is necessary for evaluation of recurrent or residual tumor. A thin, peripheral rim of enhancement can be seen surrounding the ablation zone for a few months after treatment. Recurrent or residual tumor typically shows nodular, peripheral enhancement.

4. **C.** These symptoms in addition to pain and malaise are typical of postablation syndrome. Appropriate treatment includes acetaminophen or nonsteroidal antiinflammatories plus rest. A similar phenomenon can occur after cryoablation, typically presenting with flank pain and low-grade fever.

Comment

Incidence and Classic Management

Renal tumors are being found incidentally at an increasing rate. This has allowed detection of these tumors at earlier stages while the tumors are much smaller. Surgical resection of these tumors remains the standard of care. This comprises radical and partial nephrectomy, which may be performed in an open manner or laparoscopically.

Conservative Management

Nephron-sparing therapies have gained favor in recent years for preservation of renal function. These treatments include partial nephrectomy, laparoscopic cryoablation, and percutaneous image-guided cryoablation and RF ablation. Percutaneous ablations have obvious advantages over open or laparoscopic surgical procedures including decreased morbidity and the potential for being performed under moderate sedation.

Patient Intervention

Percutaneous cryoablation was the chosen therapy for the patient in this case to treat the tumor in the left for its nephron-sparing potential and the lack of need for general anesthesia because of many comorbid conditions, placing him at increased risk for morbidity from a surgical procedure. Ultrasound or CT guidance can be used for placement of the cryoprobes (Figures S87-1 through S87-3). The freezing and thawing of the tumor are also monitored with ultrasound or CT surveillance, which can demonstrate the formation of the ice ball around the cryoprobe as well as any potential complication during the ablation (Figure S87-4).

References

Atwell TD, Farrell MA, Callstrom MR, et al. Percutaneous cryoablation of large renal masses: technical feasibility and short-term outcome. *AJR Am J Roentgenol.* 2007;188:1195–2000.

Venkatesan AM, Wood BJ, Gervais DA. Percutaneous ablation in the kidney. *Radiology.* 2011;261(2):375–391.

Cross-reference

Vascular and Interventional Radiology: The Requisites, 2nd ed, 554–561.

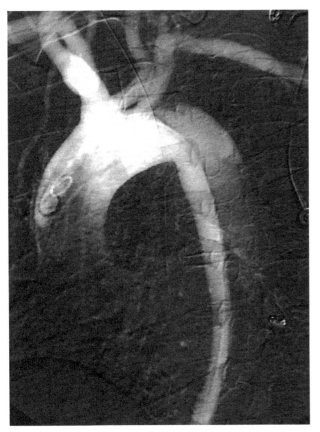

Figure 88-1

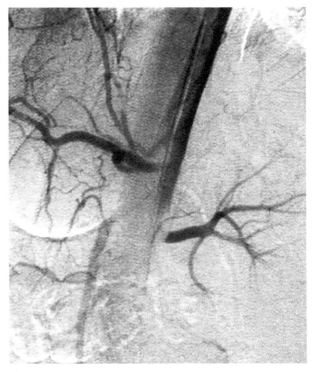

Figure 88-2

HISTORY: A 69-year-old female presents with chronic but worsening dyspnea.

1. Which of the following is the most likely diagnosis for the imaging findings presented?
   A. Congenital pulmonary valvular stenosis
   B. Chronic pulmonary embolism
   C. Hilar lymphadenopathy
   D. Cor pulmonale

2. Which of the following is *NOT* an etiology for the entity presented above?
   A. Mitral stenosis
   B. Congenital left-to-right shunts
   C. Right heart failure
   D. Lung disease

3. Which of the following imaging modalities are beneficial in the workup of this entity? (Choose all that apply.)
   A. Chest plain-film radiograph
   B. Ventilation/Perfusion (V/Q) scan
   C. Enhanced chest computed tomography (CT)
   D. Cardiac magnetic resonance imaging

4. Which of the following is a possible complication of performing pulmonary angiography in the presence of this entity?
   A. Pericardial tamponade
   B. Nephrotoxicity
   C. Transient rhythm disturbances
   D. All of the above

See Supplemental Figures section for additional figures and legends for this case.

CASE 88

Chronic Thromboembolic Pulmonary Hypertension

1. **B.** The angiography images demonstrate luminal irregularities, stenoses, occlusions, and nodular outpouchings. The constellation of findings is compatible with pulmonary hypertension secondary to chronic thromboembolism. Congenital pulmonary valvular stenosis can show similar findings with the presence of poststenotic dilatation of the pulmonary arteries. Usually, the left pulmonary artery preferentially dilates due to the orientation of the stenotic jet.

2. **C.** Right heart failure is a consequence of, not a cause of, pulmonary hypertension. All the other answer choices may be valid etiologies in the development of pulmonary hypertension.

3. **A, B, C, and D.** All of the above modalities have the ability to manifest some of the typical findings seen in pulmonary hypertension and are thus useful in establishing not just the degree or severity of the disease but also potential etiologies.

4. **D.** In the literature, mortality rates related to pulmonary angiography have been shown to be consistently low, at approximately 0.3%, with most deaths occurring from heart failure, arrhythmia induction, or severe allergic reaction (including nephrotoxicity) to contrast media. Catheter perforation of the pulmonary artery during pulmonary angiography with resultant pericardial tamponade has also been reported as a rare complication.

Comment

Clinical Presentation

In most patients with acute pulmonary embolism, the emboli resolve partially or completely within several weeks of the event. However, in some patients the emboli do not resolve, and 0.1% to 0.2% of patients develop pulmonary hypertension as a result of multiple episodes of pulmonary embolism. These patients typically present with dyspnea and fatigue that is often progressive.

Diagnostic Evaluation

In its simplest terms, pulmonary hypertension is defined as an invasively obtained mean pulmonary arterial pressure greater than or equal to 25 mm Hg at rest. It serves as an endpoint or sequela to numerous cardiopulmonary diseases and is thus found in multiple clinical conditions, chiefly left heart failure, intrinsic lung disease, and chronic pulmonary thromboembolism, among others. One of the cornerstones of evaluating a working diagnosis of pulmonary hypertension is the need to obtain a resting pulmonary capillary wedge pressure and evaluate if it is elevated (normal = 15 mm Hg). This will allow one to refine the diagnosis as either pre (normal wedge pressure) or postcapillary (elevated wedge pressure) pulmonary hypertension. This distinction is critical as treatment protocols are different for the two subclasses.

Imaging Evaluation

Angiography remains the gold standard for diagnosis. The findings are characteristic and include enlarged central pulmonary arteries, intraluminal webs, pulmonary arterial branch stenoses, luminal irregularities, and outpouchings, often with a rounded-off appearance (Figures S88-1 and S88-2) regional perfusion defects, and frank obstruction of vessels. The mean pulmonary artery pressure is typically elevated. Additionally, CT pulmonary angiography, radiography, and V/Q imaging also play a role in evaluation.

Treatment Methods

Of note, in terms of intervention, pulmonary thromboendarterectomy has been the established surgical procedure for curative intervention in patients with chronic thromboembolic pulmonary hypertension (CTEPH). In recent years, however, with the advancement in catheter technology, balloon pulmonary angioplasty has been shown to have equal efficacy and safety rates compared to PEA and should be considered as a viable treatment option for nonoperable CTEPH patients.

References

Barbosa Jr. EJ, Gupta NK, Toigian DA, et al. Current role of imaging in the diagnosis and management of pulmonary hypertension. *AJR Am J Roentgenol.* 2012;198:1320–1331.

Hoeper MM, Madani MM, Nakanishi N, et al. Chronic thromboembolic pulmonary hypertension. *Lancet Respir Med.* 2014;2:573–582.

Hofmann LV, et al. Safety and hemodynamic effects of pulmonary angiography in patients with pulmonary hypertension: 10-year single-center experience. *AJR Am J Roentgenol.* 2004;183:779–785.

Peña E, Dennie C, Veinot J, et al. Pulmonary hypertension: how the radiologist can help. *Radiographics.* 2012;32:9–32.

Taniguchi Y, Miyagawa K, Nakayam K, et al. Balloon pulmonary angioplasty: an additional treatment option to improve the prognosis of patients with chronic thromboembolic pulmonary hypertension. *EuroIntervention.* 2014;10:518–525.

Cross-reference

Vascular and Interventional Radiology: The Requisites, 2nd ed, 168–169.

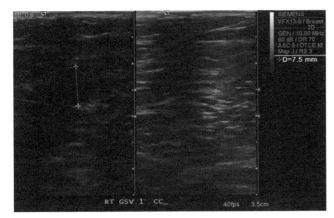

Figure 89-1. *Courtesy of Dr. Minhaj S. Khaja.*

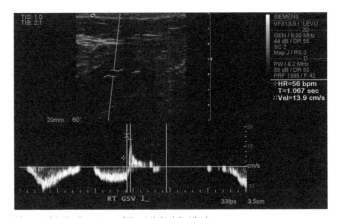

Figure 89-2. *Courtesy of Dr. Minhaj S. Khaja.*

HISTORY: A 56-year-old female presents to the office with a 2-month history of lower extremity pain and engorged veins.

1. Which of the following is the most likely diagnosis for the imaging findings presented?
   A. Deep vein thrombosis
   B. Peripheral arterial disease
   C. Varicose veins
   D. Popliteal artery aneurysm formation

2. Which vein is most typically involved in the development of the abnormalities shown in the images?
   A. Inferior vena cava
   B. Common iliac vein
   C. Femoral vein
   D. Greater saphenous vein (GSV)

3. Which therapy has been shown to be most effective for the case pictured above?
   A. Foam sclerotherapy
   B. Endovascular laser ablation
   C. Surgical stripping
   D. All therapies have the same effectiveness at 1 year

4. Which of the following tests can help distinguish between superficial and deep venous insufficiency?
   A. Straight leg raise
   B. Perthes test
   C. Allen's test
   D. Lachman's test

See Supplemental Figures section for additional figures and legends for this case.

CASE 89

Endovascular Ablation of Varicose Veins

1. **C.** These images show the development of varicose veins, which are caused by venous insufficiency of the superficial veins in the lower extremity. This chronic venous stasis leads to vessel engorgement and dilatation. Occlusion of the deep venous system can cause damage to the valves and result in reflux of blood into the superficial system via perforator veins.

2. **D.** The vein that is most often involved in the development of varicose veins is the GSV, which is the only superficial vein listed here. Both the greater and lesser saphenous veins account for a large majority of varicosity formation. The other options listed do play a role in the development of varicose veins but much less often than the great saphenous. Obstruction of the inferior vena cava or the common iliac veins may lead to very extensive varicose vein formation.

3. **D.** No randomized clinical trial has shown one method to be more effective than the other in the treatment of varicose veins. At 1 year, endovenous laser ablation, radiofrequency ablation, sclerotherapy, and surgical stripping have approximately the same outcomes.

4. **B.** The Perthes test can be used to distinguish deep venous insufficiency from the superficial system. The test is performed by placing a tourniquet to the midthigh of the patient while standing. The patient then walks for five minutes. If the veins collapse, the deep veins are patent and the etiology of the engorged veins is superficial insufficiency. If the veins, however, continue to engorge and cause the patient pain, then the deep veins are obstructed.

Comment
Pathogenesis

Varicose veins are a commonly encountered issue in the outpatient setting. Over 20% of individuals in Western populations suffer from varicose veins. Varicose veins are formed by a variety of pathophysiologic mechanisms that lead to the development of these engorged and painful vessels (Figure S89-1). These mechanisms include venous hypertension and valvular incompetence. This leads to a backflow of venous blood in dependent portions of the body (Figure S89-2). The engorged vessels then begin to develop structural changes as the inflammation from the shear stress exerted on the venous walls takes effect.

Treatment Methods

The vessel most often involved is the GSV, which has led to the development of both surgical and endovascular procedures to eliminate these varicosities. The previous standard therapy involved surgical ligation and stripping to the knee level with associated phlebectomies. Recently, however, new endovascular techniques have overtaken surgery as the most commonly utilized therapy for varicose veins. These therapies include radiofrequency ablation, laser ablation, and foam sclerotherapy (Figures S89-3 through S89-6). These endovascular procedures have found favor due to their lack of need for general anesthesia and operating room time. They also carry a lower risk of periprocedural morbidity and mortality. However, there is no difference in the effectiveness of eliminating the great saphenous vein between endovascular measures and surgical interventions at 1 year.

References

Piazza G. Varicose Veins. *Circulation*. 2014;130:582–587.

Rasmussen L, Lawaetz M, Bjoern L, et al. Randomized clinical trial comparing endovenous laser ablation, radiofrequency ablation, foam sclerotherapy and surgical stripping for great saphenous varicose veins. *Br J Surg*. 2011;98:1079–1087.

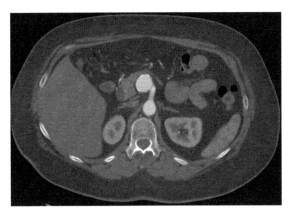

Figure 90-1. *Courtesy of Dr. Wael E. Saad.*

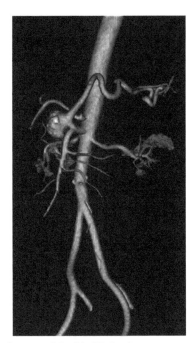

Figure 90-2. *Courtesy of Dr. Wael E. Saad.*

HISTORY: A 56-year-old female presents with vague abdominal pain.

1. Which of the following would be included in the differential diagnosis for the imaging findings presented? (Choose all that apply.)
   A. Superior mesenteric artery (SMA) aneurysm
   B. Mycotic aneurysm of the right renal artery
   C. Arteriovenous fistula
   D. Variant visceral artery anatomy

2. In which patient population are splenic artery aneurysms (SAAs) most commonly identified?
   A. 30-year-old pregnant female
   B. 50-year-old male with atherosclerosis
   C. 70-year-old female with hypertension
   D. 45-year-old male with uncontrolled diabetes

3. What is the most common location of SAAs?
   A. Proximal third of the main splenic artery
   B. Middle third of the main splenic artery
   C. Within the hilar branches of the splenic artery
   D. Within the distal intraparenchymal splenic arterioles

4. After SAAs, which visceral artery (pseudo)aneurysm is most common?
   A. SMA
   B. Inferior mesenteric arteries
   C. Renal artery
   D. Hepatic artery

See Supplemental Figures section for additional figures and legends for this case.

CASE 90

Endovascular Management of Complex Visceral Aneurysm

1. **A and D.** There is an aneurysm involving the SMA. There is variant anatomy with the splenic artery arising from the SMA, near the aneurysm.

2. **A.** True SAAs are more common in women and have been linked with pregnancy. Splenic arterial pseudoaneurysms are most commonly seen in trauma and pancreatitis.

3. **B.** SAAs most commonly occur in the mid to distal third of the main splenic artery.

4. **D.** Hepatic artery pseudoaneurysms are the next most common visceral aneurysm. These are most commonly iatrogenic.

Comment

Etiology

Visceral artery aneurysms (VAAs) are rare entities with an incidence ranging between 0.1% and 2%. They can occur in various arterial locations and have a wide range of etiologies. These are commonly found incidentally on computed tomography for some other reason (Figures S90-1 and S90-2). True SAAs are the most common type of VAA and account for approximately 60% of all VAAs. Hepatic artery aneurysms are the second most common VAA (20%) and are typically iatrogenic in etiology. The most feared complication of VAA is aneurysm rupture, which is associated with mortality rates between 10% and 70% depending on the size and location of the VAA. The annual risk of rupture also depends on the specific artery involved and size of the aneurysm, but most studies quote rupture rates of 3% to 10% annually.

Indication

The decision to employ endovascular therapy is complicated and should be made on a case-by-case basis. Generally accepted criteria for true VAAs include: (1) aneurysm growth, (2) aneurysm diameter greater than 2 cm (1.0 to 1.5 cm for SMA, gastroduodenal, and renal arteries [if symptomatic]), (3) pain, and (4) embolic or ischemic complications. On the other hand, most feel that all visceral pseudoaneurysms should be fixed because these will invariably increase in size over time and will eventually rupture. Endovascular treatment methods include embolization with coils or other agents and covered-stenting of the vessel from which the aneurysm originates, if possible (Figures S90-3 and S90-4).

Follow-up

Once an aneurysm or pseudoaneurysm is treated endovascularly, it should be followed up regularly with imaging to ensure it remains excluded and does not recanalize. If a lesion recanalizes, its risk of rupture returns. If recanalization is found, the patient's imaging should be closely evaluated for a missed feeding vessel, stent migration, or other contributing factor (Figures S90-5 and S90-6). Additionally, the patient's medications must be reviewed, as anticoagulants may contribute to persistent perfusion of the aneurysm, as was seen in this case.

References

Patel A, Weintraub JL, Nowakowski FS, et al. Single-center experience with elective transcatheter coil embolization of splenic artery aneurysms: technique and midterm follow-up. *J Vasc Interv Radiol.* 2012;23:893–899.

Yasumoto T, Osuga K, Yamamoto H, et al. Long-term outcomes of coil packing for visceral aneurysms: correlation between packing density and incidence of coil compaction or recanalization. *J Vasc Interv Radiol.* 2013;24:1798–1807.

Cross-reference

Vascular and Interventional Radiology: The Requisites, 2nd ed, 256–258.

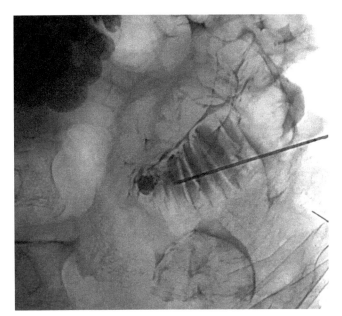

Figure 91-1

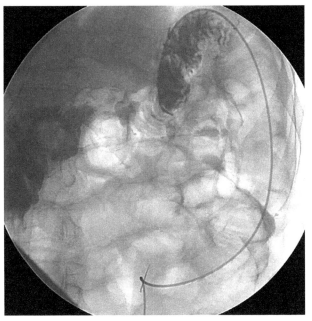

Figure 91-2

HISTORY: A 63-year-old female with gastric outlet obstruction and failure to thrive presents for enteral nutrition access.

1. Based on the images provided, what procedure has been performed?
   A. Percutaneous endoscopic gastrostomy
   B. Direct percutaneous gastrostomy
   C. Direct percutaneous gastrojejunostomy
   D. Direct percutaneous jejunostomy

2. Which of the following are potential complications of this procedure? (Choose all that apply.)
   A. Peritonitis
   B. Contrast-induced renal injury
   C. Catheter occlusion
   D. Small bowel obstruction

3. Which of the following are advantages of percutaneous fluoroscopic approach over endoscopic jejunostomy placement?
   A. Ability to traverse tight esophageal or gastric outlet strictures with small-bore catheters
   B. Ability to opacify the jejunum with contrast and reduce inadvertent puncture of other organs
   C. Lower risk of hemorrhage
   D. All of the above

4. In which of the following situations is jejunostomy tube feedings *NOT* helpful?
   A. History of tube feeding-related aspiration pneumonia
   B. Reflux esophagitis
   C. Patient with esophagectomy and gastric pull-through
   D. Distal bowel obstruction

See Supplemental Figures section for additional figures and legends for this case.

CASE 91

Direct Percutaneous Jejunostomy

1. **D.** The images demonstrate direct percutaneous jejunostomy placement under fluoroscopic guidance. There are contrast opacifying jejunal bowel loops, identified by the mucosal fold pattern. A pigtail jejunostomy tube has been placed without any endoscopic guidance. The stomach is not accessed in these images.

2. **A, C, and D.** Peritonitis may be a complication of percutaneous jejunostomy placement in the event that another loop of bowel is inadvertently punctured or there is leaking of intraintestinal contents into the peritoneum. Catheter occlusion may occur after long periods of use of a jejunostomy tube from lack of proper catheter care with flushes or administering improper or crushed medications. The jejunostomy catheter has a small bore and thus has a high propensity to occlude. Small bowel obstruction is uncommon with such a small-bore catheter.

3. **D.** All of the above are advantages of a percutaneous fluoroscopic jejunostomy placement over an endoscopic approach.

4. **D.** Enteral feeds through a jejunostomy are indicated for patients with a history of tube feeding–related aspiration pneumonia and those with reflux esophagitis. Long-term enteral access such as jejunostomy is recommended when tube feeds are required for more than 30 days. Jejunostomy placement is not recommended when there is obstruction distally.

Comment

Indication

The examination demonstrates percutaneous transabdominal placement of a jejunostomy catheter. Although surgical jejunostomy and percutaneous gastrojejunostomy represent the standard approaches for obtaining the ability to feed into the jejunum, there are occasional clinical situations in which these procedures are not possible. One common scenario is the patient who has undergone gastrectomy, esophagogastrectomy, or esophagectomy with gastric pull through, and who is also a poor operative risk.

Percutaneous Management

Because the small bowel is usually not fixed within the abdomen and can be quite mobile, direct percutaneous jejunostomy can be technically challenging to perform. Factors that help the interventionalist include: (1) The presence of an identifiable scar from a prior surgical jejunostomy, because it is likely that the adjacent loop of small bowel has been surgically tethered to the anterior abdominal wall, making it less likely to fall away during the procedure; (2) The ability to identify a suitable loop of bowel using ultrasound guidance or using fluoroscopic examination with or without injection of air through a nasogastric catheter. Although techniques vary, many interventionalists first place a T-tack into the jejunal loop under fluoroscopic guidance and use this to maintain gentle traction on the bowel while the tract is dilated to accommodate the jejunostomy catheter (Figures S91-1 through S91-3). As with gastrojejunostomy, tube feedings into the small bowel are given continuously rather than in bolus fashion.

References

Cope C, Davis AG, Baum RA, et al. Direct percutaneous jejunostomy: techniques and applications—ten years' experience. *Radiology.* 1998;209:747–754.

Hu HT, Shin JH, Son HY, et al. Fluoroscopically guided percutaneous jejunostomy with use of a 21-gauge needle: a prospective study in 51 patients. *J Vasc Interv Radiol.* 2009;20:1583–1587.

Kirby DF, Delegge MH, Fleming CR. American Gastroenterological Association medical position statement: guidelines for the use of enteral nutrition. *Gastroenterology.* 1995;108:1280.

Cross-reference

Vascular and Interventional Radiology: The Requisites, 2nd ed, 436–437.

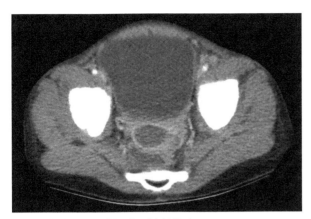

Figure 92-1. *Courtesy of Dr. Ranjith Vellody.*

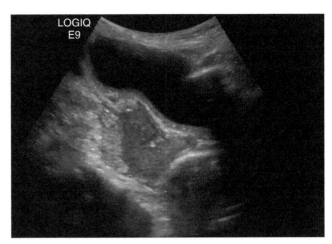

Figure 92-2. *Courtesy of Dr. Ranjith Vellody.*

HISTORY: A febrile 6-year-old male with a recent medical history of ruptured appendicitis is referred.

1. Which of the following is the most likely diagnosis for the imaging findings presented?
   A. Perirectal abscess
   B. Hemorrhoid
   C. Enterocutaneous fistula
   D. Lymphocele

2. Which of the following is *NOT* a common treatment option for the imaging findings presented?
   A. Close monitoring
   B. Blind incision through the rectal wall
   C. Ultrasound-guided drainage with a pigtail catheter
   D. Computed tomography (CT)-guided drainage with a pigtail catheter

3. What clinical picture would necessitate open laparotomy with lavage?
   A. Stable, no symptoms
   B. Multifocal abscesses with peritonitis and sepsis
   C. Single, isolated perirectal abscess
   D. Multiple abscesses that are not communicating

4. What is an advantage of a transrectal versus other percutaneous approach for drainage of a pelvic abscess?
   A. No need for antibiotics
   B. Less of a risk for postprocedural complications
   C. Reduced risk of puncture of overlying bowel loops or arteries
   D. Higher likelihood that drain will stay in place

See Supplemental Figures section for additional figures and legends for this case.

CASE 92

Transrectal Drainage of Perirectal Abscess

1. **A.** Based on the clinical history and imaging appearance, a perirectal abscess is most likely. However, in the absence of clinical history, rectal abscesses can sometimes have a similar imaging appearance to fistula and lymphoceles.

2. **A.** For perirectal abscesses, the preferred treatment is intervention. Traditionally, perirectal abscesses were drained via open laparotomy and lavage or even a blind incision through the rectal wall. However, with interventional techniques, CT and ultrasound are the choice imaging modalities for drainage.

3. **B.** Multifocal peritonitis with sepsis would necessitate urgent surgical intervention. Multifocal abscesses could, depending on the number, be managed surgically or through an interventional approach. A single abscess without sepsis is best managed without surgery.

4. **C.** A transrectal approach avoids puncture of overlying bowel loops and adjacent arteries. Many of these patients are concurrently treated with antibiotics.

Comment

Main Teaching Point

Any patient, adult or pediatric, who has had recent visceral surgical intervention with continued abdominal pain or becomes septic should have initial evaluation with CT over ultrasound. Ultrasound could miss other tiny abscesses that could easily be discovered on CT, while highlighting any other anatomic issues (Figure S92-1).

Percutaneous Management

Perirectal abscesses may be drained with ultrasound intervention. Ultrasound may be performed in pediatric patients via transabdominal route while intervention is performed transrectally (Figures S92-2 through S92-4). Alternatively, a transvaginal ultrasound transducer with needle guide may be used. Drainage in this patient was performed with a 10.2 Fr pigtail catheter (Figure S92-5).

References

Lorentzen T, Nolsøe C, Skjoldbye B. Ultrasound-guided drainage of deep pelvic abscesses: experience with 33 cases. *Ultrasound Med Biol.* 2011;37:723–728.

Sudakoff G, Lundeen S, Otterson M. Transrectal and transvaginal sonographic intervention of infected pelvic fluid collections—a complete approach. *Ultrasound Q.* 2005;21:175–185.

Cross-reference

Vascular and Interventional Radiology: The Requisites, 2nd ed, 414–415.

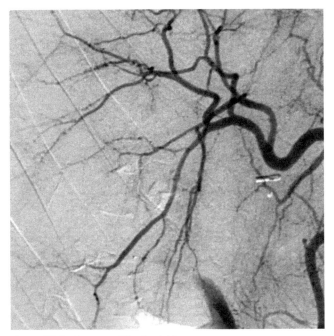

Figure 93-1. *Courtesy of Dr. Daniel Brown.*

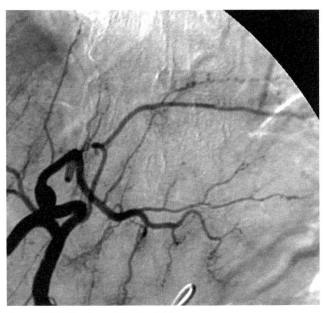

Figure 93-2. *Courtesy of Dr. Daniel Brown.*

HISTORY: A 42-year-old female presents with abdominal pain and hematuria.

1. Which of the following would be included in the differential diagnosis for the imaging findings presented? (Choose all that apply.)
   A. Polyarteritis nodosa
   B. Necrotizing angiitis secondary to methamphetamine use
   C. Hepatic artery stenosis
   D. Primary sclerosing cholangitis

2. What aspects of these images allow for the identification of the disease process?
   A. Evidence of multiple embolic phenomena
   B. Diffuse involvement of the aorta
   C. Multifocal stenoses and small aneurysms in the small and medium-size arteries
   D. The tortuosity present in the large arterioles

3. Which of the following arteries or territories is this process most likely to involve?
   A. Hepatic arteries solely
   B. Aorta and other large muscular arteries
   C. Mesenteric arteries solely
   D. Small and medium-sized muscular arteries

4. What is the most effective treatment for this patient?
   A. Conservative management with lifestyle modifications
   B. Statin therapy and blood pressure control
   C. Endovascular aneurysmal embolization
   D. Combination of corticosteroids and immunosuppressive agents

See Supplemental Figures section for additional figures and legends for this case.

CASE 93

Polyarteritis Nodosa

1. **A and B.** These two disease processes can present with identical angiographic findings found in this case. The diffuse stenotic and aneurysmal involvement of multiple small and medium-sized muscular arteries is classic for polyarteritis nodosa and necrotizing angiitis. Necrotizing angiitis is usually secondary to methamphetamine use, so a thorough history can help to differentiate the two. There are diffuse stenoses and aneurysms in these images that rule out hepatic artery stenosis and primary sclerosing cholangitis.

2. **C.** The presence of multifocal stenoses and aneurysms is classic for an angiographic diagnosis of polyarteritis nodosa. The aorta is not pictured in this image, there is no evidence of embolism, and the arteries do not show any evidence of increased tortuosity. The gold standard to diagnosis is biopsy of involved tissue.

3. **D.** Polyarteritis nodosa affects small and medium-sized vessels throughout the body. It mostly affects the renal arteries and hepatomesenteric arteries but can affect any small or medium-sized muscular arteries in the body. The disease spares the aorta and large muscular arteries.

4. **D.** The current treatment for polyarteritis nodosa is a combination of corticosteroids for acute episodes of the disease with immunosuppressive agents to prevent reemergence of symptoms. Statin therapy or conservative management would have no role in this situation. Other than hemorrhage from ruptured aneurysms, there are no endovascular interventions to treat polyarteritis nodosa.

Comment

Imaging Interpretation

The images demonstrate multifocal irregularity, stenoses, and small aneurysms in the small and medium-sized arteries of the hepatic circulation (Figures S93-1 and S93-2). This appearance is most likely due to polyarteritis nodosa. Another condition that can produce an identical appearance is necrotizing angiitis due to drug abuse (often methamphetamines). When microaneurysms are present, the possibility of mycotic aneurysms must also be considered in the appropriate clinical context (e.g., fever and/or signs of sepsis), but the angiographic appearance shown here is much less likely to represent infection.

Disease Progression

Polyarteritis nodosa is a systemic necrotizing vasculitis of small and medium-sized muscular arteries and arterioles. Patients can experience low-grade fever, myalgias and arthralgias, tender subcutaneous nodules, peripheral neuropathy, hematuria, and symptoms related to vascular involvement. The most commonly involved visceral vascular beds are the renal arteries (85%) and the hepatomesenteric circulation (50%). The large vessels, such as the aorta or major mesenteric trunks, are not likely to be involved.

References

Hernandez-Rodriguez J, Alba MA, Prieto-Gonzalez S, et al. Diagnosis and classification of polyarteritis nodosa. *J Autoimmun.* 2014; 48-49:84–89.

Stanson AW, Friese JL, Johnson CM, et al. Polyarteritis nodosa: spectrum of angiographic findings. *Radiographics.* 2001;21:151–159.

Cross-reference

Vascular and Interventional Radiology: The Requisites, 2nd ed, 260.

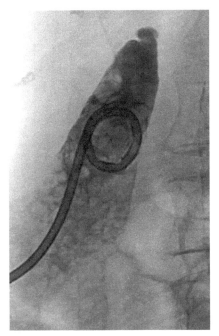

Figure 94-1

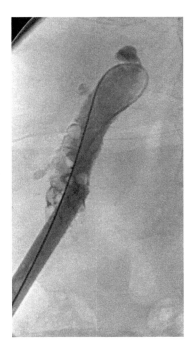

Figure 94-2

HISTORY: A 47-year-old female presents with persistent right upper quadrant pain, after cholecystostomy tube placement.

1. Which of the following is the most likely diagnosis for the imaging findings presented?
   A. Cholangiocarcinoma
   B. Cholelithiasis
   C. Normal variant
   D. Hepatocellular carcinoma

2. What is the procedure of choice for cholelithiasis?
   A. Percutaneous transhepatic cholangiogram and drainage
   B. Choledochoscopy
   C. Laparascopic cholecystectomy
   D. Open cholecystectomy

3. Which patients would optimally be treated by interventional radiology for cholelithiasis?
   A. Young, otherwise healthy patients
   B. Diabetics
   C. Patients with acalculous cholecystitis
   D. Elderly, debilitated patients

4. Which of the following reasons might favor surgery over interventional radiology treatment for cholelithiasis?
   A. Risk of recurrence
   B. Risk of anesthetic complications
   C. Poor rate of initial success
   D. Longer hospital stay

See Supplemental Figures section for additional figures and legends for this case.

CASE 94

Percutaneous Gallstone Removal

1. **B.** There are multiple filling defects in the gallbladder. There is no mass seen to suggest cholangiocarcinoma, which would be better evaluated with cross-sectional imaging. Hepatocellular carcinoma would not have this appearance and this is certainly not normal.

2. **C.** Laparoscopic cholecystectomy is the most definitive and efficient approach to permanent treatment and prevention of further episodes. Open cholecystectomy could be performed but is reserved for more complex cases. Choledochoscopy has a high rate of recurrence (up to 40 in 3 years) and drainage catheter placement will not solve the main problem of gallstones.

3. **D.** Percutaneous gallstone removal is usually reserved for patients who are unsuitable surgical candidates, usually elderly/debilitated patients who need symptomatic relief. Patients with acalculous cholecystitis may benefit from drainage without surgery. The other patients should receive laparoscopic cholecystectomy if possible.

4. **A.** Gallstone removal by interventional radiology can have up to 40% recurrence in 3 years because the gallstone-forming gallbladder remains in place. However, it is usually successful for stones up to 15 mm and can involve a shorter hospital stay. Anesthetic complications may occur with either procedure.

Comment

Main Teaching Point

Patients with biliary stones and cholangitis are often managed with catheter drainage during the initial phase. Once the acute infection and inflammation have resolved, a decision needs to be made as to what the appropriate definitive management should be. In patients with cholelithiasis (gallstones), surgical resection is the definitive treatment. Imaging may be performed with ultrasonography, computed tomography, or magnetic resonance imaging.

Percutaneous Management

Patients with significant contraindications for surgical resection are considered candidates for percutaneous methods of stone removal. After a mature transperitoneal tract has formed around the percutaneous drainage catheter (usually 2 to 4 weeks), the catheter is removed over a guidewire, the tract is dilated, and a large sheath is placed. Calculi are usually ultrasonically fragmented under endoscopic visualization, and the stone fragments are removed by aspiration and a variety of grasping devices (Figures S94-1 through S94-3). Alternatively, the stones may be fragmented and pushed through the biliary tree into the gut. Following this, a drainage catheter is left in place. Once all stones are removed (as demonstrated by cholangiography), the cystic and common bile ducts are patent, and the patient is clinically well, the tube can be capped and subsequently removed.

Outcomes

The recurrence rate of cholelithiasis following percutaneous removal is extremely high (perhaps 40% within 3 years). For this reason, this procedure is generally reserved for patients with significant surgical contraindications.

Reference

Courtois CS, Picus D, Hicks ME. Percutaneous gallstone removal: long-term follow-up. *J Vasc Interv Radiol.* 1996;7:229–234.

Cross-reference

Vascular and Interventional Radiology: The Requisites, 2nd ed, 474–480.

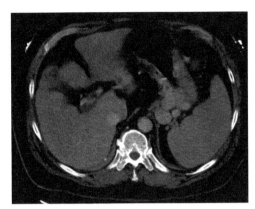

Figure 95-1. *Courtesy of Dr. Wael E. Saad.*

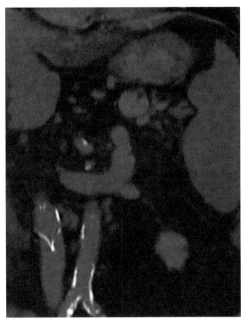

Figure 95-2. *Courtesy of Dr. Wael E. Saad.*

HISTORY: A 66-year-old male with recurrent gastrointestinal bleeding.

1. Which of the following is the most likely diagnosis for the imaging findings presented?
   A. Gastritis
   B. Gastric adenocarcinoma
   C. Gastric varices
   D. Gastrointestinal stromal tumor (GIST)

2. Which procedure(s) would help treat this condition?
   A. Transjugular intrahepatic portosystemic shunt (TIPS)
   B. Balloon-occluded retrograde transvenous obliteration (BRTO)
   C. Transarterial chemoembolization (TACE)
   D. Radiofrequency ablation (RFA)

3. In which condition would BRTO be preferred to TIPS?
   A. Hepatic encephalopathy
   B. Liver transplant candidate
   C. Bleeding from GIST
   D. Pancreatitis-induced pseudoaneurysm

4. What is a common complication after BRTO?
   A. Hepatic necrosis
   B. Diaphragmatic injury
   C. Hepatic encephalopathy
   D. Esophageal variceal bleeding

See Supplemental Figures section for additional figures and legends for this case.

CASE 95

Balloon-Occluded Retrograde Tranvenous Obliteration of Gastric Varices

1. **C.** Figures S95-1 and S95-2 demonstrate opacified, engorged vessels within the gastric wall, instead of gastric wall thickening. Adenocarcinoma and GIST are more mass-like; GISTs tend to be exophytic and adenocarcinoma often is not identified until late in the disease course.

2. **A and B.** TIPS and BRTO serve to decompress varices, albeit by differing methods. TACE and RFA are methods that interventional radiologists use to treat neoplasms.

3. **A.** Baseline hepatic encephalopathy is a relative contraindication to TIPS due to decreased filtration of blood products by the liver after an iatrogenically placed portosystemic shunt. GIST-related bleeding and pseudoaneurysms can be treated by direct embolization. Transplant candidates may receive BRTO as a temporizing measure, but it is not a first-line therapeutic procedure in these patients.

4. **D.** By shunting flow away from gastric varices, post-BRTO patients can bleed from other varices such as duodenal or esophageal varices up to 31% of the time. Hepatic necrosis may occur following TACE, diaphragmatic injury is a concern during RFA, and hepatic encephalopathy is a complication of TIPS.

Comment

Technical Concept

Balloon-occluded transvenous obliteration of gastric varices was first described in 1984 by Olson, but it became a popular treatment in Japan. The concept behind the procedure is that in order to prevent gastric variceal bleeding, the varices must be sclerosed/obliterated. However, the challenge lies in prevention of sclerosant leakage into the systemic circulation. In order to prevent systemic sclerosant leakage, balloon-occlusion is performed by placing the balloon in the venous outflow tract proximal to the connection with systemic venous circulation.

Subsequently, sclerosant is injected into the varices. Computed tomography is helpful in planning the BRTO procedure as well as in follow-up (Figures S95-1, S95-2, S95-5, and S95-6).

Procedural Technique

BRTO generally takes place via a transjugular or transfemoral approach, with catheterization of the left renal vein and subsequent balloon-occlusion of the outflow of the gastric varices, which is at the left renal vein (Figures S95-3 and S95-4). Techniques, such as those in the figures seen above, make use of Amplatzer plugs or coils instead of balloon-occlusion to prevent balloon rupture and reduce time of the procedure. Combination of BRTO with TIPS may have an even higher success rate, although more studies are forthcoming.

Outcomes/Complications

There is a fairly high technical success rate of preventing gastric bleeding with BRTO (between 91% and 100% for patients after up to three treatments). However, the complication of subsequent secondary variceal bleeding from adjacent varices (esophageal, duodenal) due to increased shunting occurs in up to 31% of patients. Simultaneous treatment with TIPS may reduce this complication rate. However, the potential for hepatic encephalopathy with TIPS placement may serve as a contraindication to TIPS in certain patients.

References

Saad W, Nicholson D. Optimizing logistics for balloon-occluded retrograde transvenous obliteration (BRTO) of gastric varices by doing away with the indwelling balloon: concept and techniques. *Tech Vasc Interv Radiol.* 2013;16:152–157.

Saad W, Simon P, Rose S. Balloon-occluded retrograde transvenous obliteration of gastric varices. *Cardiovasc Intervent Radiol.* 2014;37:299–315.

Saad W, Wagner C, Lippert A, et al. Protecting value of TIPS against the development of hydrothorax/ascites and upper gastrointestinal bleeding after balloon-occluded retrograde transvenous obliteration (BRTO). *Am J Gastroenterol.* 2013;108:1612–1619.

Cross-reference

Vascular and Interventional Radiology: The Requisites, 2nd ed, 325–326.

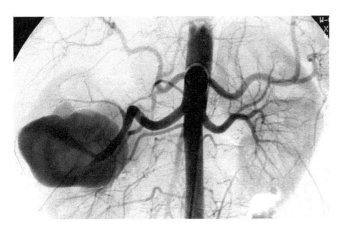

Figure 96-1

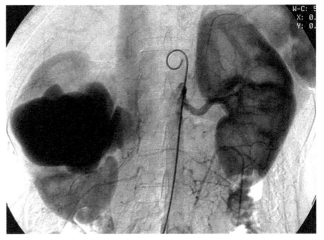

Figure 96-2

HISTORY: A 46-year-old female presents with hematuria and shortness of breath.

1. Which of the following would be included in the differential diagnosis for the imaging findings presented? (Choose all that apply.)
   A. Renal arteriovenous malformation (AVM)
   B. Renal calculus
   C. Normal
   D. Renal angiomyolipoma (AML)

2. Which of the following is/are a potential sequela of the imaging findings?
   A. Congestive heart failure
   B. Renal failure
   C. Hypertension
   D. All of the above

3. Which of the following renally-derived enzymes is involved in regulating blood pressure?
   A. Angiotensinogen
   B. Renin
   C. Angiotensin-converting enzyme (ACE)
   D. Aldosterone

4. What are the recommended initial treatment options for this imaging finding?
   A. Radiofrequency ablation or cryoablation
   B. Radical nephrectomy
   C. Embolization
   D. Lithotripsy

See Supplemental Figures section for additional figures and legends for this case.

CASE 96

Renal AVM

1. **A.** The images show an enlarged right renal artery with a large malformation and early venous filling. No mass lesion is seen to suggest AML. This is most certainly not a normal finding.

2. **D.** Congestive heart failure, hypertension, and hematuria are potential sequela of an AVM/fistula.

3. **B.** All of the mentioned enzymes are involved in the renin-angiotensin system. Renin is secreted by cells from the juxtaglomerular apparatus. It is cleaved by angiotensinogen, secreted from the liver, into angiotensinogen I. ACE in the lungs further cleaves angiotensinogen I to angiotensinogen II, which constricts blood vessels and activates the adrenal glands to release aldosterone.

4. **C.** Embolization is the first line recommended treatment option for renal AVMs/fistulas that are large and/or symptomatic (i.e., causing congestive heart failure, renal failure, hematuria). This lesion was large and the patient subsequently underwent coil embolization.

Comment

Etiology

Renal AVMs are rare lesions that may be congenital or acquired. When they are acquired, the most common cause is iatrogenic injury secondary to a renal biopsy or other intervention. The lesions often manifest with recurrent gross hematuria, and they can even produce renovascular hypertension. Successful endovascular treatment of the abnormality generally results in regression of these symptoms.

Imaging Interpretation

The selective right renal angiogram demonstrates opacification of a large AVM (Figures S96-1 and S96-2). Early filling of the venous system is a characteristic finding of such lesions and emphasizes the importance of considering whether all opacified structures are appropriate for the particular phase of the angiogram being evaluated. Opacification of venous structures should never be apparent on arterial phase images.

Endovascular Management

Endovascular therapy for simple renal AVMs (like the one pictured here) usually consists of embolization with a coil or vascular plug of the feeding artery (Figures S96-3 and S96-4). If the lesion is more complex, then particle embolization may be used to treat the abnormality while preserving the kidney for as long as possible; however, such lesions often recur following embolization, and total or partial nephrectomy is likely to be needed eventually.

Reference

Dinkel HP, Danauser H, Triller J. Blunt renal trauma: minimally invasive management with microcatheter embolization experience in nine patients. *Radiology.* 2002;223:723–730.

Cross-reference

Vascular and Interventional Radiology: The Requisites, 2nd ed, 284.

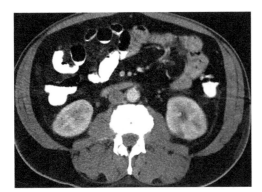

Figure 97-1. *Courtesy of Dr. David M. Williams.*

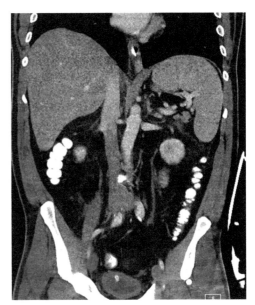

Figure 97-2. *Courtesy of Dr. David M. Williams.*

HISTORY: A 21-year-old female with history of oral contraceptive use and obesity presents with low back pain and bilateral leg swelling.

1. Which of the following is the most likely diagnosis for the imaging findings presented?
   A. Lymphadenopathy
   B. Retroperitoneal sarcoma
   C. Aortic aneurysm
   D. Inferior vena cava (IVC) thrombosis

2. What is the most common etiology of the findings demonstrated in the images above?
   A. Metastatic disease
   B. Primary neoplasm
   C. Presence of IVC filter
   D. Atherosclerosis

3. What is the preferred treatment of this condition?
   A. Recanalization
   B. IVC filter placement
   C. Surgical resection
   D. Medical management

4. What additional factors must be considered?
   A. Aortic diameter
   B. Metastatic disease
   C. Venous inflow
   D. Pulmonary reserve

See Supplemental Figures section for additional figures and legends for this case.

CASE 97

IVC Thrombosis

1. **D.** There is no mass present and the aorta is of normal caliber. The images demonstrate filling defect within the IVC.

2. **C.** IVC filters, especially those that have been in place for a prolonged period of time, increase the risk of thrombosis of the IVC, especially in hypercoagulable patients. Atherosclerosis does not typically affect the venous system and no mass is seen.

3. **A.** Recanalization of the IVC with stent placement is the preferred treatment in appropriately selected patients (see below). IVC filters can be placed during the perioperative period, but should not remain in place for a prolonged period of time. Medical management with anticoagulation should be instituted, but should not be the only treatment. Surgical resection would not treat the underlying condition.

4. **C.** Venous inflow to the IVC must be patent in order to maintain patency of the recanalized IVC. The remaining choices are simply red herrings, although pulmonary reserve may be a consideration in some patients, requiring general anesthesia for the intervention.

Comment

Main Teaching Point

Depending upon collateral formation and the extent of venous involvement, the symptoms of IVC thrombosis can include bilateral lower-extremity and lower-body wall edema and lower-extremity pain. Anticoagulation therapy is typically given to minimize the acute symptomatology and to decrease the substantial risk of pulmonary embolism. In carefully selected patients, catheter-directed thrombolysis can be used to achieve venous recanalization as well. Computed tomography or magnetic resonance venography are commonly employed for diagnosis (Figures S97-1 and S97-2).

Etiology

The etiologies of IVC thrombosis include IVC filter placement, abdominal malignancy with mass effect upon the IVC, sepsis, dehydration, and hypercoagulability. Abdominal tumors can cause IVC thrombosis via compression or outright invasion. The most common histology of such lesions is renal cell carcinoma, although other lesions such as hepatocellular carcinoma, adrenal carcinoma, nodal metastases, and IVC leiomyoma/leiomyosarcomas can cause IVC thrombosis as well. In patients with renal cell carcinoma, the presence of IVC involvement does not usually preclude surgical resection.

Endovascular Management

Certain considerations must be undertaken prior to IVC recanalization. First, the patient must be in a state of health in which she would benefit from recanalization and able to tolerate anticoagulation. The venous inflow must be interrogated and appropriately treated because inflow patency is required to maintain integrity of recanalized IVC. Placement of IVC filters above the occlusion prior to recanalization should be considered. Once access is obtained across the occlusion, balloon angioplasty and stenting are performed as necessary (Figures S97-3 and S97-4). Primary patency is between 38% and 40%, and secondary patency rates are around 79% to 86% at 54 months. Follow-up is generally performed with ultrasound or CTV although these modalities are quite technique-dependent. Repeat venography is the most accurate way to assess for in-stent stenosis with the added benefit of the ability to biopsy any filling defects.

References

Bjarnason H. Tips and tricks for stenting the inferior vena cava. *Semin Vasc Surg.* 2013;26:29–34.

Razavi MK, Hansch EC, Kee ST, et al. Chronically occluded inferior venae cavae: endovascular treatment. *Radiology.* 2000;214:133–138.

Williams DM. Iliocaval reconstruction in chronic deep vein thrombosis. *Tech Vasc Interv Radiol.* 2014;17:109–113.

Cross-reference

Vascular and Interventional Radiology: The Requisites, 2nd ed, 293–301.

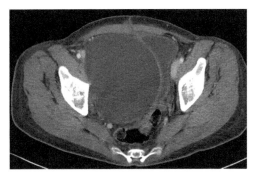

Figure 98-1. *Courtesy of Dr. Bill S. Majdalany.*

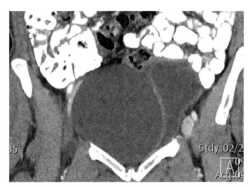

Figure 98-2. *Courtesy of Dr. Bill S. Majdalany.*

HISTORY: A 47-year-old male presents with pelvic fullness. The patient recently had a lymph node dissection.

1. Which of the following would be included in the differential diagnosis for the imaging findings presented? (Choose all that apply.)
   A. Hematoma
   B. Seroma
   C. Abscess
   D. Lymphocele

2. A drain was placed into the collection and the fluid was sent for analysis. What are the expected fluid characteristics for a pelvic lymphocele?
   A. Sterile fluid with few lymphocytes
   B. Sterile fluid with many lymphocytes
   C. Gram-negative rods with few lymphocytes
   D. Gram-negative rods with many lymphocytes

3. What is the most common cause of a pelvic lymphocele?
   A. Spontaneous
   B. Following pelvic lymph node dissection
   C. Following hip arthroplasty
   D. Following colonoscopy

4. Prior to performing ethanol sclerosis for a lymphocele, which of the following should be excluded? (Choose all that apply.)
   A. Persistent drainage from the lymphocele
   B. Colonic fistula
   C. Sterile fluid collection
   D. Infected fluid collection

See Supplemental Figures section for additional figures and legends for this case.

CASE 98

Pelvic Lymphocele

1. **A, B, C, and D.** In the setting of recent pelvic lymph node dissection, all four answer choices should be included in the differential. Analysis of the drained fluid can narrow the differential.

2. **B.** Fluid from a lymphocele is characteristically sterile with an extremely high lymphocyte concentration.

3. **B.** Pelvic lymphoceles most commonly occur following pelvic lymph node dissection. It is thought that transection of afferent lymphatic vessels during lymph node dissection causes lymphatic fluid to accumulate. Other operations with transection of lymphatic vessels may also result in a lymphocele. Spontaneous lymphoceles are rare.

4. **B and D.** Prior to performing ethanol sclerosis for a pelvic lymphocele, a fistula should be excluded. This can be done by injecting contrast into the fluid collection. Additionally, the diagnosis should be confirmed by fluid analysis prior to ethanol sclerosis. The fluid from a lymphocele is typically sterile with many lymphocytes. If the fluid is not sterile, an abscess must be considered and ethanol sclerosis should not be performed.

Comment

Main Teaching Point

The images demonstrate the typical appearance of a postoperative pelvic lymphocele (Figures S98-1 and S98-2). If the patient is symptomatic (commonly pain, fever, or leg swelling due to iliac vein compression), the intervention of first choice is percutaneous aspiration with possible drainage. The aspirated fluid should be sent for laboratory analysis as described, because the differential diagnosis is broad. If the collection is sterile and has an extremely high concentration of lymphocytes, the diagnosis of lymphocele is made.

Percutaneous Management

Although catheter drainage is sometimes successful as stand-alone therapy, a significant percentage of lymphoceles do not completely resolve with catheter drainage alone because lymphatic channels within the wall of the collection continue to produce fluid. In this situation, if the collection is not infected and no fistula is present, then periodic (usually 2 to 3 times per week) instillation of absolute ethanol or another sclerosant can produce cessation of fluid output from the collection, eventually allowing removal of the catheter (Figures S98-3 and S98-4). In general, at least several sessions of sclerosis are needed, and the entire process can take up to several months in a minority of cases.

References

Kim JK, Jeong YY, Kim YH, et al. Postoperative pelvic lymphocele: treatment with simple percutaneous catheter drainage. *Radiology.* 1999;212:390–394.

Zuckerman DA, Yeager TD. Percutaneous ethanol sclerotherapy of postoperative lymphoceles. *Am J Roentgenol.* 1997;169:433–437.

Cross-reference

Vascular and Interventional Radiology: The Requisites, 2nd ed, 416.

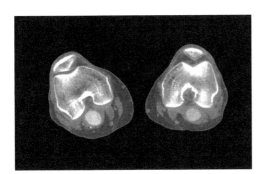

Figure 99-1

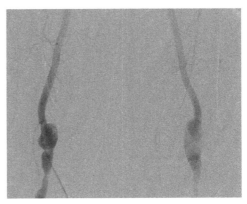

Figure 99-2

HISTORY: A 54-year-old male with a history of hyperlipidemia and smoking presents with worsening bilateral calf claudication. He was found to have palpable pulsatile masses within the bilateral popliteal fossa on physical exam.

1. Which of the following is the most likely diagnosis for the imaging findings presented?
   A. Popliteal artery rupture
   B. Popliteal artery aneurysm
   C. Popliteal artery entrapment
   D. Cystic adventitial disease of the popliteal artery

2. What is the most common complication of the imaging findings presented?
   A. Rupture
   B. Infection
   C. Paralysis
   D. Thrombosis

3. This patient should be screened for a similar disease process in which vascular territory?
   A. Brachial
   B. Renal
   C. Aorta
   D. Anterior communicating artery

4. What is a potential treatment option for this disease?
   A. Thrombin injection
   B. Compression
   C. Distal bypass
   D. Embolization

See Supplemental Figures section for additional figures and legends for this case.

CASE 99

Popliteal Artery Aneurysm

1. **B.** The computed tomography (CT) and angiographic images demonstrate bilateral popliteal artery aneurysms. There is no extravasation of contrast to suggest rupture.

2. **D.** Acute popliteal aneurysm thrombosis resulting in acute limb ischemia occurs in up to 40% of patients who are followed conservatively. Alternatively, the thrombus formed within the popliteal aneurysm may shower distal emboli.

3. **C.** Approximately 37% of patients with popliteal artery aneurysms will have an abdominal aortic aneurysm.

4. **C.** Current therapeutic interventions for popliteal artery aneurysms include surgical bypass and endovascular stent placement.

Comment

Main Teaching Point

Popliteal artery aneurysms are commonly bilateral (50%), and they often coexist with aneurysms in another location, most commonly abdominal aortic aneurysms and common femoral artery aneurysms. The most common presenting symptoms include lower-extremity ischemia and compression of adjacent nerves or other structures. Although rupture of popliteal aneurysms can occur, this complication is quite uncommon (<5% of patients). More commonly, popliteal aneurysms manifest with limb-threatening ischemia due to distal embolization (20%) or popliteal artery thrombosis (40%). The risk factors for popliteal aneurysm thrombosis have been found to include poor distal runoff, presence of thrombus, and diameter greater than or equal to 2 cm. However, even small aneurysms can produce limb-threatening ischemia. Imaging evaluation may include CT, magnetic resonance imaging, ultrasonography, or catheter-based angiography (Figures S99-1 through S99-3).

Treatment Methods

The accepted standard treatment approach for popliteal artery aneurysms is surgical aneurysm resection with distal bypass. Endovascular stent-grafting is generally of the best benefit in patients with high perioperative risk for surgery. Endovascular stent placement in patients with popliteal artery aneurysms who are not at high perioperative surgical risk is controversial and is a subject of ongoing debate. Recent literature has demonstrated that endovascular repair is associated with an increased risk of reintervention and graft thrombosis within 30 days compared to open surgery but no significant difference in primary and secondary patency rates in the long-term (12 and 72 months). Currently it is recommended that endovascular repair of popliteal artery aneurysms be considered on a case-by-case basis (Figures S99-4 and S99-5).

References

Antonello M, Frigatti P, Battocchio P, et al. Endovascular treatment of asymptomatic popliteal aneurysms: 8-year concurrent comparison with open repair. *J Cardiovasc Surg (Torino)*. 2007;48:267–274.

Joshi D, James RL, Jones L. Endovascular versus open repair of asymptomatic popliteal artery aneurysm. *Cochrane Database Syst Rev.* 2014;8:CD010149.

Piazza M, Menegolo M, Ferrari A, et al. Long-term outcomes and sac volume shrinkage after endovascular popliteal artery aneurysm repair. *Eur J Vasc Endovasc Surg.* 2014;48:161–168.

Cross-reference

Vascular and Interventional Radiology: The Requisites, 2nd ed, 354–357.

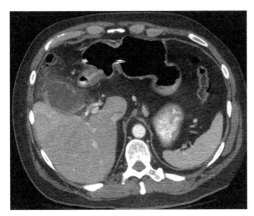

Figure 100-1

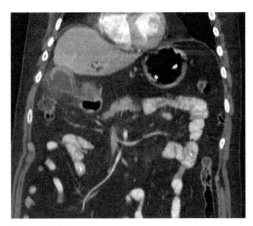

Figure 100-2

HISTORY: A 55-year-old male presents with right upper quadrant pain, emesis, and diarrhea.

1. Which of the following is the most likely diagnosis for the imaging findings presented?
   A. Portal vein thrombosis
   B. Gallbladder carcinoma
   C. Gallbladder rupture
   D. Adenomyomatosis

2. The most common route of percutaneous cholecystostomy is transhepatic. Which of the following is *NOT* a theoretical advantage of transhepatic cholecystostomy?
   A. Decreased risk of bile leak
   B. Decreased risk of colonic injury
   C. Decreased risk of pneumothorax
   D. More rapid fibrin sheath formation, facilitating subsequent removal

3. Which type of gallbladder rupture is depicted in this case?
   A. Type I
   B. Type II
   C. Type III
   D. Type IV

4. Five days following the initiation of intravenous antibiotics and percutaneous cholecystostomy, the patient remains febrile, tachycardic, and hypotensive. On physical exam, the patient has persistent right upper quadrant tenderness without rebound or guarding. What is the most likely diagnosis?
   A. Portal vein thrombosis
   B. Pericholecystic abscess
   C. Acute hepatitis
   D. Bile peritonitis

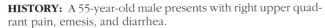

See Supplemental Figures section for additional figures and legends for this case.

CASE 100

Gallbladder Rupture with Pericholecystic Abscess

1. **C.** The computed tomography images demonstrates diffuse gallbladder wall thickening, pericholecystic fluid, and increased enhancement of the liver surrounding the gallbladder fossa. These findings are consistent with acute cholecystitis. However, there is also a focal defect within the fundus of the gallbladder that is concerning for gallbladder rupture.

2. **C.** In most cases, there is no difference in the risk of pneumothorax from a transhepatic technique versus a transperitoneal approach. The transhepatic cholecystostomy technique has the advantage of a decreased risk of bile leak, decreased risk of colonic injury, and more rapid fibrin sheath formation, which facilitates subsequent removal.

3. **B.** The image depicts a type II gallbladder perforation, localized gallbladder rupture with a pericholecystic abscess. A type I gallbladder perforation is where there is rupture of the gallbladder into the peritoneum with generalized peritonitis. A type III perforation occurs when there is a cholecystoenteric fistula. There is no type IV perforation.

4. **B.** The initial image demonstrates a pericholecystic abscess in addition to gallbladder perforation. In these cases, the abscess must also be drained in addition to the gallbladder.

This can be performed by placing additional side holes in the cholecystostomy catheter or by placing a separate abscess drain. The absence of rebound and guarding on physical exam make bile peritonitis unlikely.

Comment

Main Teaching Point

Complications of acute cholecystitis can include free rupture into the peritoneum or contained rupture with pericholecystic abscess formation (Figures S100-1 and S100-2). Historically, the presence of gallbladder rupture was an absolute indication for emergency cholecystectomy. In modern practice, however, most surgeons much prefer to operate after the acute infection and pericholecystic inflammation have subsided. For these reasons, percutaneous cholecystostomy may still be performed. However, the abscess must also be drained, either using the same drainage catheter with additional side-holes created to drain the abscess or via a separate (second) catheter (Figure S100-3).

References

Ahkan O, Akinsi D, Ozmen MN. Percutaneous cholecystostomy. *Eur J Radiol.* 2002;43:229–236.

Sato K. Percutaneous management of biliary emergencies. *Semin Intervent Rad.* 2006;23:249–257.

Cross-reference

Vascular and Interventional Radiology: The Requisites, 2nd ed, 474–480.

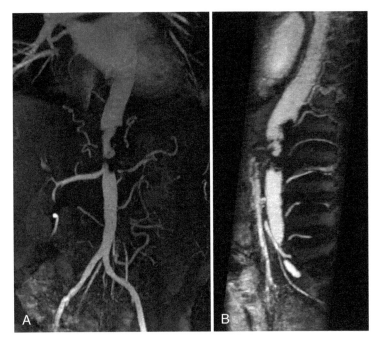

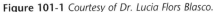

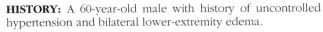

Figure 101-1 *Courtesy of Dr. Lucia Flors Blasco.*

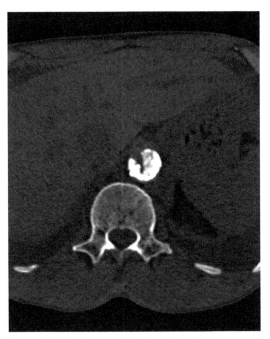

Figure 101-2. *Courtesy of Dr. Lucia Flors Blasco.*

HISTORY: A 60-year-old male with history of uncontrolled hypertension and bilateral lower-extremity edema.

1. Which of the following is the most likely diagnosis for the imaging findings presented?
   A. Aortic stenosis
   B. Abdominal aortic aneurysm
   C. Aortic dissection
   D. Penetrating ulcers within the abdominal aorta

2. The hypointense material adherent to the aortic wall seen on these images most likely represents:
   A. Intramural hematoma
   B. Fibrofatty atheromatous plaque
   C. Calcified atheromatous plaque
   D. Mycotic aneurysm

3. The most appropriate treatment for aortic stenosis secondary to focal, concentric, short lesions is:
   A. Percutaneous balloon angioplasty
   B. Aortofemoral bypass graft
   C. Endarterectomy
   D. Percutaneous balloon angioplasty followed by stent placement

4. Stent placement may be least helpful after percutaneous balloon angioplasty for treatment of aortic stenosis in which of the following circumstances?
   A. Flow-limiting dissection occurs after angioplasty.
   B. The stenosis recurs following successful angioplasty.
   C. No pressure gradient is present across the lesion after angioplasty.
   D. Angioplasty fails to reduce the stenosis to less than 30% diameter.

See Supplemental Figures section for additional figures and legends for this case.

CASE 101

Abdominal Aortic Stenosis

1. **A.** Contrast-enhanced magnetic resonance (MR) angiography shows severe stenosis of the suprarenal abdominal aorta with occlusion of the proximal celiac, superior, and inferior mesenteric arteries. No aortic aneurysm, penetrating ulcers, or intimal flap from aortic dissection are seen.

2. **C.** Calcium appears hypointense on all types of MR sequences, whereas it appears hyperdense on computed tomography (CT). Although MR is less sensitive than CT to detect small calcifications, the marked hypointensity seen on these images highly suggests the extensive calcium component of the atheromatous plaques.

3. **A.** Although aortofemoral bypass grafting is associated with high patency rates, percutaneous interventions are usually used first for appropriate lesions because of their lower morbidity rates. For focal, concentric, short lesions, percutaneous balloon angioplasty is an appropriate first treatment.

4. **C.** Postangioplasty stent placement may be performed if flow-limiting dissection occurs following angioplasty, if angioplasty fails to reduce the stenosis to less than 30% diameter, if a persistent pressure gradient (>10 mm Hg systolic) is present across the lesion after angioplasty, or if the stenosis recurs following successful angioplasty.

Comment

Clinical Presentation

Although hypertension, diabetes, and hyperlipidemia are all associated with the development of atherosclerotic lesions, patients with a history of smoking are particularly prone to develop occlusive disease in the aorta and iliac arteries as seen in this patient (Figures S101-1 and S101-2).

Management Options

Invasive therapy is only performed in patients with lifestyle-limiting claudication or rest pain. Although aortofemoral bypass grafting is associated with high patency rates, percutaneous interventions are usually used first for appropriate lesions because of their lower morbidity rates. For focal, concentric, short lesions, percutaneous balloon angioplasty is an appropriate first treatment. Patencies following aortic angioplasty are comparable to those associated with iliac artery lesions. Endarterectomy, the surgical removal of the plaque, is usually performed when there is involvement of the visceral arteries, as in the case we present (Figure S101-3).

Indications for Stent Placement

Postangioplasty stent placement may be performed if flow-limiting dissection occurs following angioplasty, if angioplasty fails to reduce the stenosis to less than 30% diameter, if a persistent pressure gradient (>10 mm Hg systolic) is present across the lesion after angioplasty, or if the stenosis recurs following successful angioplasty. Primary stent placement (placement of a stent without preceding angioplasty) is generally used for extremely calcified or eccentric lesions.

References

Sandhu C, Belli AM. Abdominal aortic stenting: current practice. *Abdom Imaging.* 2001;6:453–460.

Shih MC1, Angle JF, Leung DA, et al. CTA and MRA in mesenteric ischemia: part 2, normal findings and complications after surgical and endovascular treatment. *Am J Roentgenol.* 2007;188:462–471.

Cross-reference

Vascular and Interventional Radiology: The Requisites, 2nd ed, 209–214.

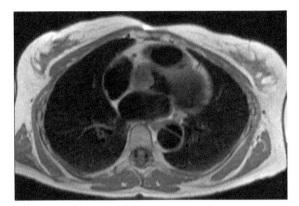

Figure 102-1. *Courtesy of Dr. Peter Liu.*

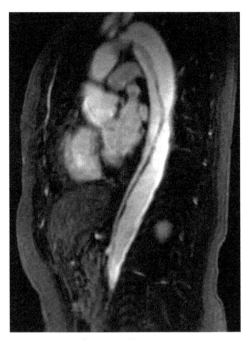

Figure 102-2. *Courtesy of Dr. Peter Liu.*

HISTORY: A 35-year-old male presents to the emergency department with chest pain radiating to his back.

1. Which of the following is the most likely diagnosis for the imaging findings presented?
   A. Aortic dissection
   B. Double aortic arch
   C. Mural thrombus
   D. Penetrating atherosclerotic ulcer

2. What other modalities are commonly used for diagnostic confirmation? (Choose all that apply.)
   A. Chest radiography
   B. Computed tomography (CT) angiography
   C. Transesophageal echocardiography (TEE)
   D. Transthoracic echocardiography

3. What is one of the major complications of this given entity?
   A. Compression of the adjacent structures
   B. Saccular aneurysm formation
   C. Abdominal organ malperfusion
   D. Septic embolism

4. Which one of the following syndromes may predispose the patient to developing this entity?
   A. Marfan syndrome
   B. Tuberous sclerosis
   C. Neurofibromatosis type I
   D. Sturge-Weber syndrome

See Supplemental Figures section for additional figures and legends for this case.

CASE 102

Magnetic Resonance Imaging of Aortic Dissection

1. **A.** The images demonstrate a dissection flap in the visualized thoracoabdominal aorta. The flap did not extend into the ascending aorta (not pictured), making this a type B aortic dissection. Penetrating atherosclerotic ulcer would show a focal, contrast, or blood-filled outpouching/crater. A mural thrombus would not be subintimal and would not show flow-related enhancement in the false lumen, as seen here.

2. **B and C.** Multiple research studies have shown an equally reliable diagnostic value of all of these three modalities for the diagnosis of aortic dissection. In fact, TEE is commonly employed during open aortic repair for aortic dissection.

3. **C.** Extension of the dissection into the visceral vessels is a well-known complication of aortic dissection. Septic embolism or compression of adjacent structures is not as well reported in the literature as dissection-related complications. Saccular aortic aneurysm is rare and can be seen with trauma or penetrating aortic ulcer. Dissections may lead to fusiform aneurysmal formation.

4. **A.** Patients with Marfan syndrome are predisposed to have connective tissue abnormalities, which make them more likely to develop aortic dissection. The other listed syndromes do not have a known increased incidence of aortic dissection.

Comment

Diagnostic Imaging

Magnetic resonance imaging (MRI) is equal or superior to helical CT and TEE for making the diagnosis of acute and chronic aortic dissection (Figures S102-1 through S102-4). The longer image-acquisition time and greater difficulty in patient monitoring in the MRI scanner have been considered relative disadvantages of its use in the acute aortic dissection setting. However, MRI and helical CT are better able than TEE to evaluate the entire aorta (including its subdiaphragmatic segment), and MRI has the advantage in not requiring iodinated contrast. In current practice, aortography is reserved for evaluating patients with clinical evidence of complications of aortic dissection for whom surgical or interventional therapy is being planned.

References

Criado FJ. Aortic dissection: a 250-year perspective. *Tex Heart Inst J.* 2011;38:694–700.

Macura KJ, Corl FM, Fishman EK, et al. Pathogenesis in acute aortic syndromes: aortic dissection, intramural hematoma, and penetrating atherosclerotic ulcer. *Am J Roentgenol.* 2003;181:309–316.

Shiga T, Wajima Z, Apfel CC, et al. Diagnostic accuracy of transesophageal echocardiography, helical computed tomography, and magnetic resonance imaging for suspected thoracic aortic dissection: systemic review and meta-analysis. *Arch Intern Med.* 2006;166:1350–1356.

Cross-reference

Vascular and Interventional Radiology: The Requisites, 2nd ed, 188–192.

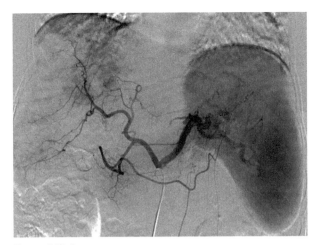

Figure 103-1

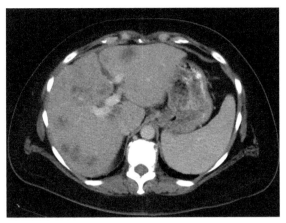

Figure 103-2

HISTORY: A 51-year-old female with known metastatic colorectal cancer.

1. A selective angiogram of which vessel is demonstrated in the first image?
   A. Celiac artery
   B. Superior mesenteric artery
   C. Common hepatic artery
   D. Proper hepatic artery

2. Transcatheter arterial radioembolization is Food and Drug Administration (FDA)-approved for which of the following? (Choose all that apply.)
   A. Colorectal metastatic disease to the liver
   B. Melanoma metastatic disease to the liver
   C. Cholangiocarcinoma
   D. Hepatocellular carcinoma

3. Which, radioisotope is used for transcatheter radioembolization and what particle type does it emit?
   A. I^{131}-beta
   B. Y^{90}-beta
   C. Tc^{99}-gamma
   D. Sa^{153}-beta and gamma

4. Reflux into which of the following extrahepatic arteries is most likely to cause a nontarget complication from an intrahepatic embolization? (Choose two.)
   A. Right gastric
   B. Left gastric
   C. Gastroduodenal
   D. Splenic

See Supplemental Figures section for additional figures and legends for this case.

CASE 103

Colorectal Metastases to Liver: Radioembolization

1. **A.** The first image demonstrates a celiac arteriogram with conventional hepatic arterial anatomy. Many normal variants are possible, but conventional hepatic arterial anatomy includes a common hepatic artery originating from the celiac artery, which becomes the proper hepatic artery and gastroduodenal arteries. The left and right hepatic arteries arise from the proper hepatic artery.

2. **A and D.** Currently, Y^{90} treatment is FDA-approved for use in patients with colorectal metastatic disease to the liver or primary hepatocellular carcinoma.

3. **B.** Y^{90} is a pure beta-emitter with a half-life of 64.2 hours. The majority of the dose (94%) is delivered within the first 11 days following treatment. The average tissue penetration distance is 2.5 mm.

4. **A and C.** Y^{90} reflux is most common into the right gastric and gastroduodenal arteries, which can lead to ischemia and/or radiation enteritis. These arteries are identified on the planning angiogram for potential optimization, either coil embolization or more distal arterial selection prior to radioembolization. Pretreatment evaluation with Tc^{99m} macroaggregate albumin (MAA) is used to identify extrahepatic deposition in the gastrointestinal and pulmonary system with subsequent modification of the radioembolization procedure and/or dose calculation.

Comment

Preprocedural Planning

Radioembolization with Y^{90} microspheres is an FDA-approved therapy for treating unresectable hepatocellular carcinoma and metastatic colorectal carcinoma to the liver. The microspheres are delivered to the tumors in a transcatheter approach through the hepatic artery and, once in place, emit radiation that acts on the tumor cells. Careful patient selection after cross-sectional imaging review and discussion with patient and referring physician is necessary to obtain optimal results (Figure S103-2).

Procedural Technique

Owing to the variation in hepatic arterial anatomy and the potential complications that can result from nontarget embolization of microspheres to the bowel, gallbladder, pancreas, and other nearby structures that derive part of their arterial supply from branches closely associated with those that supply the liver, careful mapping of the arterial supply to the intended target lesion(s) and optimization of the arterial anatomy by selective embolization of vessels is mandatory (Figure S103-1). After optimizing the arterial anatomy, the microcatheter tip is placed in the planned position for delivery of the radioembolic microspheres and approximately 5 mCi of Tc^{99m}-MAA is delivered through the microcatheter. This is followed by single-photon emission computerized tomography (SPECT) imaging to assess the activity within the liver and to detect any activity in extrahepatic abdominal structures and the lungs to evaluate for nontarget delivery and tumor arteriovenous shunting, respectively (Figure S103-3). Once the planning images are reviewed and the patient is deemed a candidate for treatment, dosimetry data are calculated. Dosimetry calculation methods vary; however, some factors that are considered include body surface area, liver volume, tumor burden, and underlying liver cirrhosis. The dose delivery must be carefully monitored under fluoroscopy to ensure optimal radioembolization (Figure S103-4). Some centers perform a follow-up positron emission tomography–computed tomography (CT) or fused SPECT-CT to assess delivery of the dose (Figure S103-5).

References

Murthy R, Kamat P, Nunez R, Salem R. Radioembolization of yttrium-90 microspheres for hepatic malignancy. *Semin Intervent Rad.* 2008;25:48–57.

Salem R, Thurston KG. Radioembolization with yttrium microspheres: a state-of-the-art brachytherapy treatment for primary and secondary liver malignancies. Part 1: technical and methodologic considerations. *J Vasc Interv Radiol.* 2006;17:1251–1278.

Cross-reference

Vascular and Interventional Radiology: The Requisites, 2nd ed, 250–252.

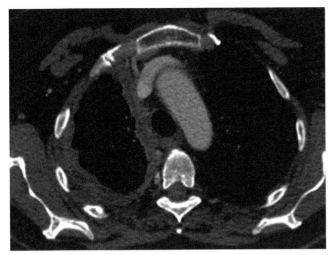

Figure 104-1. *Courtesy of Dr. Lucia Flors Blasco.*

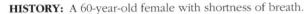

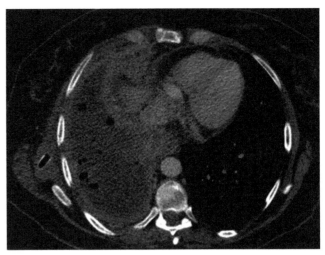

Figure 104-2. *Courtesy of Dr. Lucia Flors Blasco.*

HISTORY: A 60-year-old female with shortness of breath.

1. Which of the following is the most likely diagnosis for the imaging findings presented?
   A. Mesothelioma
   B. Parapneumonic pleural effusion
   C. Localized fibrous tumor of the pleura
   D. Transudative pleural effusion

2. What is the most common symptom in patients presenting with malignant pleural effusion?
   A. Chest pain
   B. Hemoptysis
   C. Fever
   D. Dyspnea

3. Which of the following is *NOT* a computed tomography (CT) imaging feature of malignant pleural disease?
   A. Circumferential pleural thickening
   B. Smooth pleural thickening
   C. Parietal pleural thickening greater than 1 cm
   D. Mediastinal pleura involvement

4. What is the most common treatment for prompt relief of symptomatic patients with malignant pleural effusion?
   A. Pleuroperitoneal shunt
   B. Pleurodesis
   C. Tunneled pleural catheter (TPC)
   D. Pleurectomy

See Supplemental Figures section for additional figures and legends for this case.

CASE 104

Malignant Pleural Effusion

1. **A.** Contrast-enhanced CT images show right pleural effusion and circumferential pleural thickening with mediastinal involvement, findings indicative of malignant pleural disease such as mesothelioma. Metastatic pleural involvement may present similar imaging findings. Parapneumonic pleural effusion, transudative pleural effusion—as seen on congestive heart failure—and fibrous tumor of the pleura are benign entities.

2. **D.** Dyspnea is the most common symptom in patients with pleural effusion as the lung has less space to expand. However, patients may also present with low-grade fever or cough.

3. **B.** Nodular or circumferential pleural thickening, parietal pleural thickening greater than 1 cm, and mediastinal pleura involvement are CT imaging features helpful in distinguishing malignant from benign pleural disease (smooth pleural thickening).

4. **C.** The management of malignant pleural effusion has been trending recently toward minimally invasive procedures by placement of TPCs. Ninety percent of patients experience relief of dyspnea within 48 hours.

Comment

Clinical Presentation

Pleural effusion often complicates the course of malignant pleural disease, either primary pleural neoplasm or secondary to metastatic involvement, and is a poor prognostic indicator. The impact on patients' quality of life is significant, and the most common symptom is dyspnea.

Diagnostic Imaging

CT provides detailed information on morphological changes associated with pleural effusion. Nodular or circumferential pleural thickening, parietal pleural thickening greater than 1 cm, and mediastinal pleura involvement are CT imaging features helpful in distinguishing malignant from benign pleural disease (Figure S104-1). Positron emission tomography has proven to have significantly higher diagnostic accuracy compared to CT in detecting malignant pleural disease (Figure S104-3).

Management Options

The approach to management is a palliative one and has traditionally been by thoracostomy and pleurodesis. More recently, management has been trending toward minimally invasive procedures by placement of TPCs (Figure S104-2). Ultrasound or fluoroscopic guidance is used for accessing the pleural cavity, and the catheter is placed through a peel-away sheath and subsequently tunneled in the subcutaneous tissues of the chest. The catheter has a one-way valve that prevents leakage of pleural fluid from the catheter when it is not connected to a drainage flask and also prevents the entry of air into the pleural cavity through the catheter.

Ninety percent of patients experience relief of dyspnea within 48 hours. Spontaneous pleurodesis can occur in up to 46% of patients, usually within a month of placement. Chemical sclerotherapy through the catheter can be used to increase the rate of pleurodesis. If pleurodesis is achieved, the catheter may be removed.

References

Leung AN, Müller NL, Miller RR. CT in differential diagnosis of diffuse pleural disease. *Am J Roentgenol.* 1990;154(3):487–492.

Orki A, Akin O, Tasci AE, et al. The role of positron emission tomography/computed tomography in the diagnosis of pleural diseases. *Thorac Cardiovasc Surg.* 2009;57(4):217–221.

Pollak JS. Malignant pleural effusions: treatment with tunneled long-term drainage catheters. *Curr Opin Pulm Med.* 2002;8:302–307.

Pollak JS, Burdge CM, Rosenblatt M, et al. Treatment of malignant pleural effusions with tunneled long-term drainage catheters. *J Vasc Interv Radiol.* 2001;12:201–208.

Cross-reference

Vascular and Interventional Radiology: The Requisites, 2nd ed, 418–423.

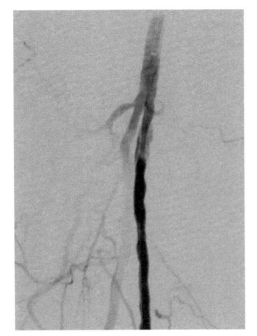

Figure 105-1. *Courtesy of Dr. Minhaj S. Khaja.*

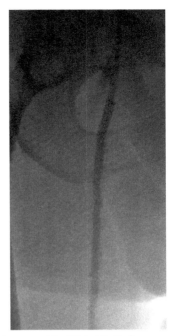

Figure 105-2. *Courtesy of Dr. Minhaj S. Khaja.*

HISTORY: A 78-year-old woman presents with right lower extremity claudication. Conventional angiography and balloon angioplasty were performed. Images were taken following balloon angioplasty.

1. Which of the following is the most likely diagnosis for the imaging findings presented?
   A. Stenosis
   B. Occlusion
   C. Dissection
   D. Aneurysm

2. Which of the following systolic (arterial) pressure gradients would represent a clinically significant gradient?
   A. 2 mm Hg
   B. 6 mm Hg
   C. 9 mm Hg
   D. 12 mm Hg

3. Which of the following techniques are *NOT* used to correct the disease shown in the image?
   A. Blood pressure control without further intervention
   B. Prolonged balloon angioplasty
   C. Balloon fenestration
   D. Stent placement

4. Which of the following are risk factors for arterial dissection?
   A. Obesity
   B. Hypertension
   C. Hypercalcemia
   D. Alcohol use

See Supplemental Figures section for additional figures and legends for this case.

CASE 105

Iatrogenic Superficial Femoral Artery Dissection

1. **C.** Digital subtraction angiography of the superficial femoral artery (SFA) demonstrates a dissection flap, which has resulted in greater than 50% decrease in flow distal to the lesion. Iatrogenic arterial dissection typically occurs at the time of needle puncture, during dilation of an arterial stenosis, or during attempts to cross high-grade stenoses or occlusions.

2. **D.** A systolic pressure gradient of 10 mm Hg or greater signifies a flow-limiting lesion.

3. **A.** The majority of arterial dissections resolve spontaneously without the need for percutaneous or surgical treatment. Flow-limiting dissections, however, require acute intervention with surgery or intervention. Shorter lesions (less than 10 cm) within the SFA are commonly managed with prolonged balloon angioplasty with or without stent placement or balloon fenestration, while longer lesions may require femoral-popliteal bypass with interposed saphenous vein stent or a graft.

4. **B.** Risk factors for arterial dissection include trauma, collagen vascular diseases (Ehler-Danlos syndrome, Marfan syndrome, cystic medial sclerosis, fibromuscular dysplasia), preexisting aneurysm, and the typical cardiovascular risk factors (hypertension, smoking, diabetes mellitus, hyperlipidemia).

Comment

Main Teaching Point

Repeat angiography is always performed immediately following angioplasty in order to assess whether the stenosis has been adequately treated and to evaluate for any complications (Figure S105-1). It is wise to perform angiography in two projections because intimal dissection flaps oriented in the coronal plane might not be appreciated on a single anteroposterior view. Postangioplasty pressure measurements across the lesion may also be obtained: If an unexplained significant (>10 mm Hg) systolic pressure gradient is still present, the presence of occult dissection should be suspected. Intravascular ultrasound, when available, can be extremely helpful in clarifying whether this is indeed the case and in assessing the entire extent of the dissection process.

Endovascular Management

Dissections caused by retrograde passage of a guide-wire in a false channel often resolve spontaneously. Anterograde dissections are more likely to extend and to occlude flow. Flow-limiting dissections (dissections resulting in >10 mm Hg systolic pressure gradient across the lesion or >50% stenosis) require urgent treatment to prevent thrombosis. Most iliac artery dissections that do not extend into the common femoral artery can be managed with balloon angioplasty and stent placement (Figures S105-2 through S105-4). Surgical bypass may be a management choice if the patient is thought to be able to tolerate a surgical procedure rather than stent placement.

References

Fornaro J, Meier T, Pfammatter T. Percutaneous balloon fenestration of flow-limiting iatrogenic dissection of the common femoral artery: report of two cases. *J Vasc Interv Radiol.* 2010;21:1115–1118.

Funaki B. Iatrogenic flow-limiting arterial dissection. *Semin Intervent Rad.* 2008;25:437–441.

Cross-reference

Vascular and Interventional Radiology: The Requisites, 2nd ed, 347–351.

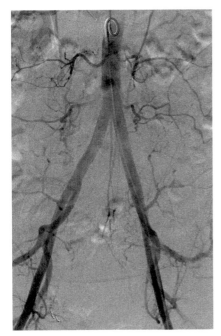

Figure 106-1 *Courtesy of Dr. Wael E. Saad.*

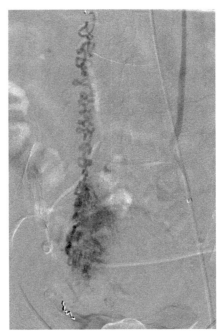

Figure 106-2 *Courtesy of Dr. Wael E. Saad.*

HISTORY: A 40-year-old woman with history of menorrhagia from fibroids presents with continued bleeding, 9 months post uterine artery embolization (UAE).

1. Which of the following is the most likely diagnosis for the imaging findings presented?
   A. Nutcracker syndrome
   B. Leriche syndrome
   C. Pelvic congestion syndrome
   D. Extrauterine arterial perfusion of fibroids

2. Which abnormal artery is depicted in the second image?
   A. Inferior epigastric artery
   B. Iliolumbar artery
   C. Ovarian artery
   D. Inferior mesenteric artery

3. Can this vessel be safely embolized for effective treatment of fibroids?
   A. Yes, patients generally have no increased side effects compared with normal UAE.
   B. Yes, but patients frequently go into premature menopause.
   C. No, because embolizing this vessel is unlikely to affect fibroid perfusion.
   D. No, because it will infarct the ovary.

4. For which symptom is UAE most effective?
   A. Menorrhagia
   B. Dysuria
   C. Constipation
   D. Sciatica

See Supplemental Figures section for additional figures and legends for this case.

CASE 106

Ovarian Artery Embolization

1. **D.** The aortogram and delay pelvic image clearly demonstrate a hypertrophied and tortuous ovarian artery with parenchymal blush in the uterus.

2. **C.** The tortuous vessel coursing inferiorly from the abdominal aorta into the pelvis is the right ovarian artery.

3. **A.** Ovarian artery embolization for fibroid treatment has been shown to be both effective and to generally have no additional symptoms above and beyond those seen with conventional UAE. Patients may enter menopause early, but not frequently.

4. **A.** Dysfunctional uterine bleeding is more likely to respond to UAE than bulk symptoms; therefore, careful patient selection is key to maximize patient satisfaction with the result.

Comment

Main Teaching Point

UAE has been shown to improve menorrhagia symptoms and pelvic pain in 85% to 90% of patients. There are several potential reasons why a patient may not demonstrate clinical response after embolization. One potential reason is incomplete bilateral embolization. The most common reason this might occur is when arterial spasm-related slow flow in the uterine artery deceives the angiographer into believing that embolization has been achieved. Another common reason is the presence of additional blood supply to the fibroid uterus. This can result from congenital variations in uterine artery anatomy or from pelvic collateral supply.

Imaging Interpretation

The images here demonstrate the most common source of extrauterine supply to the uterus: an enlarged ovarian artery. In the aortogram, there is a highly tortuous artery coursing along the right side of the aorta, the ovarian artery (Figure - S106-1). The second image demonstrates an enlarged right ovarian artery with blush of the uterine fibroid (Figure S106-2). Many interventional radiologists perform an abdominal and pelvic aortogram following UAE in order to evaluate for residual perfusion of the fibroids from an ovarian artery (Figures S106-3 through S106-5).

Endovascular Management

Fortunately, the ovarian artery can also be embolized. Most interventionalists embolize the main ovarian artery using Gelfoam, although some advance a microcatheter beyond the ovary and attempt subselective embolization of the uterine branches.

References

Bulman J, Ascher S, Spies J. Current concepts in uterine fibroid embolization. *Radiographics*. 2012;32:1735–1750.

Pelage JP, Walker WJ, Le Dref O, et al. Ovarian artery: angiographic appearance, embolization and relevance to uterine fibroid embolization. *Cardiovasc Intervent Radiol*. 2003;26:227–233.

Worthington-Kirsch RL, Andrews RT, Siskin GP, et al. Uterine fibroid embolization: technical aspects. *Tech Vasc Interv Radiol*. 2002;5:17–34.

Cross-reference

Vascular and Interventional Radiology: The Requisites, 2nd ed, 222–225.

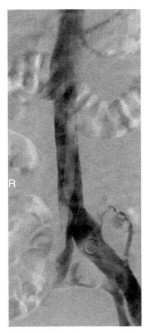

Figure 107-1

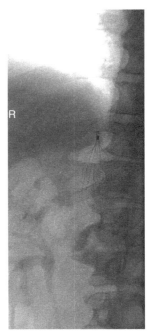

Figure 107-2

HISTORY: A 59-year-old male with recent diagnosis of lung cancer presents with shortness of breath.

1. Which of the following is the most likely diagnosis for the imaging finding presented on the left image?
   A. Thrombosed inferior vena cava (IVC) filter
   B. Chronic deep vein thrombosis (DVT)
   C. Free-floating IVC thrombus
   D. Atherosclerosis

2. Which of the following is an indication for the placement of an IVC filter?
   A. Upper-extremity DVT
   B. Factor V Leiden deficiency
   C. Free-floating iliofemoral or IVC thrombus
   D. Septic pulmonary emboli

3. If an IVC filter is being placed in this case, what access site should be used?
   A. Left common femoral vein
   B. Right common femoral vein
   C. Left internal jugular vein
   D. Right internal jugular vein

4. Where would you place an IVC filter in this patient?
   A. In the right common iliac vein
   B. In the infrarenal IVC
   C. In the suprarenal IVC
   D. There is no indication for IVC filter placement.

See Supplemental Figures section for additional figures and legends for this case.

CASE 107

Free-Floating IVC Thrombus

1. **C.** There is a large ovoid filling defect within the right iliac vein extending into the IVC, consistent with a large free-floating acute thrombus. The appearance does not suggest a chronic DVT. There is no intraluminal stenosis or narrowing to suggest atherosclerosis. No radiopaque object with the appearance of an IVC filter with thrombosis is seen in the image.

2. **C.** The presence of a free-floating iliofemoral or IVC thrombus is a valid indication for placement of an IVC filter. The other answer choices, upper-extremity DVT, Factor V Leiden deficiency, and septic pulmonary emboli, are not definite indications for placement of an IVC filter.

3. **D.** The right internal jugular vein would be the best, most straightforward access point for placement of the IVC filter. The next best options are the left common femoral vein and left internal jugular veins. The right common femoral vein would be a poor access site as catheter and guidewire manipulation could potentially cause distal embolization of the clot leading to life-threatening pulmonary embolism.

4. **C.** It is generally preferable to place the filter in the IVC at the level of the most inferior renal vein such that the apex of the filter is at or just above the lower lip of the renal vein. It is thought that the high flow from the renal veins bathes the apex and helps prevent filter thrombosis. Some postulate that endogenous substances (such as urokinase), produced in the kidneys and subsequently carried in the renal veins,

also help prevent thrombosis of the filter. However, in this case, the proximal aspect of the thrombus extends to the level of the left renal vein, preventing placement at this location. Therefore, the IVC filter should be placed between the renal veins and hepatic veins within the suprarenal IVC as is shown in the image on the right.

Comment

Main Teaching Point

The images demonstrate a large ovoid filling defect within the right iliac vein extending into the IVC, consistent with a large free-floating acute thrombus (Figure S107-1). The venographic appearance of this abnormality suggests a predilection for easy migration and embolization. This necessitates extreme care if catheter manipulations are performed in this region, either for IVC filter placement or for thrombolytic therapy (Figure S107-2). Free-floating iliac vein and/or IVC thrombus is considered an indication for filter placement, even if no other contraindications to anticoagulation exist. In appropriate clinical scenarios, more aggressive endovascular treatments options, such as catheter-directed thrombolysis and suction thrombectomy, may be employed.

References

Kinney TB. Inferior vena cava filters. *Semin Intervent Rad.* 2006; 23:230–239.

Proctor MC. Indications for filter placement. *Semin Vasc Surg.* 2000;13:194–198.

Cross-reference

Vascular and Interventional Radiology: The Requisites, 2nd ed, 293–300.

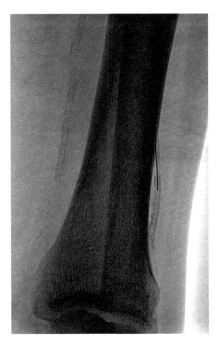

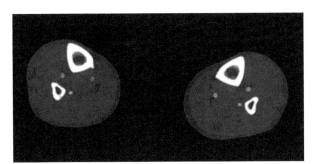

Figure 108-1. *Courtesy of Dr. Narasimham L. Dasika.*

Figure 108-2. *Courtesy of Dr. Narasimham L. Dasika.*

HISTORY: A 72-year-old male with diabetes mellitus presents with claudication.

1. Which of the following is the most likely diagnosis for the imaging findings presented?
   A. Tibial arterial atherosclerotic disease
   B. Acute lower-extremity arterial emboli
   C. Congenital absence of bilateral posterior arteries
   D. Deep venous thrombosis

2. When diagnosing this entity using computerized tomography angiography (CTA), what specifically can obscure the disease or its extent?
   A. Arrhythmia
   B. Adjacent soft tissue
   C. Calcification
   D. Breathing artifact

3. Which of the following is the main reason why endovascular or surgical treatments have a poorer response in patients with diabetic peripheral arterial disease?
   A. Worse inflow disease
   B. Worse outflow disease
   C. Poor endovascular tools
   D. Microvascular disease

4. In which of the following patients would pedal access be appropriately employed for revascularization?
   A. A 46-year-old female claudicant with short segment superficial femoral artery disease, ankle brachial index (ABI) 0.74
   B. A 54-year-old diabetic male with nonhealing great toe ulcer, ABI 0.3
   C. A 72-year-old male claudicant with popliteal artery disease, ABI 0.6
   D. All of the above

See Supplemental Figures section for additional figures and legends for this case.

CASE 108

Diabetes-Related Tibial Atherosclerosis

1. **A.** The popliteal artery generally bifurcates into the anterior tibial artery and the tibioperoneal trunk. The tibioperoneal trunk then gives rise to the peroneal artery and the posterior tibial artery. Acute lower extremity arterial emboli are exceedingly rare. The given images show the arterial anatomy, and so the diagnosis of deep venous thrombosis cannot be made. The images also demonstrate the extensive tibial artery calcifications seen on a spot radiograph during an intervention.

2. **C.** As seen in our case, calcifications can mimic endoluminal contrast, especially on three-dimensional reconstructed images. As such, the images may appear to show good flow even in the regions that are heavily calcified and occluded. Angiography as such remains the gold standard for evaluation.

3. **D.** Microvascular disease in diabetic patients is a complex process that includes autonomic nervous dysfunction, impaired inflammatory response, and impaired oxygen diffusion among other issues, all of which result in poor wound healing. These patients commonly have adequate inflow and outflow vessels and usually tibial disease.

4. **B.** Pedal access, although a very helpful access route, is usually reserved for use in patients with critical limb ischemia. It is commonly considered a salvage technique, as complications in a single tibial vessel could be devastating in a claudicant. However, many interventionalists are increasing their use and experience with pedal access and use it more frequently as sole access for infrapopliteal interventions.

Comment

Main Teaching Point

Although smoking, hypertension, and hyperlipidemia also promote atherosclerosis, a particular pattern of arterial involvement is often seen in patients with diabetes mellitus. The primary feature of this pattern is multifocal severe stenoses and/or occlusions of the distal popliteal artery, tibioperoneal trunk, and the proximal segments of the anterior tibial, posterior tibial, and peroneal arteries. This typical pattern of disease often occurs in the presence of normal or near-normal iliac and femoral arteries although diabetic patients are certainly prone to atherosclerotic lesions in the more proximal arteries. An interesting finding also seen in these patients is peroneal sparing. Many of these patients have CTA (if renal function allows), magnetic resonance angiogram, or angiography for evaluation of anatomy and potential treatment planning (Figures S108-1 through S108-4).

Disease Progression

The clinical manifestations of diabetic arteriopathy are often more severe than the angiogram might indicate, because of the presence of microvascular disease not appreciated on angiography. Because patients with diabetic neuropathy are prone to pedal trauma, the combination of arterial insufficiency and trauma leads to frequent ulceration with difficulty in healing.

Treatment Methods

Surgical arterial revascularization is commonly performed to help with ulcer healing in these patients. However, skilled interventionalists have had increasing success in treating these patients, especially with advanced techniques such as pedal access and subintimal arterial flossing with antegrade-retrograde intervention (Figures S108-5 and S108-6). Unfortunately, limb amputation owing to vascular insufficiency is a fairly common event in this patient subset.

References

Conte MS. Diabetic revascularization: endovascular versus open bypass—do we have the answer? *Semin Vasc Surg.* 2012;25:108–114.

Gibbons GW, Shaw PM. Diabetic vascular disease: characteristics of vascular disease unique to the diabetic patient. *Semin Vasc Surg.* 2012;25:89–92.

Pomposelli F. Arterial imaging in patients with lower extremity ischemia and diabetes mellitus. *J Vasc Surg.* 2010;52:81S–91S.

Sabri SS, Hendricks N, Stone J, et al. Retrograde pedal access technique for revascularization of infrainguinal arterial occlusive disease. *J Vasc Interv Radiol.* 2015;26:29–38.

Cross-reference

Vascular and Interventional Radiology: The Requisites, 2nd ed, 347–351.

CASE 109

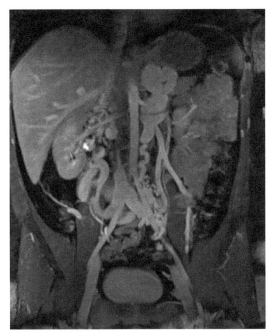

Figure 109-1. *Courtesy of Dr. Lucia Flors Blasco.*

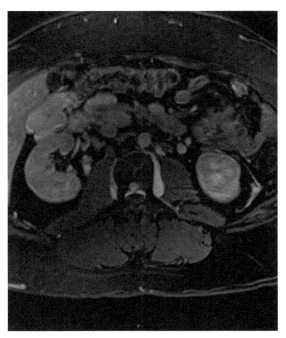

Figure 109-2. *Courtesy of Dr. Lucia Flors Blasco.*

HISTORY: A 28-year-old male with chronic low back pain.

1. Which of the following is the most likely diagnosis for the imaging findings presented?
   A. Duplicated inferior vena cava (IVC)
   B. Left-sided IVC
   C. Interruption of the intrahepatic IVC
   D. Chronic IVC occlusion

2. Which of the following imaging findings most likely indicates chronicity?
   A. Extension of the thrombosis from the iliofemoral veins
   B. Prominent retroperitoneal collaterals
   C. Enlargement of the IVC
   D. Presence of pulmonary embolism

3. Asymptomatic patients with chronic IVC occlusion are typically treated with:
   A. IVC stent
   B. Anticoagulation
   C. Lower-extremity compression
   D. Anticoagulation and lower-extremity compression stockings

4. Which of the following is the most appropriate endovascular therapy in patients with chronic IVC occlusion and severe symtpoms?
   A. Medical management
   B. Graded compression stockings
   C. Percutaneous balloon angioplasty alone
   D. Recanalization and stenting

See Supplemental Figures section for additional figures and legends for this case.

CASE 109

Chronic IVC Occlusion

1. **D.** Contrast-enhanced magnetic resonance images show occlusion of the juxtarenal and infrarenal IVC with extensive retroperitoneal collaterals. The intrahepatic IVC appears patent. No left-sided IVC is seen.

2. **B.** The visualization of a prominent collateral network usually indicates long-term occlusion.

3. **D.** Asymptomatic patients with chronic IVC occlusion are typically treated with anticoagulation and lower-extremity compression stockings.

4. **D.** In carefully selected patients with severe postthrombotic syndrome, endovascular therapy may be attempted, which consists of recanalization and stenting to re-establish flow.

Comment

Pathophysiology

The images demonstrate occlusion of the IVC with reconstitution of the intrahepatic segment and extensive collaterals from the lumbar venous plexus and azygos and hemiazygos system (Figures S109-1 through S109-3). The visualization of prominent collateral network indicates long-standing IVC occlusion. Occlusion of the IVC can be caused by extension of iliofemoral deep vein thrombosis, IVC filters, and abdominal masses. Congenital absence of infrarenal IVC with preservation of the suprarenal segment is extremely rare and it is thought to represent the sequela from intrauterine or perinatal thrombosis of the IVC rather that a truly congenital anomaly.

Patient Management

Patients with chronic IVC occlusion are typically treated with anticoagulation and lower-extremity compression stockings. Although this management is generally sufficient to prevent pulmonary embolism in all but a few cases, these patients tend to experience severe long-term postthrombotic syndrome which symptoms include chronic leg pain, swelling, redness, and ulcers. For this reason, in carefully selected patients with severe symptoms, endovascular therapy may be attempted. Endovascular therapy consists of recanalization and stenting with or without thrombolysis, as needed.

References

Bjarnason H. Tips and tricks for stenting the inferior vena cava. *Semin Vasc Surg.* 2013;26(1):29–34.

Kandpal H, Sharma R, Gamangatti S, Srivastava DN, Vashisht S. Imaging the inferior vena cava: a road less traveled. *RadioGraphics.* 2008;28:669–689.

Razavi MK, Hansch EC, Kee ST, et al. Chronically occluded inferior venae cavae: endovascular treatment. *Radiology.* 2000;214:133–138.

Cross-reference

Vascular and Interventional Radiology: The Requisites, 2nd ed, 293–296.

CASE 110

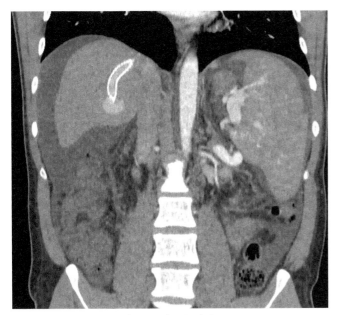

Figure 110-1. *Courtesy of Dr. Minhaj S. Khaja.*

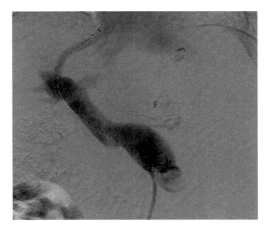

Figure 110-2. *Courtesy of Dr. Minhaj S. Khaja.*

HISTORY: A 45-year-old male with cirrhosis and portal hypertension status post transjugular intrahepatic portosystemic shunt (TIPS) and balloon-retrograde transvenous obliteration presents with persistently elevated portal pressures and ascites.

1. Which of the following would be included in the differential diagnosis for the imaging findings presented? (Choose all that apply.)
   A. Patent TIPS
   B. Splenomegaly
   C. Ascites
   D. Hepatocellular carcinoma (HCC)

2. Which of the following is an indication for partial splenic embolization (PSE)?
   A. Bleeding gastric varices in a cirrhotic patient with an in-stent TIPS stenosis
   B. Bleeding gastric varices in a cirrhotic patient with encephalopathy
   C. Hepatogenic ascites in a patient with cirrhosis without encephalopathy
   D. Hepatogenic ascites in a patient with a splenic to liver volume ratio of 0.2

3. Which of the following is true regarding PSE in the setting of portal hypertension?
   A. The success of PSE for treating bleeding esophageal varices is a direct result of the reduction of the portosystemic pressure gradient.
   B. It can effectively improve leukopenia.
   C. It can exacerbate thrombocytopenia.
   D. It cannot be used in the setting of sinistral portal hypertension.

4. Which of the following is a relative contraindication to PSE?
   A. Bleeding esophageal varices in cirrhotic patients
   B. Hepatopedal flow in the portal vein
   C. Hepatofugal flow in the portal vein
   D. Thrombosis of the superior mesenteric vein

See Supplemental Figures section for additional figures and legends for this case.

CASE 110

PSE in the Management of Portal Hypertension

1. **A, B, and C.** The images demonstrate a patent TIPS in a patient with splenomegaly and ascites. No evidence of HCC is seen on the provided images.

2. **B.** PSE can be employed for the treatment of various sequela of portal hypertension, such as gastric varices and hepatogenic ascites when TIPS is contraindicated and the spleen to liver volume ratio is 0.5 or greater. As such, the cirrhotic patient with bleeding esophageal varices in the setting of encephalopathy would be the best candidate. Additionally, PSE can be performed in patients who have had a TIPS with persistent splenomegaly and portal hypertension.

3. **B.** PSE can effectively improve leukopenia by increasing the life-cycle of white blood cells (WBCs). PSE can also decrease sequestration and improve thrombocytopenia caused by hypersplenism. The mechanism by which PSE is thought to treat varices is by altering flow within the varices, not by directly reducing portal pressures. Patients with sinistral portal hypertension may benefit more from PSE over TIPS.

4. **C.** Hepatofugal flow in the portal vein is considered a contraindication for PSE due to an increased risk of portal venous thrombosis.

Comment

Clinical Presentation

Clinically significant portal hypertension can manifest in many ways. The most common presentations include, but are not limited to, variceal hemorrhage, hepatogenic ascites, hydrothorax, and hypersplenism that can subsequently lead to significant anemia and thrombocytopenia. While TIPS placement is considered the treatment of choice for reducing portal pressures when medical therapy fails to control symptoms of portal hypertension, it is not indicated and successful as sole therapy for all patients. For example, patients with advanced liver dysfunction, encephalopathy, and those with portal vein thrombosis should not undergo a TIPS procedure. Further, if the underlying cause of variceal bleeding is secondary to sinistral portal hypertension (isolated splenic vein thrombosis, which usually occurs as a complication of pancreatitis), TIPS should not be performed as PSE artery or splenectomy may successfully treat this source of variceal bleeding.

Indication

The goal of PSE is to diminish inflow of blood into the portal vein that, in theory, would secondarily reduce the portal pressure. However, the changes in variceal flow, rather than changes in portal pressure, have been found to be more predictive of favorable outcomes and more likely account for the success of PSE in the setting of bleeding varices. PSE has also proven to be an effective treatment for hyperslenism-induced thrombocytopenia by reducing the size of the spleen and subsequently decreasing platelet sequestration. PSE can increase WBC counts in this patient population by increasing the overall WBC survival time. Additionally, recent studies have found that PSE has been helpful in treating patients with persistent ascites who have a widely patent TIPS, essentially splenomegaly with hyperdynamic portal hypertension (Figures S110-1 through S110-6).

Imaging Evaluation

Patients with a spleen-to-liver computed tomography (CT) volume ratio above 0.5 typically demonstrate a 20% decrease in portal pressures or more. Therefore a spleen-to-liver CT volume ratio above 0.5 is used as one inclusion criterion. Hepatofugal flow in the portal vein seen on Doppler ultrasound is considered a contraindication for PSE due to an increased risk of portal venous thrombosis.

References

Kirby JM, Cho KJ, Midia M. Image-guided intervention in management of complications of portal hypertension: more than TIPS for success. *Radiographics*. 2013;33:1473–1496.

Quintini C, D'Amico G, Brown C, et al. Splenic artery embolization for the treatment of refractory ascites after liver transplantation. *Liver Transpl*. 2011;17:668–673.

Smith M, Ray CE. Splenic artery embolization as an adjunctive procedure for portal hypertension. *Semin Intervent Rad*. 2012;29:135–139.

Cross-reference

Vascular and Interventional Radiology: The Requisites, 2nd ed, 326.

CASE 111

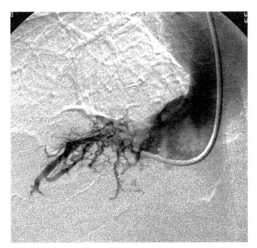

Figure 111-1. *Courtesy of Dr. Daniel Brown.*

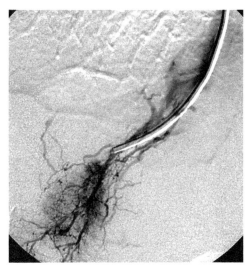

Figure 111-2. *Courtesy of Dr. Daniel Brown.*

HISTORY: A 48-year-old female taking oral contraceptives presents with vague abdominal pain and ascites.

1. Which of the following is the most likely diagnosis for the imaging findings presented?
   A. Primary sclerosing cholangitis
   B. Budd-Chiari syndrome (BCS)
   C. Cavernous transformation of the portal vein
   D. Cirrhosis

2. Which of the following imaging tests is the gold standard for diagnosis of this condition?
   A. Computed tomography (CT)
   B. Ultrasound
   C. Magnetic resonance imaging (MRI)
   D. Hepatic venography

3. Which of the following endovascular procedures is used in the management of this condition? (Select all that apply.)
   A. Balloon angioplasty and stenting
   B. Catheter-directed thrombolysis
   C. Transjugular intrahepatic portosystemic shunt (TIPS)
   D. Inferior vena cava (IVC) filter placement

4. With which of the following disease processes is this entity associated?
   A. Hypertension
   B. Congestive heart failure
   C. Hematologic disorders including polycythemia vera
   D. Hepatic metastases

See Supplemental Figures section for additional figures and legends for this case.

CASE 111

Budd-Chiari Syndrome

1. **B.** BCS refers to a group of disorders characterized by hepatic venous outflow obstruction, with hepatic venography classically demonstrating a complex spider-web-like network of collateral veins draining directly into the IVC. Cavernous transformation of the portal vein occurs as a result of portal vein thrombosis with the formation of venous collateral channels.

2. **D.** Hepatic venography allows for anatomic characterization of the venous outflow problem, hemodynamic information in the form of pressure measurements, histologic correlation via transjugular liver biopsy, and endovascular management.

3. **A, B, and C.** Balloon angioplasty and stenting may effectively treat isolated hepatic vein or IVC stenoses or occlusions, catheter-directed thrombolysis may effectively treat IVC thrombosis, and TIPS may effectively decompress the obstructed hepatic venous system if isolated hepatic vein or IVC interventions fail.

4. **C.** Approximately 75% of BCS patients have a hematologic disorder such as polycythemia vera or a thrombotic diathesis, such as pregnancy or inherited factor V Leiden mutation.

Comment

Clinical Presentation

Patients with BCS present with severe ascites (85% to 90% of patients), hepatosplenomegaly, abdominal pain, jaundice, vomiting, and lower extremity edema. If untreated, BCS patients develop progressive portal hypertension with esophageal variceal bleeding, encephalopathy, hepatic failure, and death. BCS can be caused by tumor invasion of the IVC or hepatic veins, membranous suprahepatic IVC obstruction, right atrial tumors, and hematologic disorders and thrombotic diatheses including myeloproliferative disorders such as polycythemia vera, pregnancy, postpartum state, oral contraceptive use, paroxysmal nocturnal hemoglobinuria, venoocclusive disease (in patients who have received chemotherapy and radiation), and heritable conditions such as factor V Leiden mutation.

Imaging Interpretation

CT and MRI findings in BCS include hepatomegaly, ascites, caudate lobe hypertrophy, inhomogeneous enhancement which is greater centrally, IVC compression, and nonvisualization of the hepatic veins. Duplex ultrasound can demonstrate hepatic vein flow to be absent, reversed, turbulent, or monophasic. Hepatic venography, the gold standard for diagnosis, can demonstrate webs, stenosis, or thrombus within the suprahepatic IVC or hepatic veins with abundant collaterals between the main hepatic veins (Figures S111-1 through S111-3).

Endovascular Management

Patients with BCS due to IVC or hepatic vein stenosis may be treated effectively with balloon angioplasty or stent placement (when stenosis recurs following angioplasty). Patients with IVC thrombosis may be treated with thrombolytic therapy. Patients with hepatic vein thrombosis have been successfully treated with TIPS, although this may be technically difficult to perform and the long-term results of this approaches are unknown (Figure S111-4). TIPS in these patients tend to be longer due to a hypertrophied caudate lobe and enlarged and congested liver parenchyma.

References

Brancatelli G, Vilgrain V, Federle MP, et al. Budd-Chiari syndrome: spectrum of imaging findings. *Am J Roentgenol*. 2007;188: W168–W176.

Cura M, Haskal Z, Lopera J. Diagnostic and interventional radiology for Budd-Chiari syndrome. *Radiographics*. 2009;29:669–681.

Ferral H, Behrens G, Lopera J. Budd-Chiari syndrome. *Am J Roentgenol*. 2012;199:737–745.

Mancuso A, Fung K, Mela M, et al. TIPS for acute and chronic Budd-Chiari syndrome: a single-centre experience. *J Hepatol*. 2003; 38:751–754.

Cross-reference

Vascular and Interventional Radiology: The Requisites, 2nd ed, 326–327.

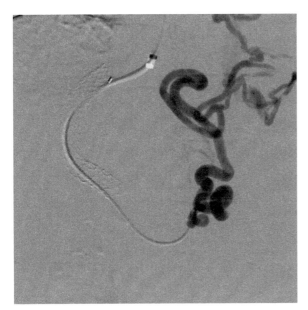

Figure 112-1. *Courtesy of Dr. Bill S. Majdalany.*

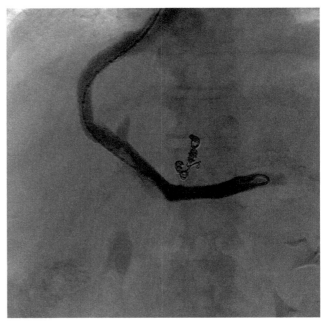

Figure 112-2. *Courtesy of Dr. Bill S. Majdalany.*

HISTORY: A 56-year-old male with presents bleeding esophageal varices.

1. Which of the following is the most likely diagnosis for the imaging findings presented?
   A. Cavernous transformation of the portal vein
   B. Esophageal varix after transjugular intrahepatic portosystemic shunt (TIPS) placement
   C. Contrast extravasation secondary to iatrogenic dissection/rupture during TIPS
   D. Hepatic arteriovenous malformation

2. In the setting of residual varices with a patent TIPS and a portosystemic pressure gradient (PSG) less than 12 mm Hg, what additional procedure may be performed as treatment of the varices?
   A. Additional stenting of the TIPS to further decrease the portosystemic gradient
   B. Infusion of nonselective beta blockers
   C. Embolization of the varices
   D. Surgical creation of a portocaval shunt

3. Which of the following are benefits of adjunctive embolotherapy of varices during TIPS?
   A. Decreased incidence of hepatic encephalopathy
   B. Decreased incidence of variceal rebleeding
   C. Decreased 6-month mortality
   D. Decreased incidence of shunt malfunction or failure

4. Which of the following statements is correct?
   A. Esophageal varices are more common than gastric varices and are associated with higher bleeding and mortality rates.
   B. Gastric varices are more common than esophageal varices and are associated with higher bleeding and mortality rates.
   C. Esophageal varices are less common than gastric varices and are associated with higher bleeding and mortality rates.
   D. Gastric varices are less common than esophageal varices and are associated with higher bleeding and mortality rates.

See Supplemental Figures section for additional figures and legends for this case.

CASE 112

Post-TIPS Variceal Embolization

1. **B.** Images are most representative of an esophageal varix that may persist status post-TIPS and that correlate with high risk of subsequent hemorrhage and mortality.

2. **C.** Embolization of the varices with metallic coils or sclerosing agents may be performed before or after TIPS as an adjunctive measure. Concurrent embolotherapy has been shown to decrease the rate of variceal rebleeding. Additional stenting of a TIPS with a PSG less than 12 mm Hg will not affect the varices. Nonselective beta-blockers are a prophylactic treatment shown to slow variceal growth and are not a definitive treatment of existing varices or variceal hemorrhage. Surgical creation of a portosystemic shunt is an alternative to TIPS, not an adjunctive treatment.

3. **B.** Recent studies have shown adjunctive variceal embolization to decrease rate of variceal rebleed and increase time between episodes of rebleeding. A meta-analysis found no significant difference between TIPS with or without adjunctive variceal embolization regarding shunt function, encephalopathy, or mortality.

4. **D.** Gastric varices are less common than esophageal varices, found in approximately 20% of patients with portal hypertension, whereas approximately 30% to 60% of patients with portal hypertension are found to have esophageal varices. Gastric varices are associated with more bleeding and higher mortality rates.

Comment

Main Teaching Point

The hemodynamic goal of TIPS is to achieve the optimal degree of reduction in the portosystemic gradient that will prevent variceal bleeding and ascites, but that will preserve hepatic perfusion (thereby preventing encephalopathy and liver failure). In most patients, reducing the portosystemic gradient to 8 to 12 mm Hg produces this effect. Likewise, in most patients, portal venography performed immediately after TIPS demonstrates markedly reduced filling of gastroesophageal varices compared to the pre-TIPS venogram. In a minority of patients, however, persistent variceal filling is observed (Figure S112-1). Visualizing the varices after the successful placement of a widely-patent TIPS is subjective, and there are no clear objective criteria as to which visualized varices need to be embolized.

Main Teaching Point

When persistent variceal filling is found post-TIPS, the presence of residual stenosis or thrombus within the TIPS tract or portal vein should first be sought and corrected by additional angioplasty. If variceal filling is still observed, or in select cases in which the patient is hemodynamically unstable due to variceal bleeding, the gastroesophageal varices can be selected from the portal venous system and percutaneously embolized using coils or sclerosant (Figure S112-2).

References

Chen S, Li X, Wei B, et al. Recurrent variceal bleeding and shunt patency: prospective randomized controlled trial of transjugular intrahepatic portosystemic shunt alone or combined with coronary vein embolization. *Radiology.* 2013;268:900–906.

Qi X, Liu L, Bai M, et al. Transjugular intrahepatic portosystemic shunt in combination with or without variceal embolization for the prevention of variceal rebleeding: a meta-analysis. *J Gastroenterol Hepatol.* 2014;29:688–696.

Tesdal K, Filser T, Weiss C, et al. Transjugular intrahepatic portosystemic shunts: adjunctive embolotherapy of gastroesophageal collateral vessels in the prevention of variceal rebleeding. *Radiology.* 2005;236:360–367.

Cross-reference

Vascular and Interventional Radiology: The Requisites, 2nd ed, 315–325.

Challenge

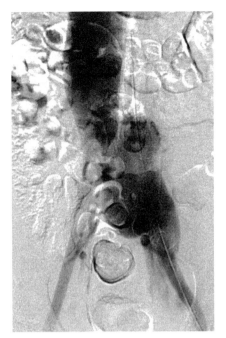

Figure 113-1

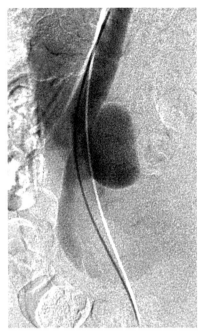

Figure 113-2

HISTORY: A 65-year-old smoker presenting with worsening dyspnea and abdominal pain. On exam, an abdominal bruit is detected and there is elevation of the jugular venous pressure.

1. Which of the following is the most likely diagnosis for the imaging findings presented?
   A. Contained rupture of aorta
   B. Arteriovenous fistula
   C. Mycotic aneurysm
   D. Aortoenteric fistula

2. Which of the following is the most common location of fistulous tract formation?
   A. Iliocaval
   B. Aortorenal
   C. Ilioiliac
   D. Aortocaval

3. All of the following statements regarding arteriovenous fistulas are considered true *EXCEPT*?
   A. Perioperative mortality for surgical treatment of arteriovenous fistula is equal to that of endovascular modalities.
   B. Etiology is usually congenital or a complication of trauma and surgery.
   C. Arteriovenous fistulas are more common in men.
   D. Incidence is rare, involving less than 1% of abdominal aortic aneurysms.

4. Which of the following is the most common complication of stent-graft placement in aortocaval fistula repair?
   A. Inferior vena cava (IVC) thrombosis
   B. Type II endoleak
   C. Graft thrombosis
   D. Persistent fistula

_____

See Supplemental Figures section for additional figures and legends for this case.

CASE 113

Aortocaval Fistula

1. **B.** The imaging demonstrates a fistulous tract between an aortic bifurcation pseudoaneurysm and the common iliac vein confluence. Computed tomography angiography is the primary modality utilized for initial diagnosis of arteriovenous fistula. Doppler sonography may demonstrate the presence of cardiac-phased high flow in the IVC. If these modalities fail, more invasive angiography and venography can be pursued. The other options listed do not have the imaging characteristics described.

2. **D.** Aortocaval is the most commonly encountered segment involved, representing the vast majority of arteriovenous fistula cases. Iliocaval, aortorenal, and ilioiliac fistulas have also been described in the literature, although they are considered more rare.

3. **A.** Compared to the complexity of open surgical repair, endovascular intervention is considered less invasive with less risk of major intraoperative hemorrhage. Perioperative mortality is documented as high as 30% in open surgical repair, markedly higher than the endovascular alternative. Though arteriovenous fistula is a rare complication of aortic aneurysm, it is more commonly observed in men and is usually congenital in etiology or a complication of trauma and surgery.

4. **B.** Type II endoleak is the most commonly reported complication of stent-graft placement and is characterized by perfusion of the residual aneurysmal sac via arterial branches arising from the excluded aortic segment. The other options have been documented but are not as common.

Comment

Clinical Presentation

Arteriovenous fistulas can occur as congenital abnormalities or as rare complications of trauma and surgery. Clinical manifestations can include high-output cardiac failure, ischemia distal to the fistula due to steal, dilated and enlarged peripheral veins, stasis dermatitis and ulceration due to increased venous pressure distal to the fistula, swelling of distal tissues, a palpable mass, an audible bruit, and a palpable thrill.

Imaging Interpretation

Angiography is useful to confirm the diagnosis of an arteriovenous fistula and delineate the anatomy, including the site of the fistula, its relationship to the involved vessels, and the presence of nearby branches that would confound endovascular repair (Figures S113-1 and S113-2). Large-volume injections in multiple projections with rapid filming are often necessary owing to the high flow volumes.

Treatment Methods

Depending upon the location of the fistula and the presence of regional side branches, stent-graft placement can be used to seal the defect in patients who are poor candidates for surgery on anatomic or medical grounds. Recent research indicates that endovascular modalities can provide a safer and more efficient alternative to open surgery.

References

Nakkad G, AbiChedid G, Osman R. Endovascular treatment of major abdominal arteriovenous fistulas: a systemic review. *Vasc Endovascular Surg.* 2014;48:388–395.

Parodi JC, Schonholz C, Ferreira LM, et al. Endovascular surgical treatment of traumatic arterial lesions. *Ann Vasc Surg.* 1999;13:121–129.

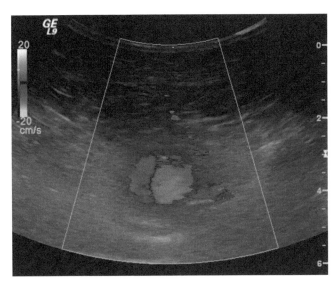

Figure 114-1. *Courtesy of Dr. Minhaj S. Khaja.*

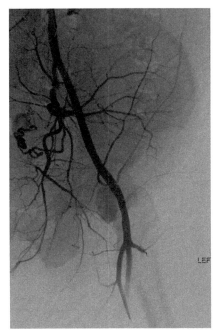

Figure 114-2. *Courtesy of Dr. Minhaj S. Khaja.*

HISTORY: A 48-year-old female, 2 weeks post cardiac catheterization, presents to the emergency department with a painful swollen lump over her left inguinal area.

1. Which of the following is the most likely diagnosis for the imaging findings presented?
   A. True aneurysm formation
   B. Arteriovenous fistula
   C. Access-site pseudoaneurysm
   D. Neoplastic lesion

2. What is the most common cause of the abnormality in the images presented?
   A. Trauma/iatrogenic
   B. Congenital wall defects
   C. Atherosclerosis
   D. Hypertension

3. What is the most common treatment option for the abnormality presented?
   A. Medical management and risk factor modifications
   B. Surgical repair
   C. Surveillance
   D. Interventions such as ultrasonography (US)-guided compression or thrombin injection

4. What differentiates a true aneurysm from a pseudoaneurysm?
   A. Location of the aneurysm
   B. Cause of the aneurysm
   C. Involvement of all three vessel wall layers
   D. Clinical sequelae of the aneurysm

See Supplemental Figures section for additional figures and legends for this case.

CASE 114

Complex Access-Site Pseudoaneurysm Management

1. **C.** The images show pseudoaneurysm formation at the proximal common femoral artery. The characteristics that allow for the identification of a pseudoaneurysm are to and fro flow within the lesion as well as the presence of a neck, which is the communication of the vessel lumen and the pseudoaneurysmal sac. A true aneurysm would not have a neck but instead would involve all three layers of the vessel wall.

2. **A.** The most common etiologies of access-site pseudoaneurysms include trauma and iatrogenic causes. These cause damage to the vessel wall leading to a false aneurysm that is contained within the vessel's adventitia. Congenital wall defects, atherosclerosis, and hypertension can lead to true aneurysm formation.

3. **D.** The most common treatment options for these abnormalities is now intervention, such as US-guided compression, thrombin injection, or, when necessary, covered stent placement. The gold standard treatment used to be open surgery with ligation, but this has since fallen out of favor in most institutions.

4. **C.** The differentiation between a pseudoaneurysm and a true aneurysm is the involvement of all three layers of the vascular wall (adventitia, media, and intima). A true aneurysm is a defect in all three layers while a pseudoaneurysm is contained within the adventitia.

Comment

Main Teaching Point

The images show a complex pseudoaneurysm following vascular access (Figures S114-1 through S114-3). As interventional procedures become more commonplace in medicine today, iatrogenic pseudoaneurysms continue to increase in both prevalence and incidence. These pseudoaneurysms classically present as a swollen, painful, and sometimes pulsatile mass. A common site is the inguinal fold due to this being a popular area for vascular access, but any vascular site can be involved. A pseudoaneurysm, or false aneurysm, is differentiated from a true aneurysm by the lack of involvement of all three vascular layers. In a pseudoaneurysm, the aneurysm is contained by the adventitia, and there is a direct communication between the arterial lumen and the aneurysmal sac. A true aneurysm is a protrusion or defect of all three arterial wall layers.

Treatment Options

Surgery used to be the gold standard for repair of these lesions, but less invasive procedures have become more popular for initial management. These procedures include US-guided compression in which the neck, or communication between the lumen and sac, is compressed and the aneurysm is clotted off; thrombin injection into the sac; and, when necessary, more complex interventions. Some pseudoaneurysms may be unsafe to inject as they have a wide neck or are difficult to directly access. As seen in this case, combination therapy with balloon occlusion of the neck with direct thrombin injection or covered stent placement may be helpful in more complex cases (Figures S114-4 and S114-5). If the patient fails initial intervention, complex techniques may be employed. However, surgical consultation is recommended in patients with pseudoaneurysms that cannot be safely managed percutaneously or in patients with large hematomas resulting in compression of the pelvic or thigh nerves.

References

Hendricks NH, Saad WE. Ultrasound-guided management of vascular access pseudoaneurysms. *Ultrasound Clin.* 2012;7:299–307.

Keeling AN, Mcgrath FP, Lee MJ. Interventional radiology in the diagnosis, management, and follow-up of pseudoaneurysms. *Cardiovasc Intervent Radiol.* 2009;32:2–18.

Cross-reference

Vascular and Interventional Radiology: The Requisites, 2nd ed, 356–357.

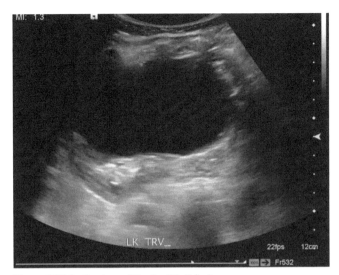

Figure 115-1. *Courtesy of Dr. Ranjith Vellody.*

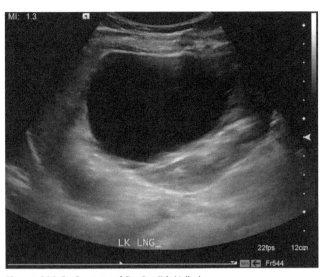

Figure 115-2. *Courtesy of Dr. Ranjith Vellody.*

HISTORY: A 7-year-old boy presents with left flank pain and hematuria after he fell from the monkey bars at school, landing on his back. An ultrasound was performed and revealed the following images.

1. Which of the following would be included in the differential diagnosis for the imaging findings presented? (Choose all that apply.)
   A. Isolated renal cyst
   B. Ureteropelvic junction obstruction
   C. Duplicated collecting system
   D. Cystic renal cell carcinoma

2. Which classification system may be used to guide management based on computed tomography (CT) characteristics of renal cysts?
   A. Wilms criteria
   B. Bosniak criteria
   C. RIFLE criteria
   D. Brodel's criteria

3. Which are potential manifestations of renal cysts? (Choose all that apply.)
   A. Hematuria
   B. Hypertension
   C. Renal insufficiency
   D. Abdominal, flank, or back pain

4. Which of the following is *NOT* an acceptable management option for symptomatic renal cysts?
   A. Open cyst unroofing
   B. Image-guided aspiration
   C. Image-guided percutaneous sclerotherapy
   D. Nonsteroidal anti-inflammatory drugs

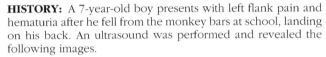

See Supplemental Figures section for additional figures and legends for this case.

CASE 115

Renal Cyst Sclerosis

1. **A, B, C, and D.** On the isolated ultrasound frames of the left kidney, a large, well-circumscribed, thin-walled anechoic structure is pictured within the renal parenchyma. Based on this single image, the differential remains broad and includes cystic lesions as well as entities leading to calyceal obstruction.

2. **B.** The Bosniak renal cyst classification system was created to help diagnose and guide management of cystic renal masses. Based upon morphologic and enhancement characteristics with CT scanning, cystic renal masses are placed into one of five different categories, with category I as the most benign.

3. **A, B, C, and D.** Although most benign renal cysts in children remain asymptomatic, manifestations such as gross or microscopic hematuria, proteinuria, pain, hypertension, renal insufficiency, and secondary infection have been reported.

4. **D.** Management of symptomatic renal cysts can be accomplished with several methods from simple aspiration to surgical excision. Image-guided aspiration with sclerotherapy is considered minimally invasive, safe, and low cost with favorable therapeutic outcomes. Ethanol is the most commonly used sclerosing agent for cyst ablation.

Comment

Main Teaching Point

The vast majority of simple renal cysts do not require any form of treatment; however, a small number of patients develop symptoms that are often associated with the presence of a large, dominant cyst. In these patients, several percutaneous treatment methods can be used. Renal cyst aspiration via image-guided percutaneous puncture may be performed. Many patients respond to this limited form of therapy, although, in a large percentage, symptoms recur. For this reason, sclerotherapy can be performed either as the first approach or after a trial of aspiration has failed.

Percutaneous Management

Under ultrasound and fluoroscopic guidance, a needle is positioned in the cyst and a drainage catheter is placed over a guide wire (Figures S115-1 through S115-4). The cyst is aspirated dry. Contrast is injected into the cyst to ensure that no communication is present with the renal collecting system and to define the volume of the cyst (Figure S115-5). The contrast is aspirated and is replaced with a smaller volume of sclerosant. Ethanol is the most commonly used sclerosing agent. Protocols vary, but in general the ethanol is allowed to dwell for 15 minutes as the patient periodically changes position. The sclerosant is then aspirated. This procedure may be repeated twice at the initial sitting. The catheter may be left to gravity drainage for a period of time following the procedure to increase cyst wall adherence. Follow-up imaging is commonly performed with ultrasound to document improvement or resolution (Figure S115-6).

References

Akinci D, Akhan O, Ozmen M, et al. Long-term results of single-session percutaneous drainage and ethanol sclerotherapy in simple renal cysts. *Eur J Radiol.* 2005;54:298–302.

Paananen I, Hellstrom P, Leinonen S, et al. Treatment of renal cysts with single-session percutaneous drainage and ethanol sclerotherapy: long-term outcome. *Urology.* 2001;57:30–33.

Skolarikos A, Laguna M, Rosette J. Conservative and radiological management of simple renal cysts: a comprehensive review. *BJU Int.* 2012;110:170–178.

Cross-reference

Vascular and Interventional Radiology: The Requisites, 2nd ed, 416.

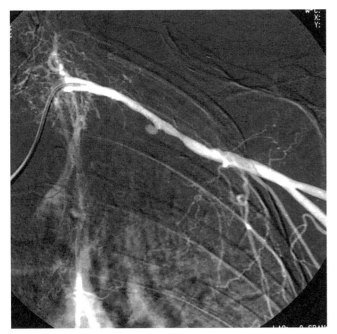

Figure 116-1

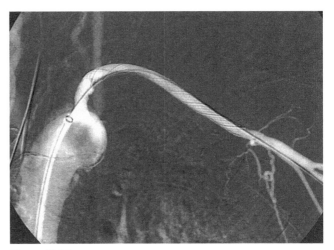

Figure 116-2

HISTORY: A 55-year-old patient with a history of metastatic nodal disease in the left axilla presents with enlarging hematoma.

1. Which of the following is the most likely diagnosis for the findings in the first image?
   A. Pseudoaneurysm
   B. Axillary artery dissection
   C. Axillary artery thrombus
   D. Arteriovenous (AV) fistula

2. What procedure precedes the second image?
   A. Axillary-carotid artery bypass
   B. Axillary artery stent-graft placement
   C. Axillary artery mechanical thrombectomy
   D. Surgical AV fistula repair

3. Which of the following is *LEAST* likely to be a direct complication of the procedure?
   A. Distal emboli
   B. Hematoma enlargement
   C. Pulmonary embolus
   D. Infection

4. Which of the following arteries usually arises from the axillary artery?
   A. Subscapular artery
   B. Thyrocervical trunk
   C. Dorsal scapular artery
   D. Costocervical trunk

See Supplemental Figures section for additional figures and legends for this case.

CASE 116

Axillary Artery Stent-Graft Placement

1. **A.** The given image of the left subclavian artery angiogram demonstrates a small outpouching from the subclavian-axillary artery junction representing a pseudoaneurysm. The metastatic nodal disease likely eroded the adjacent artery. No draining veins are seen to suggest a fistula. No filling defects are seen indicative of a thrombus. In the absence of a traumatic history or a flap, dissection is unlikely.

2. **B.** The second image demonstrates placement of a stent graft excluding the pseudoaneurysm. There is no evidence of a surgical fistula repair or a bypass formation.

3. **C.** Axillary artery stent-graft placement is a relatively uncommon procedure. The current literature details very few complications. However, similar to other endovascular stent placement procedures, hemorrhage and infection remain potential access-site risks. Additionally, in the event of a known plaque, distal emboli can also occur. Since the blood flow is toward the distal extremities, a pulmonary embolus as a direct result of this intervention is unlikely.

4. **A.** The thyrocervical trunk, costocervical trunk, and dorsal scapular artery most commonly arise from the subclavian artery before it continues as the axillary artery.

Comment

Main Teaching Point

Stent grafts are increasingly being used in the arterial and venous systems. The stent component of a stent graft enables enlargement of a vascular lumen and facilitates graft fixation. The graft component of the stent graft enables one to reline the interior of a vessel wall. Current applications for these devices include (1) atherosclerosis: the graft lining is thought to be associated with lower restenosis potential than bare stents; (2) peripheral aneurysms; (3) trauma-related vascular injury in patients with high surgical risk; and (4) AV fistulas and similar lesions. This technology often enables treatment of very difficult surgical problems in a minimally invasive manner.

Imaging Interpretation

In this case, hypervascularity is observed within the lower neck, consistent with the history of metastatic disease. A small pseudoaneurysm arises from the left subclavian-axillary artery junction (Figure S116-1). Given the patient's short life expectancy and the presence of a tumor in this area, surgical repair would be undesirable and may be impossible. For this reason, a stent graft was percutaneously inserted across the pseudoaneurysm, providing hemostasis (Figure S116-2).

References

Castelli P, Caronno R, Piffaretti G, et al. Endovascular repair of traumatic injuries of the subclavian and axillary arteries. *Injury*. 2005;36: 778–782.

DuBose JJ, Rajani R, Gilani R, et al. Endovascular management of axillo-subclavian arterial injury: a review of published literature. *Injury*. 2012;43:1785–1792.

Cross-reference

Vascular and Interventional Radiology: The Requisites, 2nd ed, 131–134.

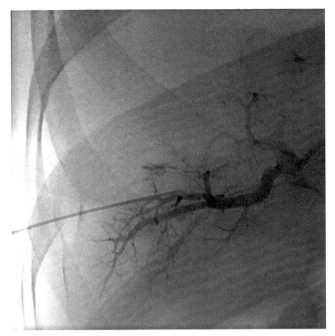

Figure 117-1. *Courtesy of Dr. Wael E. Saad.*

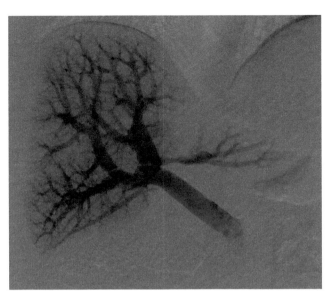

Figure 117-2. *Courtesy of Dr. Wael E. Saad.*

HISTORY: A 45-year-old man with a history of type 1 diabetes presents to interventional radiology.

1. The imaging provided demonstrates opacification of which hepatic system?
   A. Biliary tree
   B. Hepatic arteries
   C. Hepatic veins
   D. Portal veins

2. Which is *NOT* a potential reason for accessing this particular system?
   A. Portal vein embolization
   B. Islet cell transplantation
   C. Pressure measurement
   D. Balloon-occluded retrograde transvenous obliteration (BRTO) for gastric varices

3. What is the normal pressure range for this particular system?
   A. Less than 8 mm Hg
   B. 10 to 12 mm Hg
   C. 15 to 20 mm Hg
   D. 120/80 mm Hg

4. What is the projection that best delineates this vascular system within the liver?
   A. 35- to 45-degree right anterior oblique (RAO) with 10 degree cranial
   B. 20-degree RAO with 15-degree cranial
   C. 35- to 45-degree RAO with 10 degree caudal
   D. Anterior-posterior

See Supplemental Figures section for additional figures and legends for this case.

CASE 117

Portal Vein Access for Islet Cell Transplantation

1. **D.** These images demonstrate direct transhepatic access of the portal system. When obtaining portal venous access, the hepatic veins and biliary tree are commonly opacified.

2. **D.** BRTO generally involves obliteration/sclerosis of gastric varices through an acquired gastrorenal shunt via left renal vein, in a *retrograde* fashion. A balloon-occluded *antegrade* transvenous obliteration may be through a transjugular intra-hepatic portosystemic shunt (TIPS) or transhepatic access. The other three options could all involve direct portal access.

3. **B.** The normal portal pressure should be less than 8 mm Hg. Many clinicians, however, use a portosystemic gradient value of greater than 12 mm Hg at high risk for variceal hemorrhage.

4. **A.** This is the ideal projection that opens up the portal vein bifurcation. The other choices are incorrect.

Comment

Main Teaching Point

Direct portography via percutaneous catheter placement in the right portal vein for infusion of islet cells in a diabetic patient is depicted (Figures S117-1 through S117-3). This procedure is still experimental and involves harvesting islet cells from the pancreas of a deceased donor, direct transhepatic portal vein access, and transvenous administration with continuous pressure monitoring. Patients with elevated portal venous pressures are not candidates for the procedure.

Percutaneous Management

Direct portal vein access can be useful in a few additional clinical situations. When estimation of portal pressures is confounded by the presence of sinusoidal liver disease, a small catheter may be placed in the portal vein for direct pressure transduction. When transjugular portal vein access during TIPS is thought to be challenging, some physicians place a catheter within the right portal vein to provide a target for transhepatic puncture. In carefully selected patients, the percutaneous route may be used to clear thrombus from a thrombosed portal vein before placing a TIPS. Finally, portal vein embolization can be performed in a diseased liver lobe to allow hypertrophy of the remaining liver, such that a sufficient functional liver remnant will remain after hepatectomy.

References

Gaba RC, Garcia-Roca R, Oberholzer J. Pancreatic islet cell transplantation: an update for interventional radiologists. *J Vasc Interv Radiol.* 2012;23:583–594.

Goss JA, Soltes G, Goodpastor SE, et al. Pancreatic islet transplantation: the radiographic approach. *Transplantation.* 2003;76:199–203.

Lin J, Zhou KR, Chen ZW, et al. 3D contrast-enhanced MR portography and direct x-ray portography: a correlation study. *Eur Radiol.* 2003;12:1277–1285.

Cross-reference

Vascular and Interventional Radiology: The Requisites, 2nd ed, 314–315.

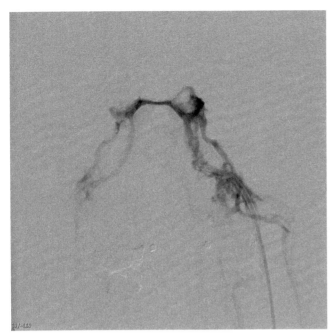

Figure 118-1. *Courtesy of Dr. J. Fritz Angle.*

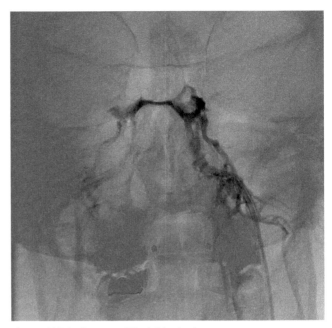

Figure 118-2. *Courtesy of Dr. J. Fritz Angle.*

HISTORY: A 40-year-old woman with central obesity, hypertension, skin thinning, and striae found to have hypercortisolemia presents for further evaluation.

1. Where are the catheter tips positioned in the images provided?
   A. Superior petrosal sinuses
   B. Cavernous sinuses
   C. Inferior petrosal sinuses (IPSs)
   D. Facial veins

2. Why was this examination performed?
   A. Preoperative venous mapping
   B. Adrenocorticotropic hormone (ACTH) venous sampling
   C. Cortisol venous sampling
   D. Manometry

3. Prophylactic administration of which medication is particularly important during catheter manipulation in patients with hypercortisolemia?
   A. Heparin
   B. Phentolamine
   C. Desmopressin
   D. Dexamethasone

4. The IPS receives tributaries draining all of the following *EXCEPT*:
   A. Medulla
   B. Pituitary
   C. Inferior cerebellum
   D. Midbrain

See Supplemental Figures section for additional figures and legends for this case.

CASE 118

Inferior Petrosal Sinus Sampling

1. **C.** The pituitary gland venous drainage begins with the hypophyseal veins, which subsequently drain into the cavernous sinuses, usually in a unilateral fashion. The IPS drains the cavernous sinus posteriorly, passes through the anterior portion of the jugular foramen, and empties into the internal jugular vein.

2. **B.** ACTH levels collected in both IPSs and in the periphery can be used to confirm and localize a hypersecretory pituitary adenoma.

3. **A.** Patients with hypercortisolemia are prone to thrombosis, and occasional thromboembolic events have been reported in inferior petrosal sinus sampling (IPSS). It is important to administer heparin once access has been obtained and prior to catheter manipulation of the internal jugular veins.

4. **D.** In addition, the IPS receives veins from the internal ear.

Comment

Main Teaching Point

Cushing syndrome is characterized by hypercortisolemia, most often due to exogenous glucocorticoid drugs. Uncommonly, Cushing syndrome may be caused by an ACTH-secreting pituitary adenoma, specifically referred to as Cushing disease. Localization of such adenomas using cross-sectional imaging remains difficult due to their small size.

Endovascular Management

IPSS is used to distinguish Cushing disease from an ectopic ACTH source. The procedure involves sampling of ACTH peripherally and from the bilateral IPSs. Access is typically obtained from a bilateral transfemoral venous approach. Administration of heparin prior to the remainder of the procedure is essential, given the hypercoagulable state of patients with Cushing disease. Angle-tipped catheters are advanced over guidewires and placed within the IPSs, bilaterally. Venography is gently performed from each catheter to confirm appropriate positioning within the IPS and reflux of control to the contralateral IPS (Figures S118-1 through S118-4). Samples are collected both before and after administering corticotropin-releasing hormone (CRH). Once sample results are obtained, the ratio of IPS to peripheral ACTH levels is measured. A baseline ratio of IPS to peripheral ACTH level greater than or equal to 2 or CRH-stimulated ratio of greater than or equal to 3 confirms the diagnosis. Sensitivity approaches 100% with CRH stimulation. Lateralization of the adenoma is often possible, as the pituitary venous drainage is primarily ipsilateral. When comparing samples from the bilateral IPSs, a ratio of greater than or equal to 1.4 is suggestive of ipsilateral location, with an accuracy ranging from 57% to 68%.

References

Deipolyi AR, Hirsch JA, Oklu R. Bilateral inferior petrosal sinus sampling. *J Neurointerv Surg.* 2012;4:215–218.

Potts MB, Shah JK, Molinaro AM, et al. Cavernous and inferior petrosal sinus sampling and dynamic magnetic resonance imaging in the preoperative evaluation of Cushing's disease. *J Neurooncol.* 2014;116:593–600.

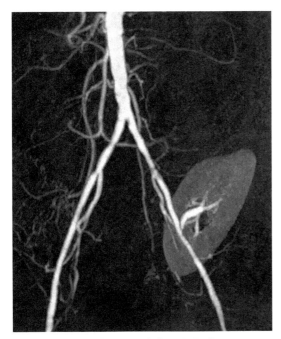

Figure 119-1. *Courtesy of Dr. Narasimham L. Dasika.*

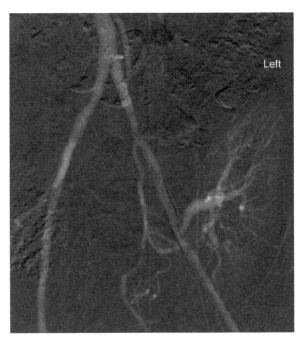

Figure 119-2. *Courtesy of Dr. Narasimham L. Dasika.*

HISTORY: A 71-year-old female with history of renal transplant presents with worsening renal function.

1. Which of the following is the most likely diagnosis for the imaging findings presented?
   A. Fibromuscular dysplasia
   B. Renal artery stenosis
   C. Renal artery aneurysm
   D. Renal artery dissection

2. Which of the following parameters is utilized in clinically suspecting the pathological entity in question?
   A. Blood urea nitrogen
   B. Platelet count
   C. Glomerular filtration rate (GFR)
   D. Renal blood flow

3. Which of the following noninvasive imaging modalities is *NOT* commonly utilized in diagnosing the pathological entity in question?
   A. Doppler ultrasound (DUS)
   B. Computed tomography (CT) angiogram
   C. Magnetic resonance imaging
   D. Radionuclide renal scans

4. What type of endovascular intervention is being shown in this case?
   A. Renal artery coil embolization
   B. Radiofrequency ablation
   C. Rheolytic renal thrombectomy
   D. Percutaneous transluminal angioplasty (PTA)

See Supplemental Figures section for additional figures and legends for this case.

CASE 119

Transplant Renal Artery Stenosis

1. **B.** The magnetic resonance angiography (MRA) image demonstrates a transplanted kidney in the left iliac fossa with a focal narrowing of the transplanted renal artery, specifically at the site of anastomosis between the donor renal artery and the recipient external iliac artery. The CO_2 angiogram confirms this finding.

2. **C.** Vascular complications in transplanted kidneys most commonly cause deterioration of renal function, decreased urine output, and hypertension. Creatinine and GFR are considered the best overall indices of renal function and degree of renal insufficiency.

3. **B.** CT angiogram has a negligible role in the workup of transplanted renal artery stenosis due to the use of iodinated intravenous contrast, which is particularly detrimental in the setting of renal insufficiency. All the other listed options are viable noninvasive diagnostic modalities.

4. **D.** Renal artery coil embolization is primarily used in the treatment of renal artery aneurysms. Radiofrequency ablation is used in the setting of a renal neoplasm or a failing transplant beyond repair. Rheolytic renal thrombectomy can be utilized in the treatment of renal artery thrombosis. The primary endovascular intervention of choice in managing transplanted renal artery stenosis is PTA with or without stent placement.

Comment

Main Teaching Point

Vascular complications after solid-organ transplantation are not an uncommon entity. These complications must be recognized in a timely manner in order to prevent graft dysfunction, and ultimately, graft loss. Most cases of transplant renal artery stenosis (TRAS) occur within the first 6 months of the posttransplant period. TRAS most commonly occurs at the anastomosis but can occur preanastomotic or postanastomotic in location as well.

Imaging Evaluation

The indications for vascular imaging of transplanted kidneys include deterioration of renal function (as evidenced by falling GFR and rising creatinine levels), decreasing urinary output, and new-onset or worsening hypertension. The noninvasive imaging modalities most frequently used in the evaluation of vascular and nonvascular complications after renal transplantation include the following: DUS, MRA, and radionuclide renal scans (Figure S119-1). The most common initial evaluation is with DUS, due to its vast availability and relatively low cost. Furthermore, the relatively superficial location of the transplanted kidney and its vasculature makes it an ideal candidate for effective and accurate sonographic evaluation. Given the advances in the technologies of DUS and magnetic resonance, nuclear studies are less commonly used in evaluating the vascular status of transplanted kidneys.

Endovascular Intervention

Catheter-based angiography remains the gold standard for the diagnosis of TRAS. CO_2 can be used in lieu of contrast dye in most cases (Figures S119-2 and S119-3). Additionally, endovascular management may include pressure measurements across the anastomosis and recipient artery. The primary endovascular intervention of choice in managing TRAS is PTA with or without stent placement (Figures S119-4 and S119-5).

References

Khaja MS, Matsumoto AH, Saad WE. Complications of transplantation. Part 1: renal transplants. *Cardiovasc Intervent Radiol.* 2014;37: 1137–1148.

Norton PT, DeAngelis GA, Ogur T, et al. Noninvasive vascular imaging in abdominal solid organ transplantation. *AJR Am J Roentgenol.* 2013;201:544–553.

Cross-reference

Vascular and Interventional Radiology: The Requisites, 2nd ed, 281–283.

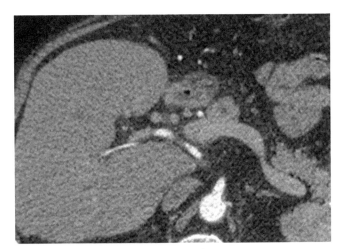

Figure 120-1. *Courtesy of Dr. Minhaj S. Khaja.*

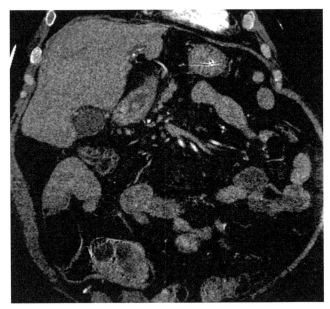

Figure 120-2. *Courtesy of Dr. Minhaj S. Khaja.*

HISTORY: A 60-year-old male presents with hematemesis and melena.

1. Which of the following is the most likely diagnosis for the imaging findings presented?
   A. Upper gastrointestinal (GI) bleed, duodenum
   B. Upper GI bleed, stomach
   C. Lower GI bleed, transverse colon
   D. Lower GI bleed, jejunum

2. What is the first-line therapy for the abnormality identified in the images above?
   A. Super-selective arteriography with embolization
   B. Endoscopy
   C. Conservative management with blood pressure control and proton pump inhibitor therapy
   D. Surgical intervention

3. What are the two most common causes of the problem shown above? (Select two.)
   A. Smoking
   B. Iatrogenic abdominal procedures
   C. Duodenal ulcer
   D. Pancreatitis

4. Which of the following arteries is *NOT* a collateral pathway between the celiac artery and superior mesenteric artery (SMA)?
   A. Pancreaticoduodenal arcade
   B. Gastroepiploic arteries
   C. Arc of Buhler
   D. Arc of Riolan

See Supplemental Figures section for additional figures and legends for this case.

CASE 120

Bleeding Duodenal Ulcer

1. **A.** The axial and coronal computed tomography images demonstrate a region of hyperdensity within the second portion of the duodenum.

2. **B.** The first-line therapy for any upper GI bleed is endoscopic investigation and therapy. If the bleeding is unable to be controlled by endoscopic means, then transcatheter arteriography and embolization are the next steps. Given that this patient has an active GI bleed, conservative management would not be recommended.

3. **C and D.** Pancreatitis and duodenal ulcers are the two most common causes of upper GI bleeding.

4. **D.** The arc of Riolan is a collateral pathway between the SMA and inferior mesenteric artery (IMA). The superior (gastroduodenal artery [GDA]) and inferior (SMA) pancreaticoduodenal arcade, right (GDA) and left (splenic) gastroepiploic arteries, and arc of Buhler are all collateral pathways between the celiac axis and SMA.

Comment

Main Teaching Point

Upper GI bleeding is typically initially evaluated and managed with endoscopy (Figures S120-3 and S120-4). However, when endoscopic therapy fails, angiography may be indicated. The GDA runs immediately behind the first part of the duodenum. Consequently, ulcers penetrating its posterior wall can cause life-threatening arterial bleeding into the GI tract. These may also be seen on computed tomography angiography (Figures S120-1 and S120-2).

Endovascular Management

Depending upon the endoscopically determined location of bleeding, patients with upper GI bleeding are evaluated with selective arteriography of either the celiac artery (most of the time) or SMA. The parent catheter or a microcatheter can then be used to subselect the bleeding artery. If contrast extravasation is observed, embolization is performed using either Gelfoam or coils (Figures S120-5 and S120-6). When using coils, it is important to be sure to embolize from distal to proximal to prevent backfilling of the ulcer from the gastroepiploic system (via the splenic artery) or the pancreaticoduodenal arcade (via the SMA). Given the intermittent nature of GI bleeding, if contrast extravasation cannot be confirmed, embolization of the GDA should still be performed if the endoscopic findings were clear or if the patient is unstable. Embolization therapy, while highly effective in producing initial cessation of bleeding and in stabilizing the patient, is less likely to provide a durable solution for large ulcers, and surgical therapy might ultimately be needed.

References

Ichiro I, Shushi H, Akihiko I, et al. Empiric transcatheter arterial embolization for massive bleeding from duodenal ulcers: efficacy and complications. *J Vasc Interv Radiol.* 2011;22:911–916.

Levkovitz Z, Cappell MS, Lookstein R, et al. Radiologic diagnosis and treatment of gastrointestinal hemorrhage and ischemia. *Med Clin North Am.* 2002;86:1357–1399.

Cross-reference

Vascular and Interventional Radiology: The Requisites, 2nd ed, 239–243.

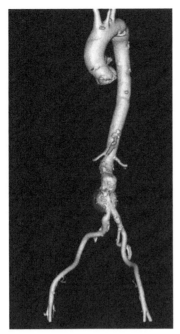

Figure 121-1. *Courtesy of Dr. John E. Rectenwald.*

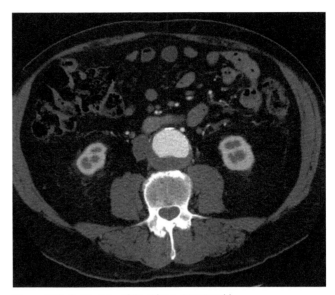

Figure 121-2. *Courtesy of Dr. John E. Rectenwald.*

HISTORY: A 68-year-old male presents with chronic abdominal and lower back pain.

1. Which of the following is the most likely diagnosis for the imaging findings presented?
   A. Infrarenal abdominal aortic aneurysm (AAA)
   B. Suprarenal AAA
   C. Abdominal aortic dissection
   D. Ruptured AAA

2. Follow-up computed tomography (CT) after endovascular aneurysm repair (EVAR) placement demonstrates contrast within the excluded aneurysm sac, apparently arising from the inferior mesenteric artery. Which type of endoleak does this likely represent?
   A. Type I
   B. Type II
   C. Type III
   D. Type IV

3. Which of the following is *NOT* an immediate procedure-related complication of EVAR?
   A. Iliac artery rupture
   B. Branch vessel occlusion
   C. Acute renal failure
   D. Aortic remodeling

4. Which of the following is an advantage of endovascular aortic repair versus open aortic repair?
   A. Decreased overall graft-related complications
   B. Decreased long-term mortality
   C. Decreased perioperative mortality
   D. No need for imaging follow-up

See Supplemental Figures section for additional figures and legends for this case.

CASE 121

Endoluminal Graft Repair of Abdominal Aortic Aneurysm

1. **A.** The images demonstrate endovascular repair of an infrarenal AAA. There is no evidence of suprarenal extension, dissection or rupture.

2. **B.** A type II endoleak is defined as aneurysm sac filling via a branch vessel. A type I endoleak is a leak at the endograft attachment site. A type III endoleak is caused by a defect in the graft, either by junctional separation or fractures/holes in the endograft material. A type IV leak is a leak through the graft fabric as a result of graft porosity.

3. **D.** All of the other choices are potential procedural-related complications, which may arise as part of the EVAR procedure. Aortic remodeling is not a complication but one of the goals of aneurysm exclusion.

4. **C.** EVAR has been shown to have a decreased rate of perioperative mortality compared to open aortic repair. However, there has been no proven difference in long-term morality between the treatments. EVAR has a higher rate of graft-related complications and requires follow-up CT imaging to evaluate for endoleak and aneurysm sac expansion.

Comment

Main Teaching Point

Endovascular repair (stent-graft placement) of AAA has been increasingly used since 1991. Endovascular repair of AAA is associated with reduced hospital stay, periprocedural morbidity, and need for blood transfusions compared with open repair. By enabling treatment of patients with significant comorbidities, this procedure has expanded the range of patients who can be offered aneurysm repair. However, strict anatomic criteria must be used to select appropriate candidates for this procedure. Computed tomography angiography is commonly obtained prior to intervention for sizing and planning the procedure (Figures S121-1 and S121-2).

Endovascular Management

Advances in device technology have made it technically feasible to perform the procedure through a percutaneous approach without the need for femoral artery cutdown. Fluoroscopic guidance is used throughout the procedure. An aortogram is performed (Figure S121-3). Over a stiff wire, a large delivery sheath is carefully advanced into the aorta and, following repeat angiography, the trunk component is deployed with its upper end just below the lowest renal artery origin (Figure S121-4). The contralateral limb is catheterized from the other femoral artery, and repeat angiography is performed to define the distal neck of the contralateral side. The contralateral component is then deployed, overlapping with the trunk component and expanded by angioplasty. Final angiography is performed to ensure that the graft limbs are patent, no endoleak is present, and all previously noted branch vessels are still patent (Figure S121-5). The groins are then closed surgically if femoral cutdown was performed, or they are closed by percutaneous arterial closure devices if the procedure was performed in a completely percutaneous manner. After the procedure, patients are followed diligently with CT angiography and abdominal x-rays to evaluate for endoleak and late endograft migration.

References

The United Kingdom EVAR Trial Investigators. Endovascular versus open repair of abdominal aortic aneurysm. *N Engl J Med.* 2010;362: 1863–1871.

Vandy F, Upchurch Jr. GR. Enodvascular aneurysm repair: current status. *Circ Cadiovasc Interv.* 2012;5:871–872.

Cross-reference

Vascular and Interventional Radiology: The Requisites, 2nd ed, 203–209.

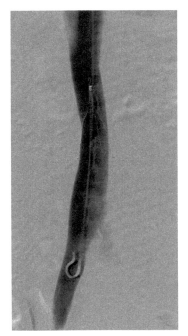

Figure 122-1. *Courtesy of Dr. Minhaj S. Khaja.*

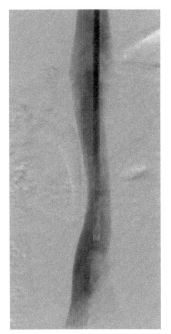

Figure 122-2. *Courtesy of Dr. Minhaj S. Khaja.*

HISTORY: A 52-year-old male with history of inferior vena cava (IVC) filter placed for PE risk presents for retrieval.

1. What procedure has been performed between the two images presented?
   A. IVC embolization
   B. IVC filter placement
   C. IVC filter retrieval
   D. Iliocaval stenting

2. Which of the following is *NOT* a risk factor for failed IVC filter retrieval?
   A. Age greater than 50 years
   B. Hook wall apposition
   C. Dwell time
   D. Gender

3. What is the major reason why IVC filter retrieval via routine techniques fails?
   A. Thrombosis of IVC filter
   B. Filter tilt with embedded hook
   C. Stenosis at filter placement
   D. Filter penetration

4. Which is *NOT* a major complication of temporary IVC filter placement after trauma?
   A. Adherence to wall of IVC
   B. Thrombosis occluding IVC filter
   C. Filter migration
   D. Displaced or tilted filter within IVC

See Supplemental Figures section for additional figures and legends for this case.

CASE 122

Inferior Vena Cava Filter Retrieval

1. **C.** The images show an inferior cavagram prior to and after IVC filter retrieval, respectively.

2. **D.** A recent retrospective study found that there are multiple risk factors for failed IVC filter retrieval including age greater than 50 years, hook wall apposition, and dwell time. However, gender, caval angulation, caval penetration, and insertion site were not associated with failed IVC filter retrieval.

3. **B.** Filter tilt with an embedded hook is a major reason why conventional retrieval methods of snaring the hook and sheathing the filter are unsuccessful. When this occurs, other advanced techniques of filter retrieval are required.

4. **C.** The major, long-term sequelae of temporary IVC filter placement are adherence to the wall of IVC, thrombus formation within the filter, and displaced filter within IVC. The risk of these complications in trauma patients increases greatly when temporary IVC filters are left in place for greater periods of time.

Comment

Main Teaching Point

The Gunther Tulip IVC filter was the first IVC filter designed specifically for retrieval, although there are now several other retrievable IVC filters including the Denali, Optease, Crux, and Option Elite, among others. Particular subsets of patients in whom these filters might be useful include trauma patients and postoperative patients who have a reason to be hypercoagulable for a defined period of time (e.g., patients undergoing orthopedic operations).

Endovascular Management

The images picture a Gunther Tulip filter, which is well positioned within the infrarenal IVC (Figure S122-1). This filter is retrievable by snaring the upper hook, provided no thrombus is present within the filter (Figures S122-3 and S122-4). Once the hook is snared, the sheath is advanced over the filter, which collapses the filter (Figure S122-5). Next, the filter is carefully removed through the sheath (Figure S122-6). A follow-up cavagram is performed to ensure no caval injury is present (Figure S122-2).

References

Al-Hakim R, Kee ST, Olinger K, et al. Inferior vena cava filter retrieval: effectiveness and complications of routine and advanced techniques. *J Vasc Interv Radiol.* 2014;25:933–939.
Avgerinos ED, Bath J, Stevens J, et al. Technical and patient-related characteristics associated with challenging retrieval of inferior vena cava filters. *Eur J Vasc Endovasc Surg.* 2013;46:353–359.
Smouse HB, Rosenthal D, Thuong VH, et al. Long-term retrieval success rate profile for the Gunter Tulip vena cava filter. *J Vasc Interv Radiol.* 2009;20:871–877.

Cross-reference

Vascular and Interventional Radiology: The Requisites, 2nd ed, 296–301.

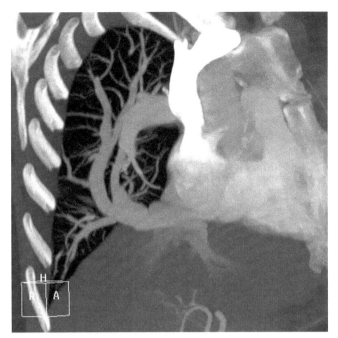

Figure 123-1. *Courtesy of Dr. Wael E. Saad.*

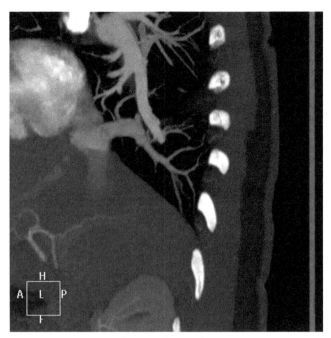

Figure 123-2. *Courtesy of Dr. Wael E. Saad.*

HISTORY: A 32-year-old male presents with shortness of breath.

1. Which of the following would be included in the differential diagnosis for the imaging findings presented? (Choose all that apply.)
   A. Atrial-septal defect (ASD)
   B. Total anomalous pulmonary venous return
   C. Partial anomalous pulmonary venous return (PAPVR)
   D. Ventricular-septal defect

2. What is the most common presentation of patients with this abnormality?
   A. Asymptomatic
   B. Cyanosis
   C. Chest pain
   D. Dyspnea on exertion

3. Which of the following is *NOT* a type of this abnormality?
   A. Supracardiac
   B. Infracardiac
   C. ASD-type
   D. Cardiac

4. Which scenario best describes the radiographic findings of scimitar syndrome?
   A. PAPVR from right upper lobe to the superior vena cava (SVC)
   B. PAPVR from left lower lobe to inferior vena cava
   C. PAPVR from right lower lobe to inferior vena cava
   D. PAPVR from right middle lobe to inferior vena cava

See Supplemental Figures section for additional figures and legends for this case.

CASE 123

Partial Anomalous Pulmonary Venous Return

1. **B and C.** The differential in this case shows pulmonary venous return from specific lobes of the lung returning to the inferior vena cava. Total anomalous venous return cannot be ruled out. Total anomalous venous return is much more likely to present early in life with cyanosis. The other two diagnoses would not show anomalous return from the pulmonary vasculature.

2. **A.** The most common presentation of patients with PAPVR is actually asymptomatic. Since there is less than 50% of the total blood flow not returning to the left-sided circulation, the patients have adequate oxygenated blood to distribute to the systemic circulation. The patients may, however, have significant shunt and may present with dyspnea, chest pain, or cyanosis, but these presentations are not very common.

3. **C.** The different subtypes of PAPVR include supracardiac, cardiac, and infracardiac, which are based upon the final anomalous venous drainage pathway.

4. **C.** Scimitar syndrome is partial anomalous venous return from the right lower lobe to the inferior cava and gains its name from the classic appearance on plain chest films. The other anomalies do not have classic appearances.

Comment

Main Teaching Point

The true incidence of PAPVR is difficult to determine because many patients are asymptomatic. Symptoms typically arise from associated congenital heart defects or from increased pulmonary flow and right heart volume overload resulting from left-to-right shunting. Symptoms are rarely seen when less than 50% of pulmonary venous blood returns to the right atrium. A number of congenital cardiac defects have been identified in association with PAPVR. The most common is an ASD, particularly when the PAPVR drains the right lung to the SVC. Other associated cardiac defects include ventricular-septal defect (VSD), tetralogy of Fallot, pulmonary valve atresia with VSD, aortic coarctation, common atrium, and single ventricle.

Classification

There are multiple forms of PAPVR: supracardiac, cardiac, infracardiac, and mixed type (Figures S123-1 through S123-5). The right lung is more commonly affected, and, rarely, both lungs are involved. The most common form of PAPVR is an anomalous connection between the right upper-lobe pulmonary vein and the SVC. PAPVR from the right lower-lobe pulmonary vein to the inferior vena cava is called scimitar syndrome because of its classic plain film appearance.

References

Dillman JR, Yarram SG, Hernandez RJ. Imaging of pulmonary venous development anomalies. *AJR Am J Roentgenol.* 2009;192:1272–1285.

Hong YK, Park YW, Ryu SJ, et al. Efficacy of MRI in complicated congenital heart disease with visceral heterotaxy syndrome. *J Comput Assist Tomogr.* 2000;24:671–682.

Cross-reference

Vascular and Interventional Radiology: The Requisites, 2nd ed, 159–164.

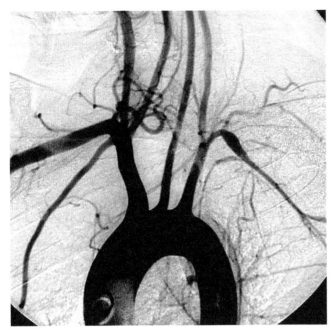

Figure 124-1. *Courtesy of Dr. Daniel Brown.*

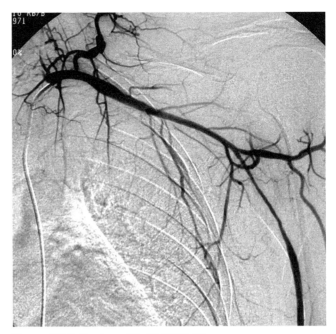

Figure 124-2. *Courtesy of Dr. Daniel Brown.*

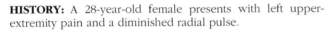

HISTORY: A 28-year-old female presents with left upper-extremity pain and a diminished radial pulse.

1. Which of the following would be included in the differential diagnosis for the imaging findings presented? (Choose all that apply.)
   A. Giant cell arteritis
   B. Atherosclerotic disease
   C. Traumatic vascular injury
   D. Takayasu's arteritis (TA)

2. Which of the following is the most common location of vascular involvement of this pathology?
   A. Pulmonary artery
   B. Descending thoracic aorta
   C. Renal artery
   D. Left subclavian artery

3. First-line therapy for active TA is which of the following medication?
   A. Methotrexate
   B. Corticosteroids
   C. Cyclophosphamide
   D. Azathioprine

4. In the consideration of endovascular intervention, which of the following is *TRUE*?
   A. Percutaneous transluminal angioplasty is the standard of therapy.
   B. Periprocedural anticoagulation is not warranted.
   C. Stent grafting is preferred over the utilization of uncovered metal stents.
   D. Endovascular intervention should ideally be considered for long-segment stenosis.

See Supplemental Figures section for additional figures and legends for this case.

CASE 124

Takayasu's Arteritis

1. **A, B, and D.** The images depict a long-segment stenosis of the left axillosubclavian artery, a characteristic appearance of TA. The left subclavian artery is most often affected, as demonstrated in this example with vessel wall thickening and resultant stenosis. Giant cell arteritis also represents a subset of granulomatous vasculitis and may be difficult to differentiate radiographically. Atherosclerotic stenosis may present similarly, though absence of calcified plaques and the clinical symptoms makes this diagnosis lower on the differential. No contrast extravasation is evident to indicate traumatic vascular injury.

2. **D.** Involvement of the aortic branch vessels and, more specifically, the left subclavian artery, is the most common manifestation of TA. Ostial stenosis and/or occlusion of the arch vessels can often be identified radiographically. Though involvement of the aorta, renal artery, and pulmonary arteries can occur, they are less common.

3. **B.** In the presence of active TA, high-dose prednisolone or its equivalent is considered standard initial therapy. Response to high-dose corticosteroids is often favorable, though immunosuppressive medications (i.e., methotrexate, cyclophosphamide, or azathioprine) can be considered in the setting of relapse or if corticosteroids are contraindicated. In cases of recalcitrant disease, studies have indicated the potential benefit of infliximab and other anti-TNF (tumor necrosis factor) agents.

4. **C.** Stent grafts are considered better options compared to uncovered metal stents in terms of patency and lower incidence of restenosis. Placement of stent grafts is thought to decrease luminal blood flow, resulting in decreased fibrotic changes and chronic inflammation that could end in restenosis. To decrease the occurrence of restenosis, antiplatelet therapy should be initiated before and after endovascular intervention. Percutaneous angioplasty is well suited for short-term relief of short-segment stenosis, though the higher incidence of restenosis makes this option less cost-effective and not ideal. In the case of long-term stenosis, surgical bypass is preferred over endovascular intervention.

Comment

Main Teaching Point

TA is a granulomatous vasculitis that primarily involves the thoracic and abdominal aorta and its large branch vessels. Because of infiltration of the adventitia with inflammatory cells, the luminal caliber of the vessel is compromised and fibrotic stenoses eventually develop. It is more common in women younger than 50 years. Patients characteristically have an elevated erythrocyte sedimentation rate, and approximately half exhibit constitutional symptoms in the acute inflammatory stage including myalgias, fatigue, low-grade fever, tachycardia, and pain adjacent to the inflamed arteries. Interestingly, there may be a 5-year to 20-year interval between the onset of acute inflammatory symptoms and the development of symptomatic arterial occlusive disease. Patients typically present with neurologic symptoms, history of stroke, or asymmetric arm blood pressure measurements and/or pulses.

Imaging Interpretation

Aortography typically shows smooth concentric narrowing of the aorta and/or branch vessel stenoses or occlusions (Figures -S124-1 and S124-2). In 75% of cases the aortic arch and branch vessels are affected. The left subclavian artery is most commonly affected (55%), followed in decreasing order of frequency by the right subclavian artery, left common carotid artery, and right common carotid artery.

Treatment Methods

The treatment of patients with TA is sometimes just as difficult as making the diagnosis. First-line therapy includes the use of high-dose corticosteroids and immunosuppression with agents such as methotrexate, azathioprine, and cyclophosphamide, among others. If patients are in the chronic phase, revascularization can be performed as needed. Studies have found that angioplasty alone has higher rates of re-stenoses. Other studies have found that stent grafts perform superiorly to bare metal stents in these patients. Surgical bypass is also an option for long regions of narrowing.

References

Keser G, Direskeneli H, Aksu K. Management of Takayasu arteritis: a systemic review. *Rheumatology.* 2014;53:793–801.

Qureshi MA, Martin Z, Greenberg RK. Endovascular management of patients with Takayasu arteritis: stents versus stent grafts. *Semin Vasc Surg.* 2011;24:44–52.

Weyand CM, Goronzy JJ. Medium- and large-vessel vasculitis. *N Engl J Med.* 2003;349:160–169.

Cross-reference

Vascular and Interventional Radiology: The Requisites, 2nd ed, 130–131.

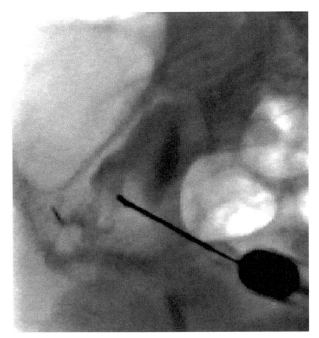

Figure 125-1. *Courtesy of Dr. Ranjith Vellody.*

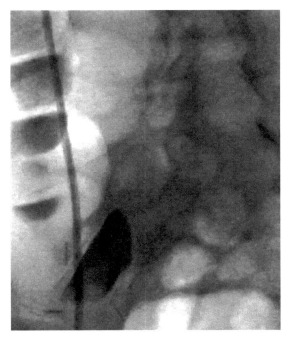

Figure 125-2. *Courtesy of Dr. Ranjith Vellody.*

HISTORY: An 8-year-old boy with history of chronic constipation has failed medical management and behavioral therapy. He is referred for procedural intervention for refractory chronic constipation.

1. Which of the following procedures was performed in the images presented?
   A. Ileostomy formation
   B. Gastrostomy tube placement for decompression
   C. Percutaneous abscess drainage
   D. Cecostomy tube placement

2. What is the most common cause of chronic constipation in the pediatric population?
   A. Hirschsprung disease
   B. Functional constipation
   C. Celiac disease
   D. Internal anal sphincter achalasia

3. Which of the following procedures is NOT appropriate to provide long-term improvement?
   A. Ileostomy or colostomy
   B. Decompressive colonoscopy
   C. Cecostomy
   D. Colonic resection

4. Trapdoor-type cecostomy catheters should be changed at what interval?
   A. Every 3 to 6 months
   B. Monthly
   C. Every 12 to 15 months
   D. Change tube only if malfunctioning

See Supplemental Figures section for additional figures and legends for this case.

CASE 125

Cecostomy Tube Placement

1. **D.** The fluoroscopic image shows percutaneous access of the cecum with a needle near a retention anchor suture with intraluminal contrast in the process of placing a cecostomy tube for antegrade continence enemas (ACE).

2. **B.** Functional constipation is the most common cause of chronic constipation in the pediatric population. The Rome III criteria are used to define functional constipation for those 4 years or older.

3. **B.** Patients with refractory constipation may be referred for procedural intervention. Viable options include a diversion procedure such as ileostomy or colostomy, cecostomy placement for ACE and, less commonly, colectomy. A decompressive colonoscopy would not provide long-term improvement.

4. **C.** The current approach to routine Chait Trapdoor Cecostomy (Cook Medical, Bloomington, IN) catheter exchange is to replace the catheter every 12 to 15 months. This interval has been shown to reduce pain and difficulty of changing catheters hardened with fecal residue.

Comment

Main Teaching Point

Chronic constipation is a common entity in the pediatric population, accounting for 25% of pediatric gastroenterology evaluations. The etiology may be from a variety of causes. The most common cause is functional constipation, which is defined by the Rome III criteria. The diagnostic evaluation may include such studies as anorectal manometry, sitz marker study, and defecography. Most cases are successfully managed with diet modifications and medications. For those with refractory constipation, surgical options may be considered.

Percutaneous Management

A percutaneous cecostomy tube provides a means to deliver antegrade enemas to evacuate the entire colon at regular controlled intervals. Preparation may include bowel prep and abdominal radiographs. Intravenous sedation or general anesthesia is typically required with antibiotic prophylaxis. Intravenous glucagon may also be considered for bowel paralysis. The colon is distended by using an insufflator through a rectal Foley catheter. The cecum is then punctured with a needle under fluoroscopic guidance. Intraluminal position is confirmed with contrast injection (Figure S125-1). Retention anchor sutures may be utilized to secure the cecum to the abdominal wall (Figure S125-2). For initial catheter insertion, a pigtail catheter may be used and eventually changed to a long-term low-profile catheter such as the Chait Trapdoor catheter (Figure S125-3).

References

Chait P, Shlomovitz E, Connolly B, et al. Percutaneous cecostomy: updates in technique and patient care. *Radiology.* 2003;227:246–250.

Christison-Lagay ER, Rodriguez L, Kurtz M, et al. Antegrade colonic enemas and intestinal diversion are highly effective in the management of children with intractable constipation. *J Pediatr Surg.* 2010;45:213–219.

Khan W, Satkunasingham J, Moineddin R, et al. The percutaneous cecostomy tube in the management of fecal incontinence in children. *J Vasc Interv Radiol.* 2015;26:189–195.

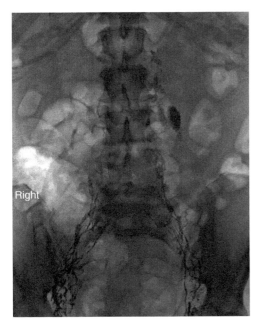

Figure 126-1 *Courtesy of Dr. Bill S. Majdalany.*

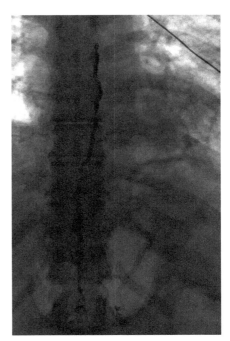

Figure 126-2 *Courtesy of Dr. Bill S. Majdalany.*

HISTORY: A 56-year-old female presents with recurrent pleural effusions.

1. What type of access is commonly used for the procedure presented in the images? (Choose all that apply.)
   A. Pedal
   B. Transhepatic
   C. Intranodal
   D. Endoscopic ultrasound guidance

2. What procedure is being performed here in Figure 126-2?
   A. Internal mammary artery embolization
   B. Thoracic duct embolization
   C. Esophageal variceal embolization
   D. Lumbar artery collateral embolization

3. What is one of the contraindications for the given procedure?
   A. Recent history of variceal bleeding
   B. Dialysis-dependent chronic kidney injury
   C. Recent myocardial infarction (MI)
   D. Pulmonary insufficiency

4. What is one of the hypothetical complications for the given procedure?
   A. Right-to-left shunt
   B. Spinal cord ischemia
   C. Pulmonary embolism
   D. Upper gastrointestinal bleed

See Supplemental Figures section for additional figures and legends for this case.

CASE 126

Lymphangiography

1. **A and C.** Image 126-1 shows contrast material outlining the bilateral inguinal lymph nodes during a lymphangiogram procedure. The pedal approach requires identifying lymphatic drainage under fluoroscopy after injection of dye (methylene blue or indigo carmine) subcutaneously. Alternatively, direct cannulation of an inguinal lymph node can also be performed using ultrasound.

2. **B.** Image 126-2 shows obliteration of the thoracic duct being performed for recurrent chylous perfusions. The other choices are incorrect as the first image clearly demonstrates the procedure being performed in the lymphatic system and not arterial.

3. **D.** Chronic lung disease remains one of the relative contraindications to the procedure due to the hypothetical risk of pulmonary embolism and subsequent pulmonary infarct, which can worsen the respiratory function. While iodinated contrast is indeed used for the procedure, further kidney damage would be meaningless in a patient already on dialysis. Recent MI or variceal bleeding does not significantly impact the outcome of the procedure.

4. **C.** The embolization agents used for thoracic duct embolization (mostly glue or coils) can enter the systemic circulation and lead to pulmonary embolism. Other more common complications are related to vascular access (hemorrhage, infection, etc.), inadvertent puncture of abdominal organs during the cannulation of cisterna chyli, or peripheral lower extremity lymphedema.

Comment

Main Teaching Point

The images here demonstrate an intranodal lymphangiogram followed by thoracic duct embolization (Figures S126-1 through S126-4). Lymphatic leakage and fistulae can occur secondary to many intrathoracic or intra-abdominal surgeries. Additionally, some patients also experience significant lymphedema after extensive lymph node dissection. For many of these patients, a lymphangiogram can be both diagnostic and even therapeutic. This is possibly secondary to lipiodol's inflammatory and granulomatous effects. A lymphangiogram will detect a cisterna chyli or an enlarged retroperitoneal lymph node, which can then be accessed under fluoroscopic guidance for thoracic duct cannulation. This will allow access for thoracic duct embolization, potentially reducing the chylous effusions.

Contraindications

Because these procedures are relatively infrequently performed, the contraindications and complications have yet to be fully examined. Some of the quoted contraindications include right-to-left cardiac shunt and pulmonary insufficiency. A right-to-left shunt may lead to accidental emboli of systemically absorbed embolization particles to end organs leading to infarcts. Pulmonary insufficiency can also be worsened since nontarget pulmonary embolization is a well-known complication. This can worsen the respiratory function.

Complications

Some of the known complications include access-site related complications (in particular infection or hemorrhage), nontarget embolization as noted above, lower-extremity lymphedema, or chronic diarrhea. Hypothetically, during the cisterna chyli access, one could also perforate visceral organs.

References

Kariya S, Komemushi A, Nakatani M, et al. Intranodal lymphangiogram: technical aspects and findings. *Cardiovasc Intervent Radiol.* 2014;37:1606–1610.

Lee EW, Shin JH, Ko HK, et al. Lymphangiography to treat postoperative lymphatic leakage: a technical review. *Korean J Radiol.* 2014;15:723–732.

Pamarthi V, Stecker MS, Schenker MP, et al. Thoracic duct embolization and disruption for treatment of chylous effusions: experience with 105 patients. *J Vasc Interv Radiol.* 2014;25:1398–1404.

Cross-reference

Vascular and Interventional Radiology: The Requisites, 2nd ed, 196–198.

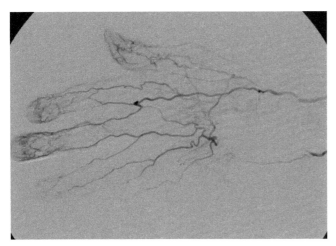

Figure 127-1

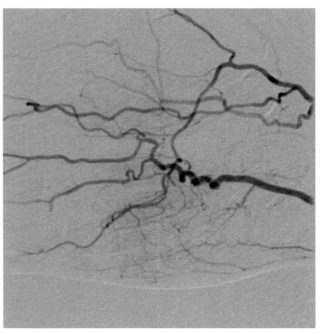

Figure 127-2

HISTORY: A 34-year-old male construction worker presents with sensitivity to cold, blue 4th and 5th digits, and pain in the medial wrist. His proximal vessels are widely patent without atherosclerotic disease.

1. Which of the following would be included in the differential diagnosis for the imaging findings presented? (Choose all that apply.)
   A. Raynaud's disease
   B. Arterial emboli from a cardiac source
   C. Hypothenar hammer syndrome
   D. Thromboangiitis obliterans

2. What anatomic location of the ulnar artery is thought to be most susceptible to injury?
   A. Division of brachial artery into ulnar and radial arteries
   B. Ulnar artery at Guyon's canal
   C. Dorsal carpal branch of ulnar artery
   D. Proximal superficial palmar arch

3. What is the gold standard for establishing the diagnosis of hypothenar hammer syndrome?
   A. Doppler ultrasonography
   B. Magnetic resonance angiography
   C. Computed tomography angiography
   D. Upper-extremity (UE) angiography

4. What is the initial management of patients with hypothenar hammer syndrome?
   A. Surgical resection and reconstruction of ulnar artery and palmar arch
   B. Conservative treatment including smoking cessation, avoidance of trauma, and cold
   C. Endovascular angioplasty and stent placement
   D. Antiplatelet therapy with sympathectomy

See Supplemental Figures section for additional figures and legends for this case.

CASE 127

Hypothenar Hammer Syndrome

1. **A, B, C, and D.** With DSA evidence of ulnar artery occlusion and a clinical history that includes symptoms such as cold, painful, or blanched digits, the differential diagnosis must include all of the choices provided. Raynaud's disease can involve the thumb and second digit, which differentiates it from hypothenar hammer syndrome. Thromboangiitis obliterans can involve both upper and lower extremities, the main symptom being pain, but ulcerations and gangrene in the extremities are also common complications.

2. **B.** The ulnar artery pathogenesis is related to the anatomy of the ulnar artery as it enters the palm. The ulnar artery crosses the surface of the hypothenar muscles for approximately 2 cm near Guyon's canal. Due to its superficial location this segment of the artery has a much higher susceptibility for damage. Repetitive trauma in these patients can result in aneurysm formation of the ulnar artery near the hamate bone.

3. **D.** UE angiography can provide the most information to support the diagnosis of hypothenar hammer syndrome. This information includes the location of vascular occlusion, the nature of the ulnar artery disturbance (vasospasm, thrombus, or aneurysm), and the evaluation of the presence of digital artery emboli. UE angiography can also define the anatomy of the palmar arch, which can be used if planning to intervene surgically.

4. **B.** Treatment for hypothenar hammer syndrome is controversial due to limited studies on this pathological condition, but most patients respond well to conservative and nonsurgical treatment options. In the setting of vasospasm with adequate collateral circulation, conservative options include smoking cessation, cold avoidance, avoidance of further trauma, calcium-channel blockers, or antiplatelet agents.

Comment

Clinical Presentation

Hypothenar hammer syndrome is an uncommon cause of digital ischemia that occurs as a result of repetitive blunt trauma or mechanical vibration or pressure to the wrist or palm. Typically it is the result of occupational trauma (e.g., jackhammer operators), and it can be seen in persons who practice martial arts. Lesser forms of trauma, including repetitive microtrauma in typists or pianists, can also lead to digital ischemia.

Imaging Interpretation

Chronic trauma produces spasm and intimal injury resulting in thrombosis and/or formation of a pseudoaneurysm. A pseudoaneurysm might serve as a source of emboli to the digital arteries. The ulnar artery is particularly vulnerable where it crosses the hamate bone and can be compressed. Angiographic features seen in the presence of hypothenar hammer syndrome include aneurysm formation, occlusion of the ulnar artery segment overlying the hook of the hamate, occluded digital arteries in an ulnar artery distribution, tortuosity of the ulnar artery with "corkscrew" appearance, and demonstration of intraluminal emboli at sites of digital obstruction (Figures S127-1 through S127-4). The degree of symptomatology depends upon vessel patency, the presence of emboli, and the degree of completeness of the palmar arch. Symptoms include evidence of digital ischemia, Raynaud's phenomenon, and/or a pulsatile mass.

References

Ablett C, Hackett L. Hypothenar hammer syndrome: case reports and brief review. *Clin Med Res.* 2008;6:3–8.

Bozlar U, Ogur T, Khaja M, et al. CT angiography of the upper extremity arterial system – part 2: clinical applications beyond trauma patients. *AJR Am J Roentgenol.* 2013;201:753–763.

Hui-Chou H, McClinton M. Current options for treatment of hypothenar hammer syndrome. *Hand Clin.* 2015;31:53–62.

Cross-reference

Vascular and Interventional Radiology: The Requisites, 2nd ed, 131–134.

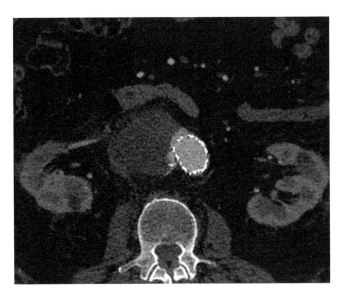

Figure 128-1. *Courtesy of Dr. Alan H. Matsumoto.*

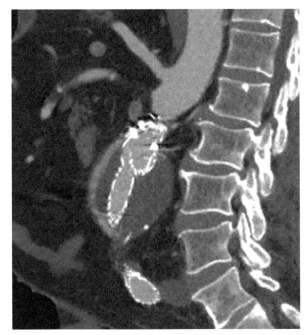

Figure 128-2. *Courtesy of Dr. Alan H. Matsumoto.*

HISTORY: A 57-year-old male with history of abdominal aortic aneurysm (AAA) status post endovascular aneurysm repair (EVAR) presents for follow-up imaging.

1. Which of the following would be included in the differential diagnosis for the imaging findings presented? (Choose all that apply.)
   A. Type I endoleak
   B. Type II endoleak
   C. AAA
   D. Aortic dissection

2. What are the key computed tomography imaging findings of a type I endoleak following EVAR?
   A. Opacification of excluded aortic branches with contrast material
   B. Presence of fracture of junctional separation of stent graft with enhancement of aneurysm sac
   C. Hyperdense collection continuous with proximal or distal stent attachment sites
   D. Focal areas of hyperattenuation extending beyond the expected contour of the aortic wall

3. The incidence of type I endoleak decreases with which of the following?
   A. Long, straight aneurysm neck
   B. Landing zone with calcification and thrombus
   C. Funnel neck (uneven size)
   D. Tortuous aorta

4. What intervention is recommended for confirmed type I endoleak?
   A. Continued surveillance with computed tomography angiography (CTA) every 6 months
   B. Immediate conversion to open repair
   C. Coil embolization of aneurysmal sac
   D. Re-ballooning of attachment sites or placement of additional aortic cuffs/stents

See Supplemental Figures section for additional figures and legends for this case.

CASE 128

Type I Endoleak

1. **A, B, and C.** Given the imaging findings, the differential diagnosis must include endoleak following EVAR and AAA. Specific imaging findings that support type I endoleak include early-phase contrast enhancement at the proximal (type IA) and/or distal (type IB) ends of the stent-graft.

2. **C.** A Type I endoleak results from an incompetent seal at the proximal or distal attachment sites of the stent graft. On CTA, opacification at proximal or distal ends of the stent graft is seen. It is important to have noncontrast, contrast-enhanced, and delayed images to evaluate the endoleak.

3. **A.** Short, angulated necks as well as the other options increase the risk of type I endoleak as the endograft may not fully appose the aortic wall at the seal zone. A straight, long neck would improve the chances of an appropriate seal.

4. **D.** A type I endoleak is considered a high-pressure leak due to aneurysm sac exposure to systemic blood pressure. Following discovery, type I endoleaks are primarily treated endovascularly, but an operation may be needed in some cases.

Comment

Main Teaching Point

An endoleak is defined as the persistence of blood flow outside the graft within the aneurysm sac following endoluminal repair and is the most common complication of EVAR. An aneurysm sac that is completely excluded from flow typically thromboses and often shrinks in diameter. The presence of perigraft flow leaves the aneurysm at risk for enlargement and/or rupture. Patients should be followed with surveillance imaging to assess for endoleaks, aneurysm sac enlargement, or other device complications. Imaging modalities commonly used are CTA, magnetic resonance imaging, and Doppler sonography (Figures S128-1 and S128-2). Aortography is commonly only employed for confirmation of endoleak and subsequent intervention.

Classification

Endoleaks are classified by type. Type I endoleaks result from flow around the ends of the endograft and are subdivided into type IA (proximal attachment site leak) and IB (distal attachment site leak). These endoleaks require urgent therapy. Type II endoleaks are the most common and result from retrograde arterial flow into the aneurysm sac from patent aortic side branches (typically lumbar, sacral, gonadal, accessory renal, or inferior mesenteric artery branches). The criteria upon which to base treatment of type II endoleaks are controversial. Some physicians treat all type II leaks via side-branch embolization or embolization of the aneurysm sac, and others believe that watchful waiting is sufficient provided the aneurysm is not enlarging. Type III endoleaks are rare and result from tears in the graft fabric or separation of graft components. Type IV endoleaks represent leakage of contrast due to porosity of the graft fabric material. Type V endoleaks are also referred to as endotension. Endotension is defined as pressure within the aneurysm sac without evidence of endoleak. Although uncommon, endotension is seen in 2% to 5% of patients following EVAR.

Treatment Methods

Type I endoleaks are commonly treated by re-ballooning of the proximal and/or distal fixation sites of the previously placed aortic graft. If persistent, aortic cuffs or stents, or extensions can be used (Figures S128-3 and S128-4). Newer methods of treatment include catheter-direct embolization of the leak or fixation with anchors (Figures S128-5 and S128-6). If refractory to endovascular options, open surgery can be performed.

References

Adams JD, Tracci MC, Sabri S, et al. Real-world experience with type I endoleaks after endovascular repair of the thoracic aorta. *Am Surg.* 2010;76:599–605.

Picel AC, Kansal N. Essentials of endovascular abdominal aortic aneurysm repair imaging: postprocedure surveillance and complications. *AJR Am J Roentgenol.* 2014;203:358–372.

White S, Stavropoulos S. Management of endoleaks following endovascular aneurysm repair. *Semin Intervent Radiol.* 2009;26:33–38.

Cross-reference

Vascular and Interventional Radiology: The Requisites, 2nd ed, 209–214.

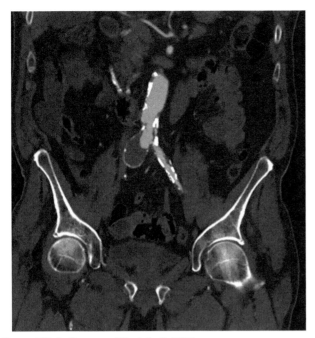

Figure 129-1. *Courtesy of Dr. Luke R. Wilkins.*

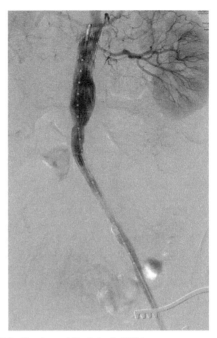

Figure 129-2. *Courtesy of Dr. Luke R. Wilkins.*

HISTORY: A 57-year-old male with a history of hypertension, diabetes, and coronary artery disease was found to have an abdominal aortic aneurysm (AAA) on recent computed tomography.

1. What procedure was formed based on the imaging findings presented?
   A. Endovascular repair of AAA with an aortouniiliac endograft
   B. Endovascular repair of AAA with a bifurcated aortic endograft
   C. Open repair of AAA with an aortouniiliac endograft
   D. Open repair of AAA with a bifurcated aortic endograft

2. What are the indications for placement of an aortouniiliac endograft? (Choose all that apply.)
   A. Complete occlusion of an iliac artery
   B. Severe tortuosity of the iliac artery on one side that precludes placement of a bifurcated aortic endograft
   C. Very small caliber of the distal aorta
   D. Severe unilateral iliac disease with calcifications and/or a stenotic lumen

3. What is the purpose of occluding the contralateral iliac artery?
   A. To increase flow through the endograft
   B. To prevent a retrograde endoleak
   C. To increase flow through the femorofemoral bypass graft
   D. To prevent turbulent flow

4. What adjunctive operation needs to be performed after endograft placement?
   A. Iliac stent placement
   B. Femorofemoral bypass
   C. Proximal extension cuff placement
   D. Angioplasty

See Supplemental Figures section for additional figures and legends for this case.

CASE 129

Aortouniiliac Endograft with Femorofemoral Bypass

1. **A.** The images demonstrate endovascular repair of an AAA with an aortouniiliac endograft.

2. **A, B, C, and D.** In all of these situations an aortouniiliac endograft would be the preferred treatment for aortic aneurysmal disease over a traditional bifurcated device due to the described technical challenges.

3. **B.** Occlusion of the contralateral iliac artery serves to prevent blood flow from recirculating and creating an endoleak following endograft placement. Additionally, occluding the contralateral iliac artery may be necessary if no seal zone is possible for a bifurcated endograft.

4. **B.** A femorofemoral bypass graft must be placed following aortouniiliac endograft placement to provide inflow to bilateral lower extremities. The other choices are potential secondary procedures that may be performed if needed but are not required adjuncts. An iliac stent may be placed in the event of significant stenosis. The proximal end of the endograft may need to be extended with a cuff if there is an endoleak, and angioplasty may be performed to relieve any stenosis within the endograft or femorofemoral bypass graft.

Comment

Main Teaching Point

AAAs have been treated endovascularly with the use of a bifurcated aortic stent graft that contains distal limbs that pass into each common iliac artery. Some patients are not suitable candidates for such a device due to their anatomy or vascular disease, particularly one common iliac artery. An iliac artery that is completely occluded or contains calcifications or severe atherosclerotic disease may make it very difficult to access and deploy a limb of an endograft or its extension (Figures S129-1 and S129-2). The same applies for very tortuous common iliac vessels. An aortouniiliac endograft has provided a solution for such patients by stenting the aneurysm from the abdominal aorta into one common iliac artery. Branch vessels may be purposefully occluded during the procedure by embolization to prevent endoleak (Figures S129-3 and S129-4). Finally, a femorofemoral bypass graft is created to allow blood flow to bilateral lower extremities (Figure S129-5). Recent studies have shown this to be a safe and effective alternative treatment with good patency rates and low complications.

References

Dortch JD, Oldenburg WA, Farres H, et al. Long-term results of aortouniiliac stent grafts for the endovascular repair of abdominal aortic aneurysms. *Ann Vasc Surg.* 2014;28:1258–1265.

Heredero AF, Stefanov S, Riera del Moral L, et al. Long-term results of femoro-femoral crossover bypass after endovascular aortouniiliac repair of abdominal aortic and aortoiliac aneurysms. *Vasc Endovascular Surg.* 2008;42:420–426.

Cross-reference

Vascular and Interventional Radiology: The Requisites, 2nd ed, 203–214.

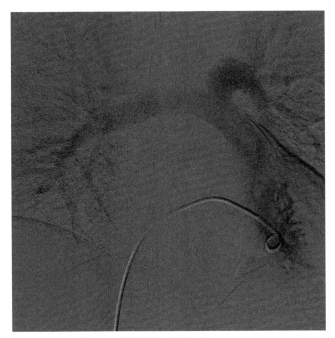

Figure 130-1. *Courtesy of Dr. Wael E. Saad.*

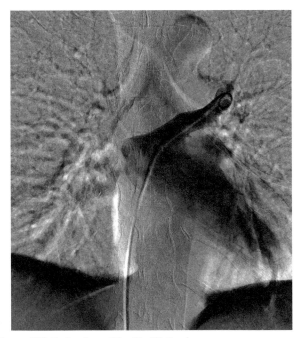

Figure 130-2. *Courtesy of Dr. Wael E. Saad.*

HISTORY: A 42-year-old woman with shortness of breath was referred for pulmonary angiography.

1. Which of the following is the most likely diagnosis for the imaging findings presented?
   A. Patent foramen ovale
   B. Patent ductus arteriosus
   C. Ventricular septal defect
   D. Partial anomalous pulmonary venous return

2. Where is the catheter tip located in the second image?
   A. Left upper lobe pulmonary artery
   B. Main pulmonary artery
   C. Left pulmonary artery
   D. Left superior pulmonary vein

3. If the catheter does not easily advance into the right ventricle during pulmonary angiography, it may have entered the:
   A. Pericardial space
   B. Inferior vena cava
   C. Right coronary artery
   D. Coronary sinus

4. During test injection into the pulmonary arteries, slow flow and delayed washout of contrast are visualized. How should the contrast injection be adjusted?
   A. Increase rate and volume.
   B. No change to the standard injection rate and volume is needed.
   C. Decrease rate and volume.
   D. Increase rate, and keep the volume the same.

See Supplemental Figures section for additional figures and legends for this case.

CASE 130

Patent Foramen Ovale

1. **A.** The catheter takes a transseptal course through a patent foramen ovale, through the left atrium, and into the left superior pulmonary vein. The ductus arteriosus is a connection between the aorta and pulmonary arterial system in the fetal circulation. A patent ductus arteriosus may be seen in patients with severe structural heart disease where it is required for oxygenation.

2. **D.** The catheter tip is positioned in the left superior pulmonary vein; however, it is in the expected location of the left pulmonary artery on fluoroscopy. Contrast injection shows opacification of the vein and flow of contrast into the left heart. Additional images demonstrate flow within the aorta.

3. **D.** Some resistance to forward catheter advancement into the right ventricle may suggest placement in the coronary sinus. Gentle contrast injection can confirm the location. The coronary sinus drains blood from the left ventricular tissue into the right atrium.

4. **C.** Slow flow and delayed washout of contrast in the pulmonary arteries suggest uncompensated pulmonary hypertension. The volume and rate of contrast injection should be decreased to avoid acute right heart failure.

Comment

Main Teaching Point

The foramen ovale remains patent in an estimated 22% to 38% of the population. Patent foramen ovalia have been implicated in paradoxical embolism and ischemic stroke. When right atrial pressure exceeds left atrial pressure, a right-to-left shunt can develop. In the basal state, the left atrial pressure is higher than the right atrial pressure. However, when a patient coughs or takes a deep breath, venous blood return to the right atrium increases, theoretically allowing venous thromboemboli to bypass the lungs and enter the systemic circulation. Pulmonary hypertension can also increase right atrial pressure and result in right-to-left shunting.

Imaging Interpretation

In the images above, pulmonary angiography was performed (Figures S130-1 through S130-5). During attempted selection of the left pulmonary artery, the catheter takes a course consistent with the left pulmonary artery (Figure S130-4). However, after injection of contrast, it was revealed that the catheter actually took an unexpected course through a patent foramen ovale in the atrial septum, through the left atrium, and into the left superior pulmonary vein (Figure S130-2). Contrast injection confirms the location with progressive filling of the left atrium, left ventricle, and thoracic aorta (Figure S130-3). An important lesson from this case is to perform a test injection in order to confirm the true location of your catheter prior to a power injected angiographic run. Additionally, it is important to be very careful to ensure there are no bubbles within your tubing or catheter whenever performing angiography, but especially when above the diaphragm to minimize the risk of embolization to the brain.

References

Reilly BK, Friedman A, Nasrallah EJ, et al. Bihemispheric stroke complicating right pulmonary angiography. *J Vasc Interv Radiol.* 2003;14:1211–1213.

Tobis J, Shenoda M. Percutaneous treatment of patent foramen ovale and atrial septal defects. *J Am Coll Cardiol.* 2012;60:1722–1732.

Cross-reference

Vascular and Interventional Radiology: The Requisites, 2nd ed, 159–164.

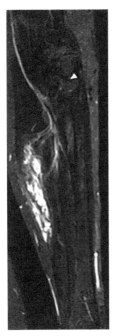

Figure 131-1. *Courtesy of Dr. Auh Whan Park.*

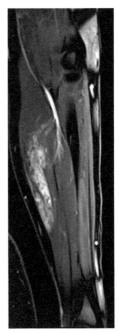

Figure 131-2. *Courtesy of Dr. Auh Whan Park.*

HISTORY: A 24-year-old female presents with left arm pain and swelling.

1. Which of the following would be included in the differential diagnosis for the imaging findings presented? (Choose all that apply.)
   A. Lymphatic malformation
   B. Intramuscular myxoma
   C. Venous malformation
   D. Infantile hemangioma

2. Of the following, which is the *LEAST* characteristic imaging feature of venous malformations?
   A. Punctate internal calcifications
   B. Tangle of serpentine channels
   C. Extension and involvement of bone
   D. Slow vascular flow

3. What is the initial therapeutic consideration in the management of this patient?
   A. Elastic compression garments
   B. Aspirin therapy
   C. Immediate surgical resection
   D. Percutaneous sclerotherapy

4. Which of the following is *NOT* considered an associated abnormality of venous malformations?
   A. Hemangiopericytoma
   B. Maffucci syndrome
   C. Klippel-Trenaunay syndrome
   D. Blue rubber bleb nevus syndrome

See Supplemental Figures section for additional figures and legends for this case.

CASE 131

Venous Malformation

1. **A, C, and D.** The images demonstrate a conglomerate of T2-hyperintense serpentine venous channels with diffuse contrast enhancement on magnetic resonance (MR), compatible with this patient's diagnosis of venous malformation. Differential consideration includes infantile hemangioma, lymphatic malformation, and arteriovenous malformation. Unlike infantile hemangiomas, venous malformations do not involute over time. Intramuscular myxomas are benign, soft-tissue neoplasms with prominent myxoid stroma, typically occurring in older patients.

2. **C.** Venous malformations present as a tangle of T2-hyperintense serpentine venous channels that enhance on postcontrast MR. Calcified phleboliths can be incidentally identified on radiography, MR, or ultrasound. Monophasic, slow waveforms are detected if evaluated by Doppler ultrasound. Involvement of bone is uncommon, however.

3. **B.** Initiation of aspirin therapy should be considered in the initial management of these patients to prevent thrombosis in the setting of venous stasis. Elastic compression garments can be considered prior to more definitive treatment, including percutaneous sclerotherapy or surgical resection.

4. **A.** Hemangiopericytomas are vascular tumors of pericytic origin. Unlike venous malformations, they more commonly occur in bones and can have malignant potential. Maffucci syndrome, Klippel-Trenaunay syndrome, and blue rubber bleb nevus syndrome are considered variant presentations of venous malformations.

Comment

Main Teaching Point

Vascular malformations are congenital lesions that grow periodically, often in relation to trauma, surgery, or hormonal stimulation (via puberty, pregnancy, or hormonal therapy). Vascular malformations are typically categorized into arterial, capillary, venous, lymphatic, and mixed subtypes. Magnetic resonance imaging (MRI) is useful to determine the depth and extent of these lesions as well as their proximity to normal structures (Figures S131-1 and S131-2). MRI is also useful in the imaging follow-up after treatment because multiple ablation sessions are often necessary.

Imaging Interpretation

Owing to the presence of an intervening capillary network, the inflow arteries to venous malformations, like the one depicted, are normal in size. Flow within these dilated abnormal veins tends to be slow or stagnant, and calcified phleboliths may be identified.

Treatment Methods

Small, asymptomatic venous malformations in the extremities are treated conservatively with compressive stockings and follow-up. Surgical resection is not indicated owing to the difficulty in extricating these delicate vascular structures from surrounding normal tissues. Sclerotherapy is the favored treatment, with absolute ethanol and sodium tetradecyl the preferred agents among many operators. After the lesion is directly punctured with a needle, contrast is injected to confirm needle placement and determine the volume necessary to fill the lesion (Figures S131-3 and S131-4). A similar volume of sclerosant is then injected and allowed to dwell in the lesion. Tourniquets are commonly applied to the extremity to occlude venous flow during the intervention. Follow-up venography is performed to confirm thrombosis of the lesion.

References

Flors L, Leiva-Salinas C, Maged I, et al. MR imaging of soft-tissue vascular malformation: diagnosis, classification, and therapy follow-up. *Radiographics*. 2011;31:1321–1340.

Flors L, Leiva-Salinas C, Norton PT, et al. Ten frequently asked questions about MRI evaluation of soft-tissue vascular anomalies. *AJR Am J Roentgenol*. 2013;201:554–562.

Legiehn GM, Heran MK. A step-by-step practical approach to imaging diagnosis and interventional radiologic therapy in vascular malformations. *Semin Intervent Radiol*. 2010;27:209–231.

Cross-reference

Vascular and Interventional Radiology: The Requisites, 2nd ed, 381–385.

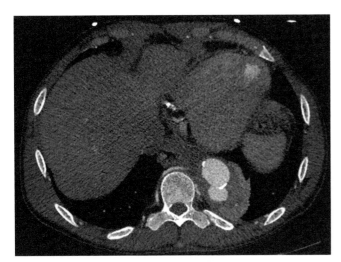

Figure 132-1. *Courtesy of Dr. David M. Williams.*

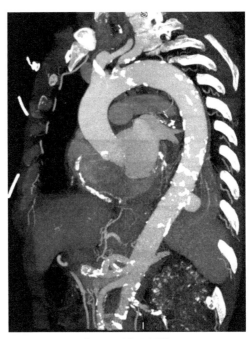

Figure 132-2. *Courtesy of Dr. David M. Williams.*

HISTORY: A 40-year-old male with a history of tuberculosis and intravenous (IV) drug abuse presents with fevers and chest pain.

1. Which of the following is the most likely diagnosis for the imaging findings presented?
   A. Dissection
   B. Atherosclerotic aneurysm
   C. Infectious (mycotic) aneurysm
   D. Ductus diverticulum

2. What is the most useful imaging technique for initial diagnosis?
   A. Computed tomography (CT) angiography
   B. Ultrasound
   C. Digital subtraction angiography (DSA)
   D. Magnetic resonance angiography (MRA)

3. In what patient population is endovascular therapy for the treatment of mycotic aneurysms preferred?
   A. Immunocompromised patients
   B. High-risk patients with significant medical comorbidities
   C. Pediatric patients
   D. Patients older than 70 years of age

4. What is the most likely organism found in mycotic aneurysms?
   A. *Candida*
   B. *Staphylococcus*
   C. *Klebsiella*
   D. *Pseudomonas*

See Supplemental Figures section for additional figures and legends for this case.

CASE 132

Mycotic Aneurysm

1. **C.** A saccular, infectious (mycotic) aneurysm is seen on cross-sectional imaging. In the presence of clinical symptoms and a possible source of infection there is a high likelihood that the imaging findings seen are an infected (mycotic) pseudoaneurysm. A dissection would commonly show narrowing of the vessel and/or medial displacement of intimal calcifications. A dissection flap may also be seen. Atherosclerosis leads to a weakening of the vessel wall and is the most common cause of aortic aneurysms. A CT can show the location, caliber of the aneurysm, degree of calcification, and presence of a mural thrombus. A ductus diverticulum is located at the site of the ductus arteriosus and is a developmental outpouching of the thoracic aorta.

2. **A.** CT angiography is the most useful modality for diagnosing infected aneurysms. MRA is a useful alternative if there is a contraindication for the use of iodinated contrast. DSA cannot reliably distinguish between infected or atherosclerotic aneurysms. The presence of an irregular lumen, perianeurysmal fluid, gas, hematoma, disruption of intimal calcification, and/or obscuring of the aortic wall can be helpful in determining the etiology of the aneurysm.

3. **B.** Primary clinical management has typically included antibiotic therapy combined with surgery. Initial empiric antibiotic therapy commonly includes coverage of both gram-positive and gram-negative organisms. Surgical intervention includes debridement with or without revascularization. In high-risk patient populations where surgery would carry unacceptable risk, endovascular interventions have proven beneficial. Endovascular repair can also be used as a palliative option in patients with significant medical comorbidities.

4. **B.** Gram-positive organisms are most commonly found in mycotic aneurysms; most commonly *Staphylococcus*, *Streptococcus*, and *Salmonella*. *Staphylococcus* infections can be seen in patients with a history of IV drug abuse. While infections due to gram-negative organisms are less common, they are still seen in 35% of cases. Fungal infections are rare but can be seen in patients with diabetes or a history of immunosuppression.

Comment

Etiology

Infectious (mycotic) aneurysms can occur anywhere in the arterial system. The usual cultured infectious organisms are *Salmonella, Streptococcus,* or *Staphylococcus* species, and the latter is commonly found in IV drug abusers. Although gram-positive organisms are predominant, gram-negative are seen in 35% of cases. Blood cultures are positive in 50% to 85% of cases.

Pathogenesis

Mycotic aneurysms represent an infection of the artery wall itself either caused by seeding of a preexisting aneurysm or by primary infection of a normal artery with subsequent dilation. The infection can be introduced from infected blood in the lumen or vasa vasorum, by spread from a neighboring soft tissue infection, or from penetrating trauma. Therefore, mycotic aneurysms can be true or false aneurysms and may be single or multiple depending upon the underlying condition of the vessel and the method of infection. The symptomatology and angiographic appearance can differentiate these from degenerative aneurysms. The mycotic aneurysm sac is typically irregular, saccular, and eccentric, and the arterial system is less likely to show chronic atherosclerosis. Computed tomography angiography or MRA are commonly employed in the diagnosis of infectious aneurysms (Figures S132-1 through S132-3).

Treatment Methods

Treatment consists of antibiotics, surgical resection of the aneurysm, debridement of infected tissues, and drainage of the infected region. In some cases the artery can be ligated, but when revascularization is necessary, an extra-anatomic bypass can often be performed to avoid the infected region. In some cases, an anatomic bypass can successfully be performed with autogenous materials (native veins) or cryopreserved allografts if success in clearing of infection with antimicrobial agents is anticipated. Prosthetic material should not be inserted into a known infected space, except in patient populations where surgery carries too high of a risk (Figures S132-4 and S132-5).

References

Brunner S, Engelmann MG, Näbauer M. Thoracic mycotic pseudoaneurysm from *Candida albicans* infection. *Eur Heart J.* 2008;29:1515.

Macedo T, Stanson A, Oderich G, et al. Infected aortic aneurysms: imaging findings. *Radiology.* 2004;231:250–257.

Patel HJ, Williams DM, Upchurch Jr. GR, et al. Late outcomes of endovascular aortic repair for the infected thoracic aorta. *Ann Thorac Surg.* 2009;87:1366–1371.

Cross-reference

Vascular and Interventional Radiology: The Requisites, 2nd ed, 217–218.

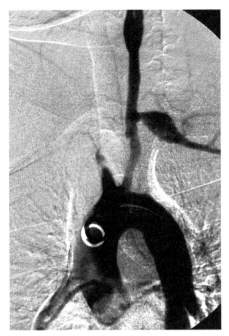

Figure 133-1

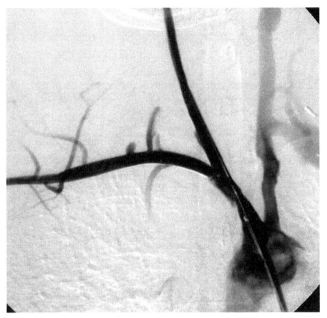

Figure 133-2

HISTORY: A 35-year-old Asian female presents with asymmetric upper-extremity blood pressures, fevers, and myalgia.

1. Which of the following is the most likely diagnosis for the imaging findings presented?
   A. Ascending aortic aneurysm
   B. Right internal carotid artery dissection
   C. Proximal brachiocephalic artery stenosis
   D. Thoracic outlet syndrome

2. What is the most likely diagnosis?
   A. Polyarteritis nodosa
   B. Kawasaki disease
   C. Granulomatosis with polyangiitis
   D. Takayasu's arteritis

3. Which type of lesion is shown for the correct pathology in question 2?
   A. Type I
   B. Type II
   C. Type III
   D. Type IV

4. A patient with Takayasu's arteritis status post multiple occluded bypass grafts presents with worsening right hand pain with elevated C-reactive protein (CRP) and erythrocyte sedimentation rate (ESR) but a good right radial pulse. What is the next best step in management?
   A. Emergent surgical bypass
   B. Observation
   C. Corticosteroid therapy
   D. Emergent endovascular intervention

See Supplemental Figures section for additional figures and legends for this case.

CASE 133

Brachiocephalic Artery Stent Placement

1. **C.** The images demonstrate focal narrowing of the brachiocephalic artery. The visualized aorta is normal in caliber. There is no abnormality of the right internal carotid artery. Thoracic outlet syndrome is caused by compression of the subclavian artery at the thoracic outlet.

2. **D.** Given the location of the stenosis and the patient's age/ethnicity, the most likely diagnosis is Takayasu arteritis. Polyarteritis nodosa and Kawasaki disease typically affect medium-sized and small-sized arteries. Kawasaki disease is also more common in children. Granulomatosis with polyangiitis primarily affects small-sized arteries.

3. **A.** Type I only affects the aortic arch branches. Type II involves the thoracic aorta. Type III involves the thoracic/abdominal aorta distal to the arch. Type IV is the isolated involvement of the abdominal aorta and/or renal arteries.

4. **C.** Given the evidence of acute inflammation (elevated ESR and CRP) and the presence of a strong radial pulse, the patient should initially be treated with steroids. Studies have shown lower success rates for surgical and endovascular intervention in the acute inflammatory stage. Additionally, arterial stenosis may improve with steroid treatment alone. Therefore, the patient should be initially treated with steroids, and then surgical or endovascular treatment should be considered when the patient is no longer in the acute inflammatory phase.

Comment

Main Teaching Point

Patients with Takayasu's arteritis can present complex management problems. Typically they are first managed with anti-inflammatory therapy until arterial symptoms develop. At this point, surgical bypass is the usual therapy employed, although angioplasty and/or stent placement can also be used for focal, short-segment lesions that are in a chronic phase. Surgery or interventional therapy in the acute inflammatory stages should be avoided owing to lower rates of long-term success.

Treatment Methods

If the brachiocephalic artery or proximal subclavian artery is occluded and the ipsilateral common carotid artery is normal, reimplantation of the subclavian artery into the carotid or carotid-subclavian bypass is the preferred operation. If the carotid artery is diseased it is replaced with graft material, and the subclavian artery is implanted into the graft or grafted to the aorta or carotid graft. In general, when treating the brachiocephalic artery, the operator should be extremely careful with the technique, as stroke may be a major complication of dissection or downstream emboli.

Imaging Interpretation

In the case presented in the unknown images, the patient had been operated on multiple times for the brachiocephalic artery occlusion and had multiple occluded bypass grafts. Because she was thought to be a poor risk for further intervention in the same operative bed, an endovascular stent was placed (Figures S133-1 and S133-2). The second case is another example with balloon-expandable stent placement (Figures S133-3 and S133-4).

References

Sharma BK, Jain S, Bali HK, et al. A follow-up study of balloon angioplasty and de-novo stenting in Takayasu arteritis. *Int J Cardiol.* 2000;75:S147–S152.

van Hattum ES, de Vries JP, Lalezari F, et al. Angioplasty with or without stent placement in the brachiocephalic artery: feasible and durable? A retrospective cohort study. *J Vasc Interv Radiol.* 2007;18:1088–1093.

Cross-reference

Vascular and Interventional Radiology: The Requisites, 2nd ed, 6–9.

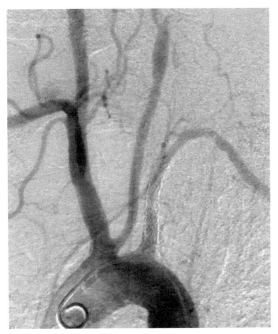

Figure 134-1 *Courtesy of Dr. Wael E. Saad.*

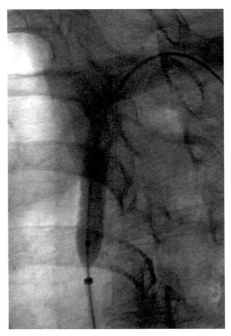

Figure 134-2 *Courtesy of Dr. Wael E. Saad.*

HISTORY: A 48-year-old female presents with history of left subclavian artery stenting with recurrent symptoms 9 months after treatment.

1. Which of the following is the most likely diagnosis for the imaging findings presented?
   A. Thoracic outlet syndrome
   B. Type B aortic dissection
   C. Left carotid artery stenosis
   D. Left subclavian artery in-stent stenosis

2. Why may the patient experience vertebrobasilar insufficiency symptoms?
   A. The stenosis of the vertebral artery is leading to reduced blood flow to the circle of Willis.
   B. The aortic dissection has spread retrograde to occlude the great vessels.
   C. The carotid artery stenosis is so severe that there are inadequate collaterals to perfuse the vertebrobasilar system.
   D. The subclavian artery in-stent stenosis is leading to subclavian steal syndrome.

3. What is the optimal initial treatment for this abnormality at this point?
   A. Endovascular balloon angioplasty
   B. Surgical carotid-subclavian artery bypass
   C. Thrombolysis
   D. Aortic endograft

4. What aspects of imaging presented here may lead to complications from an endovascular intervention in this case?
   A. The angle from the aorta to the subclavian artery is too acute for stenting.
   B. The stenosis is greater than 50% of the subclavian artery lumen, which predicts a high rate of failure for stenting.
   C. The in-stent plaque may embolize during intervention.
   D. The patient's anatomy does not have enough adequate collaterals for an endovascular intervention to be undertaken.

See Supplemental Figures section for additional figures and legends for this case.

CASE 134

Subclavian Artery In-Stent Stenosis

1. **D.** The imaging findings here clearly indicate in-stent stenosis within the subclavian artery stent. No dissection flap is identified to suggest dissection.

2. **D.** The stenosis in the left subclavian artery can lead to a syndrome called subclavian steal syndrome in which flow is reversed in the left vertebral artery to perfuse the left upper extremity via collaterals. This reversed flow is at the expense of perfusion of the vertebrobasilar system.

3. **A.** Given that a wire has crossed the lesion, balloon angioplasty is the recommended initial therapy. If the stenosis does not improve with angioplasty alone, thrombolysis could be considered. Recurrent stenosis may be managed with surgical bypass.

4. **C.** Calcified or noncalcified plaque may dislodge and send emboli to the brain during endovascular intervention. The patient should be counselled regarding this during the consent process.

Comment

Main Teaching Point

The standard treatment for a proximal subclavian artery lesion is carotid-subclavian artery bypass, which is associated with extremely high (90% to 95%) long-term patency. In selected patients, angioplasty and/or stent placement can be performed with an expectation of good short-term and mid-term results. Like atherosclerotic lesions treated with stenting in the lower extremities, aortic branch vessel and upper extremity stents may develop in-stent stenosis over time (Figures S134-1 and S134-4). These lesions may be managed by endovascular means with balloon angioplasty with or without additional stenting or thrombolysis if necessary (Figures S134-2 through S134-6). As is important in all patients with cardiovascular disease, lifestyle modification, smoking cessation, and medical management are mainstays of treatment.

References

Linn K, Ugurluoglu A, Mader N, et al. Endovascular management versus surgery for proximal subclavian artery lesions. *Ann Vasc Surg.* 2008;22:769–775.

Sixt S, Rastan A, Schwarzwalder U, et al. Results after balloon angioplasty or stenting of atherosclerotic subclavian artery obstruction. *Catheter Cardiovasc Interv.* 2009;73:395–403.

Verma A, Reilly JP, White CJ. Management of subclavian artery in-stent restenosis. *Vasc Med.* 2013;18:350–353.

Cross-reference

Vascular and Interventional Radiology: The Requisites, 2nd ed, 124–126.

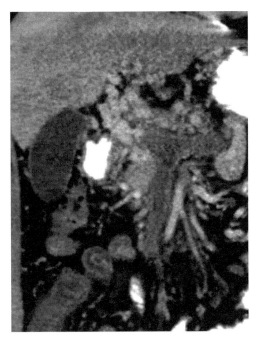

Figure 135-1. *Courtesy of Dr. Wael E. Saad.*

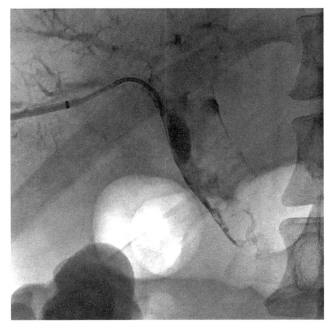

Figure 135-2. *Courtesy of Dr. Wael E. Saad.*

HISTORY: A 47-year-old male with cirrhosis presents with severe abdominal pain, vomiting, and rising lactate.

1. Which of the following would be included in the differential diagnosis for the imaging findings presented? (Choose all that apply.)
   A. Bowel edema
   B. Portal vein thrombosis (PVT)
   C. Hepatic artery dissection
   D. Occluded transjugular intrahepatic portosystemic shunt (TIPS)

2. Which of the following would *NOT* be a recommended treatment approach to improve the clot burden in this patient?
   A. Administration of anticoagulation
   B. Portal vein thrombolysis (PVT)
   C. TIPS
   D. Beta blockade

3. What is the most significant short-term complication of an acute PVT?
   A. Portal hypertension
   B. Acute liver failure
   C. Hepatic infarction
   D. Intestinal ischemia

4. Which of the following organisms, when isolated in the bloodstream, has a strong association with portal and mesenteric vein thrombosis?
   A. *Bacteroides* spp.
   B. *Klebsiella* spp.
   C. *Enterobacter* spp.
   D. *Staphylococcus* spp.

See Supplemental Figures section for additional figures and legends for this case.

CASE 135

Portal Vein Thrombosis

1. **A and B.** The images show portal and mesenteric vein thrombosis with resulting small bowel edema. A TIPS is not seen on these images.

2. **D.** Beta blockers are used prophylactically for the prevention of portal hypertension, which can develop in the setting of PVT; however, this does not treat the thrombus burden. Anticoagulation would be an acceptable management choice in a patient with an acute PVT without evidence of varices. Interventional recanalization and thrombolysis are good options in many of these patients and can be performed via a transhepatic route or through a TIPS approach.

3. **D.** If the clot extends into the superior mesenteric vein and/or the mesenteric venous arcades, reflex arteriolar vasoconstriction can occur, leading to ischemia and intestinal infarction in addition to edema from venous hypertension. Hepatic infarction and acute liver failure are less likely to occur given the dual blood supply of the liver, and acute portal hypertension necessitates a very large clot burden.

4. **A.** *Bacteroides* bacteremia has a strong association with PVT in the noncirrhotic patient.

Comment

Main Teaching Point

PVT can be caused by primary hepatic or metastatic tumor, dehydration, sepsis, transplantation, and other hypercoagulable states. Its presence is important to the interventionalist in several clinical situations, including patients with cancer in whom hepatic chemoembolization is planned. The presence of portal vein obstruction would render such patients susceptible to developing severe hepatic ischemia were the hepatic artery to be embolized. PVT is also important in patients with portal hypertension in whom TIPS is planned. In these patients, the presence of PVT would render portal vein access more difficult to obtain. However, TIPS can still be performed, either by accessing the left portal system or by recanalizing the occluded segment of the portal vein. PVT, depending on the severity and resulting symptoms, can be treated with conservative treatment, initiation of anticoagulation, and PVT (Figures S135-1 through S135-3), in the appropriate patient.

References

Hmoud B, Singal AK, Kamath PS. Mesenteric venous thrombosis. *J Clin Exp Hepatol.* 2014;4:257–263.

Sacerdoti D, Serianni G, Gaiani S, et al. Thrombosis of the portal venous system. *J Ultrasound.* 2007;10:12–21.

Uflacker R. Applications of percutaneous mechanical thrombectomy in transjugular intrahepatic portosystemic shunt and portal vein thrombosis. *Tech Vasc Interv Radiol.* 2003;6:59–69.

Cross-reference

Vascular and Interventional Radiology: The Requisites, 2nd ed, 327–330.

CASE 136

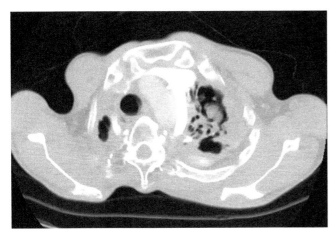

Figure 136-1

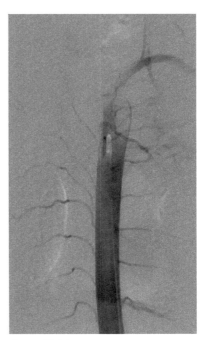

Figure 136-2

HISTORY: A 46-year-old male with acute onset hemoptysis.

1. What abnormality is visualized on the aortogram?
   A. Hypertrophied intercostal artery
   B. Hypertrophied bronchial artery
   C. Aberrant bronchial artery
   D. Aberrant left vertebral artery

2. What is the most common clinical presentation for this finding?
   A. Pleural effusion
   B. Chest pain
   C. Chronic cough
   D. Hemoptysis

3. From which spinal level do the bronchial arteries typically arise?
   A. T3 to T4
   B. T4 to T5
   C. T5 to T6
   D. T6 to T7

4. Which of the following embolic agents would you LEAST likely use for hemoptysis from bronchial arteries?
   A. Glue
   B. Coils
   C. Gelfoam
   D. Particles

See Supplemental Figures section for additional figures and legends for this case.

CASE 136

Cavitary Lung-Mass Embolization

1. **B.** There is a hypertrophied left bronchial artery, which is selectively catheterized on the third image. Horizontally oriented intercostal arteries are also noted at multiple levels.

2. **D.** Massive hemoptysis is the most typical presentation, although these patients commonly also have a cough and chest pain.

3. **C.** Most commonly, the bronchial arteries arise from the aorta at the level of T5 to T6. Significant variation exists in origin and branching pattern. However, commonly there are two left and one right bronchial arteries.

4. **B.** Particles are preferred for most distal embolization. Re-bleeding is common in these patients, and other agents such as coils can inhibit re-embolization.

Comment

Etiology and Initial Evaluation

Common causes of severe hemoptysis include cystic fibrosis, chronic obstructive pulmonary disease, bronchiectasis, and vascular tumors. Additionally, cavitary lung masses from aspergilloma, tuberculosis (TB), and squamous cell carcinoma can lead to massive hemoptysis. Bronchoscopy is routinely performed before arteriographic evaluation of hemoptysis, in order to determine which bronchial segment contains the bleeding source. This greatly helps the angiographer, because many patients have enlarged bronchial arteries bilaterally with no evidence of contrast extravasation. The angiographer can then direct therapy to the artery thought likely to be causing the bleeding based upon bronchoscopy.

Endovascular Management

As seen in the figures, this patient has a cavitary lung mass with hypertrophied left bronchial artery (Figures S136-1 to S136-3). The left bronchial arterial branches are hypertrophied and tortuous (Figure S136-3). There are multiple areas of vascular splaying suggesting necrosis. The differential diagnosis includes primary lung carcinoma, metastatic disease, and infectious lesions such as TB and fungal disease (which was the case in the patient shown). In the vast majority of cases, contrast extravasation is not visualized. In this patient, treatment was performed using embolization with polyvinyl alcohol particles, with subsequent cessation of bleeding with subsequent lobectomy (Figure S136-4).

References

Barben J, Robertson D, Olinsky A, et al. Bronchial artery embolization for hemoptysis in young patients with cystic fibrosis. *Radiology.* 2002;224:124–130.

Fernando HC, Stein M, Benfield JR, et al. Role of bronchial artery embolization in the management of hemoptysis. *Arch Surg.* 1998;133:862–866.

Cross-reference

Vascular and Interventional Radiology: The Requisites, 2nd ed, 174–176.

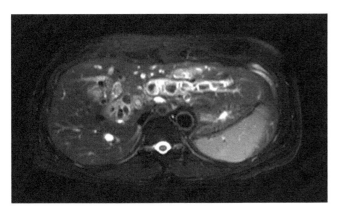

Figure 137-1. *Courtesy of Dr. Narasimham L. Dasika.*

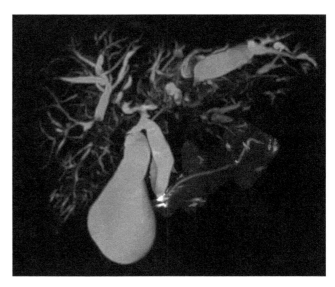

Figure 137-2. *Courtesy of Dr. Narasimham L. Dasika.*

HISTORY: A 44-year-old female with primary sclerosing cholangitis presents with recurrent right upper quadrant pain and chills.

1. Which of the following is the most likely diagnosis for the imaging findings presented?
   A. Cholangiocarcinoma
   B. Biliary stones
   C. Normal variant
   D. Hepatocellular carcinoma

2. Which noninvasive modality has the highest sensitivity in detecting the distal common bile duct disease?
   A. Ultrasound
   B. Computed tomography (CT)
   C. Magnetic resonance cholangiopancreatography (MRCP)
   D. Endoscopic retrograde cholangiopancreatography (ERCP)

3. Which of the following is the usual first-line treatment in uncomplicated cases?
   A. Cholecystectomy
   B. Whipple procedure
   C. Sphincterotomy
   D. Conservative management

4. If the first-line treatment is not successful, what can the interventional radiologist (IR) offer to help this patient? (Choose all that apply.)
   A. Percutaneous cholecystostomy
   B. Transjugular intrahepatic portosystemic shunt
   C. Percutaneous biliary drainage
   D. Percutaneous stone removal

See Supplemental Figures section for additional figures and legends for this case.

CASE 137

Complex Biliary Stone Management

1. **B.** There are multiple filling defects in the dilated biliary tree. These are discontinuous, making cholangiocarcinoma unlikely. Hepatocellular carcinoma would not have this appearance, and this is certainly not normal.

2. **C.** Although ultrasound is very useful as an initial screening method to assess biliary stones, MRCP can provide more of a global evaluation of the biliary system and surrounding structures as well as pathological conditions within the common bile duct. CT is useful in the evaluation of the liver and biliary tree but is being replaced by MRCP by many clinicians. ERCP and percutaneous cholangiography are the most specific modalities but are invasive.

3. **C.** ERCP with stone extraction and sphincterotomy, when possible, is the treatment of choice. However, in some patients this is not possible due to stone burden, stone size, and anatomy (Roux-en-Y).

4. **C and D.** IRs can assist by confirming the diagnosis with percutaneous cholangiography followed by drainage initially. Once the patient is noninfectious, the IR can perform stone extraction with many different methods, including choledochoscopy as shown in this case.

Comment

Main Teaching Point

Patients with choledocholithiasis and/or complex biliary stones can present with acute severe symptomatology (due to impaction of a mid-sized or large calculus within the common bile duct) or with chronic intermittent symptoms. Imaging commonly assists in determining the stone burden and localization of occlusion (Figures S137-1 and S137-2). Patients with symptoms suggesting the presence of cholangitis must be treated urgently with either stone removal or biliary drainage to rapidly relieve the obstruction. Afebrile patients with acute symptoms are usually managed with ERCP as the first-choice option.

Percutaneous Management

If ERCP fails or is not possible, then the patient may be referred for percutaneous biliary drainage and percutaneous management. Percutaneous treatment methods include delivery of the stone into the gut with the use of a balloon, extraction with several possible devices, fragmentation, or a combination of these methods (Figures S137-3 through S137-5).

References

Dasika NL. Percutaneous choledochoscopy: access, technique, ancillary procedures, results and complications of 174 procedures. *J Vasc Interv Radiol.* 2006;17(Suppl):S29.

Ierardi AM, Fontana F, Petrillo M, et al. Percutaneous transhepatic endoscopic holmium laser lithotripsy for intrahepatic and choledochal biliary stones. *Int J Surg.* 2013;11:S36–S39.

Peng YC, Chow WK. Alternative percutaneous approach for endoscopic inaccessible common bile duct stones. *Hepatogastroenterology.* 2011;58:705–708.

Cross-reference

Vascular and Interventional Radiology: The Requisites, 2nd ed, 471–473.

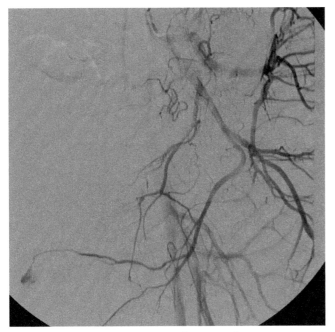

Figure 138-1. *Courtesy of Dr. Narasimham L. Dasika.*

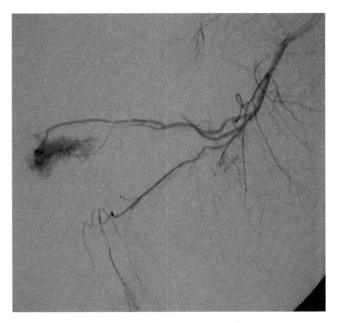

Figure 138-2. *Courtesy of Dr. Narasimham L. Dasika.*

HISTORY: A 42-year-old male presents to the emergency department with complaints of painless, penile swelling of 72 hours' duration after pelvic trauma during sexual intercourse.

1. Which of the following is the most likely diagnosis for the imaging findings presented?
   A. High-flow priapism
   B. Internal iliac artery embolism
   C. Internal pudendal artery pseudoaneurysm formation
   D. Pelvic arterial venous malformation

2. Which of the following arteries supplies the penis?
   A. Inferior gluteal artery
   B. Posterior scrotal artery
   C. Inferior rectal artery
   D. Internal pudendal artery

3. Which vessel in commonly injured in the high-flow form of this pathological condition?
   A. Internal pudendal artery
   B. Cavernous artery
   C. Interior iliac artery
   D. Inferior rectal artery

4. Which structure has its blood outflow obstructed in the low-flow form of this pathological condition?
   A. Glans penis
   B. Corpus spongiosum
   C. Corpus cavernosum
   D. Urethra

See Supplemental Figures section for additional figures and legends for this case.

CASE 138

Priapism

1. **A.** The images shown are portraying cases of high-flow priapism. There are two forms of priapism, high-flow and low-flow. It is vital to recognize this pathological condition as it can lead to permanent impotence via the development of fibrosis.

2. **D.** The artery that supplies the penis is the internal pudendal artery, which is a branch of the anterior division of the internal iliac artery. The other arteries that are listed are also branches of the internal iliac artery, but the internal pudendal is the artery that supplies the penis.

3. **B.** The injured artery that most commonly leads to a high-flow priapism is the cavernous artery. Damage to the cavernous artery via trauma to the pelvis or perineum creates an arteriolacunar fistula in which there is constant blood flow into the erectile tissue. The dorsal penile artery may also be injured in some cases, as shown in this example.

4. **C.** The pathophysiology of low-flow priapism is outflow obstruction of the corpus cavernosum. The obstruction leads to tumescence of the corpus cavernosum with sparing of the glans penis and corpus spongiosum. This leads to vascular congestion causing a lactic acidosis and eventual fibrosis leading to permanent impotence.

Comment

Main Teaching Point

High-flow priapism is a rare arterial abnormality that results from direct trauma to the perineum or penis. Laceration of the cavernous or dorsal penile artery results in development of an angiographically visible arteriolacunar fistula (Figures S138-1 through S138-3) with direct, constant entry of arterial blood into the vascular lacuna of the erectile tissue. It helps to be familiar with the normal minor arterial blush at the base of the corpus cavernosum to be able to clearly distinguish this normal finding from the more robust enhancement associated with a true arteriolacunar fistula. Low-flow priapism is caused by venous outflow obstruction of the corpus cavernosum (Figures S138-5 and S138-6). The venous congestion results in a decrease of the Po_2 of the erectile tissue. This causes a lactic acidosis and resultant fibrosis leading to permanent impotence. Thus, this condition must be treated as an emergency.

Treatment Methods

The most commonly used treatment is percutaneous embolization of the distal internal pudendal artery or feeding branch vessel (Figure S138-4). Autologous blood clot and Gelfoam, both temporary agents, have been used most extensively but have a significant rate of recurrence due to subsequent recanalization. Permanent agents, such as microcoils and bucrylate glue, have also been used. Surgical ligation of the cavernous artery is also an effective treatment, but because it produces permanent occlusion it can have damaging effects on the underlying tissues.

Complications

The feared complication of both treatment and failure to treat is the development of impotence. Although many patients report a long history of high-flow priapism with normal sexual function, long-standing persistent priapism has been reported to result in fibrosis with associated erectile dysfunction. Because it is difficult to determine which patients will develop fibrosis and impotence, the timing of intervention remains controversial.

References

Ciampalini S, Savoca G, Buttazzi L, et al. High-flow priapism: treatment and long-term follow-up. *Urology.* 2002;59:110–113.

Monkhouse SJ, Bell S. Low-flow priapism needs recognition and early treatment. *Emerg Med J.* 2007;24:209–210.

Zhao S, Zhou J, Zhang YF, et al. Therapeutic embolization of high-flow priapism 1 year follow up with color Doppler sonography. *Eur J Radiol.* 2013;82:769–774.

Cross-reference

Vascular and Interventional Radiology: The Requisites, 2nd ed, 226–227.

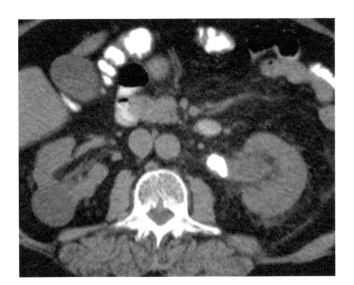

Figure 139-1

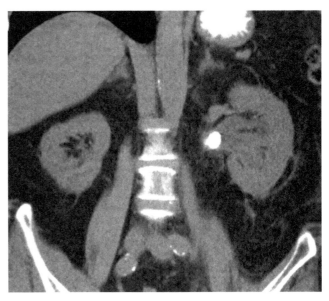

Figure 139-2

HISTORY: A 57-year-old male with left flank pain and hematuria presents for evaluation. The patient was afebrile.

1. Which of the following is the most likely diagnosis given the imaging and clinical findings presented?
   A. Pyelonephritis
   B. Renal calculus
   C. Renal cell carcinoma
   D. Angiomyolipoma

2. If the patient presented in the middle of the night with flank pain, fever, and chills, what would be the next best step in management?
   A. Nephrectomy
   B. Intravenous (IV) antibiotics and pain control
   C. Urgent nephrostomy tube placement
   D. Elective nephrostomy tube placement in the morning

3. What is the ideal puncture site for percutaneous nephrostomy tube placement?
   A. Renal pelvis
   B. Posterior calyx
   C. Anterior calyx
   D. Proximal ureter

4. Which of the following is *NOT* a potential complication of left upper pole calyx access?
   A. Pneumothorax
   B. Urothorax
   C. Renal artery pseudoaneurysm
   D. Liver injury

See Supplemental Figures section for additional figures and legends for this case.

CASE 139

Percutaneous Access for Nephrolithotomy

1. **B.** The images show a large left-sided calculus in the renal pelvis with signs of obstruction including dilated calyces. Although many patients may have signs of infection, this patient does not.

2. **B.** Administration of IV antibiotics and pain control would be the first next step in management in the patient described in this question. Nephrostomy tube placement could be performed urgently. However, antibiotics should be administered prior to needle puncture as the patient could become septic during or immediately after the procedure.

3. **B.** A zone of relative avascularity known as the avascular plane of Brodel is located posterior to the lateral convex margin of the kidney. Lower pole, posterior calyx access is commonly preferred for simple urinary drainage. Access may change based on location of stone when access is obtained for nephrolithotomy.

4. **D.** Injury may occur to the liver in upper pole access of the right kidney but would not be expected for left upper pole access. The other choices are potential complications.

Comment

Main Teaching Point

The noncontrast computed tomography images demonstrate a large calculus at the left ureteropelvic junction (Figures S139-1 and S139-2). Urgent percutaneous nephrostomy tube placement is indicated if the patient is febrile. If the patient shows no signs of infection, then percutaneous nephrostomy can be electively performed to preserve renal function and/or to facilitate percutaneous stone removal. In the setting of renal cortical thinning, the presence of significant residual function in the right kidney via renal scintigraphy may be performed before placing a nephrostomy tube in that kidney, although this is no longer commonly practiced.

Percutaneous Management

To perform percutaneous stone removal, obtaining optimal access into the renal collecting system is extremely important. Typically the collecting system is accessed and a guidewire is passed into the bladder. A balloon catheter is then used to dilate the subcutaneous tract to accommodate a large (often 26 to 30 F) sheath (Figure S139-3). Through this sheath, a nephroscope is passed into the renal collecting system, and under direct visualization the stone is fragmented and removed. A nephrostomy catheter, and sometimes a ureteral stent, is left in place after the procedure.

References

Dyer RB, Regan JD, Kavanagh PV, et al. Percutaneous nephrostomy with extensions of the technique: step by step. *Radiographics.* 2002;22:503–525.

Landman J, Venkatesh R, Lee DI, et al. Combined percutaneous and retrograde approach to staghorn calculi with application of the ureteral access sheath to facilitate percutaneous nephrolithotomy. *J Urol.* 2003;169:64–67.

Cross-reference

Vascular and Interventional Radiology: The Requisites, 2nd ed, 495–499.

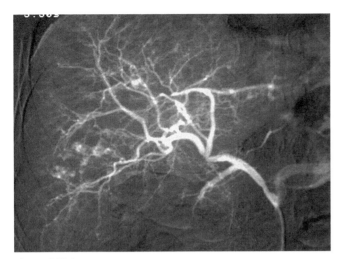

Figure 140-1

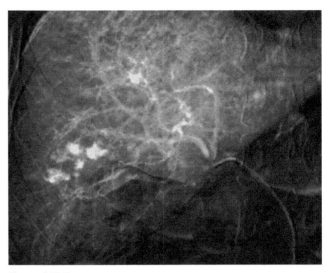

Figure 140-2

HISTORY: A 63-year-old asymptomatic female presents with a hepatic mass incidentally visualized on computed tomography (CT).

1. Which of the following would be included in the differential diagnosis for the imaging findings presented? (Choose all that apply.)
   A. Hepatocellular carcinoma (HCC)
   B. Angiosarcoma
   C. Cavernous hemangioma
   D. Hepatic adenoma

2. Which of the following hepatic tumors does *NOT* usually exhibit contrast opacification in equilibrium phase/delayed imaging?
   A. Angiosarcoma
   B. Cavernous hemangioma
   C. Cholangiocarcinoma
   D. HCC

3. Which of the following hepatic tumors has a largely idiopathic etiology?
   A. Angiosarcoma
   B. Hepatic adenoma
   C. HCC
   D. Cavernous hemangioma

4. Which of the following hepatic tumors is most likely seen in this case?
   A. Cavernous hemangioma
   B. HCC
   C. Hepatic adenoma
   D. Angiosarcoma

See Supplemental Figures section for additional figures and legends for this case.

CASE 140

Cavernous Hemangioma of the Liver

1. **A, B, C, and D.** The angiographic images demonstrate multiple foci of dense, discrete, nodular contrast opacification, scattered throughout the hepatic parenchyma. All of the above pathologies can manifest in such a manner on angiography.

2. **D.** The hallmark of 90% of cases of HCC is rapid washout, causing isointensity or hypointensity of the lesion as compared to the surrounding hepatic parenchyma on more delayed imaging. The above images demonstrate persistent contrast opacification on delayed imaging, which can be seen in all of the other mentioned answer choices.

3. **D.** Angiosarcoma, while a rare entity, has been shown to be associated with environmental risk factors such as Thorotrast, arsenic and vinyl chloride exposure. Hepatic adenomas are most frequently seen in young women who are taking oral contraceptive pills. HCC is most strongly associated with cirrhosis, either due to alcohol or viral (hepatitis B or C) etiologies. Hemochromatosis, alpha-1 antitrypsin deficiency, Wilson's disease, and exposure to aflatoxins are additional risk factors. Cavernous hemangiomas have no well-defined predisposing factors and largely occur sporadically.

4. **A.** The above angiographic images demonstrate multiple foci of dense, discrete, nodular contrast opacification, scattered throughout the hepatic parenchyma. The pattern of contrast pooling is likened to a "cotton wool" appearance. The feeding vessels are of normal caliber with no evidence of neovascularity or arteriovenous shunting. Furthermore, progressive centripedal contrast opacification with persistence of contrast fill-in beyond the venous phase is observed. This constellation of findings is typical for a hepatic cavernous hemangioma. Although hemangiomas have characteristic angiographic features, the use of angiography is not recommended in the initial diagnosis of this entity, given the diagnostic capabilities of less invasive techniques, such as CT and magnetic resonance imaging.

Comment
Main Teaching Point

Hemangiomas are the most common benign hepatic tumors and are typically found incidentally during cross-sectional imaging. Pathologically, they comprise endothelium-lined vascular spaces divided by thin septations and suspended in a loose fibroblastic stroma. They typically remain stable in size over time, but occasionally they grow quite large. When a hemangioma is present, symptoms are commonly related to the neoplasm size, but they rarely are due to rupture or platelet sequestration.

Imaging Interpretation

The arteriographic appearance is characteristic. The feeding vessels are typically normal in size unless the lesion is very large. Dense nodular opacification of the lesion starts at the periphery (Figure S140-1) and progresses inward (Figures S140-2 and S140-3). The lesions are well circumscribed and have dilated, irregular, nodule-like vascular spaces. Contrast opacification persisting well into the venous phase differentiates this lesion from other hepatic neoplasms except for the rare angiosarcoma that can mimic a hemangioma.

Differential Diagnoses

Other hepatic lesions that exhibit vascular pooling tend to be malignant tumors, including HCC and metastases. Similar to cross-sectional imaging characteristics, these can typically be differentiated by the shorter period of pooling, less uniform enhancement, enlargement of the feeding artery, and neovascularity.

Reference

Giavraglou C, Economou H, Oannidis I. Arterial embolization of giant hepatic hemangiomas. *Cardiovasc Intervent Radiol.* 2003;26:92–96.

Cross-reference

Vascular and Interventional Radiology: The Requisites, 2nd ed, 253–254.

CASE 141

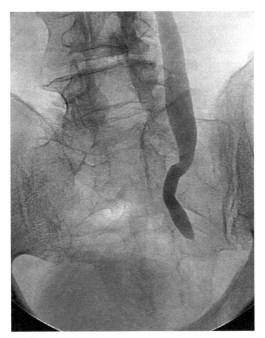

Figure 141-1

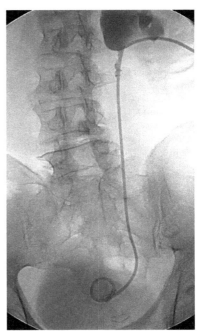

Figure 141-2

HISTORY: A 36-year-old female with history of pelvic radiation presents with left-sided flank pain.

1. Which of the following would be included in the differential diagnosis for the imaging findings presented? (Choose all that apply.)
   A. Retroperitoneal fibrosis
   B. Malignant ureteric obstruction
   C. Obstructing calculus
   D. Benign ureteric stricture

2. Which factor will have the most impact upon the likelihood of long-term success in treating a ureteral stricture?
   A. Side of stricture
   B. Grade of hydronephrosis
   C. Length of stricture
   D. Disappearance of stricture "waist" on post-procedure imaging

3. What is an indication for placement of an in situ nephrostomy catheter following ureteric balloon dilation and stenting?
   A. Hemorrhage with clot in the collecting system
   B. Post-procedure nephrostomy catheters need not be placed as the nephroureteral stent provides internal drainage
   C. Nephrostomy catheters should be placed after all ureteral dilation/stenting procedures involving strictures shorter than 2 cm
   D. Severe pre-procedure hydronephrosis

4. All of these are options for an interventional radiologist to dilate a ureteral stricture *EXCEPT*:
   A. Cryoplasty
   B. Noncutting balloon dilation
   C. Cutting balloon dilation
   D. Endoureterotomy

See Supplemental Figures section for additional figures and legends for this case.

CASE 141

Benign Ureteral Stricture

1. **B and D**. The provided case presents a column of contrast within a dilated right ureter. There is smooth tapering of contrast distally. The second image was taken after successful balloon dilation and placement of a nephroureteral stent. Differential for this appearance includes both benign malignant ureteral strictures. An obstructing calculus would produce a filling defect outlining the stone's position. Retroperitoneal fibrosis would not likely demonstrate such smooth tapering at the site of stricture.

2. **C**. The length of stricture has been found to have a large impact upon successful dilatation. Studies have found a significant difference between short (<2 cm) and long (>2 cm) segment strictures as well as a significant difference between benign and malignant strictures. Other factors including size of stricture, grade of hydronephrosis, and disappearance of "waist" of stricture have not been found to have a significant influence upon long-term outcomes.

3. **A**. A nephrostomy catheter should be placed if there was enough trauma to cause hemorrhage with clot in the collecting system. This can be left for a short period to allow for urinary drainage. The nephrostomy catheter can then safely be removed. If the procedure was relatively atraumatic, a nephrostomy catheter is not required. Preprocedure severe hydronephrosis may make the procedure more technically difficult but should not mandate a nephrostomy catheter.

4. **D**. Endoureterotomy is an open or laparoscopic surgical technique requiring an incision within the ureter. Balloon catheter dilation with both noncutting and cutting balloons has been performed. Cryoplasty is a technique in which the stricture will undergo supercooling and rewarming during dilation. This has been hypothesized to induce apoptosis rather than necrosis.

Comment

Imaging Interpretation

These images demonstrate a tight stricture of the left ureter at the ureterovesical junction, with consequent hydroureteronephrosis (Figures S141-1 and S141-2). In this patient, the stricture was due to prior radiation therapy. The benign nature of this stricture is favored by its focal, smooth appearance without evidence of mass effect. That said, the radiographic appearance is fairly nonspecific, and malignancy cannot be excluded on this basis alone. The stricture was successfully crossed, and a nephroureteral stent was placed (Figure S141-2).

Percutaneous Treatment

Balloon dilation of the ureter can be effective in treating benign strictures but is associated with high recurrence rates. Cutting balloons may also be used for difficult lesions, ones resistant to standard balloon angioplasty, and may be performed via ureteroscopic or percutaneous approach. Following intervention, a stent is typically left across the stenosis to provide a scaffold for healing while preventing collapse to an unacceptable diameter.

References

Adamo R, Saad WE, Brown D. Percutaneous ureteral interventions. *Tech Vasc Interv Radiol.* 2009;12:205–215.

Heran MK, Bergen DC, MacNeily AE. The use of cryoplasty in a benign ureteric stricture. *Pediatr Radiol.* 2010;40:1806–1809.

Lang EK, Glorioso 3rd. LW. Antegrade transluminal dilatation of benign ureteral strictures: long-term results. *AJR Am J Roentgenol.* 1988;150:131–134.

Cross-reference

Vascular and Interventional Radiology: The Requisites, 2nd ed, 499–506.

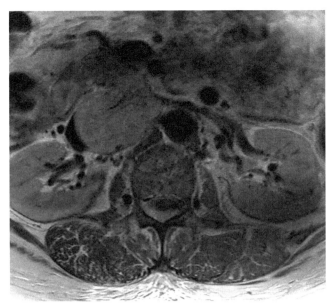

Figure 142-1. *Courtesy of Dr. Wael E. Saad.*

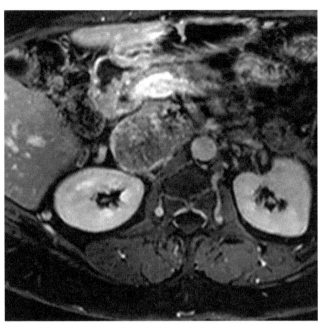

Figure 142-2. *Courtesy of Dr. Wael E. Saad.*

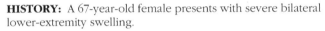

HISTORY: A 67-year-old female presents with severe bilateral lower-extremity swelling.

1. Which of the following would be included in the differential diagnosis for the imaging findings presented? (Choose all that apply.)
   A. Leiomyosarcoma
   B. Compression of inferior vena cava (IVC)
   C. Congenital anomaly of IVC
   D. Extension of tumor into IVC

2. What is the most common malignant primary IVC tumor?
   A. Sarcoma
   B. Melanoma
   C. Leiomyosarcoma
   D. Hamartoma

3. Which of the following would *MOST* suggest acute onset of disease?
   A. Venous stasis ulcers
   B. Venous collaterals on imaging
   C. Cellulitis
   D. *Phlegmasia cerulea dolens*

4. Which of the following is *NOT* a common presentation for leiomyosarcoma?
   A. Abdominal pain
   B. Arterial compromise
   C. Budd-Chiari syndrome
   D. Deep venous thrombosis (DVT)

See Supplemental Figures section for additional figures and legends for this case.

CASE 142

Infiltrating Inferior Vena Cava Tumor and Biopsy

1. **A, B, and D.** The images demonstrate a mass in the IVC. No extension to the kidneys is seen on these limited images. The differential diagnosis of an IVC mass includes leiomyosarcoma, sarcoma, thrombus, or extension of tumor into the IVC. Leiomyosarcoma and other sarcomas will enhance on post-contrast images, while bland thrombus will not enhance.

2. **C.** Leiomyosarcoma is the most common primary malignant tumor of the IVC, most frequently affecting women in the fifth and sixth decades of life.

3. **D.** *Phlegmasia cerulea dolens* (painful blue edema) is a very severe form of DVT as a result of extensive thrombosis of the deep veins and collaterals and resultant arterial compromise from swelling. Although it may not be a totally acute process, symptoms commonly surface acutely when collaterals also thrombose. These patients have painful and cyanotic lower extremities with lower-extremity edema. The other answer choices are descriptive of a chronic DVT.

4. **B.** The common presenting symptoms for leiomyosarcoma are abdominal pain, distention, Budd-Chiari syndrome, and DVT.

Comment

Main Teaching Point

Leiomyosarcoma is the most common primary tumor of the IVC. It usually occurs in women in the fifth to sixth decades of life and more commonly arises in the middle segment of the IVC. Patients affected by leiomyosarcoma usually have painful and edematous lower extremities from occlusion of the IVC. Other symptoms are reflective of level caval occlusion. Biopsy of the tumor may be performed by imaging guidance with ultrasound or computed tomography (CT) or endovascularly with forceps (Figures S142-3 through S142-5). The prognosis for leiomyosarcoma is poor, with only a 33% 5-year survival even with surgery and adjunctive and/or neoadjunctive chemoradiation.

Imaging Interpretation

On CT, leiomyosarcomas appear as low-attenuating infiltrating masses directly in the region of the IVC, usually with thrombus, internal hemorrhage, and internal necrosis. On magnetic resonance imaging, leiomyosarcomas commonly appear hypointense or isointense on T1-weighted images and hyperintense on T2-weighted images (Figure S142-1). Leiomyosarcoma commonly enhances after contrast administration, distinguishing it from bland thrombus (Figure S142-2). Either modality may show associated hepatic, intra-atrial, or pulmonary metastases.

References

Ganeshalingam S, Rajesawaran G, Jones RL, et al. Leiomyosarcomas of the inferior vena cava: diagnostic features on cross-section imaging. *Clin Radiol.* 2011;66:50–56.

Kandpal H, Sharma R, Gamangatti S, et al. Imaging of the inferior vena cava: a road less traveled. *Radiographics.* 2008;28:669–690.

Cross-reference

Vascular and Interventional Radiology: The Requisites, 2nd ed, 301–303.

CASE 143

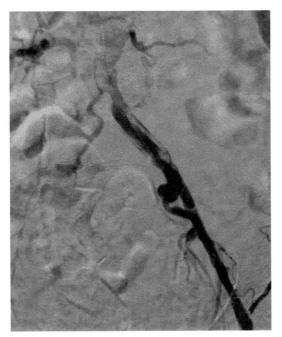

Figure 143-1

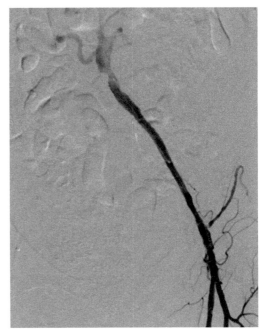

Figure 143-2

HISTORY: A 65-year-old man with hypertension presents with new-onset left buttock and leg pain following attempted angioplasty of a vascular stenosis.

1. Which of the following is the most likely diagnosis based on the imaging findings in the first image?
   A. Pseudoaneurysm
   B. Embolism
   C. Atherosclerotic stenosis
   D. Dissection

2. Which vessel is affected?
   A. Common iliac artery
   B. External iliac artery
   C. Common iliac vein
   D. Internal iliac vein

3. What is the most likely first-line treatment?
   A. Angioplasty alone
   B. Placement of a metallic stent
   C. Placement of a stent graft
   D. Surgical repair

4. In which situation is a self-expanding stent preferable to a balloon-expandable stent?
   A. When extremely precise deployment is necessary (i.e., near a critical branch point)
   B. Across a lesion that requires extremely high radial force to dilate
   C. Within a vessel that will undergo frequent motion (i.e., near a joint)
   D. When planning to over-dilate (i.e., larger than the adjacent vessel diameter)

See Supplemental Figures section for additional figures and legends for this case.

CASE 143

Stenting of Iliac Artery Dissection

1. **D.** The first image demonstrates a linear defect within the left common iliac artery with differential contrast enhancement on either side of it, compatible with a dissection. There is likely in situ thrombus as well.

2. **A.** Particularly on the second image, notice the smooth contours of the vessels with lack of visible valves, indicating these are arteries, not veins. As the abnormality occurs cephalad to the internal iliac, the affected vessel must be the common iliac artery.

3. **A.** Dissections often require the placement of a stent to hold the dissection flap against the vessel wall (otherwise the dissection will recur). However, low-pressure balloon angioplasty with a prolonged inflation is commonly the first-line treatment attempted. If this fails, most operators would place a stent. Stent grafts in this location would be reserved for the treatment of an aneurysm, pseudoaneurysm, or extravasation (conditions where the flow must stay within the stent to treat the abnormality).

4. **C.** Self-expanding stents have a predefined diameter that the stent attempts to assume and therefore can be compressed or twisted and are less likely to become permanently crushed or broken in the process.

Comment

Main Teaching Point

Stent placement has become an accepted method of treating a variety of arterial vascular abnormalities, including flow-limiting dissections, short-segment arterial occlusions, arterial stenoses refractory to angioplasty, arterial stenoses that recur following successful angioplasty, and eccentric or extremely calcified atherosclerotic lesions (Figures S143-1 and S143-2). Currently available vascular stents fall into two main categories.

Balloon-Expandable Stents

Balloon-expandable stents (prototype: Palmaz stent) are generally less than 4 cm long, although longer stents are available and are pre-mounted on an angioplasty balloon. Their primary advantage is the pinpoint accuracy with which they can be positioned, because the deployment step simply involves inflating the carrier balloon. Their primary disadvantages are the inability to treat longer lesions with a single stent and the possibility of the stent's slipping off the balloon during introduction. The latter problem has been largely remedied by stents that are securely mounted upon their carrier balloons by the manufacturer and careful deployment once the sheath has been retracted.

Self-Expandable Stents

Self-expandable stents (prototype: Wallstent) are available in longer lengths, possess greater longitudinal flexibility, and do not require balloon mounting. However, because deployment requires a carefully controlled unsheathing of the restrained stent, allowing it to expand, these stents are slightly more prone to malpositioning during deployment. However, many newer stents have easier deployment mechanisms to minimize maldeployment.

References

Funovics MA, Lackner B, Cejna M, et al. Predictors of long-term results after treatment of iliac artery obliteration by transluminal angioplasty and stent deployment. *Cardiovasc Intervent Radiol.* 2002;25:397–402.

Tsetis D. Endovascular treatment of complications of femoral arterial access. *Cardiovasc Intervent Radiol.* 2010;33:457–468.

Cross-reference

Vascular and Interventional Radiology: The Requisites, 2nd ed, 214–217.

CASE 144

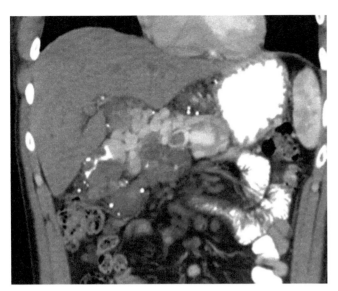

Figure 144-1. *Courtesy of Dr. Wael E. Saad.*

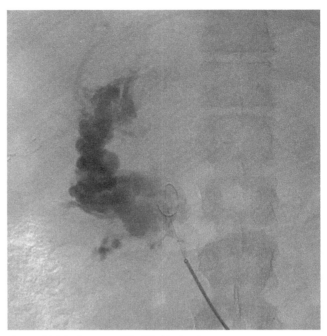

Figure 144-2. *Courtesy of Dr. Wael E. Saad.*

HISTORY: A 54-year-old male with recent diagnosis of essential thrombocythemia presents with hematemesis and melena for 1 day.

1. Which of the following is the most likely diagnosis for the imaging findings presented?
   A. Hepatoportal arteriovenous fistula
   B. Hepatocellular carcinoma (HCC)
   C. Caroli's disease
   D. Cavernous transformation of the portal vein (CTPV)

2. Which of the following is *NOT* a known underlying cause of portal vein thrombosis (PVT) that could potentially lead to the correct diagnosis in Question 1?
   A. Umbilical catheterization in children
   B. Prothrombin gene G20210A mutation
   C. Portal venous gas
   D. Pancreatitis

3. Which of the following is true regarding CTPV?
   A. CTPV becomes evident on imaging several months after the initial thrombotic event.
   B. Cirrhosis is the main risk factor for developing CTPV.
   C. CTPV often extends beyond the main portal vein and into the intrahepatic circulation.
   D. CTPV is an extensive hemodynamic adaptation that can effectively offset the development of portal hypertension.

4. Which of the following treatments is *MOST* likely contraindicated in this patient, at this time?
   A. Transjugular intrahepatic portal systemic shunt (TIPS)
   B. Liver transplant
   C. Anticoagulation
   D. Distal splenorenal shunt

See Supplemental Figures section for additional figures and legends for this case.

CASE 144

Cavernous Transformation of the Portal Vein

1. **D.** The patient has CTPV, radiographically represented as a network of intertwined periportal collateral vessels. Severe dilatation of the portovenous system secondary to portal hypertension is also seen. With the patient's history of essential thrombocythemia, which has a predilection for thrombotic complications in large abdominal vessels, he may have incurred PVT leading to CTPV. Hepatoportal arteriovenous fistula in adults most commonly occurs secondary to trauma or malignancy and will appear as a dilated hepatic artery and portal vein with early filling of the fistula and opacification of the portal venous system during the arterial phase.

2. **C.** Portal venous gas is a radiographic sign often associated with underlying abdominal disease and is not associated with development of PVT and subsequent CTPV. PVT in adults is often caused by congenital or acquired hypercoagulable states, abdominal malignancies, local inflammatory disease, cirrhosis, iatrogenic injury to the portal vein, and trauma, among other causes. PVT in children can be a sequela from sepsis or umbilical vein catheterization. CTPV does not occur in all PVT cases and may result from congenital malformation or development of hemangioma of the portal vein without a thrombotic event.

3. **C.** CTPV often occurs around the intrahepatic portal veins, well beyond the bifurcation of the portal vein. CTPV can occur only 1 to 2 weeks after the initial thrombotic event, even if the thrombosed portal vein becomes partially recanalized. Although cirrhosis may contribute to the development of PVT due to increased resistance to portal inflow, it does not have a strong predilection for developing CTPV. CTPV most commonly occurs in patients with noncirrhotic and nontumoral PVT.

4. **C.** CTPV is a relative contraindication for liver transplant and TIPS given the difficult anatomy. Other surgical options for diverting the portal blood include mesocaval, portacaval, proximal and distal splenorenal shunts. Studies suggest that early anticoagulation therapy for those with hypercoagulable state with CTPV may result in recanalization and prevention of thrombus propagation. However, in a patient with active variceal bleeding, band ligation or sclerotherapy is indicated prior to initiating anticoagulation therapy.

Comment

Etiology

CTPV is a relatively uncommon finding and is classically described as venous collateralization in response to thrombotic insult to the portal vein. Only a few days after the initial thrombotic event, collateral venous channels form in and around the intrahepatic and extrahepatic biliary channels to bypass the thrombus. Most patients with CTPV have healthy livers, and the underlying cause of PVT remains undetermined. When identifiable, the most common causes of PVT include HCC, cirrhosis, periportal inflammatory processes (e.g., pancreatitis, ascending cholangitis), and sepsis (the most common cause in children). Less common causes include hypercoagulable states and trauma.

Clinical Presentation

Many patients are asymptomatic from PVT and CTPV and present with symptoms of the underlying disease that caused the thrombosis. In symptomatic patients, upper gastrointestinal tract bleeding is the most common presentation. In advanced stages of CTPV, patients may present with decreased liver function from loss of liver mass and strictures/displacements of the biliary and main bile ducts.

Imaging Evaluation

Cross-sectional imaging modalities such as duplex ultrasound, helical computed tomography, and magnetic resonance imaging are fairly accurate in depicting PVT and CTPV. In questionable cases, definitive diagnosis of acute or partial portal vein occlusion may be identified by observing a focal filling defect within the portal vein during the venous phase of a celiac or superior mesenteric arteriogram or direct portography via transhepatic or TIPS access. CTPV is identified as enhancing serpiginous collateral veins in the porta hepatis with nonvisualization of the normal expected portal venous branching pattern (Figures S144-1 through S144-4). Patients often develop varicosities secondary to portal hypertension.

References

De Gaetano AM, Lafortune M, Patriquin H, et al. Cavernous transformation of the portal vein: patterns of intrahepatic and splanchnic collateral circulation detected with Doppler sonography. *AJR Am J Roentgenol.* 1995;165:1151–1155.

Gallego C, Velasco M, Marcuello P, et al. Congenital and acquired anomalies of the portal venous system. *Radiographics.* 2002;22:141–159.

Walser EM, Soloway R, Raza SA, et al. Transjugular portosystemic shunt in chronic portal vein occlusion: importance of segmental portal hypertension in cavernous transformation of the portal vein. *J Vasc Interv Radiol.* 2006;17:373–378.

Cross-reference

Vascular and Interventional Radiology: The Requisites, 2nd ed, 329.

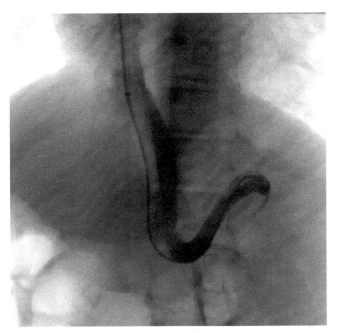

Figure 145-1. *Courtesy of Dr. Ranjith Vellody.*

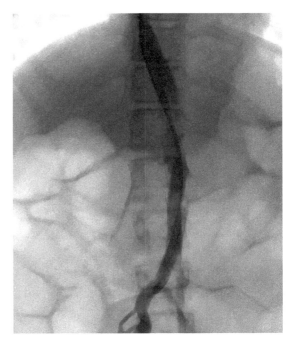

Figure 145-2. *Courtesy of Dr. Ranjith Vellody.*

HISTORY: A 12-year-old female presents with confusion and right upper quadrant pain.

1. Which of the following is the most likely diagnosis for the imaging findings presented?
   A. Normal anatomy
   B. Gastroesophageal varix
   C. Congenital absence of the portal vein (Abernethy malformation)
   D. Hypertrophied azygous vein

2. Which of the following is an associated finding in patients with the diagnosis above?
   A. Splenic cysts
   B. Pulmonary fibrosis
   C. Cardiac myxomas
   D. Hepatic tumors

3. Of the following lab abnormalities, which is the most likely cause of confusion?
   A. Low platelet count
   B. Hypokalemia
   C. Hyperammonemia
   D. Hypoammonemia

4. Which of the following subtypes of this process is surgically correctable?
   A. Type A
   B. Type I
   C. Type B
   D. Type II

See Supplemental Figures section for additional figures and legends for this case.

CASE 145

Abernethy Malformation

1. **C.** The images demonstrate injection of the splenic and superior mesenteric veins (SMVs) with flow of blood directly to the inferior vena cava and right atrium, without flow through the liver. A gastroesophageal varix may have the appearance of the venous anatomy seen with the splenic injection; however, there should be flow through the portal vein on SMV and splenic injection.

2. **D.** Hepatic tumors including adenoma, focal nodular hyperplasia, and hepatocellular carcinoma are thought to be associated with Abernethy malformation.

3. **C.** Hyperammonemia, which is more commonly seen in patients with cirrhosis and portal hypertension, is a result of the portosystemic shunting.

4. **D.** Two types of Abernethy malformations have been described; type I and II. Type I shunts occur when the portal vein is absent and the portal blood is shunted into the systemic veins. Type II shunts are described as a hypoplastic portal vein with the majority of blood diverted into the vena cava via a side-to-side connection, which may be surgically corrected.

Comment

Main Teaching Point

Abernethy malformation is a congenital shunt in which the intestinal and splenic veins bypass the liver and drain directly into the systemic veins (Figures S145-1 through S145-3). Two types have been described; type 1 occurring only in females and type II mostly in males. Type I shunts occur when the portal vein is absent and the portal blood is shunted into the systemic veins. Type I malformations are even further divided depending on whether the splenic and SMVs drain separately or as a common trunk into the systemic veins. Type II shunting is described as a hypoplastic portal vein with the majority of blood diverted into the vena cava via a side-to-side communication.

Patient Presentation

Abernethy malformation can present with a variety of clinical manifestations. These can range from remaining completely asymptomatic to having mild liver dysfunction to more serious conditions such as multiple primary hepatic tumors, pulmonary arteriovenous fistulas, and hepatic encephalopathy (Figure S145-4). These malformations can be recognized on imaging studies by only two tubular structures noted at the hepatic hilum (hepatic artery and common bile duct). Computed tomography and magnetic resonance imaging are better than ultrasound at identifying the portal vein anomaly and mapping out the portosystemic shunt. Type II shunts may be surgically corrected, whereas type 1 shunts may not.

References

Gallego C, Miralles M, Marin C, et al. Congenital hepatic shunts. *Radiographics.* 2004;24:755–772.

Lisovsky M, Konstas AA, Misdraji J. Congenital extrahepatic portosystemic shunts (Abernathy malformation): a histopathologic evaluation. *Am J Surg Pathol.* 2011;35:1381–1390.

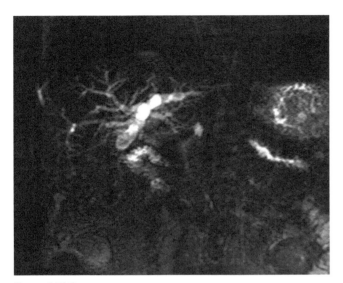

Figure 146-1

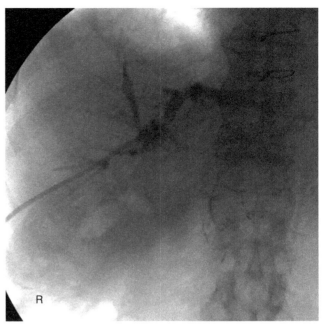

Figure 146-2

HISTORY: A 63-year-old male, status post Whipple procedure, presents with jaundice and right upper quadrant discomfort.

1. Which of the following would be included in the differential diagnosis for the imaging findings presented? (Choose all that apply.)
   A. Bile leak
   B. Primary sclerosing cholangitis
   C. Anastomotic biliary ductal stricture
   D. Ischemic bile duct injury

2. Deferral of biliary intervention should be considered in which of the following clinical scenarios?
   A. Portal hypertension
   B. Small bowel obstruction
   C. Cholangitis
   D. Localized cancer recurrence

3. Which of the following imaging modalities is most sensitive for detecting biliary ductal stricture?
   A. Magnetic resonance cholangiopancreatography (MRCP)
   B. Ultrasound
   C. Hepatobiliary scintigraphy
   D. Endoscopic retrograde cholangiopancreatography (ERCP)

4. If left untreated, biliary anastomotic strictures can result in which of the following? (Choose all that apply.)
   A. Hepatic cirrhosis
   B. Cholangitis
   C. Intrahepatic bile duct stones
   D. Biliary fistula

See Supplemental Figures section for additional figures and legends for this case.

CASE 146

Biliary-Enteric Anastomotic Stricture

1. **B, C, and D.** In this patient status post hepaticojejunostomy, MRCP and percutaneous cholangiography demonstrate moderate diffuse intrahepatic biliary dilatation to the level of the biliary-enteric anastomosis with abrupt termination at this location, compatible with biliary-enteric anastomotic stricture. Differential consideration includes ischemic bile duct injury and primary sclerosing cholangitis. Of note, primary sclerosing cholangitis will characteristically demonstrate irregular beading of intrahepatic and extrahepatic bile ducts with multifocal strictures. No contrast extravasation is observed on cholangiography to indicate a bile leak.

2. **C.** In a patient presenting clinically with cholangitis, temporary deferral of percutaneous biliary intervention may be considered until a course of antibiotics treats the infection. This can potentially avoid undesirable postintervention outcomes, including liver abscess and sepsis. However, in many cases, biliary drainage with the concurrent administration of antibiotics is the treatment necessary to decompress the system.

3. **C.** Of the modalities listed, hepatobiliary scintigraphy is the most sensitive test to detect absent biliary flow distally. Ultrasound, MRCP, and ERCP can be useful in initial evaluation of biliary dilation, though bowel contents and postoperative changes may obfuscate areas of concern. Cholangiography and ERCP are the most specific methods of confirming diagnosis but are invasive.

4. **A, B, C, and D.** Prompt intervention for biliary-enteric anastomotic strictures is mandated. Secondary biliary cirrhosis, cholangitis, intrahepatic bile duct stones, and biliary fistulas are well-documented complications of untreated biliary stricture, resulting in considerably increased morbidity. Early percutaneous intervention may circumvent these complications and avoid surgical anastomotic revision. However, surgical revision may be necessary in cases that are resistant to balloon dilation.

Comment
Main Teaching Point

A primary late complication of biliary surgery may be the development of a stricture at the biliary-enteric anastomosis. This may be diagnosed by cross-sectional imaging, cholangiography, or ERCP (Figures S146-1 and S146-2). Although surgical therapy can provide a durable treatment for this problem, the difficulty of performing repeat biliary surgery in the same operative bed is considerable.

Percutaneous Management

For this reason, percutaneous biliary drainage is usually performed initially. Balloon dilation of the anastomotic stricture can then be performed (Figures S146-3 through S146-5). An internal-external drainage catheter can be left behind for several months to serve as a scaffold of good caliber around which the anastomosis can heal. Depending upon the results of balloon dilation, definitive surgical anastomotic revision might or might not be required.

Clinical Considerations

Like other biliary interventions, antibiotic prophylaxis is recommended for biliary balloon dilation procedures. If the patient presents with cholangitis, then the balloon dilation procedure should be deferred to a future date when the patient is no longer infected. In this situation, at the initial sitting placement of a biliary drainage catheter should suffice.

References

Janssen JJ, van Delden OM, van Lienden KP, et al. Percutaneous balloon dilatation and long-term drainage as treatment of anastomotic and nonanastomotic benign biliary strictures. *Cardiovasc Intervent Radiol.* 2014;37:1559–1567.

Laasch HU, Martin DF. Management of benign biliary strictures. *Cardiovasc Intervent Radiol.* 2002;25:457–466.

Cross-reference

Vascular and Interventional Radiology: The Requisites, 2nd ed, 469–471.

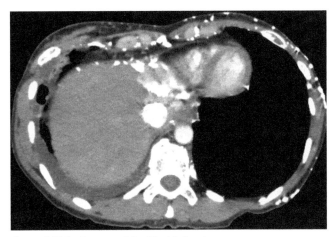

Figure 147-1. *Courtesy of Dr. Wael E. Saad.*

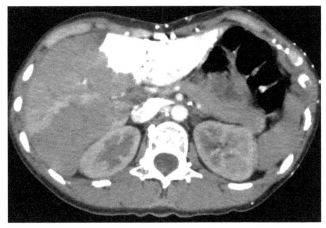

Figure 147-2. *Courtesy of Dr. Wael E. Saad.*

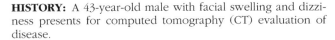

HISTORY: A 43-year-old male with facial swelling and dizziness presents for computed tomography (CT) evaluation of disease.

1. Which of the following is the most likely diagnosis for the imaging and clinical findings presented?
   A. Budd-Chiari syndrome
   B. Caval obstruction
   C. Klatskin tumor
   D. Arteriovenous malformation

2. Which of the following collateral pathways carries venous blood from the upper body through the liver in the setting of superior vena cava (SVC) obstruction?
   A. Caval-superficial-recanalized paraumbilical-portal
   B. Caval-mesenteric-portal
   C. Caval-hemiazygous-azygous
   D. Caval-retroperitoneal-portal

3. Which of the following is the *LEAST* likely etiology of SVC syndrome?
   A. Thrombosis secondary to central venous catheter
   B. Infection
   C. Extrinsic compression due to malignancy
   D. Pulmonary hypertension

4. Which of the following treatments in *NOT* commonly employed in SVC syndrome?
   A. Balloon angioplasty with or without stenting
   B. Surgical resection of the obstructed portion of the SVC
   C. Catheter thrombolysis
   D. Surgical bypass grafting

See Supplemental Figures section for additional figures and legends for this case.

CASE 147

Caval Obstruction with Collateralization: Bright Liver Sign

1. **B.** Focal hepatic enhancement involving the left lobe of the liver has been demonstrated in cases of caval obstruction and is due to development of cavoportal collateral pathways. In Budd-Chiari syndrome, hepatic venous outflow obstruction may lead to hypertrophy and hyperenhancement of the caudate lobe. Klatskin tumors cause intrahepatic biliary ductal dilatation and are not hyperenhancing. Arteriovenous malformations typically appear as a tangle of enhancing vessels.

2. **A.** Cavoportal collateral pathways carry blood to the liver in the setting of SVC obstruction including the caval-superficial-umbilical-portal pathway, which results in focal enhancement of Couinaud segment IV, and the caval-mammary-phrenic-hepatic capsule-portal pathway, which results in focal enhancement of the anterosuperior liver near the bare area. The other collateral pathways may be seen in inferior vena cava (IVC) obstruction.

3. **D.** Prior to the modern antibiotic era, infections such as tuberculosis and syphilis were the most common cause of SVC syndrome. SVC obstruction due to malignancy, whether via extrinsic compression or intrinsic involvement, is currently the most common cause, and thrombotic obstruction secondary to use of intravascular devices including central venous catheters and transvenous pacemakers is rapidly increasing. Pulmonary hypertension is not a recognized cause of SVC syndrome.

4. **B.** Endovascular procedures including balloon angioplasty with or without stenting are among the safest and most effective treatments available to relieve symptoms of SVC syndrome. Other therapies include surgical bypass grafting, catheter thrombolysis in the setting of acute thrombosis, and chemotherapy and radiotherapy in the setting of malignancy.

Comment

Etiology

Acquired caval occlusion may occur secondary to malignancy, either via direct involvement of the cava by tumor or external compression due to adjacent mass or nodal disease. Infection, though this is uncommon since the advent of antibiotics, and iatrogenic causes including central venous catheters and transvenous pacemakers, and benign conditions such as fibrosing mediastinitis are other common causes of SVC syndrome. With chronic occlusion, collateral pathways develop to facilitate venous drainage. Some are well described, including the azygous-hemiazygous, vertebral, mammary, and lateral thoracic pathways, whereas others such as the cavoportal pathways are less common.

Anatomy

The cavoportal collateral pathways include the caval-superficial-recanalized paraumbilical-portal and caval-mammary-phrenic-hepatic capsule-portal pathways, which may be seen with SVC obstruction, and the caval-renal-portal, caval-retroperitoneal-portal, and caval-mesenteric-portal pathways, which may be seen with IVC obstruction. Those seen with SVC obstruction may cause focal hepatic enhancement on CT following intravenous contrast injection into an upper extremity vein (Figures S147-1 through S147-3). The caval-superficial-paraumbilical-portal pathway is associated with hyperenhancement of Couinaud segment IV while the caval-mammary-phrenic-hepatic capsule-portal pathway is associated with hyperenhancement of an anterosuperior region near the bare area. While caval occlusion is often known or suspected in such cases, correct interpretation of these unusual hepatic enhancement patterns occasionally results in a diagnosis of previously occult obstruction.

Treatment Methods

Treatment options include chemotherapy and radiotherapy for malignant etiologies; catheter thrombolysis in the setting of soft thrombus, which should be suspected with acute symptom onset, thrombosis secondary to an intravascular catheter, or when the occlusion is easily traversed with a wire; surgical bypass grafting; and endovascular procedures including balloon angioplasty and stenting. Endovascular procedures have the advantage of low morbidity and fast onset of symptom relief and do not damage tissues in a way that would preclude subsequent sampling for pathological conditions. The occlusion is traversed with a wire and luminal patency achieved via balloon angioplasty. Stenting is commonly performed when occlusion is secondary to malignancy but is avoided if possible in patients with benign occlusion and relatively longer life expectancy due to the risk of stent occlusion.

References

Kapur S, Paik E, Rezaei A, et al. Where there is blood, there is a way: unusual collateral vessels in superior and inferior vena cava obstruction. *Radiographics*. 2010;30:67–78.

Siegel Y, Schallert E. Prevalence and etiology of focal liver opacification in patients with superior vena cava obstruction. *J Comput Assist Tomogr*. 2013;37:805–808.

Cross-reference

Vascular and Interventional Radiology: The Requisites, 2nd ed, 144–145.

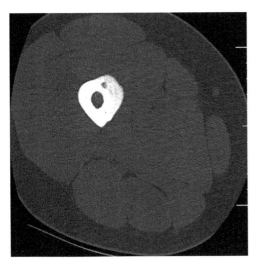

Figure 148-1. *Courtesy of Dr. Ranjith Vellody.*

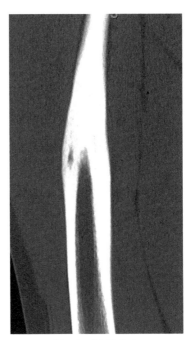

Figure 148-2. *Courtesy of Dr. Ranjith Vellody.*

HISTORY: A 15-year-old male with lower-extremity pain of 2 months, worse at night, presents for treatment.

1. Which of the following is the most likely diagnosis for the imaging findings presented?
   A. Osteomyelitis
   B. Stress fracture
   C. Osteoid osteoma
   D. Cortical desmoid

2. What is the most common region for the occurrence of this lesion?
   A. Skull
   B. Long bones of the limbs
   C. Pelvis
   D. Spine

3. Which of the following percutaneous procedures is most commonly performed for treatment of this lesion?
   A. Percutaneous aspiration
   B. Percutaneous embolization
   C. Percutaneous packing
   D. Percutaneous ablation

4. While this procedure is relatively low risk, which of the following is a known complication?
   A. Metastatic spread
   B. Growth retardation
   C. Mental retardation
   D. Superficial skin burn

See Supplemental Figures section for additional figures and legends for this case.

CASE 148

Osteoid Osteoma

1. **C.** The images show asymmetric cortical thickening with periosteal reaction and a nidus of low attenuation. Given the characterization of pain and young age, this most likely represents an osteoid osteoma; a benign bone tumor.

2. **B.** The most common locations for osteoid osteoma are in the metaphysis and diaphysis of the long bones, specifically the femur and the tibia. In the femur, the most common sites are the femoral neck and the intertrochanteric region.

3. **D.** The procedure being performed in Figures 148-1 and S148-2, as well as in Figures S148-3 and S148-4, is percutaneous radiofrequency ablation (RFA). The ablation techniques have shown to be equivalent to surgical resection in terms of treatment efficacy. Under computed tomography (CT) guidance, the nidus of the tumor is accessed with an RFA probe. The lesion then undergoes ablation for several minutes.

4. **D.** Complications related to percutaneous RFA are rare, but include superficial skin burns, cellulitis, fracture, or damage to the adjacent nerves. Case reports of fractures have been reported as well.

Comment

Main Teaching Point

Osteoid osteoma is a benign tumor of the bone most commonly found within the long bones of adolescents. It classically presents with pain and swelling, worst at night. These lesions are commonly found in the cortex of long bones of the limbs but may be found elsewhere including the phalanges and the spine. The osteoid osteoma lesion is comprised of a lucent nidus, fibrovascular rim, and adjacent reactive sclerosis (Figures S148-1 through S148-3). Diagnosis of osteoid osteoma is usually made with plain radiographs or CT. Magnetic resonance imaging or bone scintigraphy may also help in making the diagnosis.

Treatment Methods

Osteoid osteoma lesions are benign but may cause significant pain. The pain usually responds to nonsteroidal anti-inflammatory medications. However, if pain from the lesion limits the patient's activities, it can result in leg-length discrepancies, scoliosis, or disuse osteopenia. In these situations, surgical resection or curettage may be performed. Additionally, the lesions can be treated with RFA or cryoablation, which are percutaneous and avoid the potential complications of a surgical repair (Figure S148-4). The complications related to percutaneous options remain incompletely evaluated but include superficial skin burns, cellulitis, fracture, or damage to the adjacent nerves.

References

Boscainos PJ, Cousins GR, Kulshreshtha R, et al. Osteoid osteoma. *Orthopedics.* 2013;36:792–800.
Earhart J, Wellman D, Donaldson J, et al. Radiofrequency ablation in the treatment of osteoid osteoma: results and complications. *Pediatr Radiol.* 2013;43:814–819.

Cross-reference

Vascular and Interventional Radiology: The Requisites, 2nd ed, 543–544.

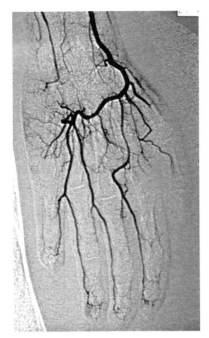

Figure 149-1

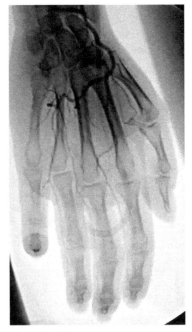

Figure 149-2

HISTORY: A 42-year-old female presents to her primary care physician with pain and paresthesias involving her hands.

1. Which of the following is the most likely diagnosis for the imaging findings presented?
   A. Traumatic injury to the radial artery
   B. Vascular manifestations of rheumatoid arthritis
   C. Systemic sclerosis
   D. Buerger's disease

2. Prior to any arterial interventions in this case, what is best test to ensure adequate collateral perfusion of the hand?
   A. Skin exam to screen for cyanosis
   B. Plain film of the hand to observe for osteonecrosis
   C. Allen's test
   D. Doppler ultrasound

3. What radiographic finding in these images allows for a confident diagnosis of the disease process?
   A. Multiple, diffuse occluded and stenotic arterial lesions
   B. The formation of pseudoaneurysms
   C. The localization of the lesions to the digits
   D. The evidence of acro-osteolysis

4. How can one best determine if there is a significant vasospastic component present?
   A. Injection of epinephrine
   B. Exposure of the digits to a cold environment
   C. Exposure of the digits to a warm environment
   D. Injection of nitroglycerin

See Supplemental Figures section for additional figures and legends for this case.

CASE 149

Scleroderma

1. **C.** The most likely diagnosis for the images presented in this case is systemic sclerosis or scleroderma. The images show multiple areas of occlusion and stenoses within the hand, which are characteristic of scleroderma. The differential should still include embolic phenomena, vasculitides, traumatic lesions, and vasospasm, but the identification of acro-osteolysis allows for a confident diagnosis of scleroderma.

2. **C.** The Allen's test is the best and most practical exam finding to ensure that there is adequate collateral perfusion of the hand. Both the ulnar and the radial artery participate in blood flow to the hand. The exam is performed by manually occluding both the radial and the ulnar artery and having the patient make a fist. While still applying pressure, have the patient open the hand and the palm should appear pallored. Release pressure on one of the arteries and color should return to the hand. Before any arterial interventions are undertaken in one of the arteries, the Allen's test should be performed to ensure that there is adequate flow from the other artery.

3. **D.** The evidence of acro-osteolysis in these images allows for a confident diagnosis of scleroderma. Acro-osteolysis is a radiographic finding that refers to terminal bony erosions due to resorption of the distal phalanges. This is a common radiographic finding in patients with vascular involvement of scleroderma. There are multiple stenotic and occluded lesions in these images, but this is not specific for scleroderma as there are many other disease processes that can present like this (embolic, vasculitis, or trauma). There is no localization to the digits in these images nor is there evidence of pseudoaneurysmal formation.

4. **D.** The injection of a vasodilator, such as nitroglycerin, would allow for the identification of a vasospastic component in this case. If the arterial lesions improve with the administration of a vasodilator, then this indicates that a sympathectomy may be beneficial for the patient (such as a patient with Raynaud's phenomenon). A vasoconstrictor, such as epinephrine, would only worsen these lesions. Exposure of the hand to warm and cold environments may elicit a response such as cyanosis of the digits, but it is not as specific as vasodilator administration.

Comment

Main Teaching Point

Small artery occlusions and stenoses in the palmar and digital arteries can produce severe pain, paresthesias, Raynaud's phenomenon, fingertip necrosis, and gangrene (Figures S149-1 through S149-4). The pathophysiology of vascular lesions in these patients often includes embolic, traumatic, vasoreactive, and inflammatory components. Diagnostic evaluation should focus upon identifying contributing factors that are treatable by medical or surgical interventions.

Endovascular Evaluation

First, the angiogram should be carefully scrutinized for any evidence of emboli. Potential sources of digital emboli include the heart (diagnosed by echocardiography and treated with anticoagulation), atherosclerotic plaques in the subclavian artery (treated with anticoagulation and/or surgical removal of the source lesion), sports-related injury to the axillary artery (subject to surgical repair), and occupational vascular injuries such as hypothenar hammer syndrome (also subject to surgical repair). Second, the presence of a significant vasospastic component to the arterial lesions should be sought during the angiographic evaluation. If the stenotic lesions improve significantly following administration of a vasodilator (such as tolazoline or nitroglycerin), then a sympathectomy may be more likely to provide some degree of symptom relief.

Disease Progression

Unfortunately, this patient has irreversible small-vessel occlusions due to scleroderma. The vascular findings mimic those seen with other small-vessel diseases. However, the diagnosis of scleroderma can confidently be made in this patient due to the clear radiographic evidence of acro-osteolysis (Figures S149-2 and S149-3).

References

Stucker M, Quinna S, Memmel U, et al. Macroangiopathy of the upper extremities in progressive systemic sclerosis. *Eur J Med Res.* 2000;5:295–302.

Taylor MH, McFadden JA, Bolster MB, et al. Ulnar artery involvement in systemic sclerosis (scleroderma). *J Rheumatol.* 2002;29:102–106.

Cross-reference

Vascular and Interventional Radiology: The Requisites, 2nd ed, 130.

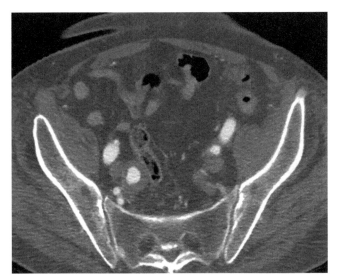

Figure 150-1

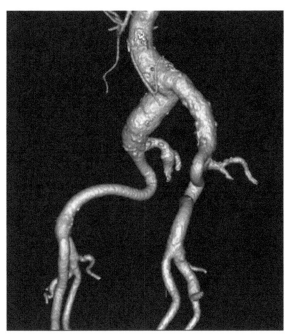

Figure 150-2

HISTORY: A 68-year-old male with abdominal aortic aneurysm presents for preoperative computed tomography angiography (CTA).

1. Which of the following would be included in the differential diagnosis for the imaging findings presented? (Choose all that apply.)
   A. Right internal iliac artery aneurysm
   B. Right common iliac artery aneurysm
   C. Right external iliac artery pseudoaneurysm
   D. Right internal iliac artery dissection

2. For asymptomatic lesions, which diameter necessitates intervention?
   A. 1.0 to 1.5 cm
   B. 2.0 to 2.5 cm
   C. 3.0 to 3.5 cm
   D. 4.0 to 4.5 cm

3. Endovascular repair is elected. Before occluding the inflow to this lesion, what step should be performed?
   A. Embolization of distal arteries arising from lesion
   B. Stent-graft placement in external iliac artery
   C. Contralateral common iliac arteriogram
   D. Thrombin injection into lesion

4. Which of the following is the most common complication of endovascular repair of this lesion?
   A. Endoleak from stent graft
   B. Buttock claudication
   C. Distal atheroembolization
   D. Colonic ischemia

See Supplemental Figures section for additional figures and legends for this case.

CASE 150

Internal Iliac Artery Aneurysm

1. **A and B.** Fusiform dilation is seen in the right common and internal iliac arteries. There is mild dilation of the left common iliac artery as well.

2. **C.** The risk of aneurysmal rupture increases dramatically with a diameter above 3 cm. Therefore asymptomatic aneurysms above 3.0 to 3.5 cm in diameter should be electively repaired.

3. **A.** In order to prevent retrograde filling of the aneurysm sac, the outflow vessels should be occluded with coils.

4. **B.** Buttock claudication occurs with a mean incidence of 21.8% in patients after endovascular repair but is usually mild and transient. Endoleak, distal arterial atheroembolization, colonic ischemia, and graft occlusion are other, less frequent complications.

Comment

Main Teaching Point

Isolated iliac artery aneurysms can rupture, embolize, or produce local compression symptoms. These may be found incidentally or as part of evaluation for other aneurysmal disease (Figures S150-1 and S150-2). The rate of rupture increases significantly between 3 and 4 cm, and therefore most surgeons recommend elective operative repair for iliac aneurysms larger than 3.0 to 3.5 cm in diameter. Because retroperitoneal dissection can be difficult when the aneurysm morphology is complex, endovascular methods to repair iliac aneurysms have gained favor. So far, the primary patencies of stent grafts for iliac artery aneurysms have been excellent (81% to 97% at 2 to 5 years), and the incidence of endoleaks has been very low.

Treatment Methods

Because of the late potential for cross-pelvic collaterals to reconstitute the aneurysm sac, it is very important to gain control of all distal vessels arising from the aneurysm, either by surgical ligation or by coil embolization (Figures S150-3 through S150-5). Once these outflow vessels are successfully occluded, the inflow to the aneurysm may be occluded by placing a stent graft across the origin of the internal iliac artery. Follow-up after endovascular repair commonly includes CTA before discharge and at 6-month intervals for the next 12 months. An increase in size greater than or equal to 5 mm requires further intervention or closer surveillance.

References

Razavi MK, Dake MD, Semba CP, et al. Percutaneous endoluminal placement of stent-grafts for the treatment of isolated iliac artery aneurysms. *Radiology.* 1995;197:801–804.

Sanchez LA, Patel AV, Ohki T, et al. Midterm experience with the endovascular treatment of isolated iliac aneurysms. *J Vasc Surg.* 1999;30:907–914.

Uberoi R, Tsetis D, Shrivastava V, et al. Standard of practice for the interventional management of isolated iliac artery aneurysms. *Cardiovasc Intervent Radiol.* 2011;34:3–13.

Cross-reference

Vascular and Interventional Radiology: The Requisites, 2nd ed, 203–209.

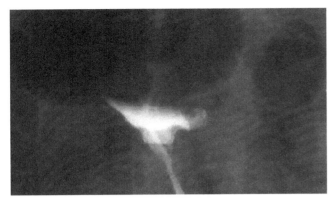

Figure 151-1. *Courtesy of Dr. David Hovsepian.*

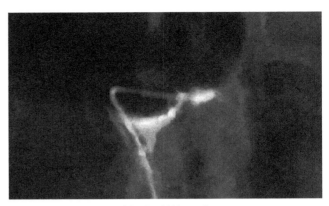

Figure 151-2. *Courtesy of Dr. David Hovsepian.*

HISTORY: A 37-year-old female presents for evaluation; remaining history is withheld.

1. What is the most common cause of the findings depicted in image 151-1?
   A. Congenital anomaly
   B. Ectopic pregnancy
   C. Pelvic inflammatory disease
   D. Endometriosis

2. For what condition would the procedure depicted in the images be performed?
   A. Pelvic congestion syndrome
   B. Infertility
   C. Ovarian torsion
   D. Uterine arteriovenous malformation

3. During which phase of the menstrual cycle is it best to perform this procedure?
   A. Follicular
   B. Ovulatory
   C. Luteal
   D. Secretory

4. Which of the following is a contraindication to performing this procedure?
   A. Fibroids
   B. Endometriosis
   C. Adenomyosis
   D. Pelvic infection

See Supplemental Figures section for additional figures and legends for this case.

CASE 151

Fallopian Tube Recanalization

1. **C.** The image demonstrates bilateral proximal fallopian tubal occlusions, for which of those listed, pelvic inflammatory disease is the most common cause.

2. **B.** Tubal disease is estimated to cause up to one-third of subfertility issues in women, with approximately 10% to 25% consisting of proximal tubal occlusions.

3. **A.** The follicular phase is the best time to perform this procedure, typically between days 6 and 11 of the menstrual cycle.

4. **D.** Active pelvic infection is a contraindication to this procedure and could result in peritonitis or bacteremia, if attempted. However, prior resolved episodes of pelvic infection are not a contraindication.

Comment

Etiology

The fallopian tube extends from the cornu of the uterine cavity to the ovary. The ovarian end is fimbriated, open to the peritoneal cavity, and adjacent to the ovary; thus allowing the ovulated egg to travel into the fallopian tube for fertilization. Approximately one-third of female infertility issues are due to tubal disease, with 10% to 20% resulting from proximal tubal occlusion. The most common cause is pelvic inflammatory disease. Hysterosalpingogram (HSG) is used to evaluate for potential causes of infertility, including uterine anatomical abnormalities and fallopian tube patency.

Procedural Technique

When HSG demonstrates proximal tubal occlusion (Figure S151-1), a selective salpingogram is performed with a small catheter through the orifice of the fallopian tube (Figure S151-2). If tubal occlusion is confirmed, a guidewire may be gently advanced in an attempt to traverse the occlusion and dislodge a mucous plug (Figure S151-3), as in this case. Repeat salpingogram then demonstrates spill of contrast into the peritoneal cavity, consistent with a patent (recanalized) fallopian tube (Figure S151-4).

Clinical Considerations

The procedure is typically performed during the follicular stage of the menstrual cycle between days 6 and 11. Active pelvic infection is an absolute contraindication. Technical success rates of the procedure are high, with reports ranging from 71% to 92%. Successful fallopian tube recanalization allows for unlimited natural attempts at conception and is less invasive and costly than other infertility treatments. The average rate of pregnancy after a successful procedure is reported as high as 60%, when the underlying tubes are normal. A few causes of failure to recanalize may be due to complete occlusions from prior infection, surgery, or endometriosis. Re-occlusion of the fallopian tubes can occur, and recanalization may be attempted. Potential complications include mild cramping, vaginal bleeding, tubal perforation (<4%), adnexal infection, and ectopic pregnancy (3%).

References

Lopera J, Suri R, Kroma GM, et al. Role of interventional procedures in obstetrics/gynecology. *Radiol Clin North Am*. 2013;51:1049–1066.

Pinto AB, Hovsepian DM, Wattanakumtornkul S, et al. Pregnancy outcomes after fallopian tube recanalization: oil-based versus water-soluble contrast agents. *J Vasc Interv Radiol*. 2003;14:69–74.

Thurmond AS. Fallopian tube catheterization. *Semin Intervent Radiol*. 2013;30:381–387.

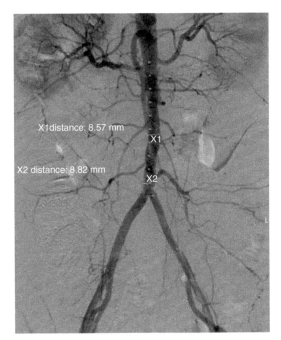

Figure 152-1. *Courtesy of Dr. Alan H. Matsumoto.*

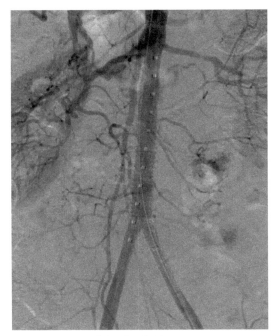

Figure 152-2. *Courtesy of Dr. Alan H. Matsumoto.*

HISTORY: A 54-year-old woman presents to her primary care physician. The remaining history is withheld.

1. Which of the following is the most likely diagnosis for the imaging findings presented?
   A. Chronic distal aortoiliac occlusive disease
   B. Infrarenal aortic dissection
   C. Occluded aortoiliac bypass graft
   D. Aortoenteric fistula

2. With what symptoms do these patients usually present?
   A. Acute-onset lower-extremity pain
   B. Lower-extremity myalgias and paresthesias
   C. Intermittent lower-extremity claudication
   D. Hematochezia

3. Which of the following procedures has been performed?
   A. Aorto-bifemoral bypass graft placement
   B. Endograft placement
   C. Percutaneous aortoiliac reconstruction
   D. Aortoiliac bypass graft placement

4. Which of the following is a complication of the intervention above?
   A. Lower-extremity microembolization
   B. Stroke
   C. Renal artery coverage
   D. Hematuria

See Supplemental Figures section for additional figures and legends for this case.

CASE 152

Percutaneous Aortoiliac Reconstruction

1. **A.** The first image demonstrates aortoiliac occlusive disease. No dissection, graft, or fistula is seen.

2. **C.** These patients commonly present with bilateral lower extremity and buttock claudication.

3. **C.** The image demonstrates percutaneous stenting of the aorta and iliac arteries. An endograft, however, was not placed nor was a bypass graft.

4. **A.** Unlike abdominal aortic aneurysm repair where the endograft is commonly advanced to the renal arteries, percutaneous stenting of the aortic bifurcation for aortoiliac occlusive disease does not require sealing of an aneurysm neck.

Comment

Main Teaching Point

Distal aortoiliac occlusive disease was historically treated with aortoiliac or aortofemoral bypass grafts. However, with the recent improvement in the endovascular technologies, a percutaneous approach is possible, in selected patients. The images demonstrate placement of aortoiliac stents with significant immediate improvement in the flow following stenting (Figures S152-1 through S152-4). Endograft placement was not possible in this case due to the small sizes of the iliac vessels and aorta.

Endovascular Management

Studies have shown that the percutaneous approach with stenting of the chronic infrarenal aortoiliac occlusive disease leads to shorter hospital stay and less morbidity. There may be slightly decreased patency rates; however, this remains controversial. With stenting, bypass can also be performed at a later date if needed. Either covered or bare stents can be used for this type of aortoiliac reconstruction. Covered stents may exclude endothelium and atheromatous plaques, hypothetically reducing the rate of re-stenosis. Because of this reason, covered stents may be more advantageous in advanced peripheral arterial disease.

References

Lun Y, Zhang J, Wu X, et al. Comparison of midterm outcomes between surgical treatment and endovascular reconstruction for chronic infrarenal aortoiliac occlusion. *J Vasc Interv Radiol.* 2015;26: 196–204.

Sharafuddin MJ, Hoballah JJ, Kresowik TF, et al. Kissing stent reconstruction of the aortoiliac bifurcation. *Perspect Vasc Surg Endovasc Ther.* 2008;20:50–60.

Cross-reference

Vascular and Interventional Radiology: The Requisites, 2nd ed, 209–214.

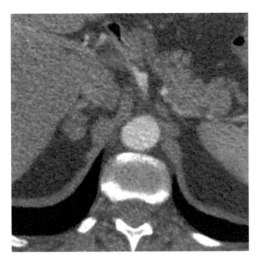

Figure 153-1 *Courtesy of Dr. Kyung J. Cho.*

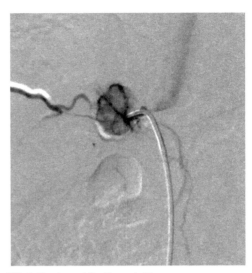

Figure 153-2 *Courtesy of Dr. Kyung J. Cho.*

HISTORY: A 62-year-old female presents with a history of hyperaldosteronism.

1. Which of the following would be included in the differential diagnosis for the imaging findings presented? (Choose all that apply.)
   A. Normal adrenal glands
   B. Adrenal metastasis
   C. Adrenal adenoma
   D. Pheochromocytoma

2. What is the most common indication for adrenal venous sampling?
   A. To identify the location of a biochemically proven pheochromocytoma without a visible source
   B. To determine whether autonomous hormone production is unilateral or bilateral
   C. To diagnose syndromes of androgen excess
   D. To diagnose adrenal Cushing's disease

3. How is the quality of an adrenal venous sample assessed?
   A. The cortisol levels of the adrenal venous sample are compared to the contralateral adrenal venous sample and should be similar.
   B. The aldosterone-cortisol ratio of the adrenal venous sample is compared to the contralateral adrenal venous sample and should be similar.
   C. The cortisol levels of the adrenal venous sample are compared to those of a peripheral blood sample and should be 2 to 3 times greater.
   D. The aldosterone-cortisol ratio of the adrenal venous sample is compared to that of a peripheral blood sample and should be 2 to 3 times greater.

4. In a unilateral adrenal adenoma, what is the contralateral normal adrenal gland aldosterone-cortisol ratio compared to a peripheral sample?
   A. Lower
   B. Equal
   C. Elevated
   D. Unpredictable

See Supplemental Figures section for additional figures and legends for this case.

CASE 153

Selective Adrenal Venous Sampling

1. **B, C, and D.** The imaging findings demonstrate a vascular mass in the region of the right adrenal gland that could represent an adrenal adenoma, metastasis, or pheochromocytoma. Based on the history, this case is most likely a right adrenal adenoma producing excess aldosterone. The left adrenal gland appears normal, but the right clearly is not.

2. **B.** The most common indication for adrenal venous sampling is to determine whether autonomous hormone production in primary hyperaldosteronism is unilateral or bilateral, as unilateral disease can be corrected surgically. Other less common indications are to diagnose syndromes of androgen excess or adrenal Cushing disease or to identify the location of a biochemically proven pheochromocytoma without a visible source.

3. **C.** Determining the quality of the adrenal venous sample involves comparing the cortisol levels of the adrenal venous sample to a peripheral blood sample. The cortisol levels in the adrenal venous sample should be 2 to 3 times greater than that in the peripheral blood.

4. **A.** Adrenal adenomas that produce excess aldosterone show an aldosterone-cortisol ratio higher than the peripheral value. To compensate for this excess production, the contralateral normal adrenal gland shows decreased aldosterone production.

Comment

Main Teaching Point

Primary hyperaldosteronism is important to identify within the hypertensive population, because most patients with a unilateral source of excess aldosterone production are amenable to surgical cure. Typically, postural hormonal testing is first performed by an endocrinologist. The diagnosis is then confirmed by selective adrenal venous sampling with measurement of aldosterone concentrations (expressed as aldosterone-to-cortisol ratio) in each adrenal vein. Selective adrenal venous sampling has been shown to be more sensitive and specific than cross-sectional imaging or scintigraphy, and endocrine surgeons are often guided by the results of the sampling study (Figures S153-1 and S153-3). Patients with unilateral disease are ideally treated by laparoscopic adrenalectomy. Patients in whom localization is not achieved usually have bilateral adrenal hyperplasia and are treated medically.

Endovascular Management

The intervention itself requires concurrent catheterization of the left and right adrenal veins with careful, controlled aspiration of blood for sampling (Figures S153-2 and S153-4). It is important to place additional side holes in the catheters to ensure appropriate sampling. The left adrenal vein is usually easier to select, given its origin from the left renal vein. The right renal vein is more difficult and may be the cause of technical failure. Once the veins are catheterized, adrenocorticotropic hormone is commonly given to stimulate cortisol and aldosterone production. Samples are obtained from the left and right adrenal veins as well as a peripheral sample, commonly from the inferior vena cava, and sent to the lab for evaluation. Once the results are available, they should be carefully analyzed for a localizing discrepancy.

References

Cho KJ. Current role of angiography in the evaluation of adrenal disease causing hypertension. *Urol Radiol.* 1981-1982;3:249–255.

Daunt N. Adrenal vein sampling: how to make it quick, easy, and successful. *Radiographics.* 2005;25:S143–S158.

Kahn SL, Angle JF. Adrenal vein sampling. *Tech Vasc Interv Radiol.* 2010;13:110–125.

Cross-reference

Vascular and Interventional Radiology: The Requisites, 2nd ed, 306–307.

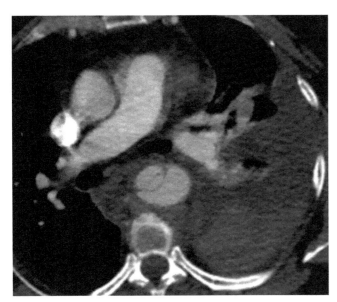

Figure 154-1. *Courtesy of Dr. David M. Williams.*

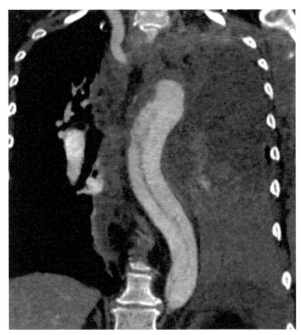

Figure 154-2. *Courtesy of Dr. David M. Williams.*

HISTORY: A 50-year-old female presents to the emergency department with severe chest and back pain.

1. Which of the following is the most likely diagnosis for the imaging findings presented?
   A. Pseudoaneurysm
   B. Thoracic aortic aneurysm
   C. Aortic dissection with rupture
   D. Penetrating atherosclerotic ulcer

2. What is the key imaging finding of intramural hematoma on a noncontrast computed tomography (CT)?
   A. Circumferential hypodensity surrounding the aorta
   B. Hypoattenuating saccular projection with direct connection to the true lumen
   C. Focal areas of hyperattenuation extending beyond the expected contour of the aortic wall
   D. Faint peripheral hyperattenuating crescent within the aortic wall

3. What is the initial management of patients with suspected thoracic aortic dissection?
   A. Pain control and blood pressure management
   B. Aortogram with fenestration of the intimal flap
   C. Surgical composite graft replacement of aortic valve, aortic root, and ascending aorta with reimplantation of coronary arteries (Bentall procedure)
   D. Endovascular stent-graft placement

4. What role does angiography currently have in the management of this disorder?
   A. Defining branch vessel anatomy and lumen of origin
   B. Confirming diagnosis of suspected acute aortic rupture in a hemodynamically unstable patient
   C. Embolization of the aortic rupture site
   D. Maintaining branch vessel patency

See Supplemental Figures section for additional figures and legends for this case.

CASE 154

Aortic Dissection with Rupture

1. **C.** The most likely diagnosis is aortic dissection with rupture. Both computed tomographic angiography (CTA) images presented here show a well-demarcated dissection flap, which starts in the descending thoracic aorta and continues distally into the abdominal aorta. Left-sided hemothorax and mediastinal hematoma are also noted. Pseudoaneurysm and aneurysm commonly present as definable dilations of the aorta, although both may be associated with dissection. Penetrating atherosclerotic ulceration tends to be a focal extension beyond the expected contour of the aortic lumen without longitudinal spread.

2. **D.** The key imaging finding of intramural hematoma (IMH) is a faint peripheral hyperattenuating crescent within the aortic wall (~40 to 50) Hounsfield units seen on noncontrast CT. IMH is thought to be due to rupture of vasa vasorum supplying the aortic wall. Within the differential one must consider an aneurysm, pseudoaneurysm, and penetrating atherosclerotic ulcer, among others.

3. **A.** Patients with suspected thoracic aortic dissection should be promptly treated with antihypertensive medications to reduce systolic blood pressure to 100 to 120 mm Hg. Surgical and endovascular treatments should only be used in confirmed cases of complicated type B aortic dissection and all cases of type A dissection. Endovascular management includes fenestration to improve visceral or lower-extremity perfusion or endograft placement across the entry tear, if visible and if anatomy allows.

4. **A and D.** Angiography may be employed to define branch vessel anatomy, patency, and lumen of origin in patients undergoing surgery or endovascular therapy, although CTA is utilized far more frequently. In patients with visceral or lower-extremity malperfusion, fenestration and stenting may be performed to maintain branch vessel patency.

Comment

Main Teaching Point

Aortic rupture is a dreaded complication of aortic dissection. Stanford type A dissections carry a moderate risk of ascending aortic rupture into the pericardial sac, producing pericardial tamponade; to prevent this, these patients are treated with immediate aortic repair. Stanford type B dissections typically are managed medically, initially with pain control and an intravenous beta-blocker unless there are signs of end-organ ischemia or continued hemorrhage into the pleural or retroperitoneal spaces. Occasionally, Stanford type B dissections progress to aortic rupture. Clinical signs that can indicate impending or completed aortic rupture are persistent or increasing chest pain, uncontrolled hypertension, development of a left-sided pleural effusion on chest radiography or CT, and/or hemodynamic instability. In the cases shown here, aortic rupture with hemothorax is clearly depicted on CT (Figures S154-1 through S154-4).

Imaging Interpretation

The majority of aortic dissections are seen in older, hypertensive patients. Connective tissue disorders including Marfan syndrome and Ehlers-Danlos syndrome are also risk factors. Modalities that assist in diagnosis include CTA, magnetic resonance imaging (MRI), and transesophageal echocardiography (TEE). The classic intimal flap is seen in approximately 70% of cases of aortic dissection. TEE has high sensitivity and specificity, but due to its invasive nature it has been largely replaced by CTA. Contrast-enhanced CT is most commonly used due to widespread availability, short acquisition time, and its noninvasive nature. For diagnosis of aortic dissection, CTA is best performed using echocardiographic gating or multidetector scanning. MRI is less commonly utilized for initial diagnosis but is very specific. Use of MRI is limited in unstable patients due to the length of study and in patients with implanted electronic devices.

Treatment Methods

The standard of care for the treatment of aortic rupture was immediate surgical aortic replacement until a relatively recent paradigm shift toward endovascular stent-graft repair. The main potential advantage of this approach is the ability to avoid thoracotomy and aortic clamping in this subset of patients who tend to have multiple comorbidities. Studies have shown improved morbidity, mortality, and length of hospitalization with similar long-term durability.

References

Braverman A. Aortic dissection: prompt diagnosis and emergency treatment are critical. *Cleve Clin J Med.* 2011;78:685–696.

McMahon M, Squirrell C. Multidetector CT of aortic dissection: a pictorial review. *Radiographics.* 2010;30:445–460.

Patel HJ, Williams DM, Upchurch Jr. GR, et al. A comparative analysis of open and endovascular repair for the ruptured descending thoracic aorta. *J Vasc Surg.* 2009;50:1265–1270.

Cross-reference

Vascular and Interventional Radiology: The Requisites, 2nd ed, 188–193.

CASE 155

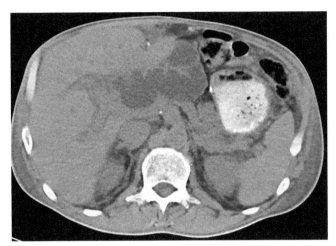

Figure 155-1

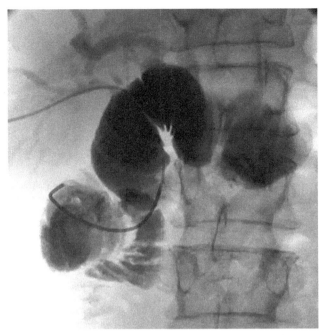

Figure 155-2

HISTORY: An 87-year-old male who had undergone a Whipple resection (pancreaticoduodenectomy) 9 months previously for pancreatic adenocarcinoma presents to the emergency department with a 10-hour history of severe epigastric pain, fever, and vomiting.

1. Which of the following is the most likely diagnosis for the clinical presentation and the imaging findings presented?
   A. Delayed gastric emptying
   B. Afferent loop syndrome (ALS)
   C. Choledocholithiasis with cholangitis
   D. Pancreatic fistula

2. Which of the following surgical techniques utilized in pancreaticoduodenectomies may have predisposed this patient to his current clinical presentation?
   A. Gastrojejunostomy placed in an antecolic position instead of a retrocolic position
   B. Jejunal portion of the afferent loop that measures less than 20 cm
   C. Pylorus preserving pancreaticoduodenectomy
   D. Laparoscopic Whipple procedure

3. Which portion of the gastrointestinal tract is most involved in the development of this syndrome?
   A. Jejunal portion proximal to the gastrojejunostomy
   B. Duodenal stump
   C. Remaining portion of the duodenum
   D. Common hepatic duct

4. Which of the following interventions can serve as a definitive treatment for this syndrome? (Choose all that apply.)
   A. Decompression with nasogastric tube and bowel rest
   B. Administration of high-dose octreotide
   C. Deconstruction of patient's previous Whipple and restoring gastrointestinal continuity with another reconstruction technique
   D. Placement of dual stents at the site of stenosis

See Supplemental Figures section for additional figures and legends for this case.

CASE 155

Afferent Loop Syndrome

1. **B.** Although delayed gastric emptying and pancreatic fistula have been reported in post pancreaticoduodenectomy patients and may present similarly, the image findings of bilateral biliary ductal dilation and pattern of small bowel dilatation make ALS the most likely diagnosis. Whipple procedure involves the removal of the gallbladder and the common bile duct, making choledocholithiasis with cholangitis unlikely.

2. **A.** ALS has been associated with antecolic gastrojejunostomy, redundant afferent loop partial omentectomy, and poor positioning of the gastrojejunostomy along the greater curvature of the stomach. Pylorus-preserving pancreaticoduodenectomy or a laparoscopic approach does not increase the risk of developing ALS.

3. **A.** A jejunal portion of the afferent loop more than 30 cm in length has been implicated in the development of internal small bowel herniation, kinking from redundancy, loop volvulus, and intussusception. The common hepatic duct, remaining duodenal length, and duodenal stump has less of an impact on development of ALS. Duodenal stump perforation or leakage from a rapidly progressing ALS is a surgical emergency.

4. **C and D.** Surgical intervention for ALS depends on the etiology of the obstruction. When the obstruction is caused by recurrent or unresectable malignancy, or immediate decompression is warranted prior to a more invasive surgical procedure, interventional radiology can provide urgent decompression via placement of a drainage catheter (Figure S155-2). This can be followed by placement of dual stents at the site of stenosis via a percutaneous transhepatic biliary drainage tract or a perioral route. For a candidate with surgically amenable disease, deconstruction of the previous Whipple and restoration of the gastrointestinal continuity with either Billroth I or Roux-en-Y is another option. Although high-dose octreotide has been shown to reduce and attenuate severe acute pancreatitis and nasogastric tube decompression with bowel rest may provide temporary relief, neither intervention can alleviate the underlying obstruction.

Comment

Etiology

ALS is a rare postoperative complication in 0.3% to 1% of patients who undergo gastrojejunal reconstructions such as Whipple procedure and Billroth II. Most of the cases are due to mechanical obstructions from adhesions, internal hernia, intussusception, volvulus, kinking of the loop, or stenosis from cancer recurrence or radiation injury. Uncommonly, preferential gastric emptying into the afferent loop or reflux of gastric content into the afferent loop due to efferent loop obstruction has been reported.

Clinical Presentation

Patients have brisk onset of symptoms and can present anywhere from a few weeks to years after their reconstructive surgery. Patients with complete obstruction will oftentimes present earlier (within a few weeks postoperatively) with severe epigastric pain, nonbilious nausea and vomiting, postprandial fullness, and rarely with obstructive jaundice. Patients with partial obstruction, considered the chronic form of ALS, will often present several months to years later. These patients will often present with projectile bilious vomiting when the distended afferent loop forcefully decompresses, pushing its content into the stomach.

Treatment Methods

Computed tomography is useful in establishing the diagnosis of ALS and will often show a severely dilated transversely oriented small bowel anterior to the spine in the mid abdomen. The first image demonstrates bilateral biliary dilation and severe dilation of a loop of bowel that courses into the hepatic hilum (Figure S155-1). Decompression of the afferent loop can be accomplished with radical reconstructive surgery (usually reserved for patients in whom the reconstructive surgery was performed for benign disease) or via percutaneous placement of a drainage catheter within the dilated loop (Figure S155-2). Once initial decompression has occurred, if a stenosis at the bowel-bowel anastomosis is detected and the patient has short life expectancy, then dual stent may be placed within the stenosis via a percutaneous transhepatic biliary drainage tract or a perioral route to relieve the obstruction in carefully selected patients.

References

Eagon JC, Miedema BW, Kelly KA. Postgastrectomy syndromes. *Surg Clin North Am*. 1992;72:445–465.

Gayer G, Barsuk D, Hertz M, et al. CT diagnosis of afferent loop syndrome. *Clin Radiol*. 2002;57:835–839.

Kim YH, Han JK, Lee KH, et al. Palliative percutaneous tube enterostomy in afferent-loop syndrome presenting as jaundice: clinical effectiveness. *J Vasc Interv Radiol*. 2002;13:845–849.

Kim DJ, Lee JH, Kim W. Afferent loop obstruction following laparoscopic distal gastrectomy with Billroth-II gastrojejunostomy. *J Korean Surg Soc*. 2013;84:281–286.

Cross-reference

Vascular and Interventional Radiology: The Requisites, 2nd ed, 437–441.

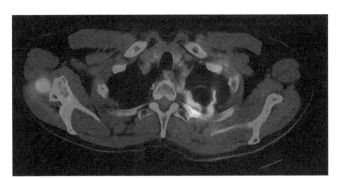

Figure 156-1. *Courtesy of Dr. Bill S. Majdalany.*

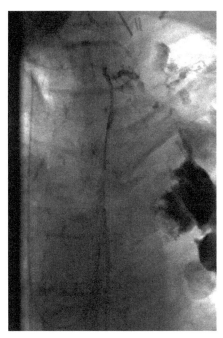

Figure 156-2. *Courtesy of Dr. Bill S. Majdalany.*

HISTORY: A 54-year-old male with history of lung cancer status post resection presents with worsening shortness of breath post-operatively.

1. Which of the following is the most likely diagnosis given the history and imaging findings presented?
   A. Myocardial infarction
   B. Malignant pleural effusion
   C. Chylous effusion
   D. Progressive malignancy

2. This patient's postoperative course was most likely complicated by which of the following?
   A. Malpositioned thoracostomy tubes
   B. Pneumothorax
   C. Elevated chest tube output
   D. Pneumonia

3. What is the most common cause of this entity?
   A. Lung resection
   B. Esophagectomy
   C. Superior vena cava thrombosis
   D. Proximal descending thoracic aortic aneurysm

4. Once access to the thoracic duct is obtained, which procedure will be performed?
   A. Pleurodesis
   B. Surgical ligation of the thoracic duct (TD)
   C. Type I thoracic duct embolization (TDE)
   D. Type II TDE

See Supplemental Figures section for additional figures and legends for this case.

CASE 156

Chylothorax-Thoracic Duct Embolization

1. **C.** The lymphangiogram depicts active extravasation of Lipiodol from the TD, confirming the diagnosis of chylothorax. The lymphangiogram was performed to aid TDE.

2. **C.** Figure 156-2 depicts active extravasation of Lipiodol from the TD with free spilling into the left pleural space, consistent with chylothorax. Typically, in the postoperative setting, chylothorax manifests with increased thoracotomy tube output. The pleural fluid is classically described as milky in appearance but is an unreliable feature of chylothorax and can also be seen in pseudochylothorax.

3. **B.** As explained further below, iatrogenic trauma is the most common cause of injury to the TD and chylothorax, with esophagectomy as the leading operation.

4. **C.** Figures S156-4 and S156-6 demonstrate coils within the TD, which is considered a type I TDE. Type II TDE describes the mechanical interruption of the lymphatic channels in the abdomen that coalesce into the TD (typically the cisterna chyli when identified), by repeatedly stabbing these channels with a needle. In addition the contrast agent used for lymphangiography, Lipiodol, is a viscous oil that has been shown to occlude the flow of lymph through the TD and thereby successfully treat chylous effusions.

Comment

Etiology

Chylous pleural effusion (chylothorax) is generically defined as the presence of chyle within the pleural space and typically occurs secondary to damage to the TD or its main branches. Chyle is composed of essential proteins, lipids, and lymphocytes from the liver, intestines, abdominal wall, and lower extremities. Thus chylous effusions can lead to immunosuppression, respiratory compromise, dehydration, cachexia, and even death. The etiologies of chylous effusions are generally grouped into traumatic and nontraumatic causes. Traumatic etiologies are by far the most common, and multiple reports suggest that intraoperative iatrogenic trauma is now the leading cause of chylothorax. This is thought to be secondary to the increasing number of oncologic thoracic procedures now being performed. Esophagectomies account for the most cases of posttraumatic chylothorax with pneumonectomies a distant second (Figure S156-1). Nontraumatic etiologies include those that obstruct lymphatic outflow (lymphoma, sarcoidosis, central venous thrombosis, Behçet's disease), diseases of the lymphatic pathways (lymphangiomyomatosis, Gorham-Stout syndrome, Noonan syndrome), increased lymph production (portal hypertension, cirrhosis), and idiopathic.

Clinical Presentation

The most common clinical symptoms of chylothorax include fatigue and dyspnea. Less commonly, patients with a chylothorax may present with pleuritic chest pain and fever. The fluid itself typically has a milky appearance, is odorless, alkaline, and typically sterile. However, the hallmark of chylous effusion is the presence of a high concentration of triglycerides within the pleural fluid (>110 mg/dL).

Treatment Methods

Conservative measures, including placing the patient on a nil per os diet with aggressive electrolyte and nutrient replacement, typically via total parenteral nutrition regimens with medium-chain triglycerides, are considered first-line therapy as this has been shown to significantly reduce the flow through the TD by inhibiting fat absorption into the lymphatic system. However, if conservative management fails, or is likely to fail (outputs greater than 1000 mL/day), invasive treatment options should be considered. While surgical ligation of the TD has been used in the past, the associated morbidity and mortality of reoperation have rendered percutaneous TDE a safe and effective alternative, with clinical success rates ranging from 70% to greater than 90% in the literature.

Endovascular Management

TDE is a minimally invasive percutaneous procedure that should be employed in the setting of chylothorax when conservative management has failed or is likely to fail (output >100 mL/day). Technical and clinical success rates of TDE are reported between 70% and 90% with a favorable safety profile when compared to open ligation of the TD. Two types of TDEs have been described: type 1, coil embolization of the TDs (Figures S156-2 through S156-6), and type 2, disruption of the cisterna chyli by mechanical (maceration with a needle) or chemical means (occlusion with Lipiodol).

References

Chen E, Itkin M. Thoracic duct embolization for chylous leaks. *Semin Intervent Radiol.* 2011;28:63–74.

Itkin M, Kucharczuk JC, Kwak A, et al. Nonoperative thoracic duct embolization for traumatic thoracic duct leak: experience in 109 patients. *J Thorac Cardiovasc Surg.* 2010;139:584–589.

Pamarthi V, Stecker MS, Schenker MP, et al. Thoracic duct embolization and disruption for treatment of chylous effusions: experience with 105 patients. *J Vasc Interv Radiol.* 2014;25:1398–1404.

Cross-reference

Vascular and Interventional Radiology: The Requisites, 2nd ed, 196–197.

CASE 157

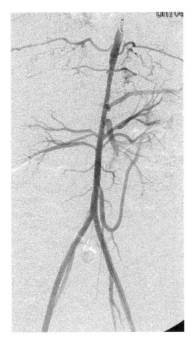

Figure 157-1. *Courtesy of Dr. Narasimham L. Dasika.*

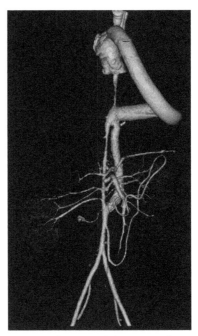

Figure 157-2. *Courtesy of Dr. Narasimham L. Dasika.*

HISTORY: An 8-year-old male with a history of coarctation/hypoplasia of the aortic arch status post repair presents with severe hypertension.

1. Which of the following would be included in the differential diagnosis for the imaging findings presented? (Choose all that apply.)
   A. Abdominal aortic aneurysm
   B. Takayasu arteritis
   C. Polyarteritis nodosa
   D. Middle aortic syndrome (MAS)

2. What is the first step in management of this patient?
   A. Balloon angioplasty
   B. Pharmacologic management of hypertension
   C. Surgical bypass
   D. Observation

3. What is the most likely etiology of hypertension in this patient?
   A. Mass effect on the kidneys
   B. Renal vasculitis
   C. Pressure gradient across the renal arteries
   D. Primary hyperaldosteronism

4. Which of the following diseases is *NOT* associated with acquired MAS?
   A. Trisomy 21
   B. Takayasu arteritis
   C. Williams syndrome
   D. Neurofibromatosis

See Supplemental Figures section for additional figures and legends for this case.

CASE 157

Middle Aortic Syndrome

1. **B and D.** The images demonstrate aortic coarctation from the level of the diaphragm to the level of the proximal renal arteries. This is consistent with MAS. Takayasu arteritis is one potential cause of acquired MAS.

2. **B.** The primary treatment of MAS is medical management of hypertension, with surgery/endovascular therapy reserved for refractory cases. Observation is not appropriate in a young patient with severe hypertension.

3. **C.** The pressure gradient across the renal arteries from the ostial narrowing results in reduced renal blood pressure. This activates the renin/angiotensin system, which results in the common clinical feature of hypertension.

4. **A.** Trisomy 21 (Down's syndrome) is not associated with MAS. The remainder of the listed diseases have an association with acquired MAS.

Comment

Main Teaching Point

First described in 1963, MAS is a rare disease that results in significant narrowing of the abdominal aorta and branches of the abdominal aorta. It typically presents as significant hypertension in a child or teenager. Additional clinical findings may include weak lower-extremity pulses, abdominal bruit, palpable superficial epigastric artery collaterals and findings associated with severe hypertension (hypertensive retinopathy, left ventricular hypertrophy, etc.). If untreated, patients will typically die by the age of 40 related to the complications of severe hypertension. It is most commonly congenital and is proposed to be due to aberrant fusion of the paired embryonic dorsal aortas. There are also acquired etiologies including neurofibromatosis, fibromuscular dysplasia, retroperitoneal fibrosis, Williams syndrome, and the giant cell arteritides.

Diagnostic Evaluation

The coarctation is typically easily identified on aortography with segmental aortic pressures demonstrating a significant systolic pressure gradient across the stenotic segment (Figures S157-1 and S157-3). Computed tomography angiography of the abdominal aorta is also an effective tool for diagnosis.

Treatment Methods

Pharmacologic hypertension control is the initial treatment of choice, with surgery and endovascular therapy reserved for severe hypertension that is refractory to medical therapy. Patients with acquired MAS related to a vasculitis should first be treated with corticosteroids or immunosuppressant therapy prior to the consideration of surgical or endovascular therapy. Surgical treatment options include aortic reconstruction with aorto-aortic bypass grafting or patch angioplasty (Figure S157-2). Cases with significant involvement of the renal arteries may require aortorenal bypass, splenorenal anastomosis, hepatorenal anastomosis or autotransplantation of the kidney into the pelvis. Balloon angioplasty with or without stent placement is the mainstay of endovascular therapy. However, only select cases are amendable to endovascular therapy.

References

Delis KT, Gloviczki P. Middle aortic syndrome: from presentation to contemporary open surgical and endovascular treatment. *Perspect Vasc Surg Endovasc Ther*. 2005;17:187–203.

Sumboonnanonda A, Robinson BL, Gedroyc WM, et al. Middle aortic syndrome: clinical and radiological findings. *Arch Dis Child*. 1992;67:501–505.

Cross-reference

Vascular and Interventional Radiology: The Requisites, 2nd ed, 219–220.

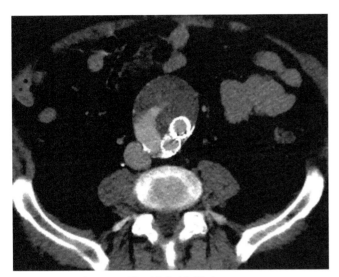

Figure 158-1. *Courtesy of Dr. Minhaj S. Khaja.*

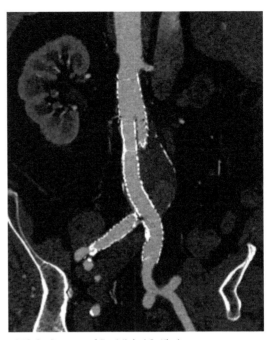

Figure 158-2. *Courtesy of Dr. Minhaj S. Khaja.*

HISTORY: A 78-year-old male with a history of endovascular aneurysm repair (EVAR) for abdominal aortic aneurysms (AAA) was referred for enlarging aneurysm sac.

1. Which of the following would be included in the differential diagnosis for the imaging findings presented? (Choose all that apply.)
   A. Type I endoleak
   B. Type II endoleak
   C. Type III endoleak
   D. Type IV endoleak

2. Which of the following test is most utilized in surveillance of patients with EVAR?
   A. Magnetic resonance imaging (MRI)
   B. Aneurysm sac pressure measurements
   C. International normalized ratio
   D. Computed tomography (CT) angiography

3. Which of the following is *NOT* recommended for persistent type II endoleak?
   A. Embolization of collateral arterial branches and aneurysm sac
   B. Surgical ligation
   C. Medical treatment with anticoagulation
   D. Continued surveillance with computed tomography angiography (CTA)

4. What are the CT features of a type II endoleak following EVAR?
   A. Increased aneurysm sac size without contrast visualization
   B. Presence of fracture or junctional separation of stent graft with enhancement of aneurysm sac
   C. Opacification of excluded aortic branches with contrast material
   D. Dense contrast collection continuous with proximal or distal stent attachment sites

See Supplemental Figures section for additional figures and legends for this case.

CASE 158

Embolization of Type II Endoleak

1. **A and B.** Specific imaging findings that support type II endoleak include late-phase contrast enhancement as well as a communication with an excluded branch artery like the inferior mesenteric artery (IMA) or lumbars. However, a type I endoleak cannot be excluded, and further investigation with angiography may be warranted.

2. **D.** The most commonly recommended imaging modality for routine follow-up after EVAR is CTA with delayed images. Delayed imaging can help distinguish between type I and type II endoleak in many cases. Acceptable alternatives if contrast use is contraindicated include Doppler ultrasonography, MRI, or unenhanced CT (only to evaluate aneurysm sac size). Aneurysm sac pressure measurement is an invasive test and should only be performed when absolutely necessary.

3. **C.** Type II endoleaks tend to resolve spontaneously and commonly do not require intervention. In the case of aneurysmal expansion, intervention is warranted. All of the above are possible methods of treatment, including continued short-term surveillance. However, studies have shown that continuation or initiation of anticoagulation inhibits resolution of endoleaks.

4. **C.** Type II endoleaks result from retrograde flow through collaterals that communicate with the aneurysm sac, most commonly IMA or lumbar arteries. Following stent-graft placement, occlusion of collateral vessels occurs. On CTA, opacification of excluded aortic branches is a common finding in type II endoleaks. Late-phase enhancement of the aneurysm sac is also more commonly seen in type II endoleaks.

Comment

Main Teaching Point

Patients who undergo endoluminal repair of AAA typically receive close surveillance with CT angiography. Endoleaks are a complication unique to EVAR and can occur in up to 25% of patients, with type II endoleak occurring most frequently. When extraluminal contrast is seen within the aneurysm sac on CT, the presence of an endoleak is confirmed (Figures S158-1 and S158-2). Precise characterization of the type and etiology of endoleak is critical in planning treatment and usually requires angiography, as described in Case 128.

Pathogenesis

Type II endoleaks involve retrograde blood flow traveling through collateral branches that communicate with the aneurysm sac. Commonly involved vessels include the inferior mesenteric artery and intercostal/lumbar arteries (Figures S158-3 through S158-5). Type II endoleaks are further subdivided into two categories based on flow through the number of vessels involved. A type IIA (simple) endoleak involves a single vessel, while a type IIB (complex) endoleak involves flow through two or more vessels.

Disease Progression

Patients with type II endoleaks and evidence of aneurysm enlargement on serial CT scans require treatment due to the risk of aneurysm rupture. The criteria upon which to base treatment of type II endoleaks in the absence of aneurysm enlargement are highly controversial, in part because more than 50% tend to close spontaneously. Hence, some physicians treat all type II endoleaks, some treat only endoleaks that are first detected several months after the procedure, and others believe that close CT follow-up is sufficient.

Treatment Methods

Treatment options include embolization of collateral vessels using coils or liquid embolic agents such as *n*-butyl cyanoacrylate, thrombin, or ethylene vinyl alcohol (Onyx, Covidien, Minneapolis, Minnesota) (Figures S158-5 and S158-6). Embolization can be performed percutaneously through a transabdominal/translumbar approach using CT or fluoroscopic guidance. Conversion to open surgery is rare and is considered a last resort only used when endovascular repair fails.

References

Baum R, Stavropoulos S, Fairman R, Carpenter J. Endoleaks after endovascular repair of abdominal aortic aneurysms. *J Vasc Interv Radiol.* 2003;14:1111–1117.

Khaja MS, Park AW, Swee W, et al. Treatment of type II endoleak using Onyx with long-term imaging follow-up. *Cardiovasc Intervent Radiol.* 2014;37:613–622.

Uthoff H, Katzen BT, Gandhi R, et al. Direct percutaneous sac injection for postoperative endoleak treatment after endovascular aortic aneurysm repair. *J Vasc Surg.* 2012;56:965–972.

White S, Stavropoulos S. Management of endoleaks following endovascular aneurysm repair. *Semin Intervent Radiol.* 2009;26:33–38.

Cross-reference

Vascular and Interventional Radiology: The Requisites, 2nd ed, 208–209.

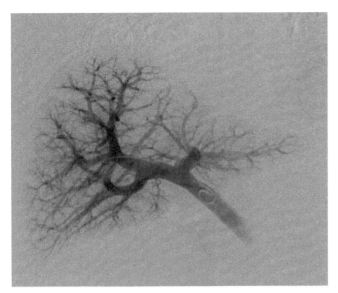

Figure 159-1. *Courtesy of Dr. Wael E. Saad.*

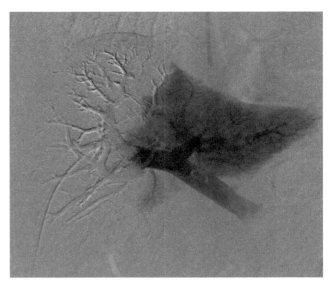

Figure 159-2. *Courtesy of Dr. Wael E. Saad.*

HISTORY: A 59-year-old female with cholangiocarcinoma presents before right hepatectomy.

1. Based on the images provided, what procedure has this patient undergone?
   A. Transjugular intrahepatic portosystemic shunt
   B. Transcatheter arterial chemoembolization (TACE)
   C. Right portal vein embolization (PVE)
   D. Y-90 embolization

2. What embolization agent has been used?
   A. Polyvinyl alcohol (PVA) particles
   B. *n*-butyl cyanoacrylate (*n*-BCA)
   C. Gelfoam
   D. Coils

3. What functional liver remnant/total liver volume (FLR/TLV) ratio is recommended for patients before planned major hepatic resection?
   A. 10% to 20%
   B. 20% to 40%
   C. 40% to 60%
   D. 60% to 80%

4. Which is an absolute contraindication to this procedure?
   A. Overt portal hypertension
   B. Biliary dilation of the FLR
   C. Extrahepatic metastatic disease
   D. Renal insufficiency

See Supplemental Figures section for additional figures and legends for this case.

CASE 159

Portal Vein Embolization

1. **C.** The patient is undergoing right PVE. TACE and Y-90 embolization are arterial interventions, and no hepatic artery is visualized here.

2. **B.** *n*-BCA casts can be seen within the right portal venous system. Coils are not seen and Gelfoam and PVA particles would not be seen; rather diminished flow can be seen during embolization.

3. **B.** An FLR of 20% to 40% is recommended before planned major hepatic resection.

4. **A.** Overt clinical portal hypertension is an absolute contraindication to portal vein hypertension as this may increase portal pressure and lead to bleeding complications. The other choices are relative contraindications and not absolute contraindications.

Comment

Main Teaching Point

Major hepatic resection is being performed at an increasing rate in the treatment of primary and secondary hepatobiliary malignancy. One of the potential postoperative complications associated with this type of surgery is fatal liver failure. This can result from the inability of the remaining liver parenchyma after resection to provide adequate function to sustain life. Preresection measures to increase the volume of the FLR have been employed to make some patients eligible for this type of surgery. This has been achieved by surgical ligation of the contralateral portal vein in the past, and, more recently, it is achieved with contralateral PVE.

Imaging Interpretation

Preprocedural cross-sectional imaging is obtained to evaluate the TLV and the estimated FLR volume (Figure S159-5). An FLR/TLV ratio of 20% to 40% is recommended for patients before planned major hepatic resection. An ipsilateral or contralateral approach is used. Follow-up cross-sectional imaging with calculation of the liver volume is obtained in 2 to 4 weeks to assess the degree of FLR hypertrophy (Figure S159-5).

Endovascular Management

Various embolic materials have been used for PVE including NBCA, PVA particles, Gelfoam, and coils (Figures S159-1 and S159-2). Quantitative, color-coded angiography, processed by syngo iFlow prototype software (Siemens AG, Forchheim, Germany) is demonstrated here, which may aid in evaluating relative perfusion in the portal system (Figures S159-3 and S159-4).

References

Madoff DC, Abdalla EK, Vauthey JN. Portal vein embolization in preparation for major hepatic resection: evolution of a new standard of care. *J Vasc Interv Radiol*. 2005;16:779–790.

Madoff DC, Hicks ME, Vauthey JN, et al. Transhepatic portal vein embolization: anatomy, indications, and technical considerations. *Radiographics*. 2002;22:1063–1076.

Saad WE, Anderson CL, Kowarschik M, et al. Quantifying increased hepatic arterial flow with test balloon occlusion of the splenic artery in liver transplant recipients with suspected splenic steal syndrome: quantitative digitally subtracted angiography correlation with arterial Doppler parameters. *Vasc Endovascular Surg*. 2012;46:384–392.

Cross-reference

Vascular and Interventional Radiology: The Requisites, 2nd ed, 331–332.

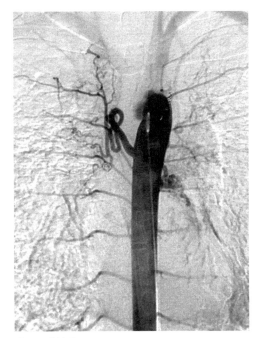

Figure 160-1

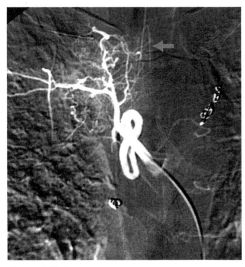

Figure 160-2

HISTORY: A 68-year-old male presents for evaluation of hemoptysis.

1. Which of the following is the most likely diagnosis for the imaging findings presented?
   A. Normal thoracic aortography
   B. Dilated and tortuous bronchial arteries with hypervascularity
   C. Pulmonary arteriovenous malformations (AVM)
   D. Neovascularity related to spinal neoplasm

2. Which vessel is marked by the arrow on Figure 160-2?
   A. Vertebral artery
   B. Lingual artery
   C. Spinal artery
   D. Superior thyroidal artery

3. What is the significance of identification of a spinal artery on angiography in most situations?
   A. Absolute contraindication to embolization or coverage
   B. Relative contraindication to embolization or coverage
   C. Alters procedural technique but is not a contraindication to embolization or stent graft coverage
   D. No clinical or procedural significance

4. Adjunctive procedural techniques associated with decreased incidence of and/or improved symptoms of spinal ischemia include which of the following? (Choose all that apply.)
   A. Monitoring of spinal cord function via motor evoked potentials
   B. Use of spinal drain to decrease cerebrospinal fluid pressure
   C. Increasing systemic mean arterial pressure
   D. No such adjunctive techniques have been described in the literature.

See Supplemental Figures section for additional figures and legends for this case.

CASE 160

Spinal Artery

1. **B.** The images demonstrate hypervascularity in the right upper lobe with dilated bronchial arteries bilaterally, right greater than left. The second image is an image from selective right bronchial artery injection revealing a spinal artery marked by the arrow. No pulmonary AVM is seen and this is not normal.

2. **C.** The image demonstrates a spinal artery arising from the right bronchial artery. Although spinal arteries do arise from the vertebral artery, this is not the vertebral artery itself.

3. **C.** Occlusion of spinal arteries or proximal supplying arteries, such as in embolization or aortic stent-graft placement, can result in spinal ischemia and associated neuromuscular deficits or paraplegia. While presence of a spinal artery or supplying artery on angiography is not a procedural contraindication (and their presence should be assumed despite nonvisualization on angiography), great care should be taken in arterial mapping, evaluation of collateral supply, procedural technique, and risk assessment.

4. **B and C.** Monitoring of motor evoked potentials has not been associated with significant improvement in spinal ischemia. See comment below for more details regarding spinal cord ischemia.

Comment

Main Teaching Point

Identification of spinal arteries during arteriography is of extreme importance. Special attention should be paid to these vessels in planned embolization procedures involving the bronchial, intercostal, and lumbar arteries from where these arise (Figures S160-1 through S160-4). Also, whereas in the past embolization was performed from the main bronchial artery through a 4- to 5-F catheter placed in the proximal segment of the bronchial artery, most interventionalists now place a microcatheter distally in the bronchial artery in order to avoid nontarget embolization of any proximal spinal or intercostal branches that may be present. For these reasons, the incidence of neurologic complications following bronchial arteriography is extremely low.

Clinical Considerations

Additionally, operators should be concerned of paraplegia in aortic endografts covering several vertebral body levels. Spinal cord perfusion pressure is defined as the difference between mean arterial blood pressure and the cerebrospinal fluid pressure. Increased spinal cord perfusion pressure, as achieved by increased mean arterial pressure and decreased cerebral fluid pressure, has been reported in association with decreased incidence of and improved symptoms of spinal ischemia.

References

Buth J, Harris PL, Hobo R, et al. Neurologic complications associated with endovascular repair of thoracic aortic pathology: incidence and risk factors (a study from the European Collaborators on Stent/Graft Techniques for Aortic Aneurysm Repair (EUROSTAR) registry). *J Vasc Surg.* 2007;46:1103–1110.

Lam CH, Vatakencherry G. Spinal cord protection with a cerebrospinal fluid drain in a patient undergoing thoracic endovascular aortic repair. *J Vasc Interv Radiol.* 2010;21:1343–1346.

Sopko DR, Smith TP. Bronchial artery embolization for hemoptysis. *Semin Intervent Radiol.* 2011;28:48–62.

Cross-reference

Vascular and Interventional Radiology: The Requisites, 2nd ed, 174–176.

CASE 161

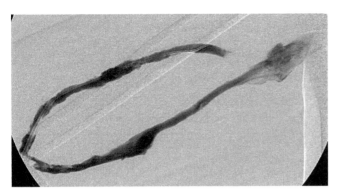

Figure 161-1

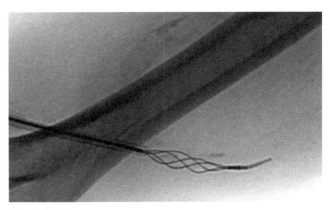

Figure 161-2

HISTORY: A 68-year-old female on hemodialysis presents with arm swelling and loss of thrill within her dialysis graft.

1. Which of the following is the most likely diagnosis for the imaging and clinical findings presented?
   A. Graft stenosis
   B. Graft thrombosis
   C. Aneurysm formation
   D. Graft rupture

2. Which of the following would be the most appropriate initial treatment for this patient?
   A. Creation of a new graft on the contralateral arm
   B. Surgical thrombectomy
   C. Percutaneous declotting
   D. Introduction of a central venous catheter

3. Which location is the most common site of stenosis in a prosthetic arteriovenous graft?
   A. At the venous anastomosis
   B. Within the graft itself
   C. At the arterial anastomosis
   D. In the parent artery

4. Which of the following is *LEAST* likely a presenting symptom for graft stenosis or thrombosis?
   A. Excessive bleeding from puncture sites
   B. Arm swelling
   C. High venous pressure during dialysis sessions
   D. Ischemia to the ipsilateral digits

See Supplemental Figures section for additional figures and legends for this case.

CASE 161

Thrombosed Dialysis Graft

1. **B.** Although all of the answer choices are possible in a patient with a hemodialysis access graft, thrombosis is the most likely in this patient as she has arm swelling and loss of thrill. Stenosis is the next most likely diagnosis.

2. **C.** Fistulography followed by attempt at declotting the graft would be the most appropriate initial treatment. The other answer choices are possible interventions but would not be the initial treatment in most patients. A central venous catheter may be placed in a patient whose graft could not be declotted as a short-term access for dialysis.

3. **A.** The most common location for stenosis is at the venous anastomosis. This is due to the large increase in shear stress in the thin-walled outflow vein leading to fibromuscular hyperplasia and fibrosis.

4. **D.** Ischemia to the digits is usually seen in patients with dialysis-access-related steal syndrome. All of the other choices are likely presenting symptoms.

Comment

Main Teaching Point

A dialysis graft is a surgically created arteriovenous fistula using prosthetic materials to the bridge the gap between an artery and a vein. There are a variety of configurations, with the most common being loop grafts in the forearm and C grafts in the upper arm. Because the outflow veins are exposed to "arterial" pressures and flows, and because of the frequent needle punctures needed for dialysis, dialysis grafts are prone to eventual failure. This failure can manifest by high venous pressures during dialysis sessions, excessive bleeding from the puncture sites, arm swelling, high recirculation values, or, ultimately, graft thrombosis.

Treatment Methods

The goals of treatment are to clear the thrombus from the graft and to treat the underlying cause of the thrombosis. The thrombus may be cleared by percutaneous declotting using pharmacologic thrombolysis or a mechanical thrombectomy device (Figures S161-1 through S161-4). The underlying cause of graft thrombosis is diagnosed by venography performed during the percutaneous declotting procedure, and it is typically treated using angioplasty and/or stent placement (Figure S161-4). Unfortunately, a thrombosed graft with completely occluded outflow veins or long-segment stricture of these veins might not be amenable to percutaneous reestablishment of flow. In these cases, surgical revision or creation of new access may be necessary.

References

Mercado C, Salman L, Krishnamurthy G, et al. Early and late fistula failure. *Clin Nephrol.* 2008;69:77–83.

Vesely TM. Mechanical thrombectomy devices to treat thrombosed hemodialysis grafts. *Tech Vasc Interv Radiol.* 2003;6:35–41.

Cross-reference

Vascular and Interventional Radiology: The Requisites, 2nd ed, 151–157.

CASE 162

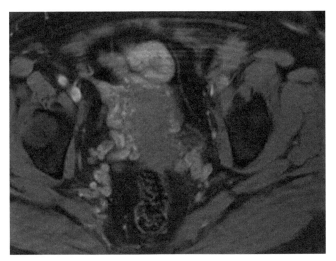

Figure 162-1

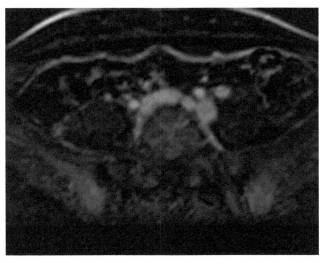

Figure 162-2

HISTORY: A 35-year-old female presents with chronic, dull pelvic pain.

1. Which of the following is the most likely diagnosis given the clinical and imaging findings presented?
   A. Uterine arteriovenous malformation
   B. Ovarian vein thrombosis
   C. Nutcracker syndrome
   D. Pelvic congestion syndrome

2. What is the diagnostic gold standard modality used to diagnose pelvic congestion syndrome?
   A. Doppler ultrasound
   B. Magnetic resonance venography (MRV)
   C. Catheter-based venography
   D. Laparoscopy

3. Which of the following is a contraindication to embolization therapy for pelvic congestion syndrome?
   A. Dyspareunia
   B. Pelvic inflammatory disease
   C. Urinary frequency
   D. Vulvar varicosities

4. Of the following, which is the most worrisome complication of transcatheter embolization in these patients?
   A. Nontarget embolization
   B. Ovarian vein perforation
   C. Postembolization syndrome
   D. Infection

See Supplemental Figures section for additional figures and legends for this case.

CASE 162

Pelvic Congestion Syndrome

1. **D.** The images demonstrate dilated parauterine veins and a dilated left ovarian vein. The presence of at least four parauterine veins (one at least 4 mm in diameter), or an ovarian vein greater than 8 mm, in a patient with pelvic pain symptoms qualifies as imaging criteria consistent with pelvic congestion syndrome. Nutcracker syndrome may result in an asymmetrically dilated gonadal vein. However, it typically occurs on the left, as it is secondary to left renal vein compression.

2. **C.** Catheter-based venography is generally accepted as the best diagnostic imaging study and route for treatment. Findings on venography include retrograde flow into the ovarian vein and/or congestion, ovarian vein diameter greater than 8 to 10 mm, and filling of pelvic veins and varicosities. MRV and ultrasound are commonly utilized in screening and diagnosis only, but neither is considered a gold standard.

3. **B.** Active pelvic inflammatory disease is considered a contraindication to embolization therapy until the infection has been treated. Dyspareunia, urinary frequency, and vulvar varicosities are all common clinical manifestations of pelvic congestion syndrome.

4. **A.** Nontarget coil embolization, particularly of the pulmonary arteries, would be considered a severe complication of the procedure. Postembolization syndrome is a relatively mild and common complication.

Comment

Patient Presentation

Chronic pelvic pain can result from problems in the reproductive organs or it may be neurologic, musculoskeletal, urologic, or gastrointestinal in nature. However, the association of ovarian and pelvic varices with chronic pelvic pain has been known for many years. Pelvic venous incompetence may be suspected when a woman reports pelvic pain in the upright position, during or after intercourse, or when varicosities are visualized in the thigh, buttocks, or perineum. Noninvasive imaging modalities such as sonography or MRV may aid in diagnosis (Figures S162-1 and S162-2).

Endovascular Management

Analogous to a male varicocele, ovarian and pelvic varices are amenable to treatment by transcatheter embolization of the refluxing ovarian veins. For this procedure, each ovarian vein is catheterized and examined with venography to determine whether significant reflux is present (Figures S162-3 and S162-4). If reflux is present, the ovarian vein and internal iliac veins may be embolized (Figure S162-5). Embolization of the internal iliac vein is recommended because of the well-documented communications between the ovarian veins and the internal iliac veins. Embolization therapy may be expected to produce some degree of symptomatic improvement in 70% to 90% of women undergoing the procedure, provided a rigorous clinical and imaging screening process is used to select patients initially.

References

Ignacio EA, Dua R, Sarin S, et al. Pelvic congestion syndrome: diagnosis and treatment. *Semin Intervent Radiol.* 2008;25:361–368.

Phillips D, Deipolyi AR, Hesketh RL, et al. Pelvic congestion syndrome: etiology of pain, diagnosis, and clinical management. *J Vasc Intervent Radiol.* 2014;25:725–733.

Venbrux AC, Chang AH, Kim HS, et al. Pelvic congestion syndrome (pelvic venous incompetence): impact of ovarian and internal iliac vein embolotherapy on menstrual cycle and chronic pelvic pain. *J Vasc Intervent Radiol.* 2002;13:171–178.

Cross-reference

Vascular and Interventional Radiology: The Requisites, 2nd ed, 304–306.

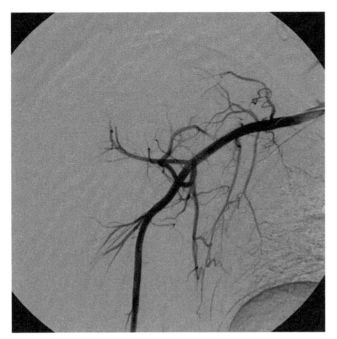

Figure 163-1

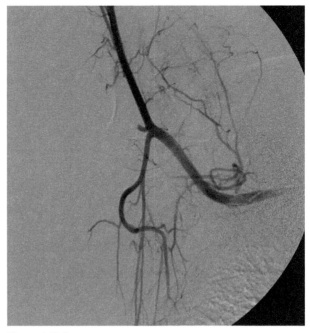

Figure 163-2

HISTORY: A 30-year-old female professional volleyball player presents with cramping of her right arm and forearm and tingling of her lateral shoulder with exertion.

1. Which of the following is the most likely diagnosis given the clinical and imaging findings presented?
   A. Arterial thoracic outlet syndrome
   B. Rotator cuff syndrome
   C. Quadrilateral space syndrome (QSS)
   D. Impingement syndrome

2. Magnetic resonance (MR) imaging of the affected limb may show which of the following? (Choose all that apply.)
   A. Teres minor atrophy
   B. Initial atrophy of the supraspinatus and infraspinatus followed by the deltoid
   C. Deltoid atrophy
   D. Narrow acromiohumeral, coracohumeral, and coracoclavicular intervals

3. Which physical exam finding is most characteristic of this syndrome?
   A. Poorly localized pain in a nondermatomal pattern when the arm is abducted and externally rotated
   B. Shoulder pain with forced flexion, when arm is fully pronated
   C. Reproduction of shoulder pain with axial load placement on the spine while neck is extended and rotated toward the affected shoulder
   D. Shoulder pain with forced internal rotation when the arm is forward elevated to 90 degrees

4. When nonsurgical management has failed, what is the management of choice?
   A. Partial myotomy of the surrounding muscles to decompress the space
   B. Lysis of fibrous tissue using a posterior approach, sparing the deltoid and teres minor muscles
   C. Intraarticular and subacromial corticosteroid injection
   D. Removal of scar tissue and spur from the subacromial space

See Supplemental Figures section for additional figures and legends for this case.

CASE 163

Quadrilateral Space Syndrome

1. **C.** The diagnosis of QSS can be made with occlusion of the posterior humeral circumflex artery (PHCA) when the symptomatic extremity is abducted and externally rotated, motion often seen in overhead athletes. Arterial thoracic outlet syndrome results in compression of the subclavian artery, most commonly by a cervical rib or scalene muscle. Rotator cuff syndrome and impingement syndrome are better evaluated through MR imaging, which may show rotator cuff tendon tears and reduced subacromial distance, respectively.

2. **A and C.** Compression of the axillary nerve and the PHCA seen in QSS results in focal atrophy of the teres minor muscle, with or without involvement of the deltoid muscle. Atrophy of the supraspinatus and infraspinanus followed by the deltoid is often seen with Parsonage-Turner syndrome. A narrow interval for acromiohumeral, coracohumeral, and coracoclavicular distances describes findings of impingement syndrome.

3. **A.** Patients with QSS often complain of poorly localized shoulder pain, paresthesia in the affected extremity in a nondermatomal distribution, and discrete point tenderness in the lateral aspect of the quadrilateral space. Symptoms often subside only a few minutes after stopping the offending overhead movements. Neer's test (choice B) and Hawkin's test (choice D) are used in the clinical diagnosis of impingement syndrome. Spurling's test (choice C) is often used in diagnosis of cervical disc disease.

4. **B.** Initial treatment of QSS is nonsurgical, consisting of analgesics, physiotherapy, and avoidance of athletic activities. Surgical decompression is reserved for those who are suffering acute or chronic symptoms not responsive to nonsurgical management. Operative management of choice is a posterior approach, sparing the deltoid and teres minor muscles and decompressing the quadrilateral space by lysing the offending fibrous tissue. Myotomy has no place in surgical management of QSS. Intraarticular and subacromial corticosteroid injection is used to treat impingement syndrome or rotator cuff tears. Removal of scar tissue and spur from the subacromial space is a treatment of subacromial impingement syndrome.

Comment

Anatomy

The quadrilateral space is bounded by the teres minor superiorly, the surgical neck of the humerus laterally, the long head of the triceps medially, and the upper border of the teres major inferiorly. It contains the axillary nerve and the posterior circumflex humeral artery. QSS is a rare condition in which the contents of the quadrilateral space are compressed, leading to vague symptoms of shoulder pain, tenderness over the quadrilateral space on palpation, and teres minor and deltoid denervation.

Etiology

The most commonly cited cause of compression of quadrilateral space structures is fibrous bands. Other causes include glenoid labral cysts, a ganglion, muscle hypertrophy, and a spike of bone after a scapular fracture.

Imaging Interpretation

The prevalence of QSS is unknown. On angiography, a position of abduction and external rotation may demonstrate significant compression of the contents of the quadrilateral space (Figures S163-1 through S163-4). Nerve conduction studies and electromyography have also been used to investigate QSS, although they often produce inconsistent results and are considered nonspecific. The appearance of denervation changes on MRI affecting the teres minor muscle with or without the deltoid muscle is often seen. Treatment is centered on surgical decompression of the contents of the quadrilateral space.

References

Chautems RC, Glauser T, Waeber-Fey MC, et al. Quadrilateral space syndrome: case report and review of the literature. *Ann Vasc Surg.* 2000;14:673–676.

Cothran Jr. RL, Helms C. Quadrilateral space syndrome: incidence of imaging findings in a population referred for MRI of the shoulder. *AJR Am J Roentgenol.* 2005;184:989–992.

Zurkiya O, Walker TG. Quadrilateral space syndrome. *J Vasc Interv Radiol.* 2014;25:229.

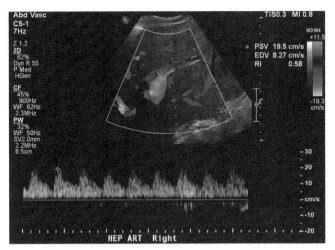

Figure 164-1. *Courtesy of Dr. Wael E. Saad.*

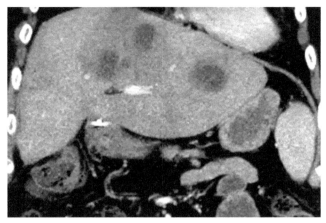

Figure 164-2. *Courtesy of Dr. Wael E. Saad.*

HISTORY: A 65-year-old male status post liver transplantation 6 years ago presents with worsening liver function tests (LFTs).

1. Which of the following would be included in the differential diagnosis for the imaging findings presented? (Choose all that apply.)
   A. Biliary stricture with biloma formation
   B. Portal vein thrombosis
   C. Hepatic artery thrombosis
   D. Acute cholecystitis

2. Which of the following studies should be the initial study performed when a liver transplant patient has elevated LFTs?
   A. Angiogram
   B. Liver ultrasound with Doppler
   C. Abdomen magnetic resonance imaging
   D. Pelvis computed tomography (CT)

3. Which of the following is *NOT* ultrasound evidence of hepatic artery stenosis?
   A. Parvus tardus waveform
   B. Arterial resistive index (RI) less than 0.50 (<50%)
   C. Aliasing in the portal vein
   D. Peak systolic velocity greater than 200 cm/s

4. Which of the following is the definitive treatment for hepatic artery thrombosis?
   A. Intravenous anticoagulation
   B. Surgical revision or retransplantation
   C. Angioplasty
   D. Biliary drainage

See Supplemental Figures section for additional figures and legends for this case.

CASE 164

Hepatic Artery Thrombosis with Biliary Strictures

1. **A and C.** The images demonstrate a hepatic arterial RI of greater than 0.50 (which usually signifies a patent hepatic artery) but with CT findings of bilomas and parenchymal ischemic necrosis within the liver. These findings are concerning for hepatic artery thrombosis, which is commonly associated with biliary stricturing and biloma formation. It is important to note that a "normal" Doppler study does not rule out hepatic artery thrombosis.

2. **B.** When a transplant patient presents with elevated LFTs, there could be many causes for dysfunction of the graft. However, the initial screening test should be the least invasive, an ultrasound of the liver with Doppler evaluation of the hepatic vasculature. The other choices may be helpful in providing further clarification about the disease entity but are not commonly the initial exam performed.

3. **C.** The remaining answer choices may be seen in patients with hepatic artery thrombosis. However, keep in mind that you may see patients with normal arterial resistive indices that do in fact have hepatic artery thrombosis, as seen in this case.

4. **B.** Although catheter-directed thrombolysis, angioplasty, and stenting may be successful in treating these patients; only surgical revision or retransplantation is the definitive treatment.

Comment

Patient Presentation

A variety of anatomic complications can occur in patients who have undergone liver transplantation: biliary anastomotic leak, stenosis of the biliary anastomosis, stenosis at the inferior vena caval anastomosis, and hepatic artery anastomotic stenosis with subsequent thrombosis. Patients who experience hepatic artery thrombosis are prone to develop biliary strictures and/or necrosis (Figures S164-2 and S164-6). The biliary endothelium in liver transplant is the most susceptible to ischemia. When this occurs, the strictures are usually centrally located and may be quite extensive and irregular in appearance. Other, less typical, biliary appearances can be seen in the initial cholangiographic findings.

Diagnosis and Treatment Methods

Patients with evidence of transplant malfunction usually undergo sonographic evaluation (Figure S164-1). When elevated velocities are observed near the arterial anastomosis, a stenosis is suspected and the patient is usually referred for confirmatory angiography. An arterial RI of 0.50 has a high sensitivity for hepatic artery stenosis or thrombosis. However, a 0.50 arterial RI can occur in the setting of hepatic artery thrombosis (Doppler ultrasound pitfall) due to reconstitution of the intrahepatic arteries by porta hepatic collaterals (Figures S164-3 through S164-5). Angioplasty can be performed to treat such stenoses, or surgical anastomotic revision may be performed. When hepatic artery thrombosis is present, surgical therapy is commonly needed, although thrombolysis may be attempted to improve arterial flow. Biliary drains are commonly placed to decompress the ischemia biliary tree.

References

Crossin JD, Muradali D, Wilson SR. US of liver transplants: normal and abnormal. *Radiographics*. 2003;23:1093–1114.

Orons PD, Sheng R, Zajko AB. Hepatic artery stenosis in liver transplant recipients: prevalence and cholangiographic appearance of associated biliary complications. *AJR Am J Roentgenol*. 1995;165: 1145–1149.

Saad WE, Saad NE, Davies MG, et al. Transhepatic balloon dilation of anastomotic biliary strictures in liver transplant recipients: the significance of a patent hepatic artery. *J Vasc Interv Radiol*. 2005;16: 1221–1228.

Cross-reference

Vascular and Interventional Radiology: The Requisites, 2nd ed, 254–255.

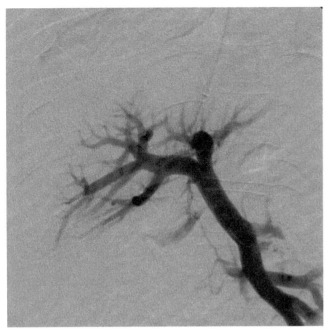

Figure 165-1 *Courtesy of Dr. Wael E. Saad.*

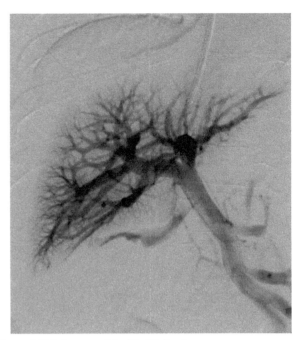

Figure 165-2 *Courtesy of Dr. Wael E. Saad.*

HISTORY: A 56-year-old male with alcoholic cirrhosis and variceal bleeding presents for transjugular intrahepatic portosystemic shunt (TIPS).

1. Which of the following is the most likely diagnosis for the imaging findings presented?
   A. Conventional portal venous anatomy
   B. Anomalous portal venous anatomy
   C. Arterial injury
   D. Portal venous injury

2. Which of the following is the access and procedure likely being performed?
   A. Transhepatic; portal vein embolization (PVE)
   B. Transjugular; PVE
   C. Transjugular; TIPS
   D. Transhepatic; portal vein angioplasty

3. How would one initially correct the issue addressed in Question 1?
   A. Coil embolization
   B. Particle embolization
   C. Open surgical repair
   D. Covered stent placement (TIPS)

4. Which of the following is the *LEAST* likely complication of TIPS?
   A. Biliary fistula
   B. Hepatic artery pseudoaneurysm
   C. Portal venous bleeding
   D. Duodenal varices

See Supplemental Figures section for additional figures and legends for this case.

CASE 165

Portal Venous Injury During TIPS

1. **D.** The images demonstrate extravasation along the caudal of the liver during portal venous injection. Arterial injury may be seen during attempted cannulation of the portal vein but would likely not be seen increasing during portal venous injection.

2. **C.** The images demonstrate transjugular access being performed as part of a TIPS procedure. No stenosis is seen in the portal vein to suggest the need for angioplasty. PVE is likely not being performed as the patient is experiencing variceal hemorrhage and TIPS would be indicated.

3. **D.** TIPS placement with a covered stent would allow for decompression of the portal venous system and likely cover the site of portal injury. Embolization may only be necessary in situations where decompression and stent placement are not successful.

4. **D.** Biliary fistula, portal venous, and arterial injury are complications reported during TIPS. Duodenal varices may be present in patients with portal hypertension but not as a result of the TIPS procedure itself.

Comment

Main Teaching Point

The ideal target of the portal vein in TIPS is the proximal right portal vein or confluence of the main portal vein. In approximately 50% of patients, the confluence is intrahepatic, otherwise extrahepatic. Portal venous injury may occur during multiple attempts at portal vein cannulation leading to portal venous extravasation (Figures S165-1 and S165-2). Even in cirrhotic patients with an extrahepatic portal vein confluence, tough fibrotic tissue at the porta hepatis usually contains the portal venous bleeding/rupture.

Endovascular Management

Treatment for portal vein injury is rapidly establishing the TIPS to decompress the high-pressure portal venous system and diversion of portal vein flow away from the site of injury and placement of a covered stent across the site of injury (Figures S165-3 and S165-4). Covering the site of injury usually requires that the covered portion of the TIPS stent is placed deeper into the portal venous system than usual. Embolization of the portal venous injury may only be necessary in situations where decompression and stent placement are not successful.

References

Uflacker R, Reichert P, D'Albuquerque LC, et al. Liver anatomy applied to the placement of transjugular intrahepatic portosystemic shunts.

Cross-reference

Vascular and Interventional Radiology: The Requisites, 2nd ed, 318–325.

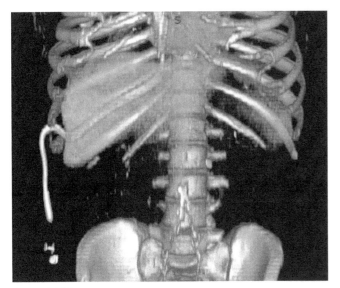

Figure 166-1

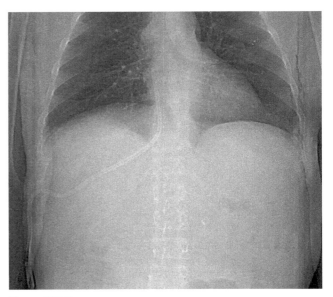

Figure 166-2

HISTORY: A 68 year-old African-American patient on chronic dialysis with a nonfunctioning left femoral tunneled catheter and history of right jugular and subclavian thrombosis presents for establishment of functioning venous access.

1. Which of the following procedures was performed based on the imaging findings presented?
   A. Percutaneous cholecystostomy
   B. Transhepatic central venous access
   C. Inferior vena cava thrombolysis
   D. Percutaneous drainage of a pleural effusion

2. Indications for transhepatic central venous access placement include all of the following *EXCEPT*:
   A. Inability to access the jugular, femoral, or subclavian veins
   B. Inability to recanalize venous occlusions
   C. Initial central venous access in patients with enlarged hepatic veins
   D. Preservation of a final remaining peripheral site for arteriovenous access

3. The most common transhepatic catheter-related complication is which of the following?
   A. Thrombosis
   B. Sepsis
   C. Hepatic hematoma
   D. Catheter migration

4. In the prevention of retroperitoneal or hepatic hematoma from transhepatic tract creation post catheter placement, which of the following can be considered? (Choose all that apply.)
   A. Coil embolization
   B. Plug embolization
   C. Gelfoam
   D. No intervention

See Supplemental Figures section for additional figures and legends for this case.

CASE 166

Transhepatic Central Venous Catheter

1. **B.** The imaging depicts a transhepatic approach of central venous access with distal tip of the catheter projecting to the right atrium. None of the other options coincides with the imaging provided.

2. **C.** Transhepatic catheter placement is indicated in all of the other choices. Most commonly, patients are often dialysis-dependent and have undergone multiple access interventions and encountered multiple failed permanent access procedures. In the pediatric population, patients with congenital heart defects and prior surgical exclusion of the superior vena cava, transhepatic approach presents an alternative option for central venous access.

3. **D.** Though all the complications listed have been reported with transhepatic catheter placement, migration of the catheter is the most common. This is often secondary to buckling outside the vein as the patient moves.

4. **A, B, C, and D.** The need to close the transhepatic tract post catheter placement is controversial. Though utilization of detachable coils, vascular plugs, and Gelfoam can be considered and is often institution dependent, the incidence of retroperitoneal or hepatic hematoma post intervention is low, and thus closure of the tract is often not necessitated.

Comment

Main Teaching Point

Adults and children who undergo placement of multiple long-term central venous catheters are prone to develop chronic occlusions of these veins. After the jugular, subclavian, and femoral veins are all exhausted, limited options exist for further central venous access in these patients. When this occurs, a few approaches may be used: (1) percutaneous recanalization of occluded central veins using angioplasty and/or stents might create enough of a channel through which a new long-term catheter can be placed; (2) transhepatic venous access may be obtained as depicted here (Figures S166-1 through S166-3); (3) in extreme cases, translumbar access to the inferior vena cava may be obtained. Unfortunately, the first option may be extremely difficult or impossible, depending upon the chronicity of the occlusion. The last two options can usually be accomplished technically, but the catheter remains at some risk of migrating peripherally due to buckling outside the vein as the patient moves.

References

Johnson KL, Fellows KE, Murphy JD. Transhepatic central venous access for cardiac catheterization and radiologic intervention. *Cathet Cardiovasc Diagn.* 1995;35:168–171.

Younes H, Pettigrew C, Anaya-Ayala J, et al. Transhepatic hemodialysis catheters: functional outcome and comparison between early and late failure. *J Vasc Interv Radiol.* 2011;22:183–191.

Cross-reference

Vascular and Interventional Radiology: The Requisites, 2nd ed, 145–150.

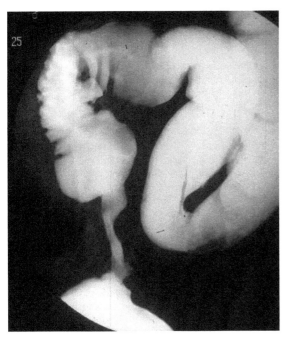

Figure 167-1. *Courtesy of Dr. Narasimham L. Dasika.*

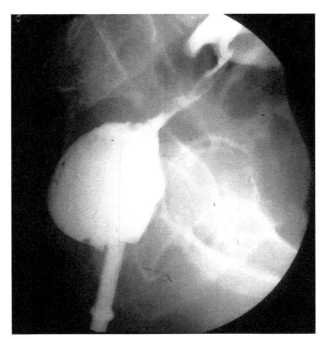

Figure 167-2. *Courtesy of Dr. Narasimham L. Dasika.*

HISTORY: A 72-year-old male poor surgical candidate presents with obstructing sigmoid adenocarcinoma.

1. What are the indications for colonic stenting in patients with malignant colorectal obstructions? (Choose all that apply.)
   A. Palliation of obstructing tumors not suitable for curative surgical resection
   B. To alleviate symptoms mainly in patients with obstruction occluding more than 90% of the lumen
   C. To facilitate reversal of Hartmann's procedure
   D. Preoperative decompression prior to elective colonic resection at a later time

2. Which of the statements is true regarding malignant colonic obstructions?
   A. Mortality in patients undergoing emergent surgery vs. elective surgery for malignant colonic obstruction is comparable.
   B. Perforation is the most common complication from colonic stenting.
   C. Stenting of distal rectal tumors can result in tenesmus and/or fecal incontinence.
   D. After stent placement, additional balloon dilatation is often performed to facilitate the expansion of the stent.

3. Which is the self-expanding metal stent of choice when treating malignant colonic obstructions?
   A. Elgiloy stents
   B. Nitinol stents
   C. Stainless steel stents
   D. Biodegradable stents

4. Which of the following is an absolute contraindication to colorectal stenting?
   A. A long segment of obstructing tumor
   B. Peritoneal carcinomatosis
   C. Documented perforation with free intraperitoneal gas
   D. Obstructing mass proximal to the splenic flexure

See Supplemental Figures section for additional figures and legends for this case.

CASE 167

Colonic Stent Placement

1. **A and D.** Major indications for colonic stents include palliative nonsurgical therapy for malignant colorectal obstruction, initial decompression to avoid emergent surgery, allowing time for a complete colonoscopy screening to detect any synchronous malignant neoplasm near the obstruction, and to buy time for patients who may benefit from chemoradiation prior to surgery. Stenting is more difficult in complete obstructions and often results in more complications. Stenting has been shown to decrease the rate of stoma creation but has not been shown to affect the reversal of the stoma.

2. **C.** Stent placement across distal rectal tumors can results in severe tenesmus and fecal incontinence. In comparison to elective intervention, emergent surgery for acute colonic obstruction is associated with significant increase in morbidity and mortality. Although perforation is the most feared complication, migration of the stent is the most common complication. Balloon dilation post stent insertion can provide more rapid expansion and earlier decompression but also increases the risk of perforation.

3. **B.** Nitinol stents are the most commonly used colonic stents and have largely replaced Elgiloy and stainless steel stents. Nitinol stents boast shape memory, superior elasticity, and are magnetic resonance imaging compatible. Biodegradable stents have varied degradation rates depending on their environment, providing inconsistent results.

4. **C.** Absolute contraindication to colonic stenting is evidence of acute perforation of the colon. All other choices are relative contraindications and may result in increased postoperative complications.

Comment

Epidemiology

Colorectal cancer is one of the most common malignancies in developed countries, and 7% to 29% of all cases will develop partial to total obstruction. Most colonic obstructions occur on the left side of the colon. At the time of presentation, the malignancy causing obstruction is usually at an advanced stage, and less than half of the patients are candidates for emergency surgery. Most commonly utilized surgical intervention is the creation of stoma with or without primary resection of obstructing tumor, which is associated with significant morbidity and mortality.

Treatment Methods

Gastrointestinal tract stent placement has been used as a minimally invasive method of relieving large-bowel obstruction in two main subsets of patients (Figures S167-1 through S167-6). Those who present with acute symptoms may receive stent placement and then undergo treatment planning instead of high-risk emergency surgery. Patients with unresectable and metastatic disease might not require operation at all but might simply be treated palliatively by stent placement. This approach has the potential to spare patients the discomfort and morbidity of surgical bowel resection under inauspicious circumstances when quality of life should be the primary concern. Colonic obstruction resolves in the majority of the patients who undergo colonic stenting, and most experience return of bowel movements within 24 hours. Major complications from colonic stent placement are migration (11%), perforation (3.5% to 4%), and reobstruction (7% to 12%).

References

Angel de Gregorio M, Mainar A, Rodriguez J, et al. Colon stenting: a review. *Semin Intervent Radiol.* 2004;21:205–216.

Nandakumar S, Richard AK. Stents for colonic strictures: materials, designs, and more. *Tech Gastrointest Endosc.* 2014;16:100–107.

Tilney HS, Lovegrove RE, Purkayastha S, et al. Comparison of colonic stenting and open surgery for malignant large bowel obstruction. *Surg Endosc.* 2007;21:225–233.

Todd HB. Technique of colonic stenting. *Tech Gastrointest Endosc.* 2014;16:108–111.

Cross-reference

Vascular and Interventional Radiology: The Requisites, 2nd ed, 437–449.

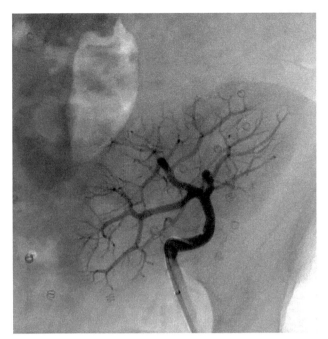

Figure 168-1. *Courtesy of Dr. Minhaj S. Khaja.*

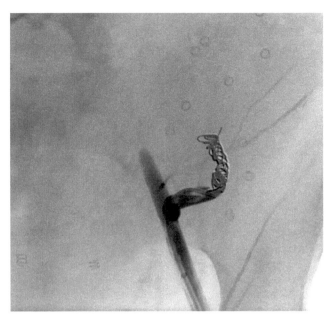

Figure 168-2. *Courtesy of Dr. Minhaj S. Khaja.*

HISTORY: A 43-year-old female with end-stage renal disease status post left pelvic renal transplant presents with hypertension, rising creatinine, and proteinuria.

1. Which of the following would be indications for performing this procedure? (Choose all that apply.)
   A. Uncontrolled hypertension
   B. Nephrotic syndrome
   C. Autosomal dominant polycystic kidney disease
   D. Secondary hyperparathyroidism

2. Which of the following techniques would *NOT* be helpful to prevent reflux of ethanol into the parent vessel?
   A. Use of a balloon occlusion catheter
   B. Rapid manual injection of ethanol
   C. Preablation identification of the adrenal, gonadal, and phrenic renal arteries
   D. Continuous fluoroscopy during ethanol injection

3. Which of the following is *NOT* a symptom of postembolization syndrome?
   A. Nausea, vomiting
   B. Fever
   C. Pain
   D. Edema

4. What are alternatives to transcatheter renal ablation for the treatment of resistant hypertension or nephrotic syndrome? (Choose all that apply.)
   A. Surgical nephrectomy
   B. Hemodialysis
   C. Radiofrequency ablation
   D. Medical renal ablation

See Supplemental Figures section for additional figures and legends for this case.

CASE 168

Renal Ablation for Hypertension/ Nephrotic Syndrome

1. **A, B, and C.** Uncontrolled hypertension, nephrotic syndrome, and autosomal dominant polycystic kidney disease are accepted indications for transarterial renal ablation. Renal ablation is not indicated for the treatment of secondary hyperparathyroidism secondary to renal disease.

2. **B.** Ethanol is cytotoxic and causes renal infarction, which is why it is very important to deliver it only to the target tissue, avoiding reflux into other vessels. Use of a balloon occlusion catheter and identification of the adrenal, gonadal, and phrenic renal arteries prior to the procedure help in preventing reflux. Continuous fluoroscopy during manual ethanol injection is another helpful technique. Rapid manual injection of ethanol is not advisable as it may increase the risk of reflux.

3. **D.** Postembolization syndrome is a common side effect of transarterial embolization. The main symptoms that may occur include pain, fever, and nausea and vomiting. Edema or swelling is not a common symptom. It is self-limiting and treatment is symptomatic relief with analgesics, antiemetics, and intravenous fluids. The incidence of postembolization syndrome increases with increased size of tumors or fibroids. Pretreatment with antipyretics or antiemetics may be helpful for patients undergoing embolization of such lesions.

4. **A and D.** Surgical removal of the kidney is an alternative to transcatheter renal ablation in treating resistant hypertension or nephrotic syndrome. It is associated with increased morbidity and complications. Medical renal ablation to halt proteinuria has also been attempted with agents such as mercury salts, angiotensin II, cyclosporine, and prostaglandin synthesis inhibitors. Case reports of renal ablation through laparoscopic bilateral ureteral ligation have also been successful. Hemodialysis must be maintained for these patients who have poor renal function and will require continued dialysis after renal ablation using any technique.

Radiofrequency ablation is not a known alternative for complete renal ablation.

Comment
Main Teaching Point

Hypertension affects 80% of patients with end-stage renal disease and can sometimes be refractory to medical treatment. Surgical nephrectomy has been performed in the past in an attempt to treat uncontrolled hypertension in this patient population. Recently, transarterial renal ablation with absolute ethanol has been adopted by some centers as a less invasive alternative therapy. Renal ablation can also be performed in patients with failing renal transplants or those with debilitating nephrotic syndrome, rather than nephrectomy, as seen in this case (Figures S168-1 through S168-3).

Endovascular Management

Ethanol in its concentrated form delivered selectively into the renal artery is cytotoxic and thrombogenic. Extreme care must be taken while infusing the ethanol to avoid reflux into other vessels. Infusion through a balloon occlusion catheter may be performed to safeguard against this potentially devastating complication. The dilution effect that occurs once it traverses the renal parenchyma into the venous system renders it harmless, thus avoiding systemic complications.

References

Golwyn Jr. DH, Routh WD, Chen MY, et al. Percutaneous transcatheter renal ablation with absolute ethanol for uncontrolled hypertension or nephrotic syndrome: results in 11 patients with end-stage renal disease. *J Vasc Interv Radiol.* 1997;8:527–533.

Keller FS, Coyle M, Rosch J, et al. Percutaneous renal ablation in patients with end-stage renal disease: alternative to surgical nephrectomy. *Radiology.* 1986;159:447–451.

Tikkakoski T, Leppänen M, Turunen J, Anderson S, Södervik H. Percutaneous transcatheter renal embolization with absolute ethanol for uncontrolled nephrotic syndrome. *Case Reports Acta Radiol.* 2001;42:80–83.

Cross-reference

Vascular and Interventional Radiology: The Requisites, 2nd ed, 284.

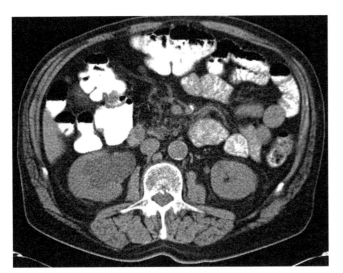

Figure 169-1

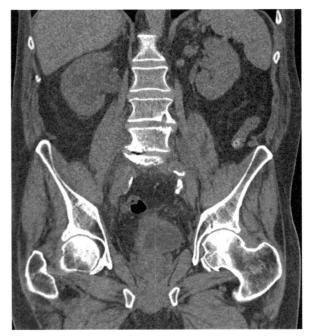

Figure 169-2

HISTORY: A 52-year-old female with bladder cancer presents with right flank pain.

1. Which of the following would be included in the differential diagnosis for the imaging findings presented? (Choose all that apply.)
   A. Urolithiasis
   B. Primary megaureter
   C. Malignant ureteral stricture
   D. Retroperitoneal fibrosis

2. A 48-year-old female with a history of treated ovarian carcinoma presents with right upper quadrant discomfort. Cross-sectional imaging and ultrasound confirm hydronephrosis and proximal hydroureter, though no evidence of cancer recurrence or obstructive disease is visualized. Pyelography confirms ureteral stricture distally. Which of the following is pertinent from the patient's history and is most likely contributing to the patient's presentation?
   A. Episode of urinary tract infection as a child
   B. Previous renal calculi that passed spontaneously
   C. Radiation therapy for pelvic malignancy
   D. Neurogenic bladder

3. Of the interventions listed, which should be avoided in the treatment of benign ureteral stricture?
   A. Percutaneous nephrostomy
   B. Placement of metallic stents
   C. High-pressure balloon ureteral dilatation
   D. Nephroureteral catheter placement

4. You are consulted on a patient with uterine cancer and confirmed malignant ureteral stricture. A nephroureteral catheter is placed percutaneously with no complications intraoperatively. Later that evening, the patient reports hematuria, and the on-call clinical service turns to you for instruction. What is the most appropriate recommendation based on this history?
   A. Cross-sectional imaging to further evaluate
   B. Angiography to exclude vascular injury
   C. Initiate empiric antibiotic treatment
   D. Reassure the clinical service and continue to monitor the patient

See Supplemental Figures section for additional figures and legends for this case.

CASE 169

Malignant Ureteral Stricture

1. **A, C, and D.** Cross-sectional imaging shows right-sided hydroureteronephrosis and focal bladder wall thickening at the ureterovesical junction, compatible with this patient's diagnosis of urinary bladder carcinoma and secondary malignant ureteral stricture. Obstructive urolithiasis and retroperitoneal ureteral fibrosis can present with ureteral dilatation and abrupt termination at the location of obstruction. In contrast, primary hydroureter is a rare condition with enlargement of calyces and/or ureter in the absence of obstruction or reflux.

2. **C.** Iatrogenic stricture is the most common etiology of ureteral stricture. History of instrumentation (i.e., lithotomy, ureteroscopy) or pelvic radiation therapy must be considered in a patient who presents with ureteral stricture. Postoperative stricture can occur at the site of anastomosis of ureter to bladder, ileal conduit, or neobladder.

3. **B.** Though the technical success rate of metallic stent placement is high, the 1-year primary patency rates are poor (~33%) and often require reinstrumentation. Placement of metallic stents should thus be considered palliative and more appropriate in patients with short life expectancy. The other interventions listed are better options for the treatment of benign ureteral stricture.

4. **D.** Transient hematuria is common post percutaneous genitourinary intervention and typically resolves in 24 to 48 hours. Angiography can be considered if bleeding persists to exclude vascular injury, including pseudoaneurysm or arteriovenous fistula formation.

Comment

Etiology

The most common etiology of ureteral stricture is iatrogenic, often presenting post lithotomy or ureteroscopy or post radiation. However, pyelography alone is often not sufficient to determine the etiology of a ureteral stricture. In these cases, knowledge of the patient's history and correlation with cross-sectional imaging modalities (to visualize a calculus, pelvic mass, or other lesion) may be helpful, as seen in this patient (Figures S169-1 and S169-2).

Treatment Methods

The treatment of malignant ureteral strictures depends largely upon the exact etiology and the overall extent of the disease. In many patients with bladder carcinoma and selected patients with other pelvic malignancies, total cystectomy with ileal conduit formation may be performed, obviating the need for percutaneous intervention. In many other patients, hydroureteronephrosis develops and is not likely to be relieved surgically. In these patients, percutaneous nephrostomy placement is usually performed, often followed by ureteral stent placement if bladder function is adequate. In the postintervention image, the stenosis was successfully crossed and a nephroureteral stent was placed (Figures S169-3 and S169-4).

References

Adamo R, Saad W, Brown DB. Percutaneous ureteral interventions. *Tech Vasc Interv Radiol.* 2009;12:205–215.

Adamo R, Saad W, Brown DB. Management of nephrostomy drains and ureteral stents. *Tech Vasc Interv Radiol.* 2009;12:193–204.

Blandino A, Gaeta M, Minutoli F, et al. MR urography of the ureter. *AJR Am J Roentgenol.* 2002;179:1307–1314.

Cross-reference

Vascular and Interventional Radiology: The Requisites, 2nd ed, 499–506.

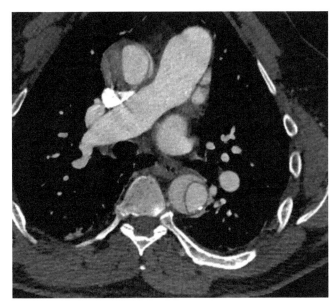

Figure 170-1. *Courtesy of Dr. David M. Williams.*

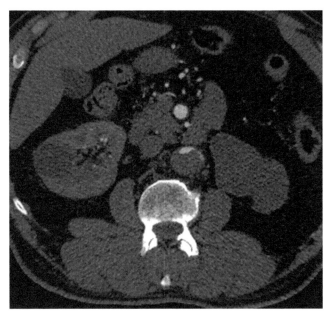

Figure 170-2. *Courtesy of Dr. David M. Williams.*

HISTORY: A 64-year-old male smoker with hypertension presents to the emergency department with abdominal and right lower extremity pain with rising lactate levels.

1. Which of the following is the most likely diagnosis, given the imaging and clinical findings presented?
   A. Aortoiliac occlusive disease
   B. Aortic dissection with malperfusion
   C. Embolic occlusion of the right common iliac artery
   D. Aortic aneurysm

2. What endovascular procedure could assist in treating the above entity?
   A. Kissing iliac stents
   B. Endograft of the descending thoracic aorta
   C. Aortic arch open repair
   D. Balloon fenestration of aortic dissection

3. What is the indication for the correct endovascular intervention from Question 3?
   A. The false lumen has stabilized and needs to be reduced.
   B. The patient has coexistent aortoiliac occlusive disease.
   C. The patient is experiencing malperfusion syndrome.
   D. The patient is actively exsanguinating.

4. All of the following complications of aortic dissection would preclude fenestration *EXCEPT*:
   A. Cardiac tamponade
   B. Coronary artery involvement
   C. Right lower extremity thrombosis
   D. Extension of dissection into the left common carotid artery

See Supplemental Figures section for additional figures and legends for this case.

CASE 170

Percutaneous Balloon Fenestration of Aortic Dissection

1. **B.** The images clearly show a type A aortic dissection. The clinical information including abdominal pain, right lower-extremity pain, and rising lactate levels suggest malperfusion.

2. **D.** Balloon fenestration of aortic dissection may aid in improving flow within the malperfused tissues. Kissing iliac stents may be placed in patients with dissection extending into the lower extremities, although this is commonly performed with fenestration and would not treat the gut malperfusion. Placing an endograft in the descending thoracic aorta would not be a primary treatment in this patient as there is a tear in the ascending aorta.

3. **C.** Balloon fenestration aims to increase blood flow to tissues perfused by the true lumen, which are ischemic as a result of the dissection.

4. **C.** The right lower extremity may be thrombosed due to extension of the dissection flap, which may be treated with thrombolysis, fenestration, and stenting. The other choices are indications for emergent surgical repair.

Comment

Main Teaching Point

Type A dissection is a surgical emergency and patients are traditionally treated with open repair of the affected aorta and aortic valve, if necessary. However, in patients with prolonged malperfusion, correction of the malperfusion prior to surgical repair may result in improved survival. Similarly, patients with malperfusion and type B dissection (complicated type B dissection) may benefit from correction of the malperfusion. Computed tomography angiography is the current initial imaging modality employed to diagnose aortic dissection, although echocardiography and magnetic resonance imaging may also be used (Figures S170-1 and S170-2).

Endovascular Management

Patients with acute dissection complicated by visceral or peripheral arterial ischemia are at high risk for death and paraplegia during surgical aortic repair. For this reason, several percutaneous methods have been used to relieve organ ischemia in these patients. Stents can be placed in branch vessels that are dissected. In addition, patients with true lumen collapse and organ ischemia due to poor inflow to a true lumen-supplied branch artery can be treated with percutaneous balloon fenestration or aortic stent placement; in early studies, perfusion was successfully restored to tissue beds that were more than 90% ischemic using these methods (Figures S170-3 through S170-6). Another endovascular approach involves placement of a stent graft across the primary intimal dissection tear in the thoracic aorta in type B dissections. Completely endovascular methods for repair of the ascending aorta and arch are currently under investigation.

References

Deeb GM, Patel HJ, Williams DM. Treatment for malperfusion syndrome in acute type A and B aortic dissection: a long-term analysis. *J Thorac Cardiovasc Surg.* 2010;140:S98–S100.

DiMusto PD, Williams DW, Patel HJ, et al. Endovascular management of type B aortic dissections. *J Vasc Surg.* 2010;52:26S–36S.

Midulla M, Renaud A, Martinelli T, et al. Endovascular fenestration in aortic dissection with acute malperfusion syndrome: immediate and late follow-up. *J Thorac Cardiovasc Surg.* 2011;142:66–72.

Cross-reference

Vascular and Interventional Radiology: The Requisites, 2nd ed, 188–192.

Supplemental Figures

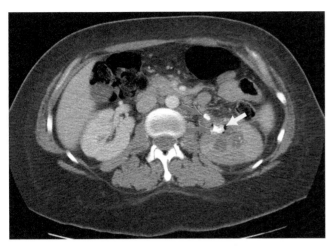

Figure S1-1 Axial contrast-enhanced CT image demonstrates a dilated left renal collecting system with multiple large calculi (red arrows), collecting system gas (yellow arrow), and delayed heterogeneous enhancement of the left kidney.

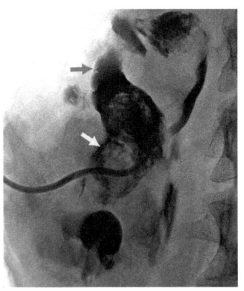

Figure S1-2 Fluoroscopic image taken during left percutaneous nephrostomy catheter placement demonstrates a dilated left renal collecting system with multiple irregular filling defects (yellow arrow). Additionally, there was extravasation of contrast from the upper pole (red arrow).

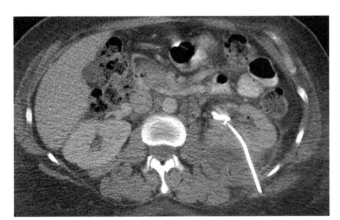

Figure S1-3 Axial contrast-enhanced CT image following placement of a left percutaneous nephrostomy catheter. There is a new left posterior subcapsular fluid collection concerning for a perinephric abscess (arrow).

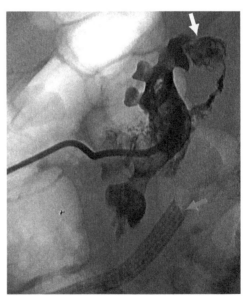

Figure S1-4 Fluoroscopic image taken during subsequent nephrostomy tube change demonstrates persistent extravasation of contrast from the upper pole (yellow arrow). There has been interval placement of a surgical drain into the previously identified perinephric abscess (red arrow).

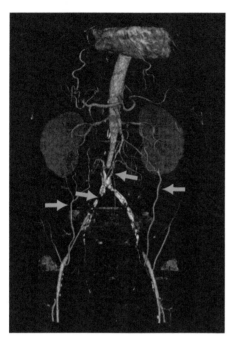

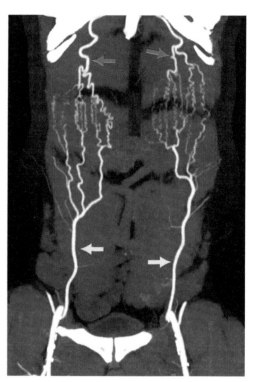

Figure S2-1 3D reconstruction from CTA shows the aortoiliac occlusion with heavy atherosclerotic burden of the infrarenal aorta and iliac arteries (green arrows) with collateral pathways (blue arrows). *Courtesy of Dr. Klaus D. Hagspiel.*

Figure S2-2 Maximum intensity projection (MIP) coronal reconstruction shows the Winslow collateral pathway of the superior epigastric (red arrows) feeding the inferior epigastric (yellow arrows) and thus retrograde filling of the external iliac arteries. *Courtesy of Dr. Klaus D. Hagspiel.*

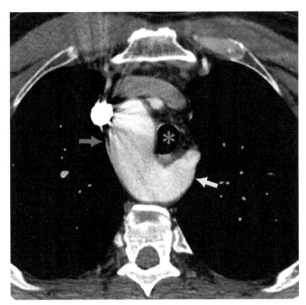

Figure S3-1 Contrast-enhanced CT showing a right-sided aortic arch (red arrow) with aberrant left subclavian artery (yellow arrow) coursing behind the trachea (asterisk).

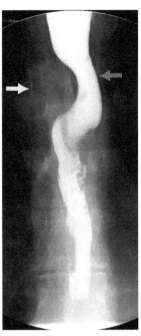

Figure S3-2 Thoracic esophagogram demonstrating leftward displacement of the barium-filled esophagus (red arrow) by the right-sided aortic arch (yellow arrow) without compression.

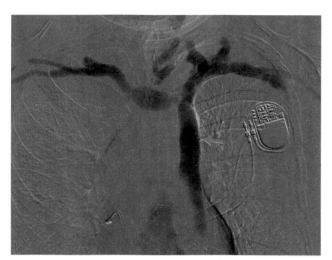

Figure S4-1 CO_2 upper extremity venogram demonstrates a persistent left SVC (arrow). *Courtesy of Dr. Minhaj S. Khaja.*

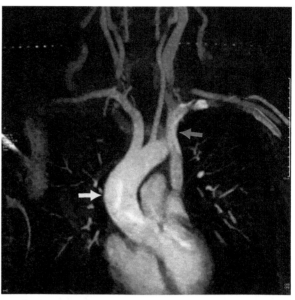

Figure S4-2 MR venogram in a different patient demonstrates a normal aortic arch (yellow arrow) and a persistent left superior vena cava (red arrow). Note its close relationship with the aorta. No right superior vena cava is seen. *Courtesy of Dr. Minhaj S. Khaja.*

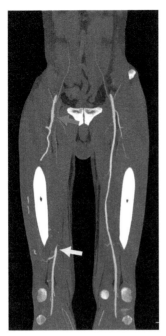

Figure S5-1 Coronal reconstruction of a CTA showing abrupt occlusion of the superficial femoral artery (red arrow) with distal reconstitution (yellow arrow). Left side is normal.

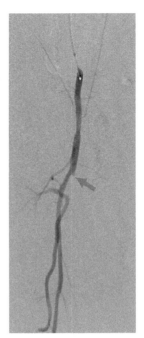

Figure S5-2 Image from digital subtraction angiogram with catheter tip in the distal external iliac artery redemonstrating abrupt occlusion of the SFA (arrow).

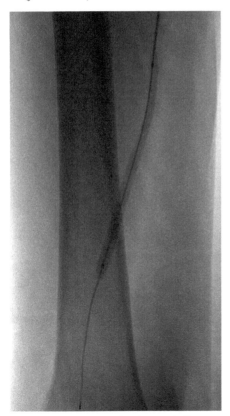

Figure S5-3 Image from angiography showing balloon angioplasty of the SFA once the lesion was crossed.

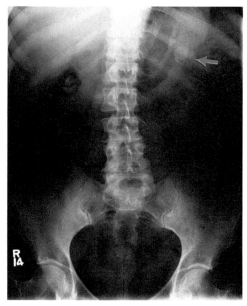

Figure S6-1 Abdominal radiograph demonstrating left upper quadrant calcifications concerning splenic artery aneurysm (arrow).

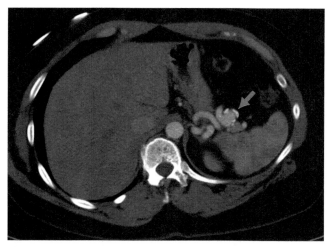

Figure S6-2 Axial image from CTA showing saccular aneurysm arising from the splenic artery with calcifications (arrow).

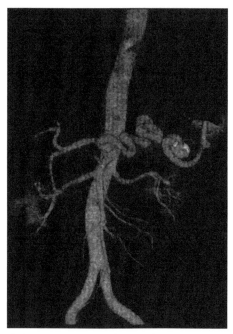

Figure S6-3 3D reconstruction of CTA redemonstrating the saccular aneurysm of the mid-splenic artery.

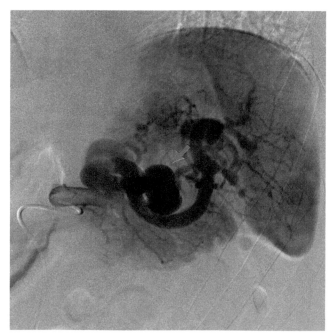

Figure S6-4 DSA image with catheter in proximal splenic artery showing saccular aneurysm from the mid-splenic artery.

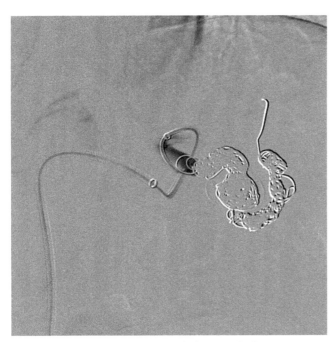

Figure S6-5 DSA image after coil embolization of splenic artery aneurysm with no flow beyond the coils or within the aneurysm.

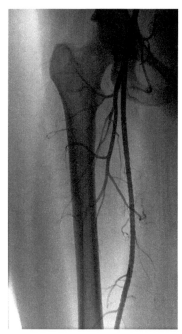

Figure S7-1 Native image from lower extremity angiogram demonstrating corrugated appearance of the proximal superficial femoral artery (SFA). *Courtesy of Dr. Alan H. Matsumoto.*

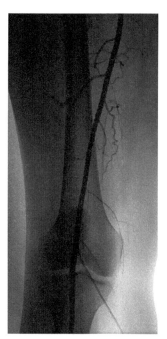

Figure S7-2 Native image from the same lower extremity angiogram demonstrating corrugated appearance of the distal SFA and popliteal artery. *Courtesy of Dr. Alan H. Matsumoto.*

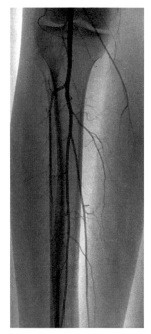

Figure S7-3 Additional native image from lower extremity angiogram demonstrating standing waves in the tibial vessels. *Courtesy of Dr. Alan H. Matsumoto.*

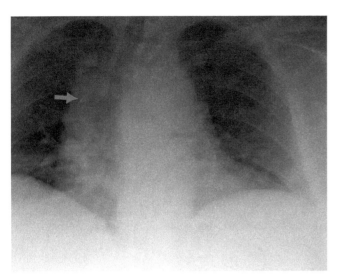

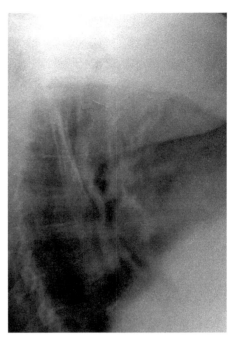

Figures S8-1 PA chest radiograph demonstrates a left PICC which courses through the SVC with the distal aspect of the catheter curved, likely due to azygous vein placement (red arrow).

Figure S8-2 Lateral chest radiograph confirms that the distal aspect of the catheter is curved posteriorly on the lateral view (red arrow). This is consistent with azygous vein placement.

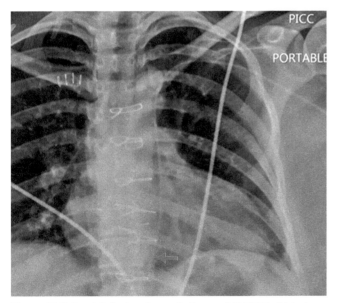

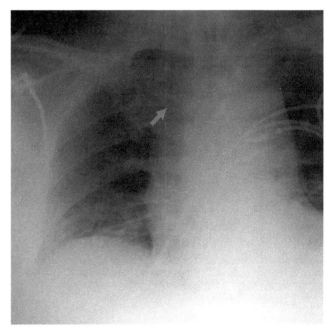

Figure S8-3 Frontal chest radiograph shows a left PICC which does not cross the midline and courses caudally within the left hemithorax, terminating over the cardiac silhouette (red arrow). This is consistent with either a left-sided SVC or a duplicated SVC.

Figure S8-4 Frontal chest radiograph reveals a right PICC, which is looped within the right internal jugular vein, with the tip at the confluence of the right brachiocephalic vein and the superior vena cava (red arrow).

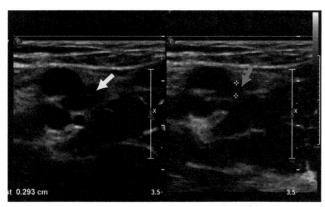

Figure S9-1 Gray-scale ultrasound image depicting a non-compressible (red arrow) right distal common femoral vein with a partially hypoechoic lumen (yellow arrow). *Courtesy of Dr. Minhaj S. Khaja.*

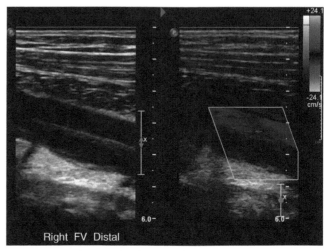

Figure S9-2 Color Doppler ultrasound image demonstrating absence of flow in the involved vein. Arterial flow is readily depicted in the adjacent right femoral artery. *Courtesy of Dr. Minhaj S. Khaja.*

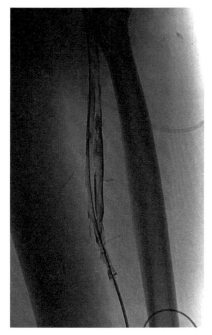

Figure S9-3 Fluoroscopic image from venogram confirming an intraluminal filling defect, peripherally outlined by contrast within an enlarged right common femoral vein. There is an absence of collateral vessel formation. *Courtesy of Dr. Minhaj S. Khaja.*

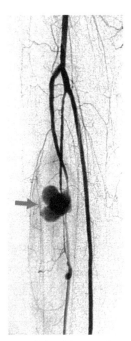

Figure S10-1 DSA image of the right runoff vessels demonstrating a lobulated pseudoaneurysm arising from the mid anterior tibial artery (arrow).

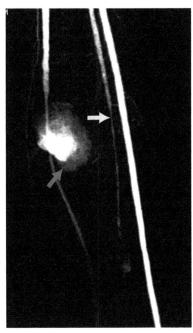

Figure S10-2 Inverted DSA image in RAO view redemonstrating pseudoaneurysm with adjacent hematoma (red arrow). Also noted is displacement of the peroneal artery by the hematoma (yellow arrow).

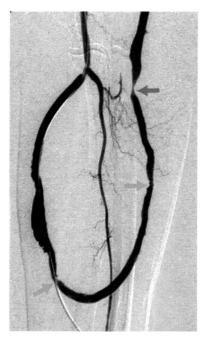

Figure S11-1 DSA image from dialysis-access fistulagram showing three distinct stenosis: a tight stenosis at the venous anastomosis (red arrow) and two mild stenoses within the graft itself (blue arrows). *Courtesy of Dr. Thomas Vesely.*

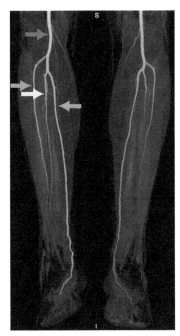

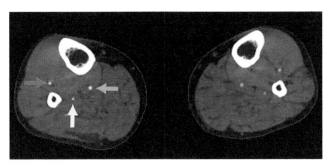

Figure S12-1 Coronal reformat MIP from a CTA with lower extremity runoff shows bilateral three vessel patency of the calf arterial circulation with normal branching anatomy. Popliteal (red arrow), anterior tibial (green arrow), posterior tibial (blue arrow), and peroneal (yellow arrow) arteries are seen. *Courtesy of Dr. Minhaj S. Khaja.*

Figure S12-2 Single axial slice from the same study demonstrates the expected branching pattern of the popliteal artery just below the knee with three-vessel patency. Anterior tibial (red arrow), posterior tibial (blue arrow), and peroneal (yellow arrow) arteries are seen. *Courtesy of Dr. Minhaj S. Khaja.*

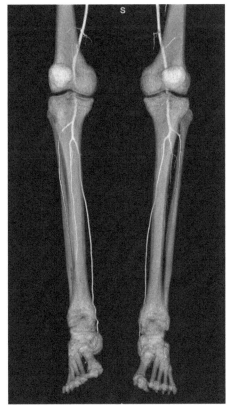

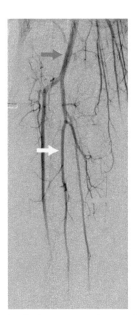

Figure S12-3 Volume-rendered 3D image from same study as Figure S12-1 with same anatomy. *Courtesy of Dr. Minhaj S. Khaja.*

Figure S12-4 DSA of right lower extremity in a different patient illustrating the conventional branch pattern of the tibial arteries. Popliteal (red arrow), anterior tibial (green arrow), posterior tibial (blue arrow), and peroneal (yellow arrow) arteries are seen. *Courtesy of Dr. Minhaj S. Khaja.*

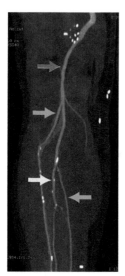

Figure S12-5 Coronal MIP of right lower extremity from a CTA shows high takeoff of the right anterior tibial artery (green arrow). Popliteal (red arrow), posterior tibial (blue arrow), and peroneal (yellow arrow) arteries are seen. This patient has atherosclerosis, with moderate narrowing at the branching of the right tibioperoneal trunk into the posterior tibial and peroneal arteries. *Courtesy of Dr. Minhaj S. Khaja.*

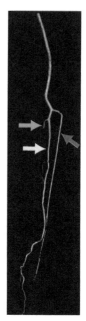

Figure S12-6 Volume-rendered reconstruction of the left lower extremity from a CTA shows peroneal arteria magna, with a normal-sized anterior tibial artery (red arrow), hypoplastic posterior tibial artery (blue arrow), and dominant peroneal artery (yellow arrow). *Courtesy of Dr. Minhaj S. Khaja.*

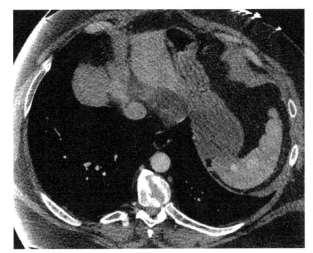

Figure S13-1 Axial contrast-enhanced CT image demonstrating foci of hyperdensity within the splenic parenchyma (red arrows). *Courtesy of Dr. Wael E. Saad.*

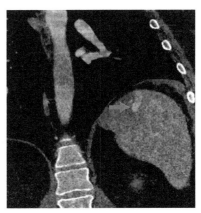

Figure S13-2 Coronal contrast-enhanced CT image demonstrating focus of hyperdensity within the splenic parenchyma (red arrow). *Courtesy of Dr. Wael E. Saad.*

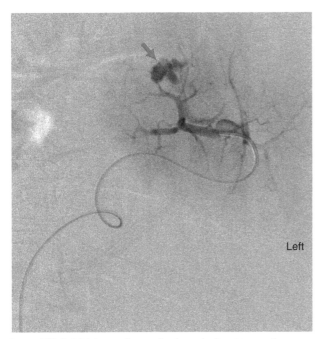

Figure S13-3 DSA image from selective splenic artery angiogram demonstrating a multilobed pseudoaneurysm (red arrow). *Courtesy of Dr. Wael E. Saad.*

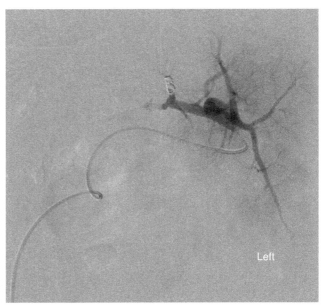

Figure S13-4 DSA image from splenic artery angiogram demonstrating coil embolization of the pseudoaneurysm without further evidence of bleeding. *Courtesy of Dr. Wael E. Saad.*

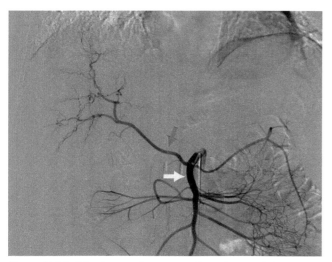

Figure S14-1 Selective superior mesenteric angiogram demonstrates a replaced right hepatic artery (red arrow) arising from the SMA (yellow arrow). *Courtesy of Dr. Minhaj S. Khaja.*

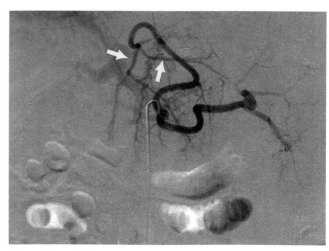

Figure S14-2 Selective celiac arteriogram illustrating a replaced left hepatic artery (yellow arrows) arising from the left gastric artery (red arrow). *Courtesy of Dr. Minhaj S. Khaja.*

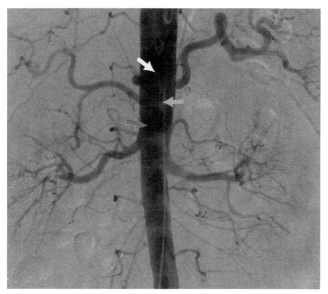

Figure S14-3 AP aortogram showing variant hepatic arterial anatomy. Celiac trunk (yellow arrow), replaced common hepatic artery (blue arrow), and SMA (red arrow) all arise directly from the aorta. *Courtesy of Dr. Minhaj S. Khaja.*

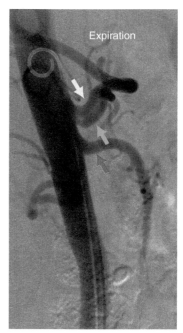

Figure S14-4 Lateral aortogram in the same patient as Figure S14-3 demonstrating the same findings. Celiac trunk (yellow arrow), replaced common hepatic artery (blue arrow), and SMA (red arrow) all arise directly from the aorta. *Courtesy of Dr. Minhaj S. Khaja.*

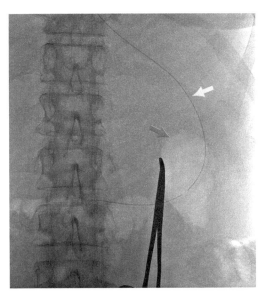

Figure S15-1 Fluoroscopic image of the left upper quadrant with metallic clamp in place. The stomach is small and underdistended (red arrow). A nasogastric tube has been placed for insufflation (yellow arrow).

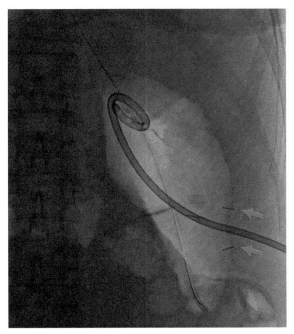

Figure S15-2 Fluoroscopic image of the left upper quadrant with gastrostomy tube within the stomach. Note the two metallic T-fasteners, placed for gastropexy (arrows).

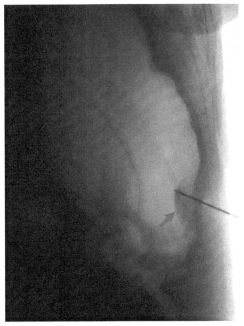

Figure S15-3 A needle has been placed through the skin under fluoroscopic guidance and is tenting the wall of the stomach (arrow).

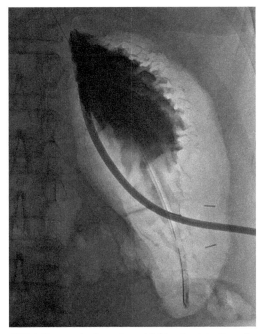

Figure S15-4 Demonstration of rugal folds after injection of contrast through the tube helps confirm intraluminal placement.

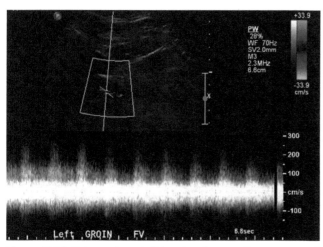

Figure S16-1 Color and spectral Doppler ultrasound image centered on the femoral vein demonstrating arterialized flow within the femoral vein. *Courtesy of Dr. Luke R. Wilkins.*

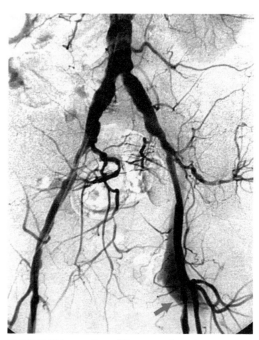

Figure S16-2 DSA image in a different patient demonstrating early venous filling of the left common femoral and external iliac veins (arrow).

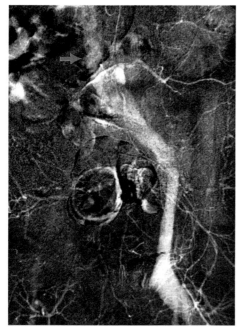

Figure S16-3 Delayed image from DSA in the same patient as in Figure S16-2 highlighting the venous drainage to the level of the IVC (arrow).

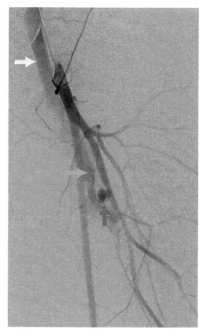

Figure S16-4 DSA image in a different patient after motor vehicle collision demonstrating a left profunda pseudoaneurysm (red arrow) with early venous filling in the profunda femoral vein (blue arrow) and common femoral vein (yellow arrow) confirming AVF. *Courtesy of Dr. Luke R. Wilkins.*

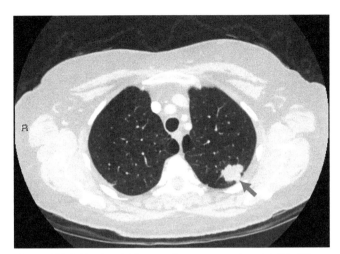

Figure S17-1 Single axial image of a contrast-enhanced CT of the chest in lung windows demonstrating a 3-cm spiculated mass in the apicoposterior segment of the left upper lobe (arrow).

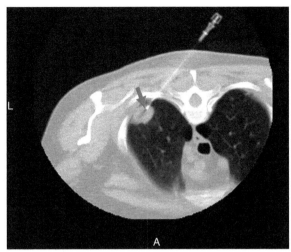

Figure S17-2 Single prone image from CT-guided coaxial core needle biopsy of the left upper lobe mass. The acute angle through the midline was chosen secondary to the presence of a rib immediately posterior to the mass. Trocar needle tip is within the mass (arrow).

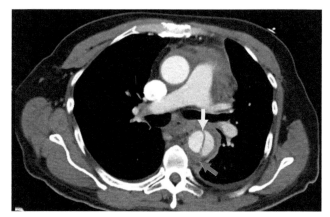

Figure S18-1 Axial image from CTA of the chest demonstrating dissection flap (yellow arrow) in the descending aorta with mediastinal hemorrhage (red arrow) suggestive of leaking. *Courtesy of Dr. David M. Williams.*

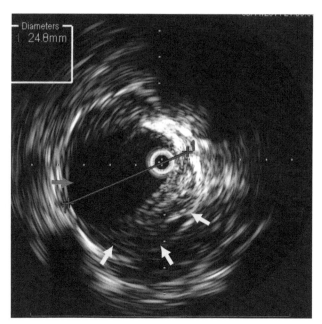

Figure S18-2 Intravascular ultrasound in the same patient shows a compressed patent true lumen (red arrow) and a thrombosed false lumen (hyperechoic crescent-shaped lumen located posterior and to the left, yellow arrows). IVUS also allows the operator to accurately measure the true and false lumens prior to stent graft placement, if indicated. *Courtesy of Dr. David M. Williams.*

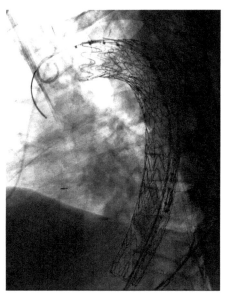

Figure S18-3 Angiographic image demonstrating deployed stent-graft. *Courtesy of Dr. David M. Williams.*

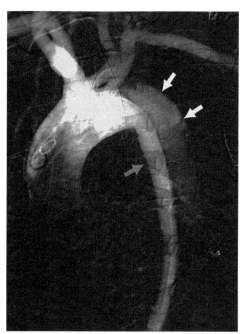

Figure S18-4 Thoracic aortogram in a different patient illustrating the true (red arrow) and false (yellow arrows) lumen appearance.

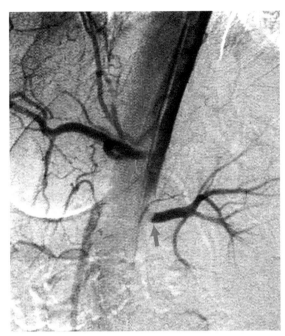

Figure S18-5 Abdominal aortogram in the same patient as in Figure S18-4 demonstrating the "floating viscera" sign with minimal opacification of the aorta while there is some flow seen in visceral and renal branches (arrows).

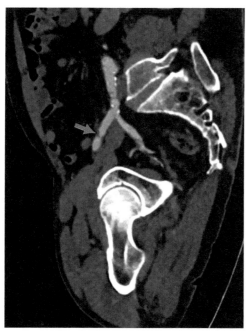

Figure S19-1 CTA MPR oblique showing focal area of right common iliac artery stenosis (arrow). *Courtesy of Dr. Saher S. Sabri.*

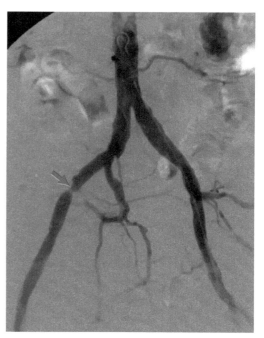

Figure S19-2 Digital subtraction pelvic angiogram in the RPO position demonstrates a high-grade focal stenosis of the right external iliac artery (arrow). *Courtesy of Dr. Saher S. Sabri.*

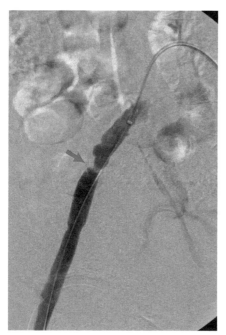

Figure S19-3 Digital subtraction angiogram in the RPO position after up and over selection of the right external iliac artery redemonstrating a high-grade focal stenosis of the right external iliac artery (arrow). *Courtesy of Dr. Saher S. Sabri.*

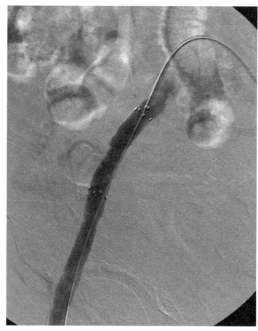

Figure S19-4 Digital subtraction angiogram in the RPO position following stenting of the external iliac artery stenosis with a widely patent lumen (arrow). *Courtesy of Dr. Saher S. Sabri.*

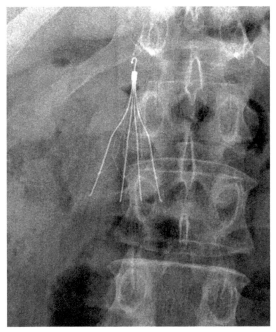

Figure S20-1 Radiograph showing the successful placement of a Gunther Tulip IVC filter.

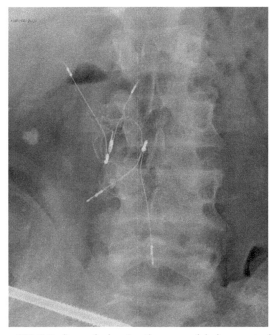

Figure S20-2 Radiograph showing the successful placement of a Bird's Nest IVC filter.

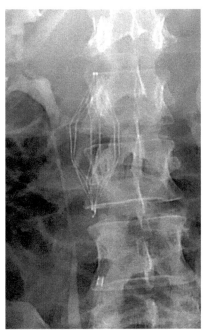

Figure S20-3 Radiograph showing the successful placement of an Optease IVC filter.

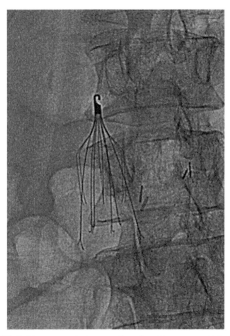

Figure S20-4 Fluoroscopic image showing the successful placement of a Denali IVC filter.

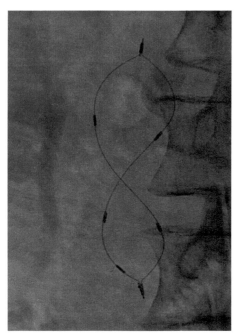

Figure S20-5 Radiograph showing the successful placement of a Crux IVC filter.

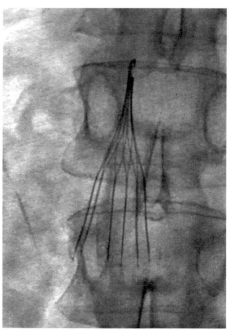

Figure S20-6 Radiographic image showing the successful placement of an Option IVC filter.

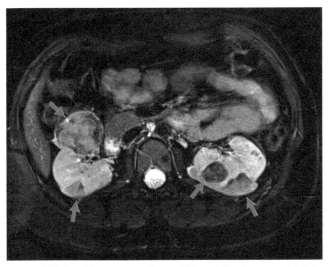

Figure S21-1 Axial contrast-enhanced T1-weighted image with fat suppression demonstrating multiple bilateral lesions with areas of enhancement and signal dropout (arrows). *Courtesy of Dr. J. Fritz Angle.*

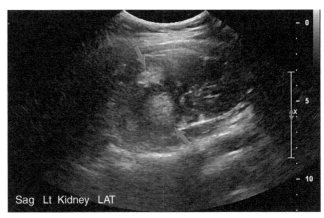

Figure S21-2 Longitudinal ultrasound image of the left kidney showing two echogenic masses (arrow). *Courtesy of Dr. J. Fritz Angle.*

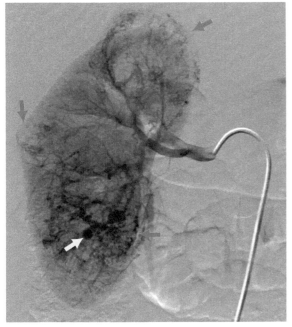

Figure S21-3 Right renal angiogram shows three separate hypervascular lesions (red arrows) with associated small pseudoaneurysm formation (yellow arrow). *Courtesy of Dr. J. Fritz Angle.*

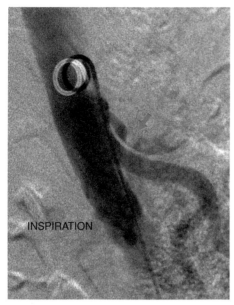

Figure S22-1 Lateral aortogram of the celiac axis during inspiration demonstrating compression of the celiac artery approximately 1 cm from its origin (arrow). *Courtesy of Dr. Minhaj S. Khaja.*

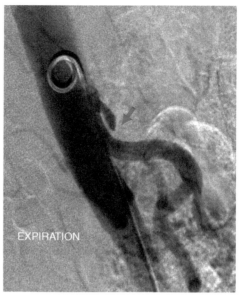

Figure S22-2 Lateral aortogram of the celiac axis in the same patient during expiration demonstrating occlusion of the celiac artery approximately 1 cm from its origin (arrow). *Courtesy of Dr. Minhaj S. Khaja.*

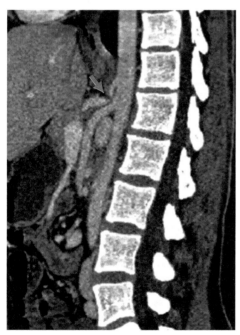

Figure S22-3 Sagittal CTA image of the abdominal aorta axis showing significant stenosis of the celiac axis (arrow) with poststenotic dilation without any evidence of atheromatous plaque. *Courtesy of Dr. Minhaj S. Khaja.*

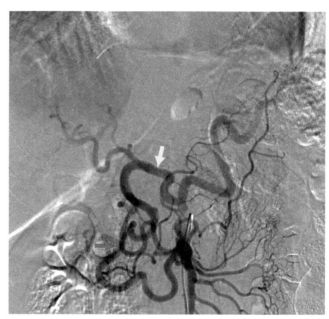

Figure S22-4 AP selective angiography of the SMA showing retrograde filling of the common hepatic (yellow arrow) and celiac artery via pancreaticoduodenal collaterals (red arrow) due to the celiac trunk stenosis. *Courtesy of Dr. Minhaj S. Khaja.*

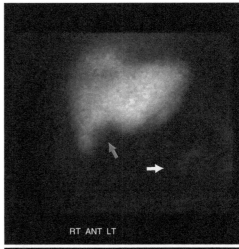

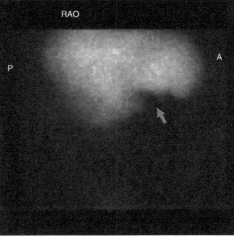

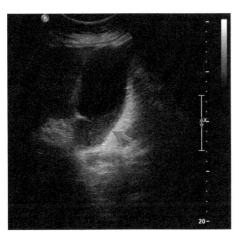

Figure S23-1 Gray-scale ultrasound image of the right upper quadrant demonstrating a dilated gallbladder with layering echogenic material (sludge) (arrow). *Courtesy of Dr. Minhaj S. Khaja.*

Figure S23-2 Planar frontal (top) and right lateral (bottom) images from a nuclear medicine hepatobiliary scan confirming obstruction of the cystic duct with no radiotracer within the gallbladder after 4-hour delay. In fact, a void is noted (red arrow). Radiotracer is seen within the gut (yellow arrow). *Courtesy of Dr. Minhaj S. Khaja.*

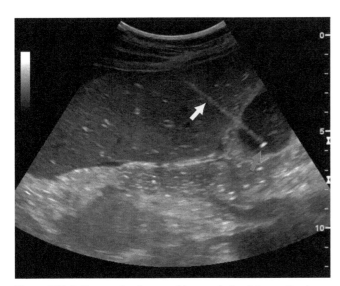

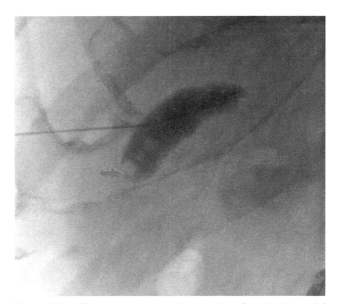

Figure S23-3 Gray-scale ultrasound image during intervention in a different patient confirming needle tip in the gallbladder (red arrow) via transhepatic approach (yellow arrow). *Courtesy of Dr. Minhaj S. Khaja.*

Figure S23-4 Fluoroscopic image after injection of contrast material confirming presence of needle within the gallbladder. Filling defects within gallbladder represent gallstones (arrow). *Courtesy of Dr. Minhaj S. Khaja.*

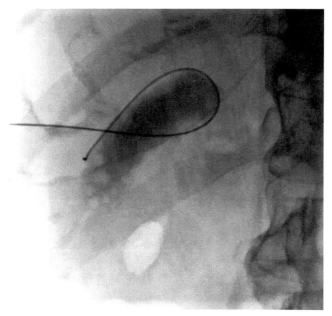

Figure S23-5 Fluoroscopic image of the right upper quadrant with wire delineating the shape of the gallbladder. *Courtesy of Dr. Minhaj S. Khaja.*

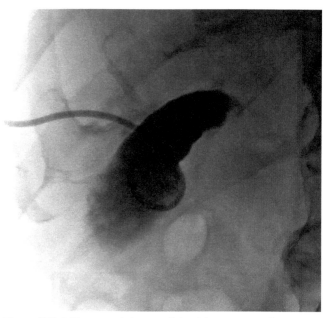

Figure S23-6 Fluoroscopic image of the right upper quadrant after tube placement confirming position within the gallbladder. Several filling defects again noted. *Courtesy of Dr. Minhaj S. Khaja.*

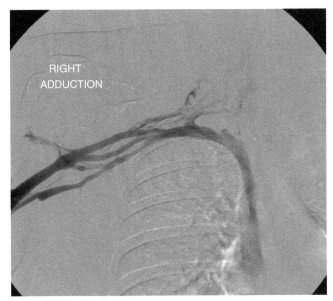

Figure S24-1 Digital subtraction venogram with the right upper extremity in adduction demonstrates mild stenosis of the subclavian vein as well as a few small venous collaterals extending toward the neck.

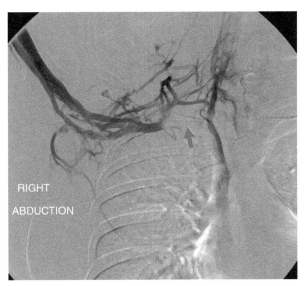

Figure S24-2 Digital subtraction venogram with the right upper extremity in abduction demonstrates occlusion of the subclavian vein (arrow) and increased filling of numerous small venous collaterals extending toward the neck.

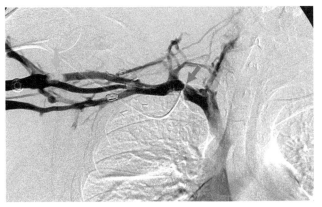

Figure S24-3 Digital subtraction venogram of the right upper extremity following first rib resection demonstrates persistent subclavian vein stenosis (red arrow). A complication of subclavian vein occlusion is present—thrombus within the axillary vein, which appears as a filling defect (blue arrow). A surgical drain is present.

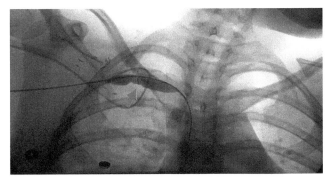

Figure S24-4 Native fluoroscopic image demonstrating balloon angioplasty at the site of subclavian vein stenosis. The site of first rib resection is well visualized at the site of stenosis (arrow). A surgical drain is present.

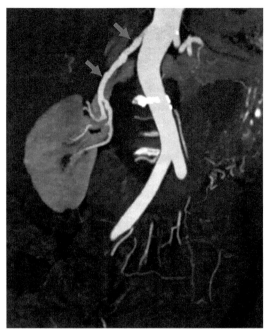

Figure S25-1 Curved multiplanar reconstruction image from CTA demarcating the irregular, "beaded" appearance of mid right renal artery (arrows). No ostial narrowing seen. *Courtesy of Dr. Alan H. Matsumoto.*

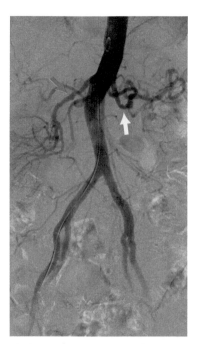

Figure S25-2 DSA image from aortogram demonstrating the same beaded appearance of the right mid right renal artery (red arrow). Also seen is a similar appearance of the left renal artery (yellow arrow). *Courtesy of Dr. Alan H. Matsumoto.*

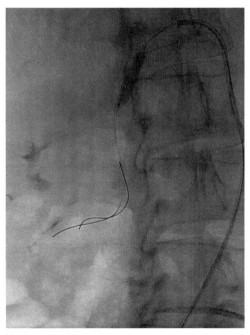

Figure S25-3 Native image from right renal angiogram with angioplasty balloon in place. *Courtesy of Dr. Alan H. Matsumoto.*

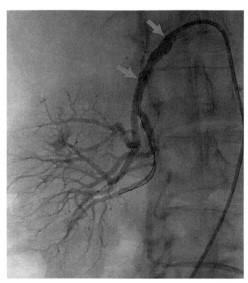

Figure S25-4 Native image after balloon angioplasty demonstrating improved appearance of right renal artery (arrows). *Courtesy of Dr. Alan H. Matsumoto.*

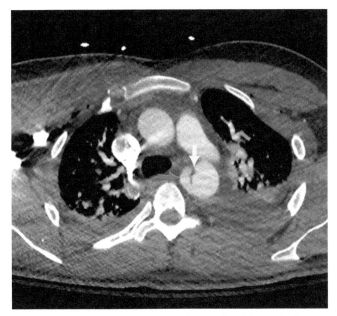

Figure S26-1 Axial image from CTA shows a focal discontinuity along the medial wall of the aortic arch (yellow arrow), with an outpouching of contrast beyond the aortic lumen (red arrow) and adjacent fluid. *Courtesy of Dr. David M. Williams.*

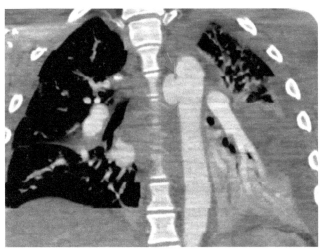

Figure S26-2 Coronal reconstruction from CTA better displays the pseudoaneurysm and its sharp margins with the aortic wall (arrows). *Courtesy of Dr. David M. Williams.*

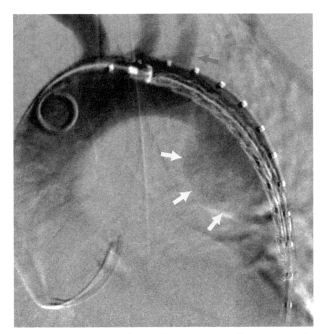

Figure S26-3 DSA image from LAO aortogram redemonstrates the pseudoaneurysm (yellow arrows) prior to endograft deployment. Note its origin begins just distal to the left subclavian artery (red arrow). *Courtesy of Dr. David M. Williams.*

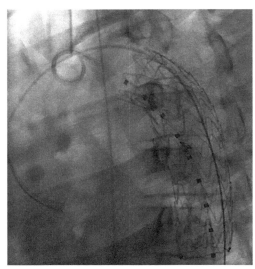

Figure S26-4 Native image in LAO projection after endograft deployment. *Courtesy of Dr. David M. Williams.*

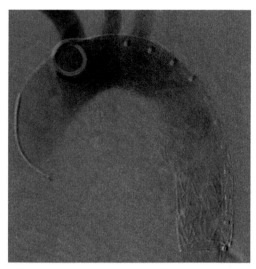

Figure S26-5 DSA image from LAO aortogram postdeployment with exclusion of the pseudoaneurysm. *Courtesy of Dr. David M. Williams.*

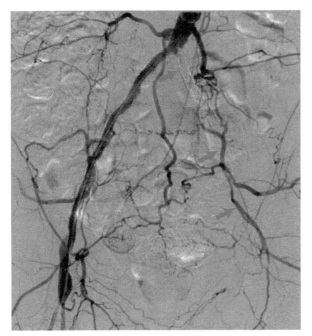

Figure S27-1 DSA image obtained at the level of the aortic bifurcation reveals kissing aortoiliac stents, with occlusion of the left common iliac artery stents (arrows).

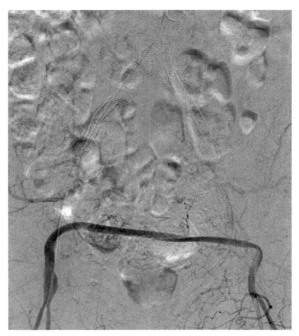

Figure S27-2 Delayed DSA image obtained during the same run reveals flow across the femorofemoral bypass graft with filling of the bilateral common femoral, proximal superficial femoral, and profunda femoris arteries.

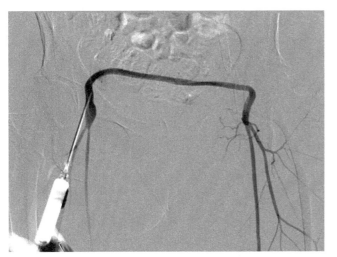

Figure S27-3 Direct manual graft injection again demonstrates flow across the femorofemoral bypass graft into patent common femoral, superficial femoral, and profunda femoris arteries, bilaterally.

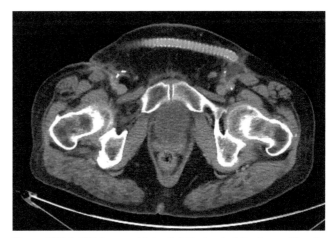

Figure S27-4 CTA image obtained at the level of the femoral heads demonstrates contrast filling the tunneled femorofemoral bypass graft which courses anteriorly along the ventral abdominal infrapubic superficial soft tissues.

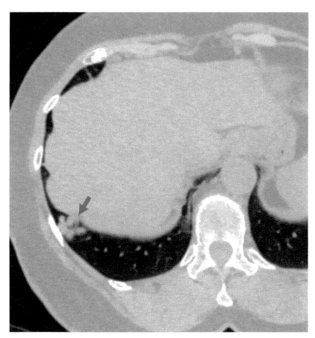

Figure S28-1 Axial image from unenhanced chest CT in the lung window demonstrates a well-defined, serpiginous lesion within the right lung base (red arrow). *Courtesy of Dr. Bill S. Majdalany.*

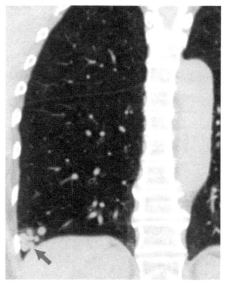

Figure S28-2 Coronal image from the same chest CT also in the lung window re-demonstrates aforementioned lesion within the right lung base (red arrow). *Courtesy of Dr. Bill S. Majdalany.*

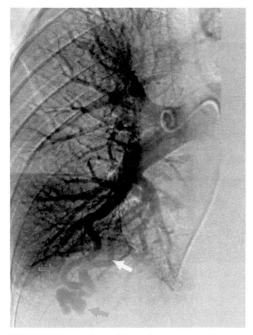

Figure S28-3 DSA image from right pulmonary arteriogram reveals a serpentine feeding artery (red arrow) traveling to and a draining vein (yellow arrow) emanating from a central aneurysmal nidus (blue arrow) within the right lung base. *Courtesy of Dr. Bill S. Majdalany.*

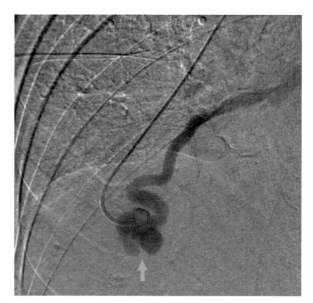

Figure S28-4 Coned down, selective DSA image of the lesion in question better delineates its nodular central aneurysmal nidus (blue arrow) with the presence of a dilated draining vein (red arrow) *Courtesy of Dr. Bill S. Majdalany.*

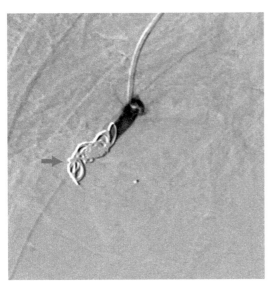

Figure S28-5 Postembolization DSA image of the same region demonstrates successful placement of coils (red arrow) and vascular plug (blue arrow) without flow through the lesion. *Courtesy of Dr. Bill S. Majdalany.*

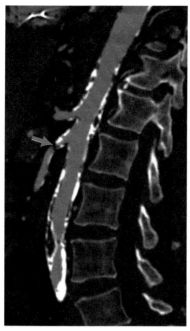

Figure S29-1 Parasagittal oblique reconstruction of CTA demonstrates high-grade stenosis near the origin of the SMA (arrow). Note also heavy atherosclerotic calcification of the abdominal aorta. *Courtesy of Dr. Alan H. Matsumoto.*

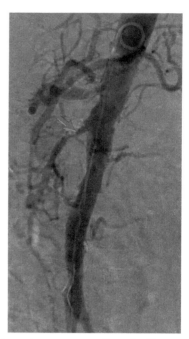

Figure S29-2 Lateral aortogram confirms significant stenosis near the origin of the SMA (arrow). *Courtesy of Dr. Alan H. Matsumoto.*

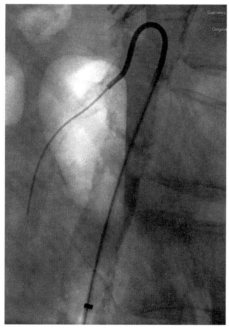

Figure S29-3 Lateral fluoroscopic image during selection of the highly calcified SMA using a wire and reverse-curve catheter shape. *Courtesy of Dr. Alan H. Matsumoto.*

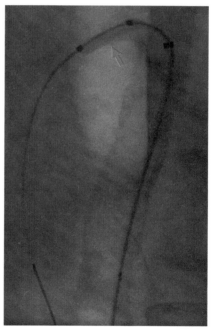

Figure S29-4 Lateral fluoroscopic image illustrates balloon angioplasty (arrow) of the SMA. Note that a sheath has been advanced. *Courtesy of Dr. Alan H. Matsumoto.*

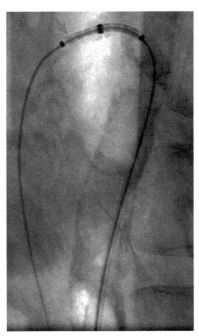

Figure S29-5 Lateral fluoroscopic image demonstrates stent placement (red arrow) and retraction of the sheath (yellow arrow). *Courtesy of Dr. Alan H. Matsumoto.*

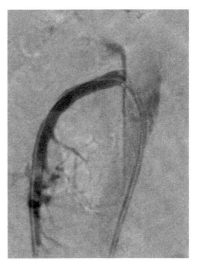

Figure S29-6 DSA image demonstrates improvement in the caliber of the proximal SMA following stent placement. *Courtesy of Dr. Alan H. Matsumoto.*

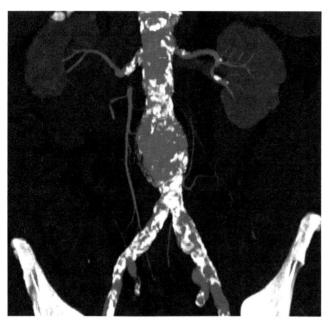

Figure S30-1 Maximum intensity projection (MIP) coronal CT reconstruction demonstrates fusiform infrarenal abdominal aortic aneurysm. *Courtesy of Dr. Klaus D. Hagspiel.*

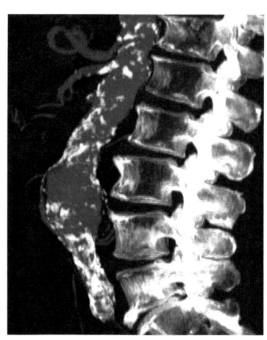

Figure S30-2 Sagittal MIP CT reconstruction demonstrates fusiform infrarenal abdominal aortic aneurysm. *Courtesy of Dr. Klaus D. Hagspiel.*

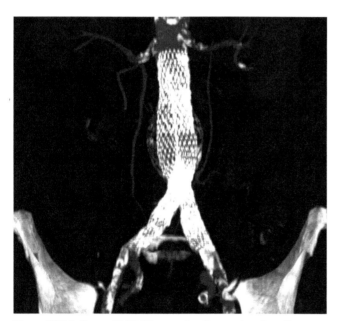

Figure S30-3 Coronal MIP CT reconstruction post-endograft placement with no increase in aneurysm sac size. *Courtesy of Dr. Klaus D. Hagspiel.*

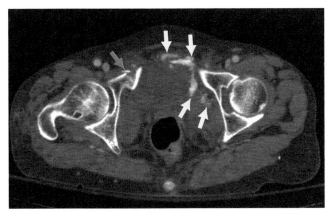

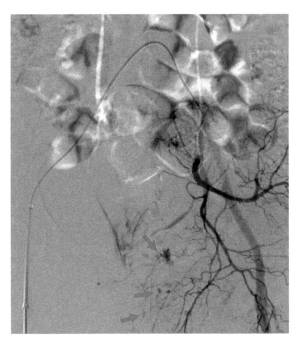

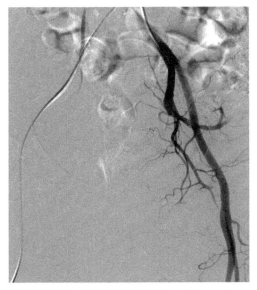

Figure S31-1 Axial contrast-enhanced CT image demonstrating region of active extravasation near the left superior pubic ramus (yellow arrows). Also noted is a fracture of the right superior pubic ramus (red arrow).

Figure S31-2 Selective DSA of the left internal iliac angiogram revealing multiple foci of active extravasation and pseudoaneurysm formation (arrows).

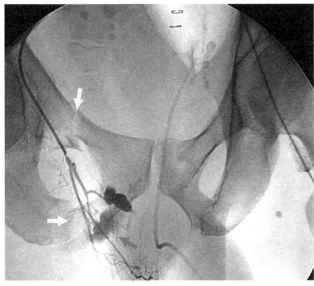

Figure S31-3 Selective DSA of the left internal iliac angiogram status post Gelfoam embolization; the treated arteries demonstrate a pruned appearance.

Figure S31-4 Native image from right internal pudendal artery angiogram in a different patient demonstrating extravasation and pseudoaneurysm formation (red arrows). Superior and inferior pubic ramus fractures are seen (yellow arrows).

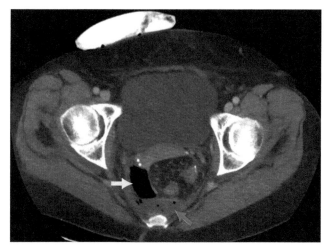

Figure S32-1 Axial contrast-enhanced CT image within the pelvis demonstrates a complex fluid collection (red arrow) with a large amount of gas (yellow arrow) in the pre-sacral region.

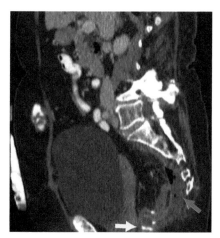

Figure S32-2 Sagittal reformatted image of the same exam as Figure S32-1 which re-illustrates the complex fluid collection (red arrow). Suture material is noted in the rectal region from recent low anterior resection (yellow arrow).

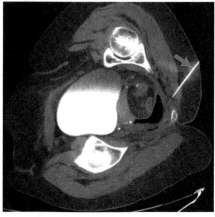

Figure S32-3 Representative image demonstrating CT-guided puncture of the pre-sacral fluid collection with an 18-gauge needle (arrow).

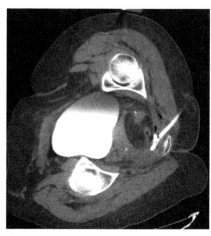

Figure S32-4 Representative image from the same procedure as in Figure S32-3, demonstrating placement of a 14-French pigtail drain.

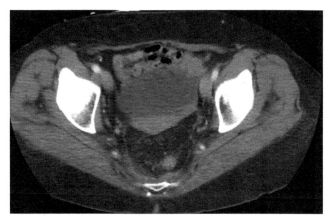

Figure S32-5 Axial contrast enhanced CT image performed 2 weeks after drain placement showing resolution of the pre-sacral fluid collection.

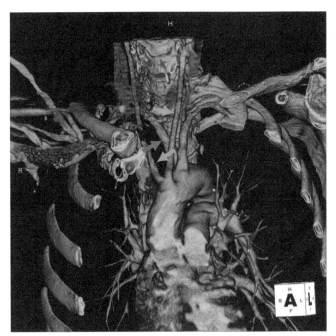

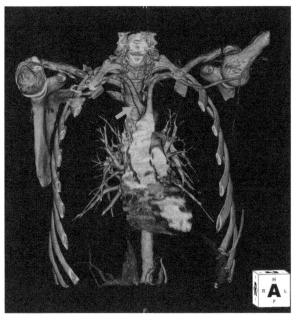

Figure S33-1 CTA volumetric MPR demonstrates an aberrant right subclavian artery (red arrow), which is the last branch of the aortic arch arising just distal to the origin of the left subclavian artery. The bilateral common carotid arteries originate from the aortic arch and share a common origin (green arrows). *Courtesy of Dr. Klaus D. Hagspiel.*

Figure S33-2 CTA volumetric multiplanar reconstruction (MPR) demonstrates an aberrant origin of the right subclavian artery (arrow). The carotid artery origins were excluded from the imaging by postprocessing to highlight the finding. *Courtesy of Dr. Klaus D. Hagspiel.*

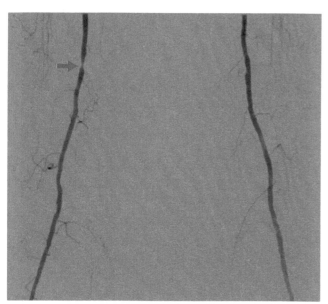

Figure S34-1 DSA image of the left and right lower extremities demonstrates a focal, moderate-to-severe concentric stenosis of the proximal right superficial femoral artery (red arrow). Left SFA with no flow-limiting stenosis seen.

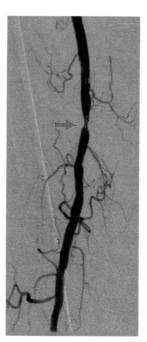

Figure S34-2 DSA image of the proximal right superficial femoral artery again demonstrates moderate-to-severe focal short-segment stenosis. A guidewire has been passed across the stenosis (arrow).

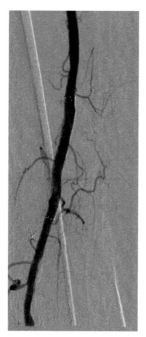

Figure S34-3 DSA image with significantly improved luminal size and flow after stent placement. Iatrogenic dissection (not imaged) was noted following angioplasty; therefore the stent was placed.

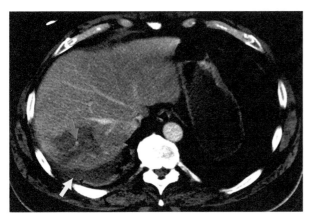

Figure S35-1 Axial image from CTA (delayed phase) showing a region of hypodensity in hepatic segment 7 consistent with contusion/laceration. There is a focus of hyperdensity in the center representing pseudoaneurysm (red arrow). There is a small amount of perihepatic fluid consistent with hemorrhage (yellow arrow).

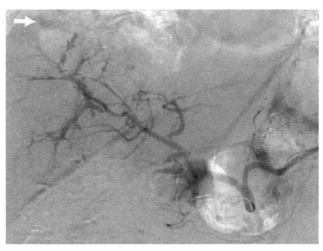

Figure S35-2 Celiac angiogram in the same patient demonstrating two areas of abnormality within hepatic segment 7. More centrally, there is a pseudoaneurysm (red arrow). Near the dome, there is a faint area of blush consistent with extravasation (yellow arrow).

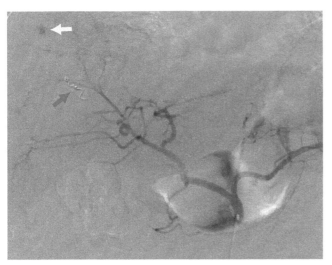

Figure S35-3 Repeat celiac angiogram after coil embolization of branch leading to pseudoaneurysm (red arrow). Again noted is the blush near the dome suggesting continued bleeding (yellow arrow).

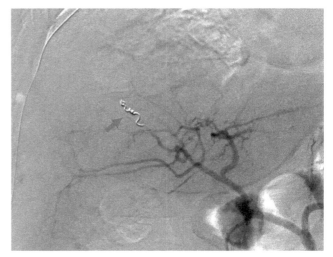

Figure S35-4 Final post-treatment celiac angiogram after coil (arrow) and Gelfoam embolization reveals no evidence of active hemorrhage.

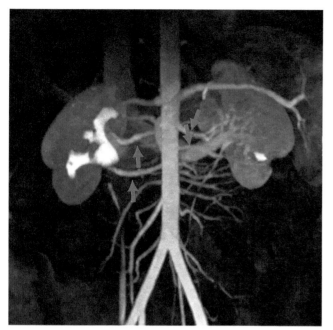

Figure S36-1 Coronal MIP from a T1-weighted post-contrast MRA reveals bilateral duplication of the renal arteries (red arrows). Evaluation is limited due to numerous lumbar artery branches. *Courtesy of Dr. J. Fritz Angle.*

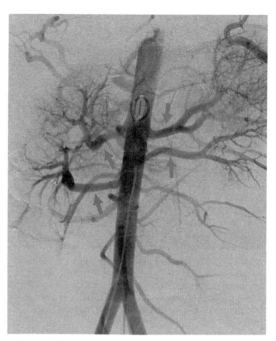

Figure S36-2 DSA image from flush aortogram re-demonstrates the presence of bilateral renal artery duplication (red arrows). *Courtesy of Dr. J. Fritz Angle.*

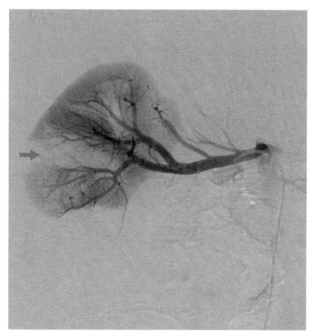

Figure S36-3 DSA image from selective catheterization of the right superior pole renal artery confirms the presence of right renal artery duplication as only the upper portion of the kidney opacifies without evidence of FMD or renal artery stenosis (RAS). Area of apparent hypoperfusion may represent scarring or boundary between arterial territories (red arrow). *Courtesy of Dr. J. Fritz Angle.*

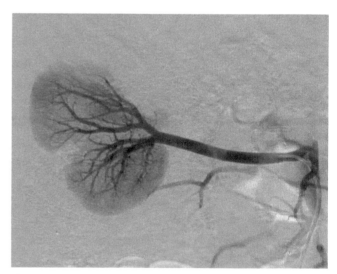

Figure S36-4 Selective catheterization of the right inferior pole renal artery showing perfusion of the lower pole without FMD or RAS. *Courtesy of Dr. J. Fritz Angle.*

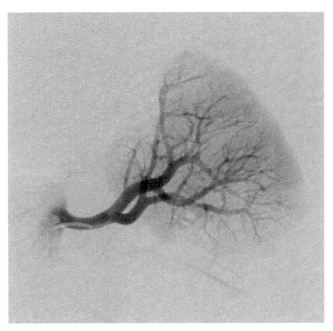

Figure S36-5 Selective catheterization of the left superior pole renal artery showing perfusion of the upper pole without FMD or RAS. *Courtesy of Dr. J. Fritz Angle.*

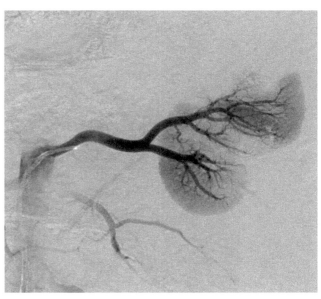

Figure S36-6 Selective catheterization of the left inferior pole renal artery showing perfusion of the lower pole without FMD or RAS. *Courtesy of Dr. J. Fritz Angle.*

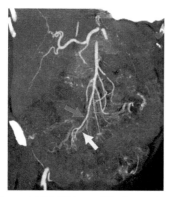

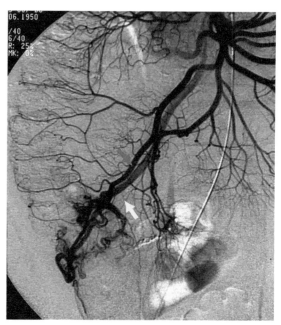

Figure S37-1 Coronal 3D MIP from CTA demonstrates the SMA (red arrow) and tangle of vessels in the RLQ with early draining vein (yellow arrow).

Figure S37-2 Selective digital subtraction angiogram of the SMA (red arrow) demonstrates the typical tangle of vessels with early draining vein (yellow arrow). No contrast extravasation was noted in the adjacent bowel. *Courtesy of Dr. Thomas Vesely.*

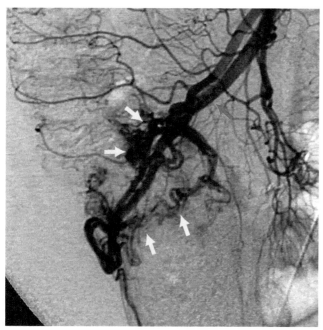

Figure S37-3 Magnified delayed phase image from the same patient as in Figure S37-2 redemonstrates the tangle of vessels (yellow arrows) and draining veins (red arrow). *Courtesy of Dr. Thomas Vesely.*

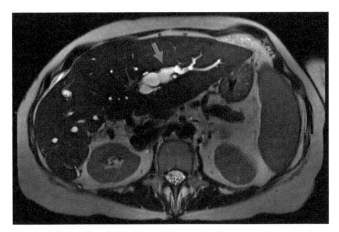

Figure S38-1 T2-weighted axial MR image demonstrating grossly dilated left-sided biliary ducts (arrow). *Courtesy of Dr. J. Fritz Angle.*

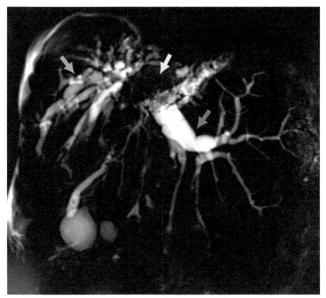

Figure S38-2 Coronal magnetic resonance cholangiopancreatography (MRCP) image illustrating grossly dilated left (red arrow) and right (blue arrow) biliary ducts. Also noted is a signal void suggesting large central obstructing mass (yellow arrow). *Courtesy of Dr. J. Fritz Angle.*

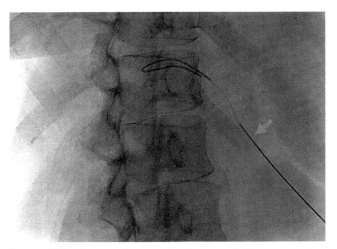

Figure S38-3 Fluoroscopic image showing a needle (arrow) accessing a peripheral left hepatic duct and passage of a wire. *Courtesy of Dr. J. Fritz Angle.*

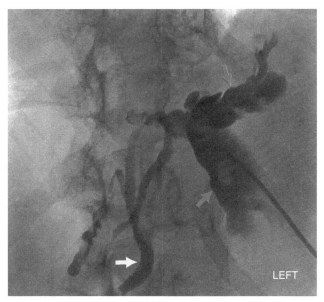

Figure S38-4 Initial cholangiogram demonstrating markedly dilated left intrahepatic bile ducts (red arrows) with passage of contrast through a non-dilated common bile duct (yellow arrow). *Courtesy of Dr. J. Fritz Angle.*

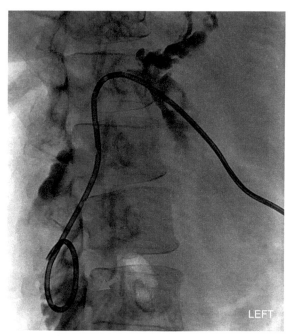

Figure S38-5 Fluoroscopic imaging following placement of an internal-external percutaneous biliary drain. There is contrast identified within the duodenum (arrow). The pigtail has been formed in the duodenum, which facilitates appropriate positioning of the drain. *Courtesy of Dr. J. Fritz Angle.*

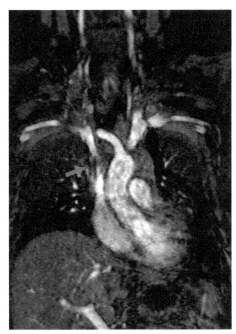

Figure S39-1 Coronal image from MRV demonstrates an area of stenosis at the mid to lower SVC (red arrow). *Courtesy of Dr. David M. Williams.*

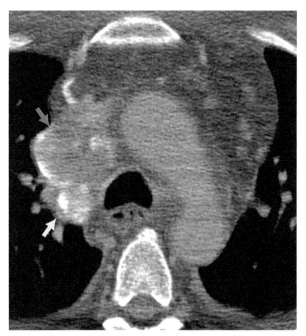

Figure S39-2 Axial contrast-enhanced CT demonstrates a heterogeneous mediastinal mass (red arrow) causing luminal narrowing in the SVC through which contrast still passes (yellow arrow). *Courtesy of Dr. David M. Williams.*

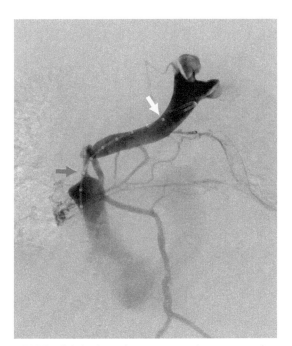

Figure S39-3 Digital subtraction venogram demonstrates short-segment circumferential stenosis of the upper SVC (red arrow). The left innominate vein is patent (yellow arrow). *Courtesy of Dr. David M. Williams.*

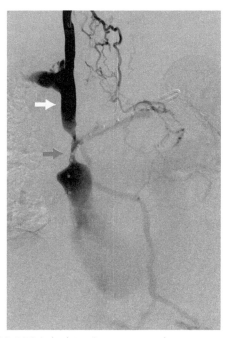

Figure S39-4 Digital subtraction venogram demonstrates short-segment circumferential stenosis of the upper SVC (red arrow). The right innominate vein is patent (yellow arrow). *Courtesy of Dr. David M. Williams.*

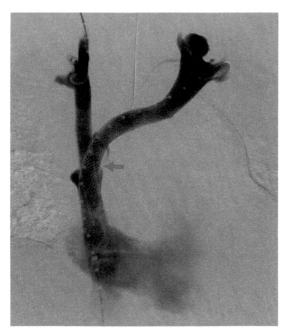

Figure S39-5 Digital subtraction venogram after endovascular placement of two stents, both in the SVC extending out to each innominate vein. No evidence of stenosis in the SVC (red arrow). *Courtesy of Dr. David M. Williams.*

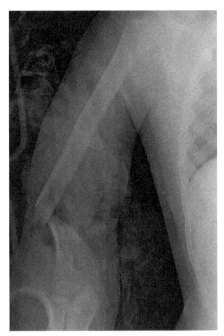

Figure S40-1 AP radiograph of the right humerus demonstrating a comminuted, spiral fracture with apex lateral angulation and mild foreshortening. There is no evidence of other osseous pathology. Presence of soft tissue gas is consistent with an open fracture.

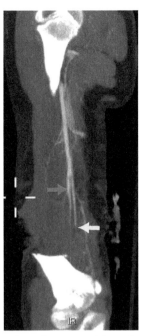

Figure S40-2 Coronal MIP from CTA of the right upper extremity demonstrating an acute occlusion of the brachial artery (red arrow) in the setting of a comminuted spiral fracture of the right humerus. There is an early branching right radial artery (yellow arrow), which is a common anatomic variant, which was also traumatically involved.

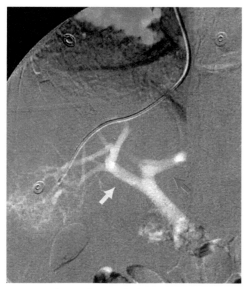

Figure S41-1 DSA image from right hepatic vein-wedged CO_2 venogram revealing the left (red arrow) and right (yellow arrow) portal veins.

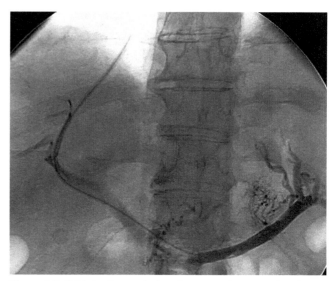

Figure S41-2 Native image during direct portal venography after access obtained from the right hepatic vein.

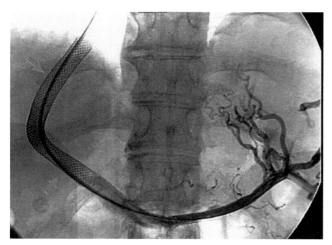

Figure S41-3 Native image from portography after TIPS placed using a Wallstent (red arrows).

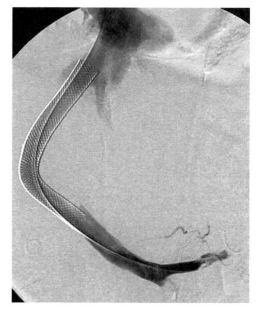

Figure S41-4 DSA image confirming flow through the newly placed TIPS.

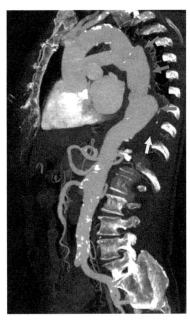

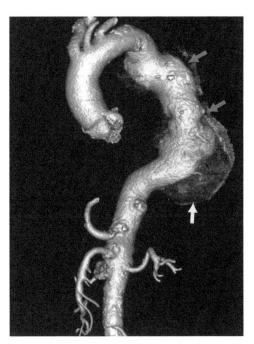

Figure S42-1 Sagittal "candy cane" MIP from a CT angiogram demonstrating an aneurysmal descending thoracic aorta (red arrows). Also denoted is the mural thrombus within the aneurysm (yellow arrow). *Courtesy of Dr. Narasimham L. Dasika.*

Figure S42-2 Volume-rendered image from the same exam as Figure S42-1 with TAA (red arrows) and mural thrombus (yellow arrow). *Courtesy of Dr. Narasimham L. Dasika.*

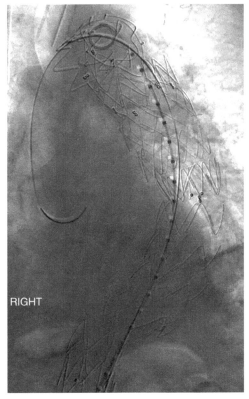

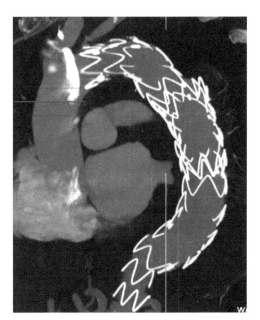

Figure S42-3 Fluoroscopic view in LAO projection demonstrating deployment of the endograft. *Courtesy of Dr. Narasimham L. Dasika.*

Figure S42-4 Sagittal MIP from follow-up CTA in same patient demonstrating endovascular repair of the descending thoracic aorta and decreased overall diameter of the contrast-filled aorta. No evidence of endoleak was seen. *Courtesy of Dr. Narasimham L. Dasika.*

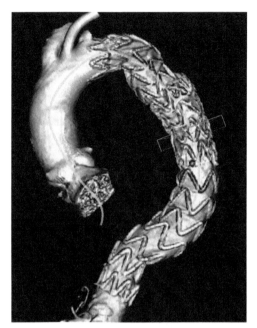

Figure S42-5 Volume-rendered image from the same exam as Figure S42-4. *Courtesy of Dr. Narasimham L. Dasika.*

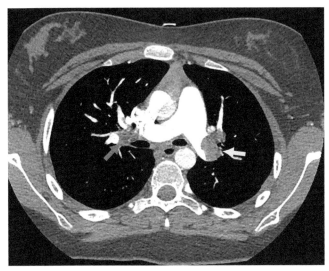

Figure S43-1 Axial image from CT pulmonary angiogram (CTPA) study demonstrates large bilateral central intraluminal filling defects within the right truncus anterior branch of the right pulmonary artery (red arrow) and within the left main pulmonary artery (yellow arrow), consistent with acute pulmonary emboli. *Courtesy of Dr. Wael E. Saad.*

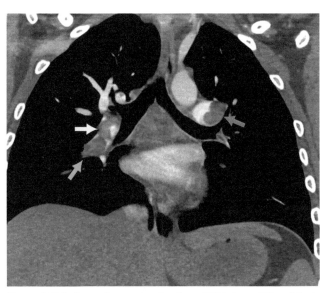

Figure S43-2 Coronal reconstruction from CTPA shows filling defects within the right pulmonary (yellow arrow), right interlobar (blue arrow), and left pulmonary arteries (red arrow). *Courtesy of Dr. Wael E. Saad.*

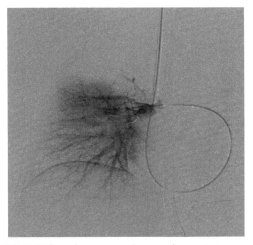

Figure S43-3 Right pulmonary angiogram demonstrates complete absence of perfusion to the superior trunk of the right pulmonary artery (truncus anterior) and its segmental branches, consistent with pulmonary embolism. *Courtesy of Dr. Wael E. Saad.*

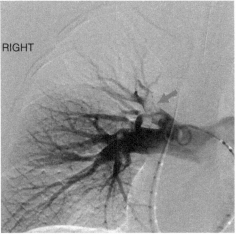

Figure S43-4 Right pulmonary angiogram after catheter-directed thrombolysis demonstrates partial recanalization of the thromboembolic lumen with some perfusion reestablished within the truncus anterior branch. Note, however, the presence of residual filling defects, suggestive of incomplete resolution of embolic foci (arrow). *Courtesy of Dr. Wael E. Saad.*

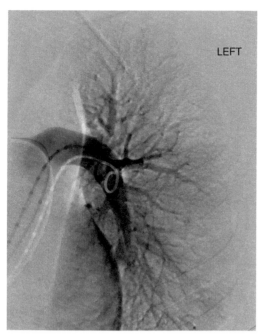

Figure S43-5 Left pulmonary angiogram after catheter-directed thrombolysis demonstrates opacification of the main artery and its segmental branches, with no residual filling defects seen. *Courtesy of Dr. Wael E. Saad.*

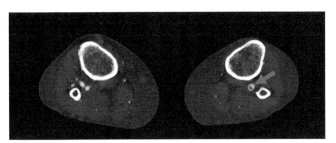

Figure S44-1 Axial image from CTA of the lower extremities demonstrating a filling defect in the distal left popliteal artery (red arrow). The defect is central, hypodense, and nearly occlusive.

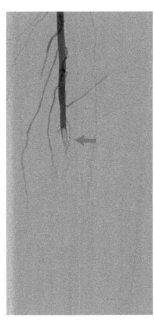

Figure S44-2 Single image from DSA demonstrating occlusion of the distal popliteal artery with a filling defect and abrupt termination of the column of contrast (red arrow). The defect has a meniscus sign, and there is only minimal atherosclerotic disease of the popliteal artery.

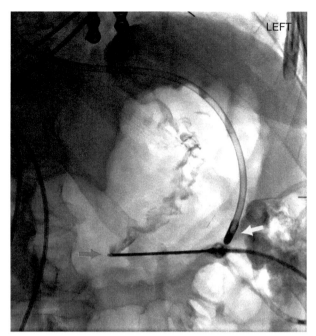

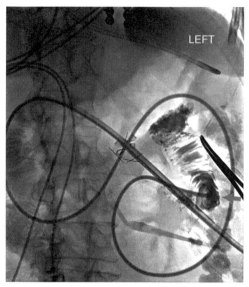

Figure S45-1 Fluoroscopic image taken during percutaneous gastrojejunostomy placement demonstrates a needle within the gastric lumen and injection of contrast, which confirms intragastric placement (red arrow). There is a nasogastric tube with tip in the stomach for the purposes of gastric distention (yellow arrow).

Figure S45-2 Fluoroscopic image taken following percutaneous gastrojejunostomy placement demonstrates contrast injection into the jejunal port, confirming appropriate tube position within the small bowel (arrow).

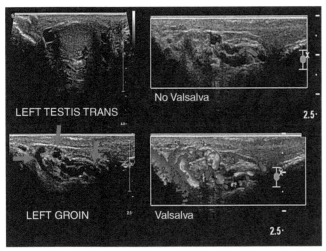

Figure S46-1 Left scrotal ultrasound. **Top left:** Dilated anechoic structures are noted around a grossly normal testicle. **Bottom left:** Better visualization of the dilated pampiniform plexus or varicocele (red arrows). **Top right:** Varicocele without valsalva shows minimal flow on color Doppler. **Bottom right:** Varicocele with valsalva shows increase in color Doppler flow and size. *Courtesy of Dr. C. Matthew Hawkins.*

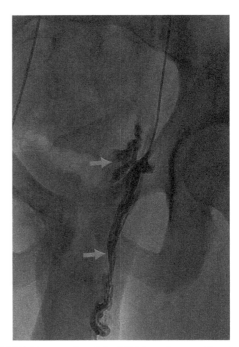

Figure S46-2 Venography of the left internal spermatic vein shows a dilated tangle of vessels in the left scrotum, consistent with varicocele (red arrows). *Courtesy of Dr. C. Matthew Hawkins.*

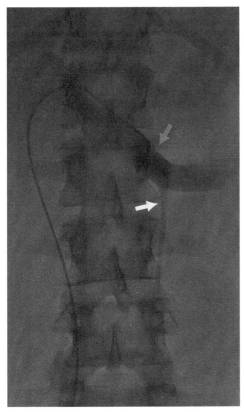

Figure S46-3 Catheter injection of the left renal vein (red arrow) reveals the left gonadal vein (yellow arrow), the access to embolize the varicocele. *Courtesy of Dr. C. Matthew Hawkins.*

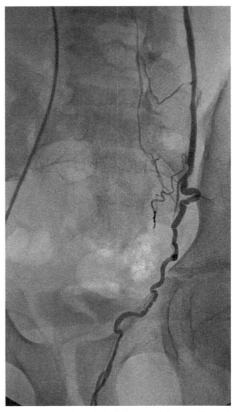

Figure S46-4 Venography of the left gonadal vein shows its dilated and tortuous course, all of which must be treated to prevent varicocele recurrence. *Courtesy of Dr. C. Matthew Hawkins.*

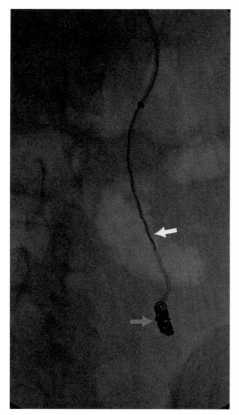

Figure S46-5 Coil embolization of the left gonadal vein after more inferior sclerotherapy (red arrow). An undeployed coil is seen within the catheter (yellow arrow). *Courtesy of Dr. C. Matthew Hawkins.*

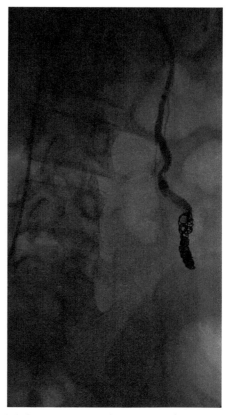

Figure S46-6 Contrast venography after partial embolization and sclerotherapy confirming complete occlusion of the left gonadal vein and no filling of the previously seen varicocele. *Courtesy of Dr. C. Matthew Hawkins.*

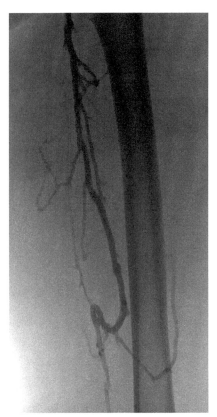

Figure S47-1 Venography of the left femoral vein at the mid-thigh demonstrates contracted vessels, synechiae, and venous collaterals. *Courtesy of Dr. Minhaj S. Khaja.*

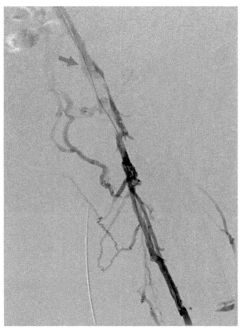

Figure S47-2 DSA image of the left femoral vein near the hip again demonstrates wall adherent thrombus (red arrow), synechiae, and venous collaterals. *Courtesy of Dr. Minhaj S. Khaja.*

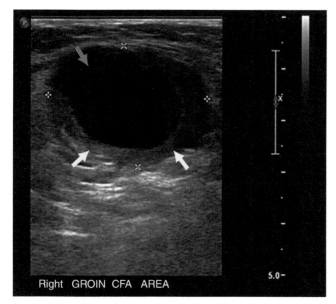

Figure S48-1 Grayscale ultrasound demonstrates an anechoic pseudoaneurysm (red arrow) which measures 3 cm with a hypoechoic rim of thrombus (yellow arrows). *Courtesy of Dr. Minhaj S. Khaja.*

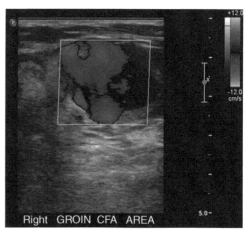

Figure S48-2 Color Doppler ultrasound highlights internal blood flow in the pseudoaneurysm, with early "yin-yang" sign indicating bidirectional flow within the sac. *Courtesy of Dr. Minhaj S. Khaja.*

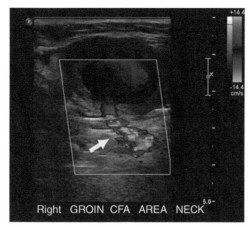

Figure S48-3 Color Doppler ultrasound shows a long, narrow neck of the pseudoaneurysm (arrow). *Courtesy of Dr. Minhaj S. Khaja.*

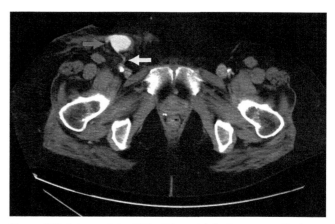

Figure S48-4 Image from CTA of the pelvis in the same patient demonstrates avid contrast filling of the aneurysm sac (red arrow) and neck (yellow arrow). *Courtesy of Dr. Minhaj S. Khaja.*

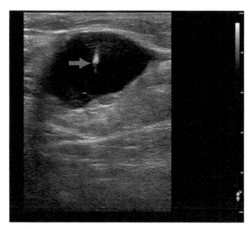

Figure S48-5 Grayscale ultrasound demonstrates insertion of needle (arrow) into aneurysm sac. *Courtesy of Dr. Minhaj S. Khaja.*

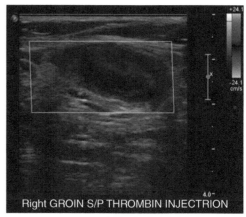

Figure S48-6 Color Doppler ultrasound following thrombin injection demonstrates thrombosis with cessation of flow. *Courtesy of Dr. Minhaj S. Khaja.*

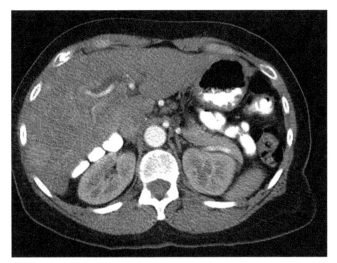

Figure S49-1 Contrast-enhanced axial CT image demonstrating arterially enhancing mass in the right hepatic lobe prior to chemoembolization (red arrow). *Courtesy of Dr. Bill S. Majdalany.*

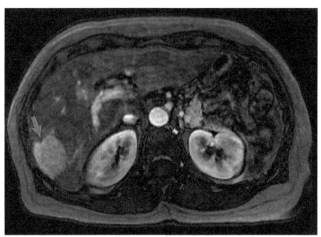

Figure S49-2 Contrast-enhanced axial MR image showing arterially enhancing mass in the right hepatic lobe prior to chemoembolization (red arrow). *Courtesy of Dr. Bill S. Majdalany.*

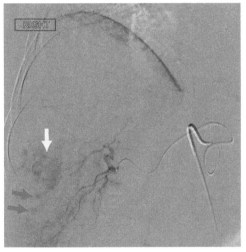

Figure S49-3 DSA image from right hepatic arteriogram confirming arterially enhancing mass in the right hepatic lobe prior (yellow arrow) with adjacent satellite lesions (red arrows). *Courtesy of Dr. Bill S. Majdalany.*

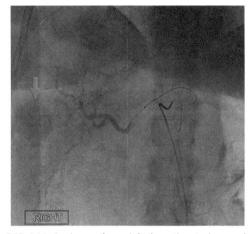

Figure S49-4 Native image from right hepatic arteriogram better illustrating the dominant arterially enhancing mass in the right hepatic lobe (red arrow). *Courtesy of Dr. Bill S. Majdalany.*

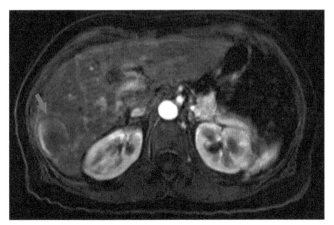

Figure S49-5 Contrast-enhanced axial MR image showing minimal marginal enhancement post embolization (red arrow). *Courtesy of Dr. Bill S. Majdalany.*

CASE 50

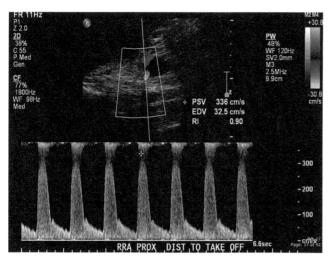

Figure S50-1 Color and spectral Doppler sonographic image obtained at the proximal right renal artery demonstrates an elevated peak systolic velocity of 336 cm/sec with aliasing of the waveform, concerning proximal right renal artery stenosis.

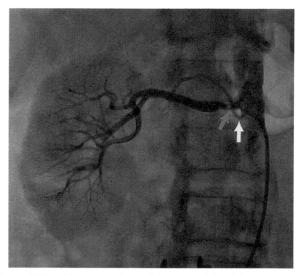

Figure S50-2 Selective angiographic image of the right renal artery showing a high-grade stenosis of the right renal artery (red arrow). An accessory right renal artery supplying the superior pole is also noted (yellow arrow).

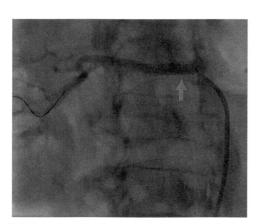

Figure S50-3 Angiographic image in the same patient obtained after balloon angioplasty and stent placement demonstrates restoration of flow with minimal residual stenosis (arrow).

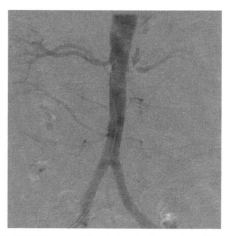

Figure S50-4 DSA image of the abdominal aorta in a different patient shows severe stenosis of the proximal left renal artery (arrow).

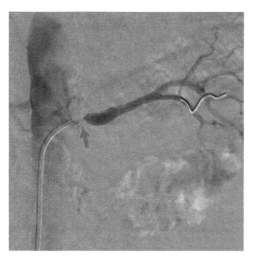

Figure S50-5 Selective left renal artery DSA image again illustrating high-grade stenosis of the proximal left renal artery (arrow) in the same patient as in Figure S50-4.

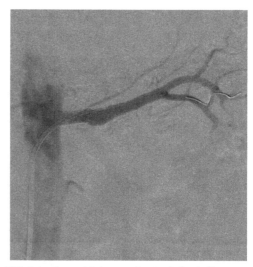

Figure S50-6 Angiographic image obtained after balloon angioplasty and stent placement demonstrates restoration of flow without residual stenosis.

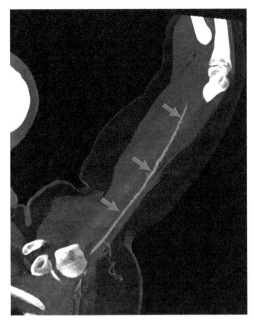

Figure S51-1 Coronal reconstruction from CT angiogram of the left upper extremity showing areas of beaded brachial artery (red arrows). *Courtesy of Dr. Alan H. Matsumoto.*

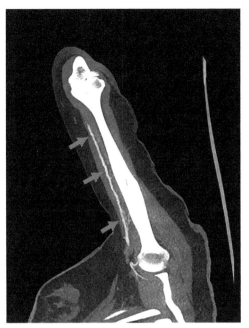

Figure S51-2 Sagittal reconstruction from CT angiogram of the left upper extremity re-demonstrating areas of beaded brachial artery (red arrows). *Courtesy of Dr. Alan H. Matsumoto.*

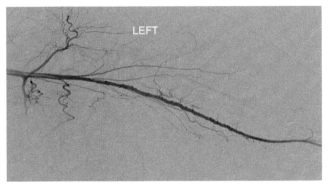

Figure S51-3 DSA image of left upper extremity angiogram in the same patient as Figure S51-1 and S51-2 demonstrating the classic "string of beads" appearance associated with fibromuscular dysplasia. *Courtesy of Dr. Alan H. Matsumoto.*

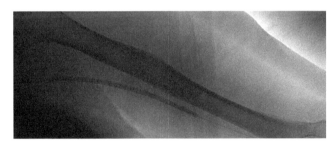

Figure S51-4 Single-shot image of balloon angioplasty of the left brachial artery. *Courtesy of Dr. Alan H. Matsumoto.*

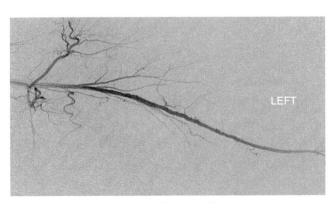

Figure S51-5 Post-angioplasty DSA image illustrating persistent, but improved luminal irregularity. *Courtesy of Dr. Alan H. Matsumoto.*

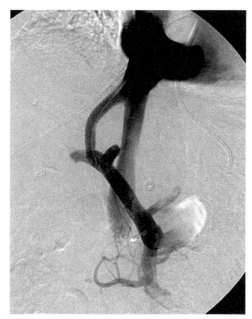

Figure S52-1 DSA image from completion portogram demonstrating patency of TIPS with a Viatorr Endoprosthesis. *Courtesy of Dr. Wael E. Saad.*

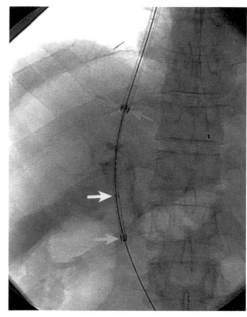

Figure S52-2 Fluoroscopic image during a TIPS procedure where a coaxial system has been advanced to the portal system. The outer sheath in the right hepatic vein is demarcated by red arrows. The yellow arrow signifying the beginning of the covered portion of the stent is noted by an open white arrow. The blue arrow demarcates the distal end of the inner sheath. *Courtesy of Dr. Wael E. Saad.*

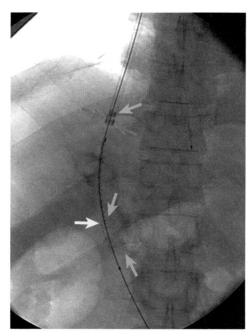

Figure S52-3 Fluoroscopic image during a TIPS procedure. The outer sheath in the right hepatic vein is demarcated by red arrows. The blue arrow demarcates the distal end of the inner sheath, which has been retracted. The radiopaque marker signifying the beginning of the covered portion of the stent is noted by a yellow arrow. The green arrows outline the uncovered, bare metal portion of the stent. *Courtesy of Dr. Wael E. Saad.*

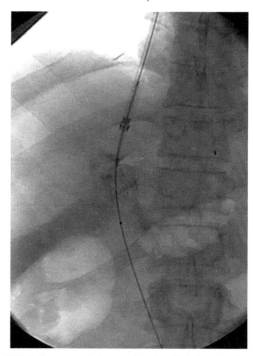

Figure S52-4 Fluoroscopic image showing that the stent has been retracted to the portal vein entry site. The red arrow confirms a waist at this site. *Courtesy of Dr. Wael E. Saad.*

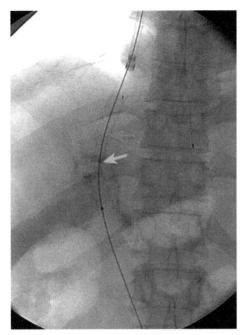

Figure S52-5 Fluoroscopic image after deployment of TIPS stent showing waists at the portal venous entry (blue arrow) and hepatic venous exit (red arrow) sites. *Courtesy of Dr. Wael E. Saad.*

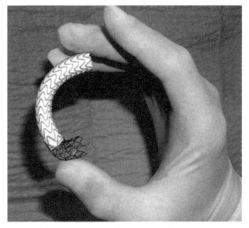

Figure S52-6 Photograph showing the flexibility of the Viatorr Endoprosthesis. The PTFE portion is noted in white and is to be deployed within the newly created intraparenchymal tract while the bare metal portion remains in the portal vein. *Courtesy of Dr. Wael E. Saad.*

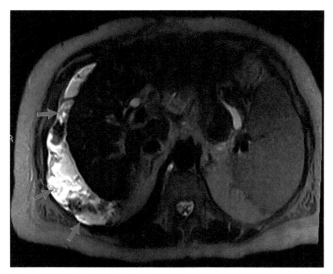

Figure S53-1 Axial T2-weighted MRI image demonstrates a shrunken liver with a nodular contour and ascites (arrows).

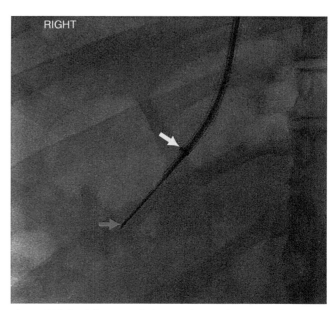

Figure S53-2 AP fluoroscopic image of a core biopsy needle (red arrow) obtaining a sample via right hepatic vein sheath (yellow arrow). Right hepatic venogram is shown in Figure S53-3.

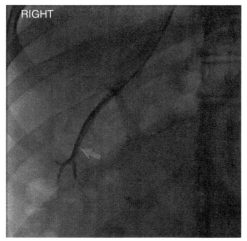

Figure S53-3 AP fluoroscopic image from right hepatic venogram, which is performed prior to obtaining core biopsy to confirm presence within a patent right hepatic vein (arrow).

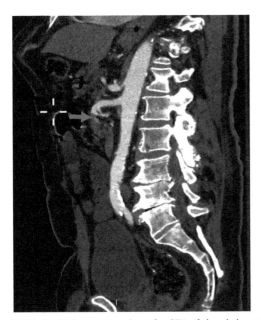

Figure S54-1 Sagittal reconstruction of a CTA of the abdomen demonstrating an occlusive filling defect in the proximal superior mesenteric artery with a meniscus (red arrow). There is no distal perfusion within the superior mesenteric artery. Absence of severe atherosclerotic disease and the thrombus morphology strongly favor a thromboembolic source.

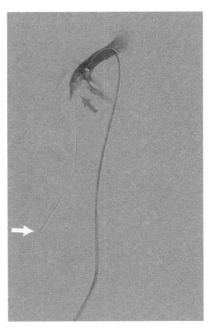

Figure S54-2 Lateral DSA image confirming an occlusive thrombus in the proximal superior mesenteric artery (red arrow). Note the meniscus sign and absent atherosclerotic disease in the proximal artery, which is consistent with thromboembolic disease. A 0.035″ wire has been advanced through the soft thrombus into the distal superior mesenteric artery in an attempt to access the vessel for thrombolysis (yellow arrow).

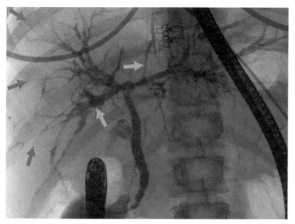

Figure S55-1 Image from ERCP demonstrates the characteristic "beading" appearance of both the intra- and extrahepatic biliary tree resulting in multifocal strictures and dilatation (blue arrows). Also present on this image is the "pruned-tree" appearance with more prominent opacification of the central ducts and smaller diminutive ducts in the periphery (red arrows).

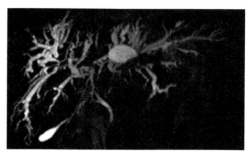

Figure S55-2 Single composed MRCP image in the same patient as in Figure S55-1 also shows diffuse segmental stricturing and irregular dilation affecting the entire biliary tree.

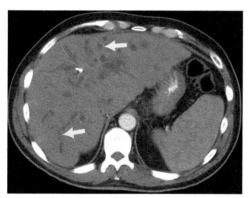

Figure S55-3 Contrast-enhanced CT in a different patient reveals, diffuse irregular intrahepatic biliary dilation and narrowing (yellow arrows). A portion of an internal biliary stent is seen in the right hepatic lobe (red arrow). The liver demonstrates cirrhotic features with caudate lobe hypertrophy and a right posterior notch sign.

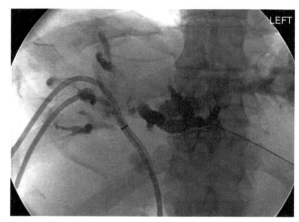

Figure S55-4 Left-sided percutaneous transhepatic cholangiogram was performed in the patient from Figure S55-3. Contrast injection demonstrates predominant dilation and stricture of the left biliary tree with "pruning" of the small peripheral ductal branches. Right-sided drainage catheters noted.

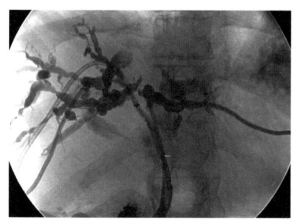

Figure S55-5 Image from cholangiography after placement of biliary drainage catheter demonstrating decompression of the left biliary system. Redemonstration of right-sided biliary strictures and dilatation.

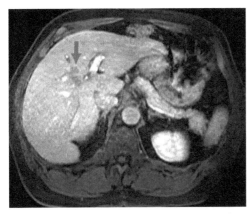

Figure S56-1 Axial image from contrast-enhanced MRI during portal venous phase shows washout of mass in right hepatic lobe (red arrow).

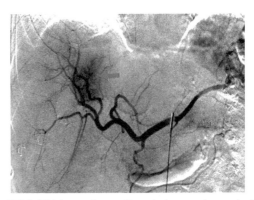

Figure S56-2 DSA image from celiac arteriogram demonstrating contrast-blush in the right hepatic lobe (red arrow).

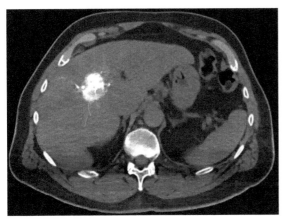

Figure S56-3 Axial image from intraprocedural CT shows complete tumor enhancement from microcatheter position prior to TACE (red arrow).

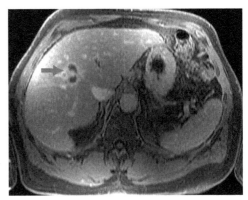

Figure S56-4 Axial image from contrast-enhanced MRI 1 month following TACE demonstrates greater than 90% tumor necrosis (red arrow) following TACE.

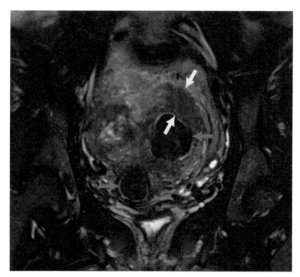

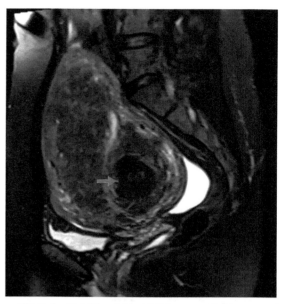

Figure S57-1 Coronal T2-weighted MR image with fat-suppression demonstrating well circumscribed, T2 hypointense fibroids within the uterus (red arrows). Also noted is thickening of the junctional zone with a heterogeneous appearance, consistent with adenomyosis (between the yellow arrows). *Courtesy of Dr. Alan H. Matsumoto.*

Figure S57-2 Sagittal T2-weighted MR image with fat-suppression demonstrating well circumscribed, T2 hypointense fibroid within the uterus (red arrow). *Courtesy of Dr. Alan H. Matsumoto.*

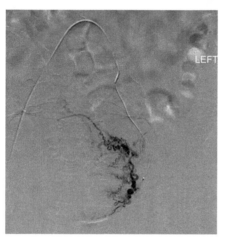

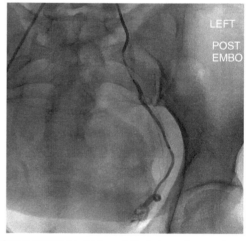

Figure S57-3 DSA image from left uterine artery angiogram demonstrating hypervascularity and early parenchymal blush prior to embolization. *Courtesy of Dr. Alan H. Matsumoto.*

Figure S57-4 Native image from left uterine artery angiogram postembolization confirming pruning of the left uterine artery. *Courtesy of Dr. Alan H. Matsumoto.*

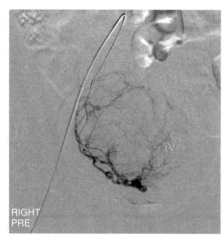

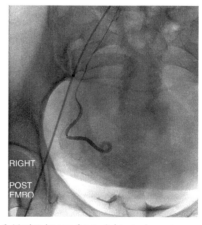

Figure S57-5 DSA image from right uterine artery angiogram demonstrating hypervascularity and early parenchymal blush prior to embolization. *Courtesy of Dr. Alan H. Matsumoto.*

Figure S57-6 Native image from right uterine artery angiogram postembolization confirming pruning of the left uterine artery. *Courtesy of Dr. Alan H. Matsumoto.*

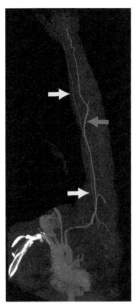

Figure S58-1 MIP image from CTA of the left upper extremity demonstrates an extremely high origin of the radial artery (yellow arrows), which travels alongside the brachial artery (red arrow). *Courtesy of Dr. Narasimham L. Dasika.*

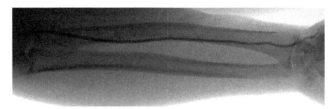

Figure S58-2 Native image from left upper extremity angiogram following selection of the radial artery, confirming a patent radial artery. *Courtesy of Dr. Narasimham L. Dasika.*

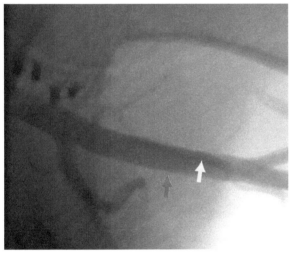

Figure S58-3 Magnified native image of the axillary artery with catheter positioned in the proximal axillary artery demonstrates a subtle finding of a vessel originating from (yellow arrow) and projecting directly over the axillary artery (red arrow). Upon further inspection, this was confirmed to be the radial artery. *Courtesy of Dr. Narasimham L. Dasika.*

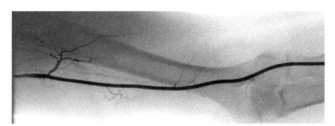

Figure S58-4 Native image from left upper extremity angiogram centered at the elbow following selection of the radial artery demonstrates a patent radial artery. *Courtesy of Dr. Narasimham L. Dasika.*

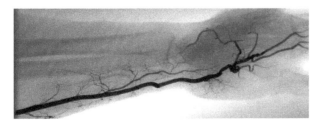

Figure S58-5 Native image from left upper extremity angiogram with catheter positioned in the midbrachial artery revealing a patent ulnar artery; however, the radial artery is not seen. *Courtesy of Dr. Narasimham L. Dasika.*

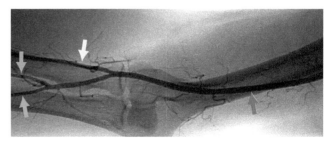

Figure S58-6 Native image from right upper extremity angiogram in a different patient demonstrating the conventional branching pattern of the brachial artery (red arrow) into the radial (yellow arrow), ulnar (blue arrow), and interosseus (green arrow) arteries. *Courtesy of Dr. Narasimham L. Dasika.*

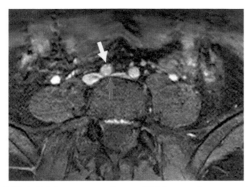

Figure S59-1 Axial contrast-enhanced T1 image demonstrating significant narrowing of the left common iliac vein (red arrow) as it courses deep to the right common iliac artery (yellow arrow). *Courtesy of Dr. David M. Williams.*

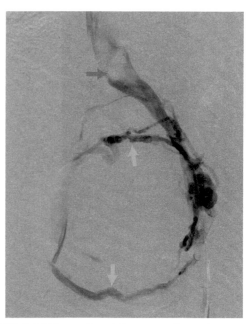

Figure S59-2 DSA image from left common femoral venogram confirming left common iliac compression (red arrow) with cross-pelvic collaterals (blue arrows). *Courtesy of Dr. David M. Williams.*

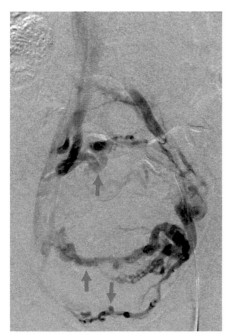

Figure S59-3 Late-phase DSA image from left common femoral venogram showing more cross-pelvic collateralization (red arrows) and flow in the right common iliac vein (blue arrow). *Courtesy of Dr. David M. Williams.*

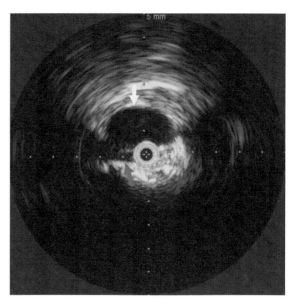

Figure S59-4 Intravascular ultrasound image redemonstrating compression of the left common iliac vein (red arrow) by the right common iliac artery (yellow arrow). Subsequent images demonstrated complete occlusion (not shown). *Courtesy of Dr. David M. Williams.*

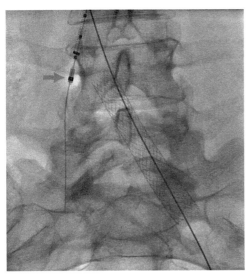

Figure S59-5 Native image after stent placement with IVUS confirming position (red arrow). *Courtesy of Dr. David M. Williams.*

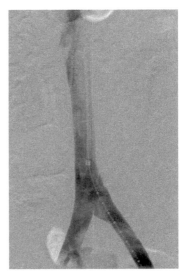

Figure S59-6 DSA image from completion venogram demonstrating patency of the stent and IVC. *Courtesy of Dr. David M. Williams.*

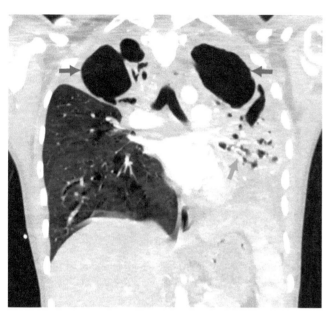

Figure S60-1 Coronal reconstruction from CTA of the chest in lung windows illustrating bilateral apical cavitation (red arrows) and left sided bronchiectasis (blue arrow). *Courtesy of Dr. Luke R. Wilkins.*

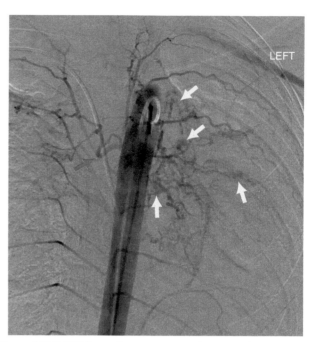

Figure S60-2 DSA image from aortogram demonstrating tortuous and hypertrophied right bronchial artery (red arrow) with abnormal left-sided hypervarscularity and parenchymal blush (yellow arrows). *Courtesy of Dr. Luke R. Wilkins.*

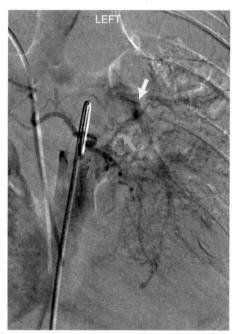

Figure S60-3 DSA image from bronchial artery trunk selection demonstrating hypertrophied bilateral bronchial arteries (red arrows) with early opacification of the left pulmonary artery (yellow arrow) and fistulous connection (blue arrow). *Courtesy of Dr. Luke R. Wilkins.*

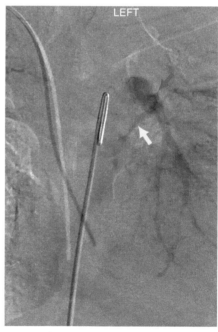

Figure S60-4 Late phase DSA image from bronchial artery trunk redemonstrating left pulmonary artery opacific (red arrow) and fistulous connection (yellow arrow). *Courtesy of Dr. Luke R. Wilkins.*

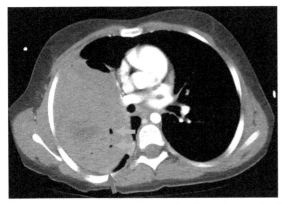

Figure S61-1 Axial image from CECT of the thorax in a pediatric patient reveals a large right-sided fluid collection with locules of gas (blue arrows). There is also enhancement of the pleura (red arrow).

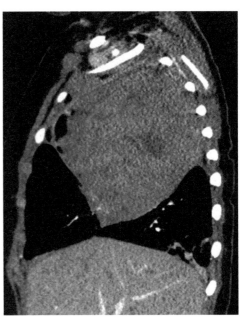

Figure S61-2 Sagittal reformat from the same CT redemonstrates a right-sided empyema, which has locules of gas within it.

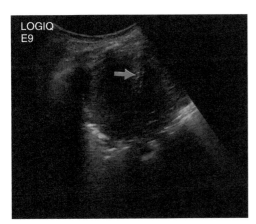

Figure S61-3 Intraprocedural ultrasound image in the same patient shows a complex fluid collection with hypoechoic and isoechoic areas within it, corresponding to the empyema seen on comparison CT. There is a catheter coursing through the midportion of this collection (red arrow).

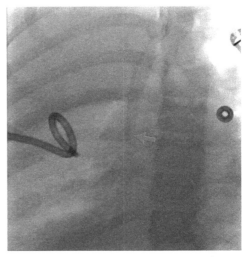

Figure S61-4 Postprocedure fluoroscopic image confirms successful placement of a pigtail drainage catheter in the right midthorax. A left-sided PICC line is also noted (red arrow).

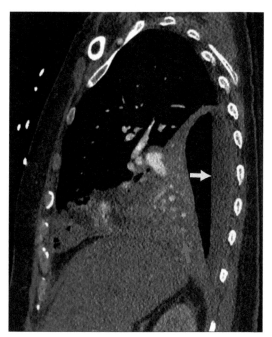

Figure S61-5 Sagittal reformat from a contrast-enhanced CT of the thorax in a different patient reveals a large dependent air/fluid level (yellow arrow) with enhancing pleura, representing the "split pleura" sign and suggestive of empyema. There is adjacent atelectasis, which enhances and has vessels coursing though it (red arrow)—this further supports the diagnosis of empyema.

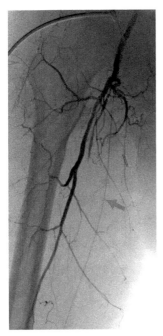

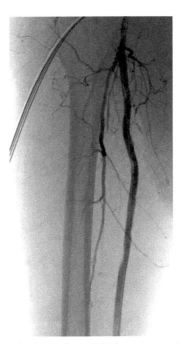

Figure S62-1 Native image from right lower extremity angiogram demonstrating the stump of an occluded right femoropopliteal artery bypass graft with a wire traversing the bypass (red arrow). *Courtesy of Dr. Minhaj S. Khaja.*

Figure S62-2 Native image from right lower extremity angiogram after three day thrombolysis demonstrating reestablishment of flow through the bypass graft. *Courtesy of Dr. Minhaj S. Khaja.*

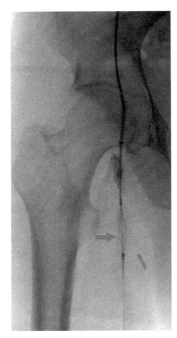

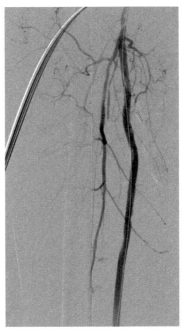

Figure S62-3 Fluoroscopic image showing percutaneous thrombolysis device within the graft (red arrow). *Courtesy of Dr. Minhaj S. Khaja.*

Figure S62-4 DSA image postthrombolysis demonstrating patency of the proximal bypass graft. *Courtesy of Dr. Minhaj S. Khaja.*

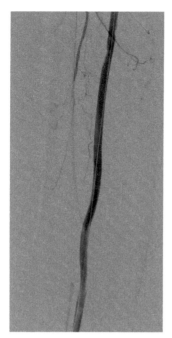

Figure S62-5 DSA image postthrombolysis demonstrating patency of the midbypass graft. *Courtesy of Dr. Minhaj S. Khaja.*

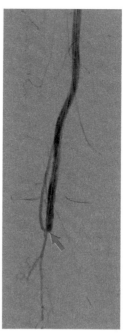

Figure S62-6 DSA image postthrombolysis demonstrating patency of the distal bypass graft and anastomosis (red arrow). *Courtesy of Dr. Minhaj S. Khaja.*

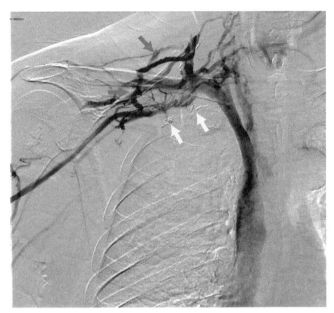

Figure S63-1 Still image from right upper extremity venogram demonstrating chronic occlusion of the right axillary and subclavian veins (blue arrow) in a patient with thoracic outlet syndrome. There are multiple collaterals (red arrows) and no true filling defect in the occluded segments. The surgical clips (yellow arrows) and absent first rib indicate a prior thoracic outlet release, with persistent obstruction.

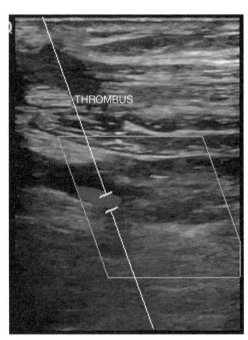

Figure S63-2 Color Doppler still image from a right upper extremity ultrasound evaluation in the same patient demonstrating an occlusive, chronic thrombus in the right axillary vein.

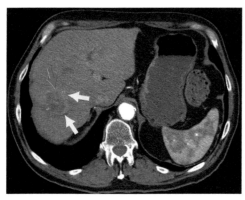

Figure S64-1 Arterial phase axial CT image demonstrates a hypoattenuating mass within the right hepatic lobe (red arrow) with heterogeneous contrast enhancement (yellow arrows). Subsequent biopsy confirmed metastatic colonic adenocarcinoma.

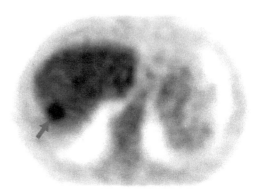

Figure S64-2 Axial image from a PET scan demonstrates a hypermetabolic lesion with the right hepatic lobe (red arrow).

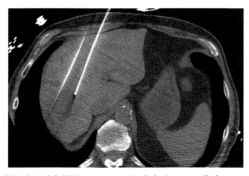

Figure S64-3 Axial CT image acquired during a radiofrequency ablation of the mass identified on PET. Two RF electrodes were placed at the superior portion of the mass and a single ablation needle was placed at the inferior portion of the lesion.

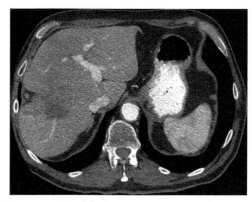

Figure S64-4 Arterial axial phase CT image 2 months postablation with hypoattenuation of ablation zone (red arrowhead) without enhancing rim or focal lesion.

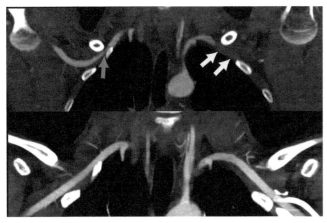

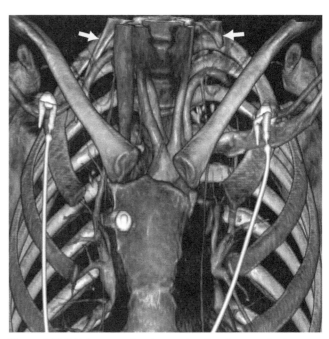

Figure S65-1 Contrast-enhanced CTA maximal intensity projection, performed with the arms abducted over the head (top) reveals high-grade stenosis in the proximal right subclavian artery (red arrow) and complete occlusion of the left subclavian artery (yellow arrows) at the thoracic inlet. These findings regress with the arms in neutral position (bottom) showing wide patency of the bilateral subclavian arteries. *Courtesy of Dr. Lucia Flors Blasco.*

Figure S65-2 Volume-rendered reconstruction from contrast-enhanced CTA in the same patient above shows the presence of bilateral cervical ribs (arrows). *Courtesy of Dr. Lucia Flors Blasco.*

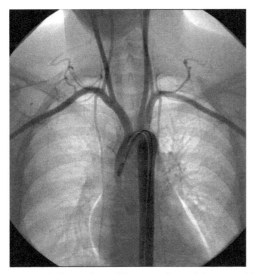

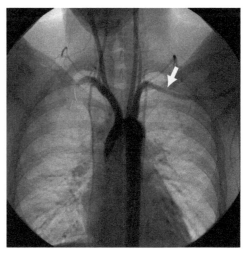

Figure S65-3 DSA image in a different patient with arms adducted demonstrating patency of the subclavian arteries bilaterally. *Courtesy of Dr. J. Fritz Angle.*

Figure S65-4 DSA image with arms abducted (same patient as in Figure S65-3) demonstrating occlusion of the right subclavian artery (red arrow) and mild compression of the left subclavian artery (yellow arrow). *Courtesy of Dr. J. Fritz Angle.*

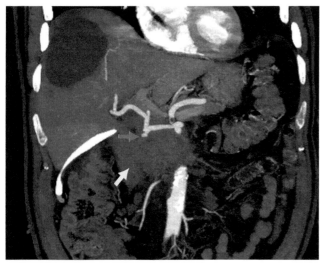

Figure S66-1 Coronal MIP image from CTA demonstrating a focal pseudoaneurysm (red arrow) from a GDA stump. Also noted is a large heterogeneous hematoma surrounding the pseudoaneurysm (yellow arrow). *Courtesy of Dr. Bill S. Majdalany.*

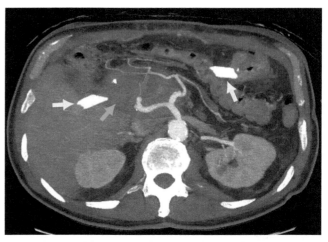

Figure S66-2 Axial MIP image from CTA showing the pseudoaneurysm (red arrow), hematoma (blue arrow), and surgical drains (yellow arrows). *Courtesy of Dr. Bill S. Majdalany.*

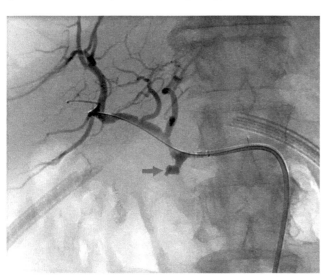

Figure S66-3 Native image from angiogram confirming GDA stump pseudoaneurysm (red arrow). *Courtesy of Dr. Bill S. Majdalany.*

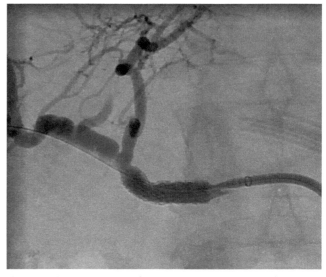

Figure S66-4 Native image from angiogram after covered stent placement excluding the pseudoaneurysm. *Courtesy of Dr. Bill S. Majdalany.*

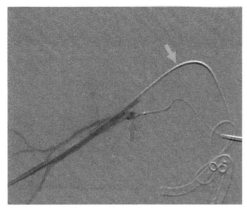

Figure S66-5 Superselective microcatheter DSA of an injured right hepatic arterial branch in a different patient demonstrating a pseudoaneurysm (red arrow). The biliary drain was removed over a wire (blue arrow) in order to visualize the pseudoaneurysm. *Courtesy of Dr. Bill S. Majdalany.*

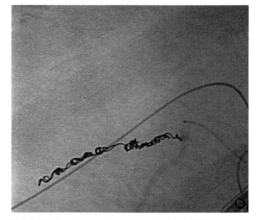

Figure S66-6 Native image of a superselective RHA branch arteriogram, in the same patient as in Figure S66-5, after coil embolization demonstrating occlusion of the involved vessel with coils deployed both distal and proximal to the injury. *Courtesy of Dr. Bill S. Majdalany.*

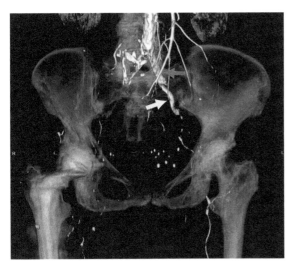

Figure S67-1 VR image from CTA demonstrating occlusion of the right common, external, and internal iliac arteries. The left common (red arrow) and internal iliac (yellow arrow) arteries are patent. The left external iliac artery is occluded as well. *Courtesy of Dr. Minhaj S. Khaja.*

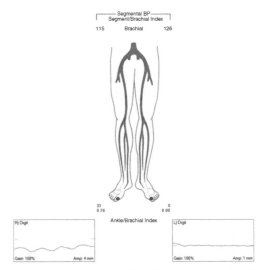

Figure S67-2 Lower extremity ABI with no flow in the left lower extremity and critical limb ischemia of the right lower extremity prior to intervention. *Courtesy of Dr. Minhaj S. Khaja.*

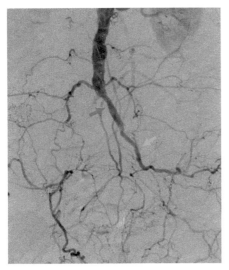

Figure S67-3 Oblique DSA image from aortogram confirming occlusion of the same vessels as seen in Figure S67-1. The left common (red arrow) and internal iliac (blue arrow) arteries are patent. Numerous collateral vessels are seen. *Courtesy of Dr. Minhaj S. Khaja.*

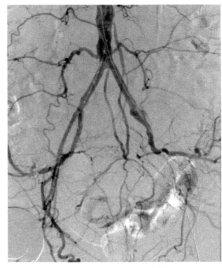

Figure S67-4 DSA image from aortogram following revascularization with angioplasty and thrombolysis revealing reestablishment of flow within the right common, external, and internal iliac arteries. *Courtesy of Dr. Minhaj S. Khaja.*

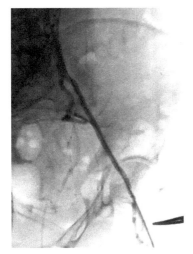

Figure S67-5 Native image from aortogram following revascularization with angioplasty and thrombolysis revealing reestablishment of flow within the left external iliac artery. *Courtesy of Dr. Minhaj S. Khaja.*

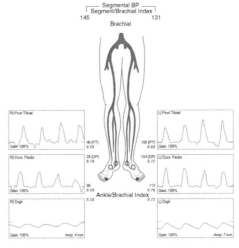

Figure S67-6 Lower extremity ABI 1 day postintervention with significant improvement in left lower extremity ABI from 0 to 0.72. *Courtesy of Dr. Minhaj S. Khaja.*

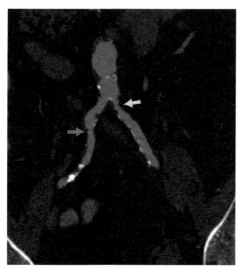

Figure S68-1 Coronal reconstruction from CTA demonstrates bilateral common iliac artery stenosis, left (yellow arrow) greater than right (red arrow). *Courtesy of Dr. Saher S. Sabri.*

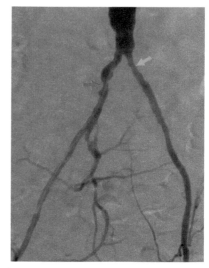

Figure S68-2 DSA image from pelvic aortogram confirms bilateral common iliac artery stenosis, left (blue arrow) greater than right (red arrow). *Courtesy of Dr. Saher S. Sabri.*

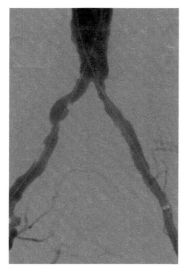

Figure S68-3 DSA image from pelvic angiogram through bilateral femoral arterial sheaths shows crossing wires in place prior to stent advancement. *Courtesy of Dr. Saher S. Sabri.*

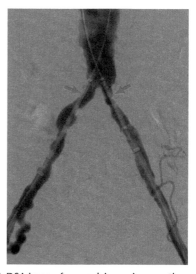

Figure S68-4 DSA image from pelvic angiogram through bilateral femoral arterial sheaths confirms stent placement (red arrows) prior to deployment. *Courtesy of Dr. Saher S. Sabri.*

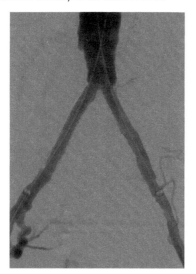

Figure S68-5 DSA image from pelvic angiogram through bilateral femoral arterial sheaths reveals improved flow through the common iliac arteries after kissing stent deployment. *Courtesy of Dr. Saher S. Sabri.*

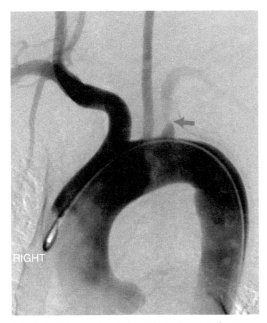

Figure S69-1 DSA image from thoracic aortogram demonstrating a focal, high-grade stenosis of the proximal left subclavian artery (red arrow) with poor opacification distally. *Courtesy of Dr. Wael E. Saad.*

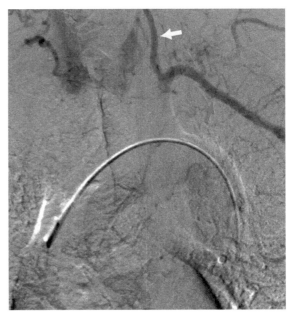

Figure S69-2 DSA image from the same aortogram, later in the run, revealing filling of the left subclavian artery (red arrow) via retrograde flow from the left vertebral artery (yellow arrow). *Courtesy of Dr. Wael E. Saad.*

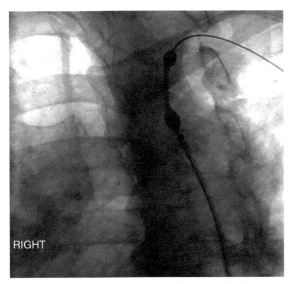

Figure S69-3 Spot radiograph from deployment of balloon-expandable stent across the left subclavian artery lesion. *Courtesy of Dr. Wael E. Saad.*

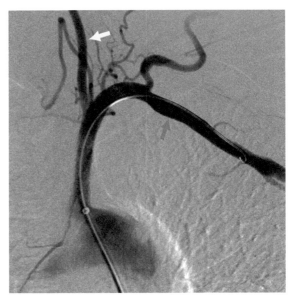

Figure S69-4 DSA image from angiogram poststent deployment showing appropriate filling of the left subclavian artery (red arrow) and vertebral artery (yellow arrow). *Courtesy of Dr. Wael E. Saad.*

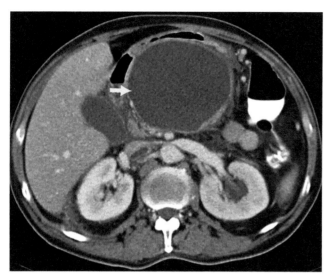

Figure S70-1 Axial CECT image demonstrating a large pancreatic pseudocyst (yellow arrow) posterior to the stomach.

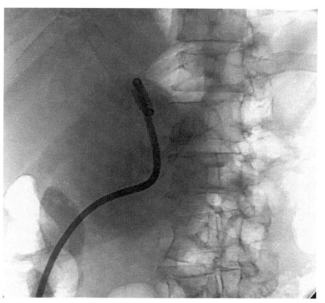

Figure S70-2 Spot fluoroscopic image confirming placement of a pigtail catheter within the pancreatic pseudocyst.

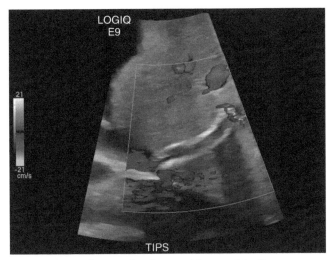

Figure S71-1 Color Doppler ultrasound image of the liver demonstrates no flow within the TIPS.

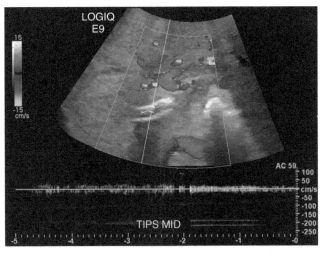

Figure S71-2 Color Doppler and spectral ultrasound reveals minimal flow within the TIPS.

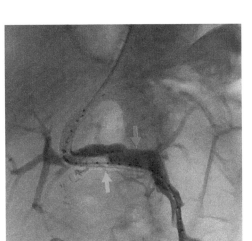

Figure S71-3 Native image from TIPS revision confirming flow within the portal venous end of the TIPS (elongated by a bare-metal stent) (red arrow). There is however no flow within the remainder of the stent (blue arrow). *Courtesy of Dr. Minhaj S. Khaja.*

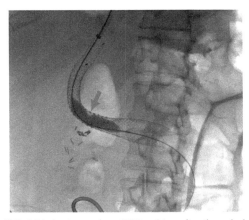

Figure S71-4 Native image from TIPS revision after thrombolysis (not shown) demonstrating balloon angioplasty with small focus of residual thrombus (red arrow). *Courtesy of Dr. Minhaj S. Khaja.*

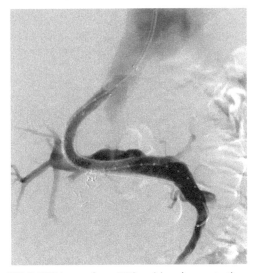

Figure S71-5 DSA image from TIPS revision demonstrating patency of the TIPS after pharmacomechanical thrombolysis and balloon angioplasty. *Courtesy of Dr. Minhaj S. Khaja.*

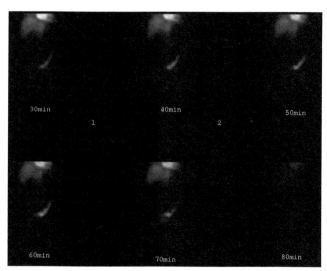

Figure S72-1 Tc-99m labeled RBC scan shows radioisotope accumulation in the left lower abdomen, at a site of active bleeding in the descending or sigmoid colon.

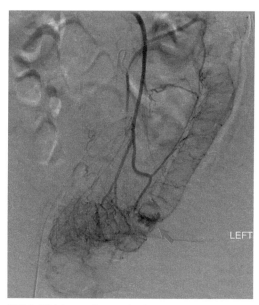

Figure S72-2 DSA image from selective IMA angiogram with demonstration of active extravasation arising from a sigmoid branch of the IMA (red arrow).

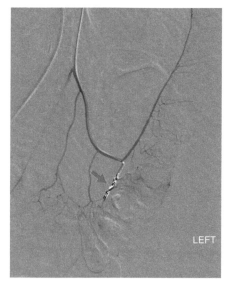

Figure S72-3 DSA image postcoil embolization (red arrow) with no evidence of contrast extravasation to suggest further active hemorrhage.

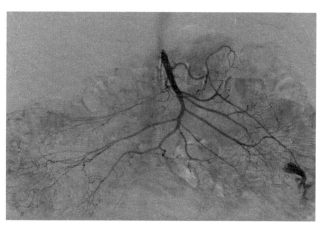

Figure S72-4 DSA image from selective SMA angiogram with demonstration of active extravasation arising from a jejunal branch of the SMA (red arrow).

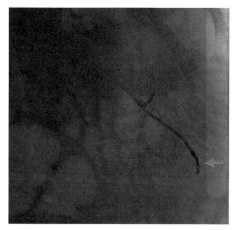

Figure S72-5 Fluoroscopic image from selective IMA angiogram after coil embolization (red arrow).

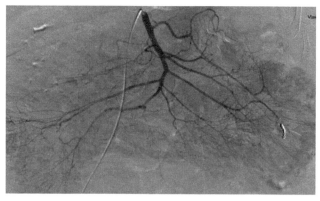

Figure S72-6 DSA image postcoil embolization (red arrow) with no evidence of contrast extravasation to suggest further active hemorrhage.

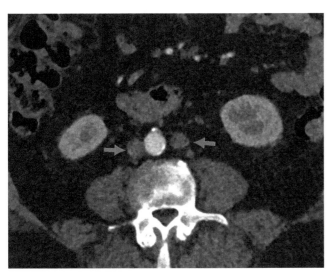

Figure S73-1 Axial image from contrast-enhanced abdominal CT, axial image demonstrating nonopacified left and right inferior vena cavae (arrows). *Courtesy of Dr. Lucia Flors Blasco.*

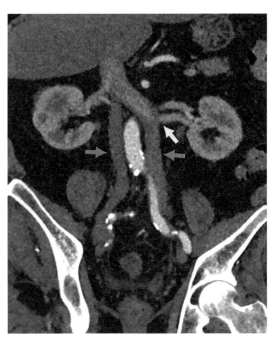

Figure S73-2 Coronal image from the same patient's CT showing the double IVCs (red arrows) with the left renal vein draining into the left IVC (yellow arrow). *Courtesy of Dr. Lucia Flors Blasco.*

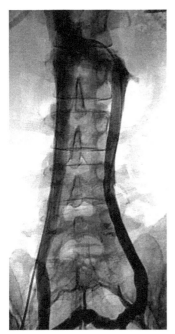

Figure S73-3 Image from digital subtraction venography in a different patient demonstrating duplicated IVCs.

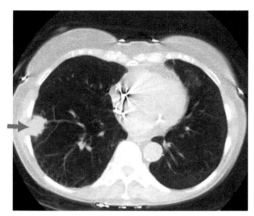

Figure S74-1 Contrast-enhanced CT of the chest demonstrating a 2.5 cm peripheral pulmonary nodule in the right lower lobe (red arrow). Note the significant emphysematous changes in the lungs. There are also cardiac pacemaker leads noted, which suggest underlying heart disease. *Courtesy of Dr. Bill S. Majdalany.*

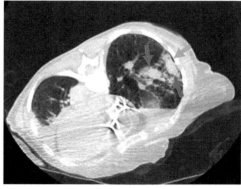

Figure S74-2 Postablation CT of the chest with the patient in the prone position demonstrating a tiny pneumothorax (blue arrow) and groundglass changes (red arrows) in the right lung representing the margins of the kill-zone. *Courtesy of Dr. Bill S. Majdalany.*

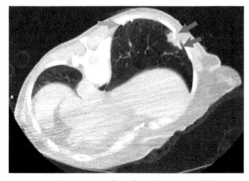

Figure S74-3 Axial CT image after the placement of the cryoablation probes (red arrows). Note the chest tube (blue arrow) in the posterior pleural space that was placed to maintain lung inflation during placement of the probes into this peripheral tumor. *Courtesy of Dr. Bill S. Majdalany.*

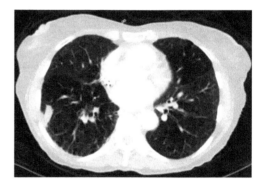

Figure S74-4 Axial CT image 12-months later demonstrates regression of the ablation zone, indicative of a successful treatment. *Courtesy of Dr. Bill S. Majdalany.*

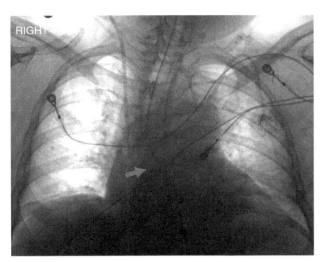

Figure S75-1 Chest radiograph shows an esophageal stent projecting over the midline (red arrow). Numerous life support devices are also in place.

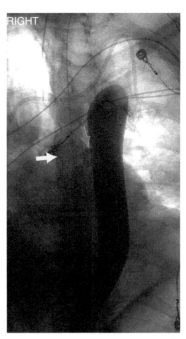

Figure S75-2 Native image from thoracic aortogram revealing a pseudoaneurysm in the descending thoracic aorta (red arrow) adjacent to the proximal end of the esophageal stent (yellow arrow).

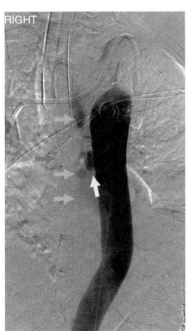

Figure S75-3 DSA image from later in the thoracic aortogram redemonstrating the pseudoaneurysm in the descending thoracic aorta (yellow arrow) adjacent to the proximal end of the esophageal stent (red arrow). However, now seen is contrast blush within the esophagus (blue arrows).

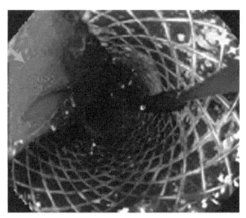

Figure S75-4 Image from EGD showing blood and clot within the esophagus near the proximal end of the esophageal stent (blue arrow).

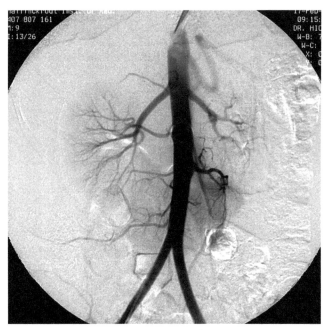

Figure S76-1 Aortogram shows abnormal rotation of the kidneys, which are medialized and fused in the lower poles.

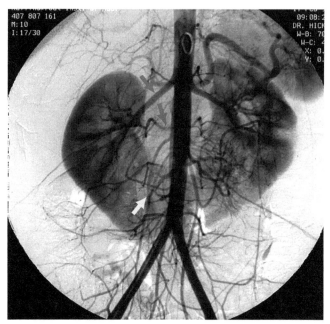

Figure S76-2 Delayed phase within the aortogram shows at least three right renal arteries (red arrows), one left renal artery, and at least one artery perfusing the isthmus (yellow arrow).

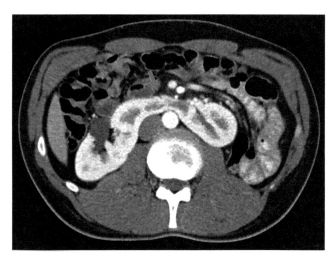

Figure S76-3 CT image from a different patient demonstrates the classic appearance of a horseshoe kidney with parenchyma (arrow) or fibrous isthmus crossing midline and fusing the lower poles.

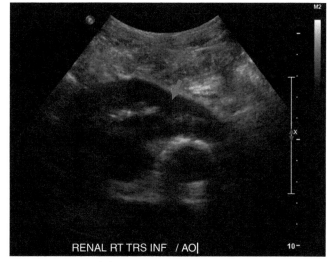

Figure S76-4 Renal ultrasound image demonstrating the midline isthmus (arrow).

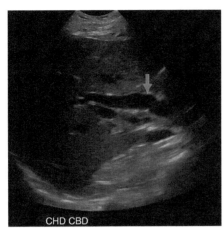

Figure S77-1 Gray-scale US image of the liver demonstrates a dilated common bile duct (red arrow) and intrahepatic biliary ducts. *Courtesy of Dr. James Shields.*

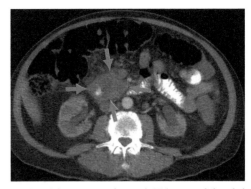

Figure S77-2 Axial contrast-enhanced CT image of the abdomen reveals a heterogeneous mass in the pancreatic head (red arrows) and extending into the pancreaticoduodenal groove. *Courtesy of Dr. James Shields.*

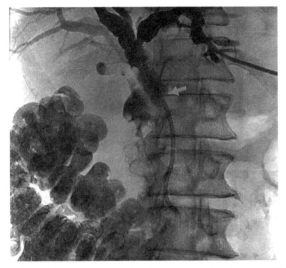

Figure S77-3 Fluoroscopic cholangioram near completion of biliary drain placement confirms obstruction of the distal common bile duct with abrupt cutoff at the level of the midcommon bile duct (red arrow) and associated moderate upstream biliary duct dilatation. *Courtesy of Dr. James Shields.*

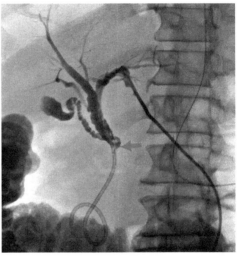

Figure S77-4 Fluoroscopic image during contrast injection of the biliary drain once again demonstrates abrupt cutoff of the midcommon bile duct (red arrow) with nonopacification of the distal common bile duct consistent with obstruction. Intrahepatic biliary duct dilation is improved following PTC placement compared to Figure S77-3. *Courtesy of Dr. James Shields.*

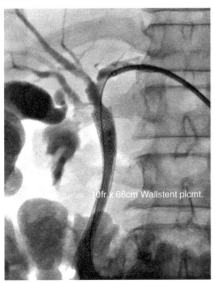

Figure S77-5 Fluoroscopic image demonstrates a newly placed Wallstent in the common bile duct with transit of contrast through the stent. *Courtesy of Dr. James Shields.*

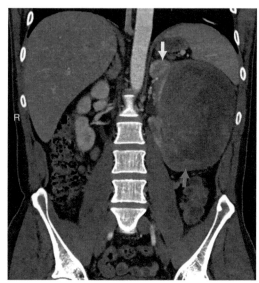

Figure S78-1 Coronal reconstruction of CECT showing a heterogeneously enhancing large left renal cell carcinoma (red arrow), which has hemorrhaged into itself and is exerting mass effect on adjacent normal renal parenchyma (yellow arrow). *Courtesy of Dr. Luke R. Wilkins.*

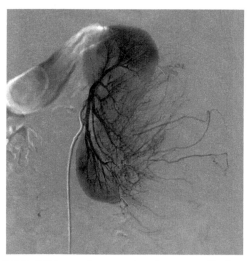

Figure S78-2 DSA image from renal angiogram confirming innumerable, abnormal parasitic arteries extending into a mass lesion of the left kidney. There is distortion of normal renal parenchyma (red arrows) as the RCC hemorrhaged into itself. *Courtesy of Dr. Luke R. Wilkins.*

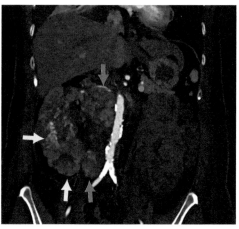

Figure S78-3 Coronal reconstruction from a CTA in a different patient showing a heterogeneous, arterially enhancing large right renal mass (yellow arrows) with extension beyond the kidney (red arrows). *Courtesy of Dr. Luke R. Wilkins.*

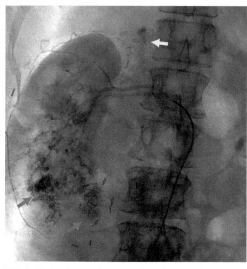

Figure S78-4 Native image from renal angiogram (same patient as in Figure S78-3) confirming parenchymal blush and distortion in the lower pole of the right kidney (red arrows). Additionally noted is tumor blush beyond the kidney (yellow arrow). *Courtesy of Dr. Luke R. Wilkins.*

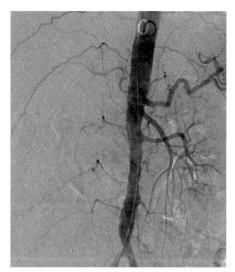

Figure S78-5 DSA image from aortogram (same patient as in Figure S78-3) after particle embolization of the right kidney. No flow noted within the right kidney. *Courtesy of Dr. Luke R. Wilkins.*

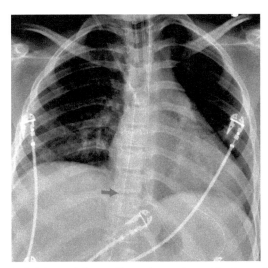

Figure S79-1 Frontal chest radiograph reveals a guidewire projecting in the location of the vena cava traveling through the right atrium (red arrow).

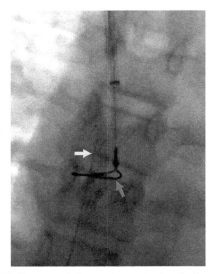

Figure S79-2 Fluoroscopic image demonstrating the introduction of a loop snare device (red arrow) around the guidewire (yellow arrow).

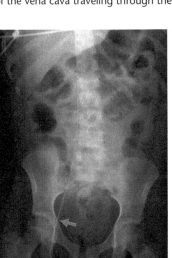

Figure S79-3 Abdominal radiograph showing continuation of the guidewire from the chest to the level of the common femoral vein (red arrow).

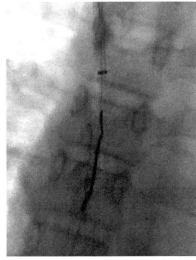

Figure S79-4 Fluoroscopic image showing the grasping of the guidewire with the loop snare technique.

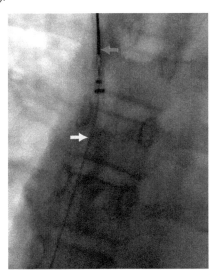

Figure S79-5 Fluoroscopic image confirming successful retrieval of the foreign body guidewire (yellow arrow) with loop-snare (red arrow) technique; the guidewire was retracted through the sheath.

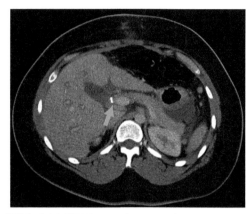

Figure S80-1 Axial CECT image demonstrating a "pseudogallbladder" related to a biloma in the gallbladder fossa (red arrow). A surgical clip is noted adjacent to the biloma (blue arrow). *Courtesy of Dr. Bill S. Majdalany.*

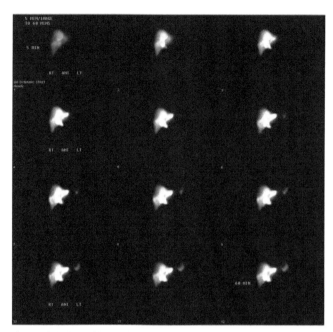

Figure S80-2 Tc-99m HIDA scan showing extrahepatic radiotracer accumulation along the left subhepatic space and in the gallbladder fossa, without bowel opacification. *Courtesy of Dr. Bill S. Majdalany.*

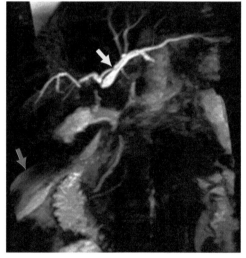

Figure S80-3 Coronal MRCP image confirming dilated intrahepatic biliary tree (yellow arrow) with an abrupt interruption of the common duct with a thin tract of increased T2 signal arising from this region and terminating in a subhepatic fluid collection (red arrow), compatible with bile leak. *Courtesy of Dr. Bill S. Majdalany.*

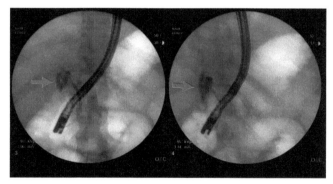

Figure S80-4 Fluoroscopic images from ERCP allowing visualization of the leak from the CHD (red arrows), which could not be treated endoscopically. *Courtesy of Dr. Bill S. Majdalany.*

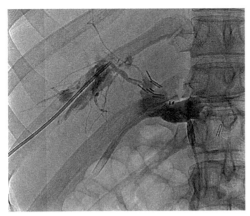

Figure S80-5 Fluoroscopic image from PTC demonstrating contrast extravasation from the common duct into the subhepatic space (red arrow). *Courtesy of Dr. Bill S. Majdalany.*

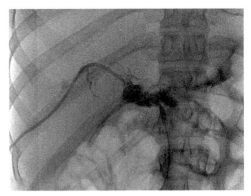

Figure S80-6 Fluoroscopic image demonstrating an external biliary drain in the right hepatic duct. *Courtesy of Dr. Bill S. Majdalany.*

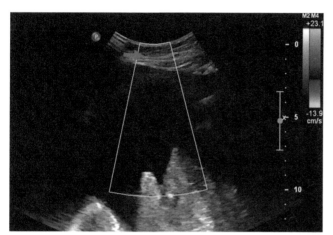

Figure S81-1 Single ultrasound image shows a large volume of anechoic fluid consistent with ascites. No Doppler flow is seen in the overlying abdominal wall (arrow). Doppler was used to evaluate for collateral vessels prior to peritoneal access and tunneling.

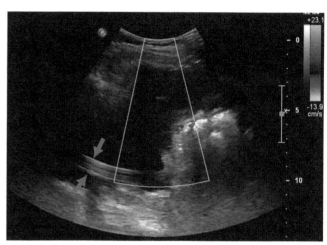

Figure S81-2 Postprocedure imaging shows a decrease in fluid and a catheter lying in the deep portion of the ascites (arrows).

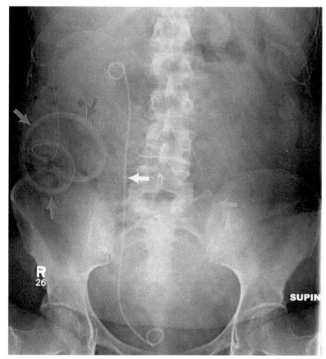

Figure S81-3 Postprocedure plain film shows percutaneous peritoneal drainage catheter tip in the left pelvis (blue arrow) and coiled external catheter over the right lower quadrant (red arrows). A right double J nephroureteral stent is also visualized (yellow arrow).

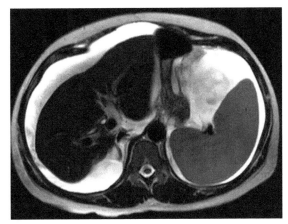

Figure S82-1 Axial T2-weighted MRI image demonstrating diffuse low signal-intensity within the liver. There is also high signal-intensity surrounding the liver, which represents ascites.

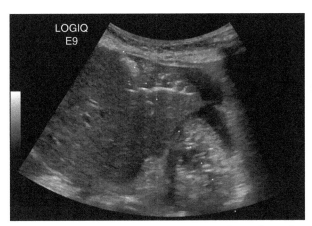

Figure S82-2 Gray-scale US image of the liver with needle-guide setting on.

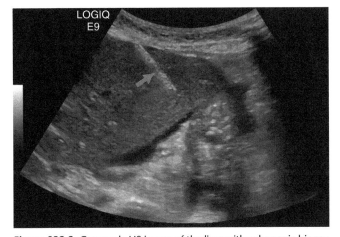

Figure S82-3 Gray-scale US image of the liver with echogenic biopsy needle in place (red arrow).

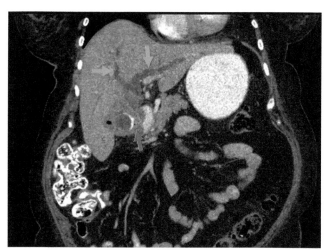

Figure S83-1 Coronal reconstruction from contrast-enhanced CT demonstrates diffuse intrahepatic biliary dilatation (blue arrows). There is a large mass replacing the gallbladder that compresses the common bile duct (red arrow).

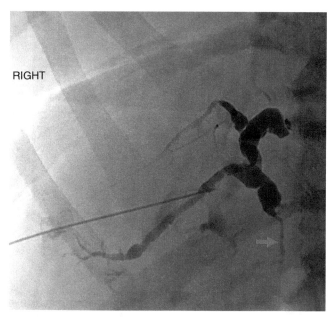

Figure S83-2 Native image from cholangiogram reveals marked biliary dilatation with an elongated, irregular stricture of the common hepatic duct (red arrow).

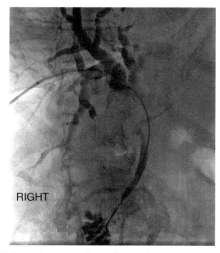

Figure S83-3 Native image from cholangiogram shows a diagnostic catheter placed across the biliary stricture via a percutaneous transhepatic approach, with opacification of the duodenum (red arrow).

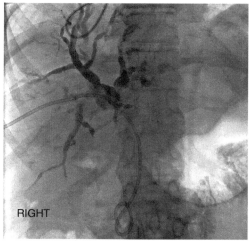

Figure S83-4 An internal/external biliary drainage catheter has been placed across the stenosis, with internal tip in the duodenum.

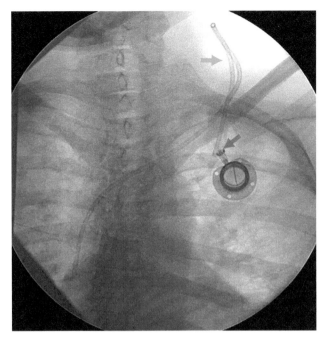

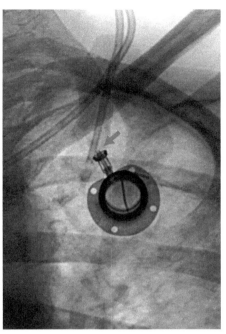

Figure S84-1 Fluproscopic image showing a left-sided subcutaneous implantable port catheter showing separation of the two attachable components (red arrow). Additionally noted is the apex cephalad displaced catheter, which may be partially extravascular (blue arrow).

Figure S84-2 Zoomed-in fluoroscopic image more clearly showing the separation of the two components of the attachable implantable port (red arrow).

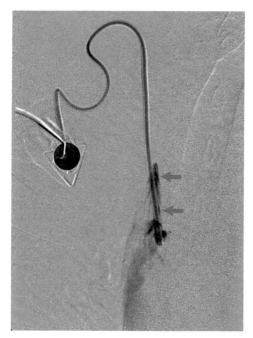

Figure S85-1 Image from digital subtraction venogram through port demonstrating reflux of contrast material along the tip (arrows).

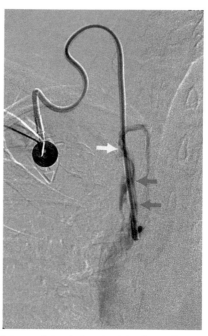

Figure S85-2 Image later during the injection redemonstrating the contrast refluxing between the catheter and fibrin sheath (red arrows) before escaping into the vein more superiorly (yellow arrow).

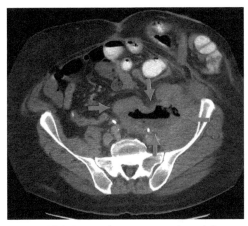

Figure S86-1 Axial CT image demonstrates a large inflammatory soft tissue mass in the pelvis extending from the midline to the left iliopsoas muscle containing a collection of fluid and gas (red arrows).

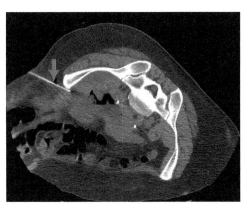

Figure S86-2 Intraprocedural CT image with the patient in the right lateral decubitus position demonstrates passage of an 18-gauge Chiba needle into the fluid collection via a transabdominal approach (red arrow).

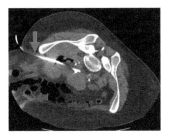

Figure S86-3 Intraprocedural CT image with the patient in the right lateral decubitus position demonstrates a 12 French catheter within the fluid collection (red arrow). One hundred milliliters of bloody fluid was aspirated.

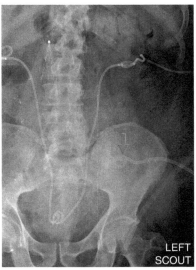

Figure S86-4 Abdominal radiograph confirming position of the pelvic drainage catheter (red arrow). Also noted are bilateral nephroureteral stents.

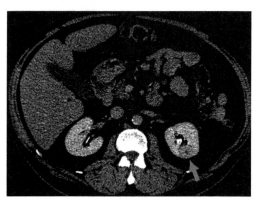

Figure S87-1 Enhanced CT shows a 2.3 cm enhancing mass in the posterior interpolar region of the left kidney (arrow). *Courtesy of Dr. Shane A. Wells.*

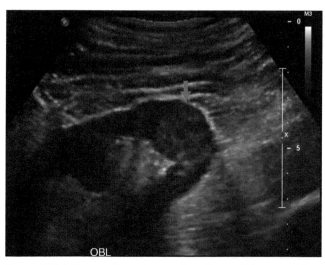

Figure S87-2 Preprocedure ultrasound confirms solid nature of the lesion (arrow) and was used for ablation planning. *Courtesy of Dr. Shane A. Wells.*

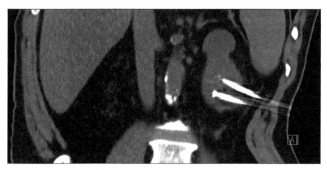

Figure S87-3 CT image during ablation procedure shows two parallel cryoablation probes within the renal mass. *Courtesy of Dr. Shane A. Wells.*

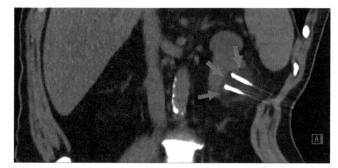

Figure S87-4 Immediate postablation CT shows uniform hypodensity within ablation zone (arrows). *Courtesy of Dr. Shane A. Wells.*

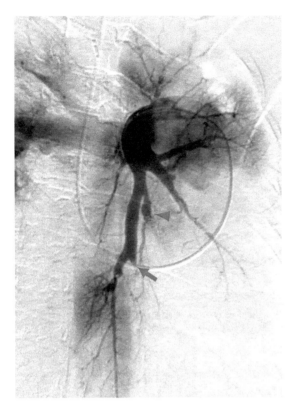

Figure S88-1 DSA image from left pulmonary angiogram revealing occluded (arrow) and rounded off (arrowhead) segmental pulmonary arteries. Note distal hypoperfusion.

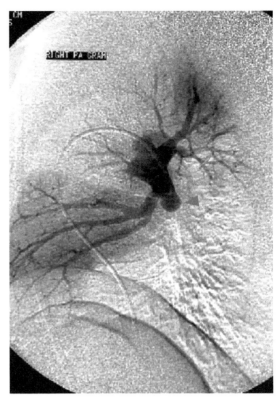

Figure S88-2 DSA image from right pulmonary angiogram showing a rounded off occlusion of the lower lobe pulmonary artery (arrowhead). Again note multiple regions of hypoperfusion.

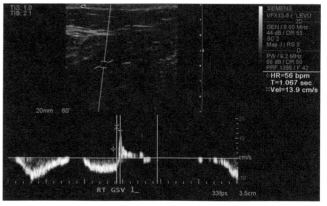

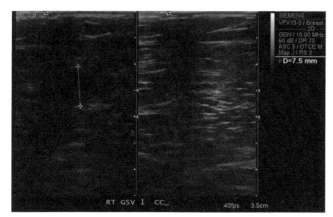

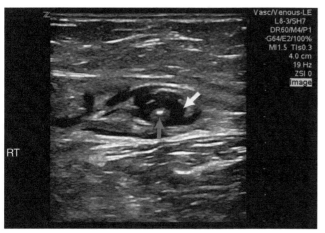

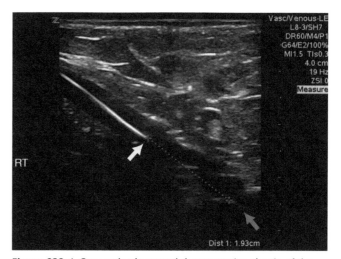

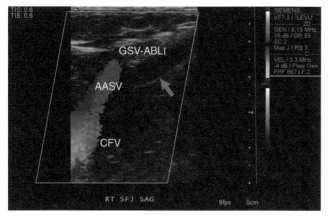

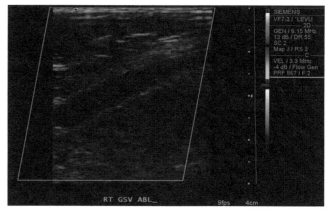

Figure S89-1 Gray-scale ultrasound without (left) and with compression of the GSV. GSV size greater than 5 mm has a high positive-predictive value for reflux.

Figure S89-2 Gray-scale and spectral ultrasound of the GSV. Spectral waveform demonstrates reflux in the GSV with valve closure time of greater than 1 second. Valve closure time greater than 0.5 second is considered by many as abnormal reflux.

Figure S89-3 Gray-scale ultrasound after the administration of tumescent anesthesia. A ring of hypoechoic fluid is noted (yellow arrow) around the GSV. Note the hyperechoic catheter within the vein (red arrow). *Courtesy of Dr. Minhaj S. Khaja.*

Figure S89-4 Gray-scale ultrasound demonstrating the tip of the ablation catheter (yellow arrow) 1.9 cm from the saphenofemoral junction. The femoral vein is noted by the red arrow. *Courtesy of Dr. Minhaj S. Khaja.*

Figure S89-5 Color ultrasound image 1 week following ablation with no flow within the GSV as it drains into the common femoral vein (red arrow). *Courtesy of Dr. Minhaj S. Khaja.*

Figure S89-6 Color ultrasound 1 week following ablation demonstrating no flow within the GSV. *Courtesy of Dr. Minhaj S. Khaja.*

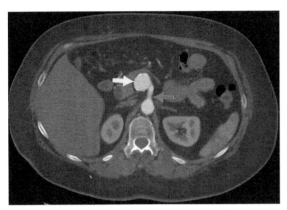

Figure S90-1 Axial CTA image demonstrating a well-circumscribed enhancing vascular structure with discontinuous peripheral calcifications (yellow arrow) arising from the SMA (red arrow). *Courtesy of Dr. Wael E. Saad.*

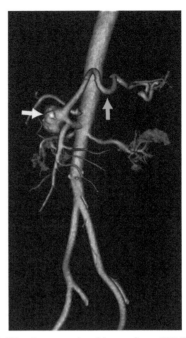

Figure S90-2 3D volume-rendered image from CTA illustrating an aneurysm arising from the SMA (yellow arrow) with variant splenic artery origin from the proximal SMA (blue arrow). *Courtesy of Dr. Wael E. Saad.*

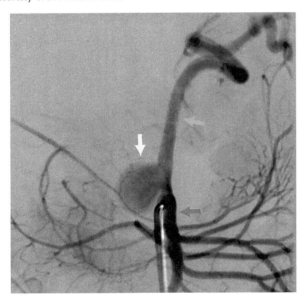

Figure S90-3 DSA image of the SMA (red arrow) confirming the aneurysm (yellow arrow) and variant splenic artery origin (blue arrow). *Courtesy of Dr. Wael E. Saad.*

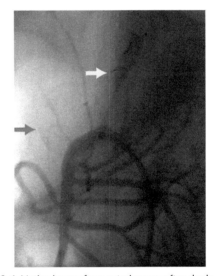

Figure S90-4 Native image from arteriogram after deployment of a covered stent in the proximal splenic artery. Note the rim of calcification around the aneurysm (red arrow). Also noted is a vascular plug at the base of the splenic artery (yellow arrow). *Courtesy of Dr. Wael E. Saad.*

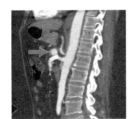

Figure S90-5 Sagittal reformat from CTA 1 month poststenting and embolization which reveals continued filling of the SMA aneurysm (red arrow). *Courtesy of Dr. Wael E. Saad.*

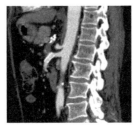

Figure S90-6 Sagittal reformat from CTA 3 months postdiscontinuation of anticoagulation confirming that the aneurysm is thrombosed and excluded. *Courtesy of Dr. Wael E. Saad.*

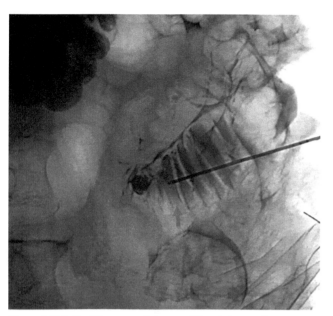

Figure S91-1 Spot fluoroscopic image of the abdomen demonstrates percutaneous needle access and opacification of a jejunal loop in preparation for jejunostomy tube placement (red arrow).

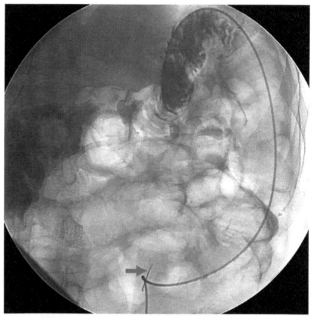

Figure S91-2 Spot fluoroscopic image demonstrates advancement of a wire into the loop of jejunum opacified with contrast. A pexy t-fastener is also in place (red arrow).

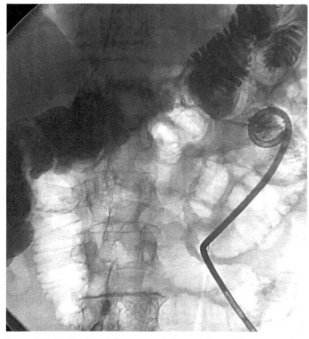

Figure S91-3 Final spot fluoroscopic image shows placement of a pigtail jejunostomy catheter with progression of contrast through the jejunum and into the distal bowel.

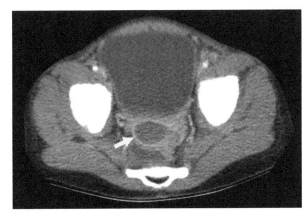

Figure S92-1 Axial image from contrast-enhanced CT of the pelvis shows a small perirectal abscess in the rectovesicular space (yellow arrow). *Courtesy of Dr. Ranjith Vellody.*

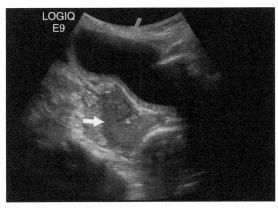

Figure S92-2 Transabdominal gray-scale ultrasound image confirms a heterogeneous, hyperechoic collection (yellow arrow) behind the bladder (red arrow). *Courtesy of Dr. Ranjith Vellody.*

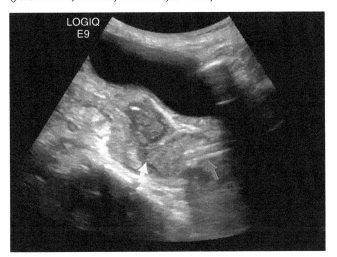

Figure S92-3 Transabdominal gray-scale ultrasound image demonstrates advancement of a needle-guide through the rectum (red arrow) near the fluid collection (yellow arrow). *Courtesy of Dr. Ranjith Vellody.*

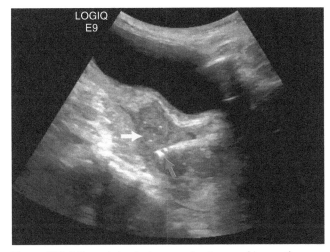

Figure S92-4 Transabdominal gray-scale ultrasound image shows advancement of a needle (red arrow) into the fluid collection (yellow arrow). *Courtesy of Dr. Ranjith Vellody.*

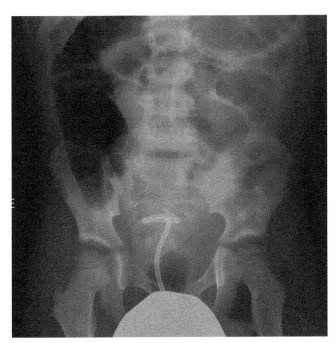

Figure S92-5 Abdominal radiograph confirms tube position postplacement. *Courtesy of Dr. Ranjith Vellody.*

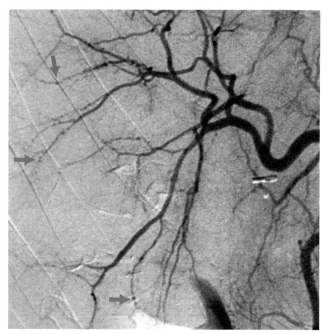

Figure S93-1 DSA image from right hepatic angiogram demonstrating multifocal irregularity with stenosis and small aneurysms in the distal hepatic artery branches (red arrows). *Courtesy of Dr. Daniel Brown.*

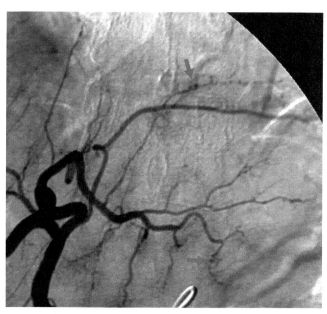

Figure S93-2 DSA image from left hepatic angiogram demonstrating multifocal irregularity with stenosis and small aneurysms in the distal hepatic artery branches (red arrows). *Courtesy of Dr. Daniel Brown.*

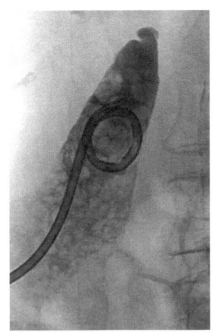

Figure S94-1 Fluoroscopic image from cholangiogram demonstrating a tube in place and numerous filling defects which are gallstones.

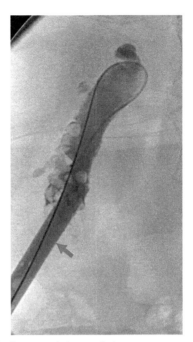

Figure S94-2 Fluoroscopic image during percutaneous gallstone removal with a sheath (red arrow) and wire in place.

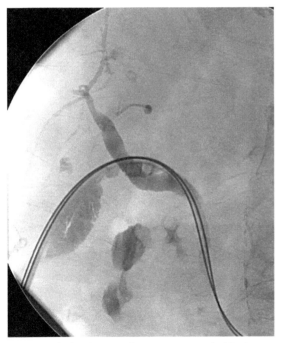

Figure S94-3 Cholangiogram after stone removal with clearance of the gallstones.

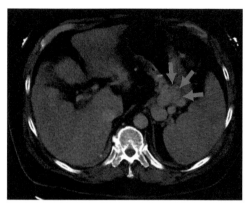

Figure S95-1 Axial contrast-enhanced CT demonstrating large gastric varices (arrows). *Courtesy of Dr. Wael E. Saad.*

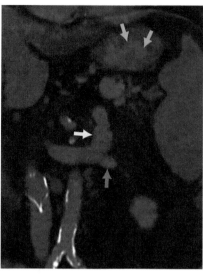

Figure S95-2 Coronal reconstruction from contrast-enhanced CT demonstrating the left renal vein (red arrow) and corresponding gastrorenal shunt (yellow arrow) leading to large gastric varices (blue arrows). *Courtesy of Dr. Wael E. Saad.*

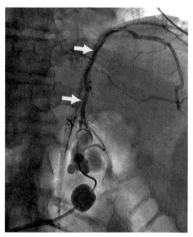

Figure S95-3 Angiographic image demonstrating balloon-occlusion (red arrow) of the gastric varices seen on CT, with inferior phrenic (yellow arrows) and retroperitoneal veins decompressing the varices. *Courtesy of Dr. Wael E. Saad.*

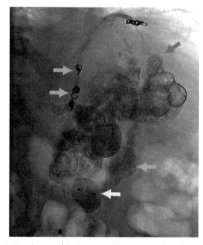

Figure S95-4 Angiographic image demonstrating Amplatzer occlusion device (yellow arrow) taking place of the occlusive balloon. True varices are noted in the right and left apices (red arrows). The posterior gastric vein is the main gastric feeder vessel (blue arrow). There are coils in the inferior phrenic draining vein (green arrows). *Courtesy of Dr. Wael E. Saad.*

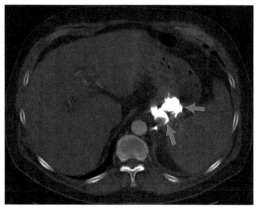

Figure S95-5 Axial contrast-enhanced CT status post-BRTO demonstrating high attenuation sclerosant in the previously identified gastric varices (arrows). *Courtesy of Dr. Wael E. Saad.*

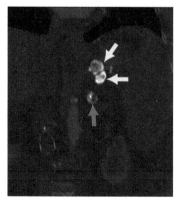

Figure S95-6 Coronal contrast-enhanced CT status post-BRTO showing sclerosed gastric varices (yellow arrows) and Amplatzer device (red arrow). *Courtesy of Dr. Wael E. Saad.*

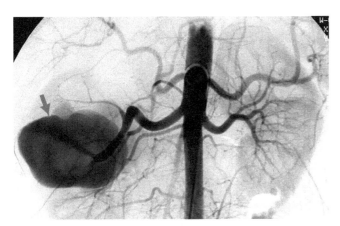

Figure S96-1 Arterial-phase DSA image from aortogram demonstrating an enlarged right renal artery with an arteriovenous malformation (red arrow) from a distal branch.

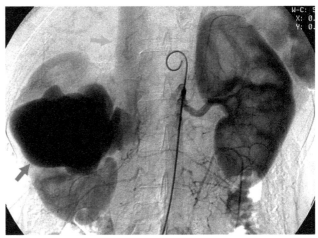

Figure S96-2 Late arterial-phase DSA image redemonstrating an arteriovenous malformation (red arrow) with early venous filling of the IVC (blue arrow).

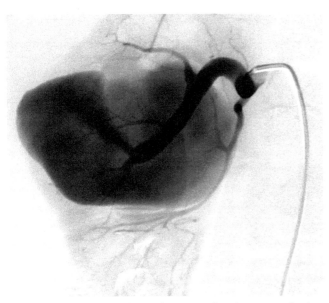

Figure S96-3 DSA image from selective renal angiogram confirming origin of renal AVM.

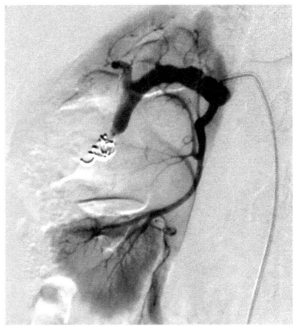

Figure S96-4 DSA image from selective renal angiogram postcoil embolization of the renal AVM.

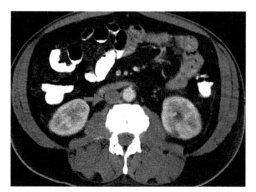

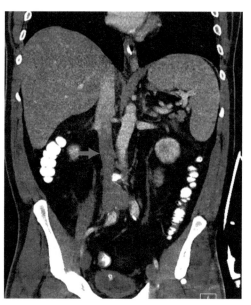

Figure S97-1 Axial image from CECT demonstrating occlusion of the IVC (red arrow). *Courtesy of Dr. David M. Williams.*

Figure S97-2 Coronal reconstruction from CECT showing occlusion of the IVC (red arrow) up to the level of the renal veins. No mass is seen. *Courtesy of Dr. David M. Williams.*

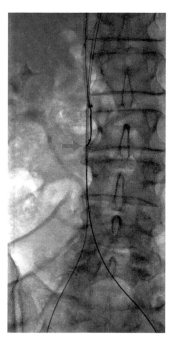

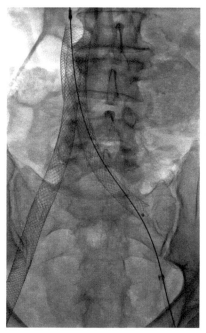

Figure S97-3 Native image from IVC recanalization showing bilateral femoral venous access and snaring of the wire from the right IJ access (red arrow). *Courtesy of Dr. David M. Williams.*

Figure S97-4 Native image from IVC recanalization after the placement of bilateral iliac vein stents. *Courtesy of Dr. David M. Williams.*

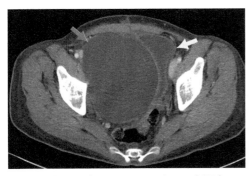

Figure S98-1 Axial image from contrast-enhanced CT demonstrates a large, low-attenuation fluid collection in the pelvis (red arrow), which is compressing and displacing the bladder (yellow arrow). *Courtesy of Dr. Bill S. Majdalany.*

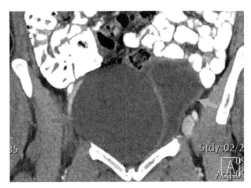

Figure S98-2 Coronal reconstruction from contrast-enhanced CT confirming the large fluid collection in the pelvis (red arrow), which is compressing and displacing the bladder (blue arrow). *Courtesy of Dr. Bill S. Majdalany.*

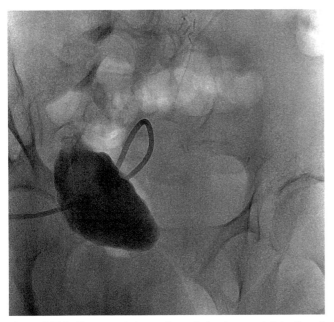

Figure S98-3 Fluoroscopic image from drain placement. Injection of contrast into the drain under fluoroscopy demonstrates filling of the fluid collection in the right hemipelvis. *Courtesy of Dr. Bill S. Majdalany.*

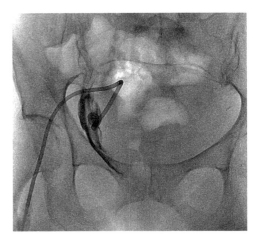

Figure S98-4 Fluoroscopic image 2 weeks after sclerosis. Injection of contrast reveals significantly decreased size of lymphocele. The drain was subsequently removed (not shown). *Courtesy of Dr. Bill S. Majdalany.*

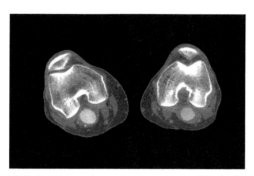

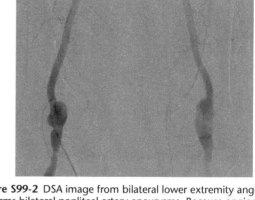

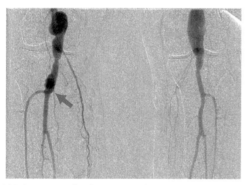

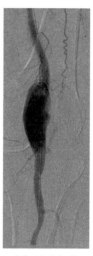

Figure S99-1 Axial image from a lower extremity CTA obtained at the level of the popliteal fossae demonstrates fusiform aneurysmal dilatation of the bilateral popliteal arteries. There is no significant mural thrombus.

Figure S99-2 DSA image from bilateral lower extremity angiogram confirms bilateral popliteal artery aneurysms. Because angiography only portrays the patent arterial lumen, cross-sectional imaging is necessary to determine true aneurysm size as popliteal artery aneurysms often demonstrate a significant amount of mural thrombus.

Figure S99-3 A more distal angiographic run reveals that while the left popliteal aneurysm (blue arrow) tapers to normal vessel caliber at the distal left popliteal artery, the right popliteal artery (red arrow) is ectatic distally to the takeoff of the right anterior tibial artery, providing no distal landing zone for endovascular stent placement.

Figure S99-4 DSA image of the LLE further delineating the left popliteal artery aneurysm.

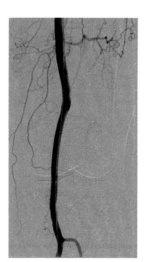

Figure S99-5 DSA image of the LLE after covered stent placement demonstrates successful exclusion of the aneurysm sac without evidence of persistent filling.

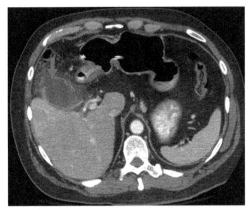

Figure S100-1 Axial contrast-enhanced CT image demonstrates pericholecystic fluid and fat stranding with a focal defect in the wall of the gallbladder fundus (red arrow), consistent with a gallbladder rupture.

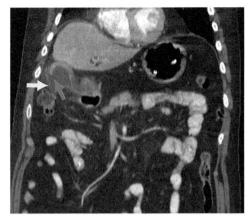

Figure S100-2 Coronal reconstruction shows wall thickening, pericholecystic fluid and a focal defect in the wall of the gallbladder fundus (red arrow), consistent with a gallbladder rupture. Adjacent enhancing fluid also noted (red arrowhead).

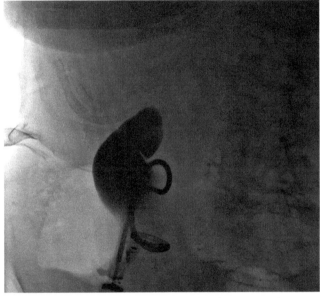

Figure S100-3 Fluoroscopic image after tube placement and contrast injection. Additional sideholes were placed to drain adjacent abscess (not shown).

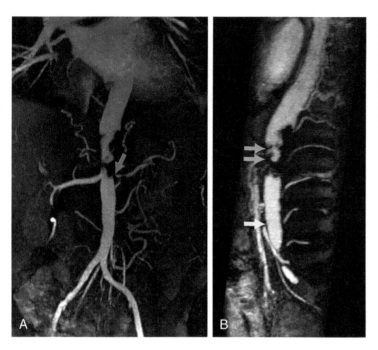

Figure S101-1 Contrast-enhanced MR angiography, coronal (A) and sagittal (B), shows severe stenosis of the suprarenal abdominal aorta caused by extensive "coral reef" atherosclerotic plaque extending from the diaphragmatic hiatus through the renal arteries (hypointensity representing calcium). Proximal occlusion of the celiac (green arrow), superior mesenteric (blue arrow), and inferior mesenteric arteries (yellow arrow) is seen on the sagittal image (B). Severe stenosis at the origin of the left renal artery is also seen (red arrow) (A). *Courtesy of Dr. Lucia Flors Blasco.*

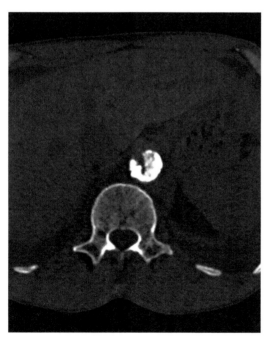

Figure S101-2 Unenhanced abdominal CT image shows near complete occlusion of the abdominal aorta caused by severe calcified atherosclerosis. Bilateral pleural effusion is also seen. *Courtesy of Dr. Lucia Flors Blasco.*

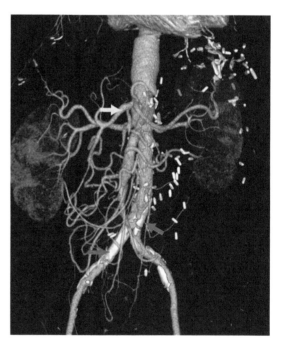

Figure S101-3 Volume-rendered reconstruction of contrast-enhanced CTA shows excellent result after endarterectomy. Note the presence of multiple surgical clips as well as the diffuse calcification of the distal abdominal aorta and bilateral common iliac arteries (arrows). *Courtesy of Dr. Lucia Flors Blasco.*

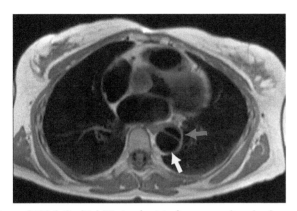

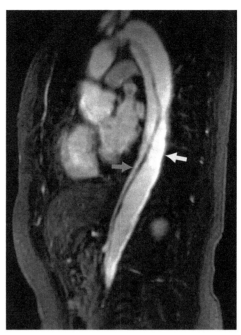

Figure S102-1 Sagittal 3D steady state free procession cine image demonstrates a dissection flap extending from the distal aortic arch to the subdiaphragmatic aorta. The flap did not extend to the ascending aorta (not pictured). The larger lumen is the false lumen (yellow arrow) with the smaller, anteriorly compressed true lumen (red arrow). *Courtesy of Dr. Peter Liu.*

Figure S102-2 Axial T1-weighted black blood image demonstrates a dissection flap in the descending aorta. The larger lumen is the false lumen (yellow arrow) with the smaller, anteriorly compressed true lumen (red arrow). *Courtesy of Dr. Peter Liu.*

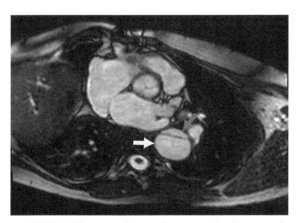

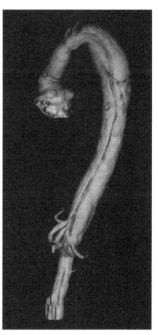

Figure S102-3 Oblique steady state free procession image at the aortic root demonstrates a dissection flap in the descending aorta. The larger lumen is the false lumen (yellow arrow) with the smaller, anteriorly compressed true lumen (red arrow). *Courtesy of Dr. Peter Liu.*

Figure S102-4 3D volume-rendered image shows aortic dissection flap throughout the thoracoabdominal aorta. *Courtesy of Dr. Peter Liu.*

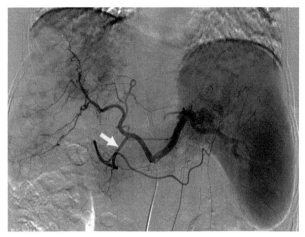

Figure S103-1 DSA image from celiac arteriogram demonstrating conventional hepatic arterial anatomy. The gastroduodenal (yellow arrow) and right gastric arteries (red arrow) are also identified.

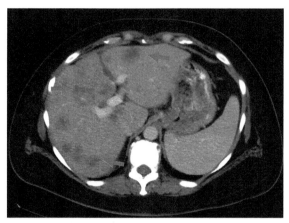

Figure S103-2 Preprocedure-enhanced CT shows numerous hypodense lesions in all lobes of the liver (arrows). No significant extrahepatic disease was found.

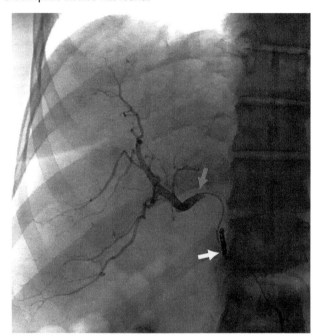

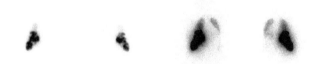

Figure S103-3 Tc^{99m} macroaggregate albumin was injected to evaluate for extrahepatic uptake. Planar nuclear medicine imaging shows no significant gastrointestinal uptake and a low lung shunt fraction (<10%). Radiotracer uptake noted in the numerous metastatic lesions.

Figure S103-4 Treatment angiogram demonstrating successful coil embolization of the right gastric artery (yellow arrow). A microcatheter was used to subselect the right hepatic artery (red arrow).

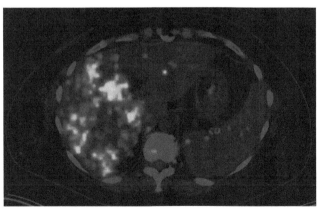

Figure S103-5 Posttreatment SPECT-CT shows focal radio-isotope uptake in the right hepatic lobe. No significant uptake was seen in the remaining chest and abdomen (not shown).

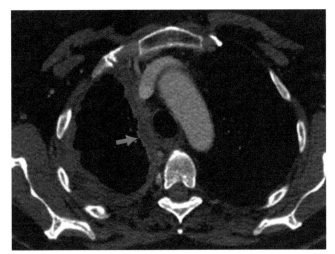

Figure S104-1 Contrast-enhanced CT image of the chest shows circumferential pleural thickening with mediastinal involvement (arrow). Parietal pleural thickening is greater than 1 cm in maximal width. *Courtesy of Dr. Lucia Flors Blasco.*

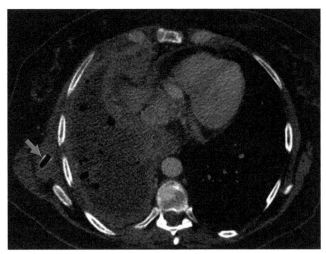

Figure S104-2 Contrast-enhanced CT lower in the chest shows right-sided pleural effusion and gas bubbles, related to recent pleural catheter placement (arrow). Pleural biopsy revealed epithelial mesothelioma. *Courtesy of Dr. Lucia Flors Blasco.*

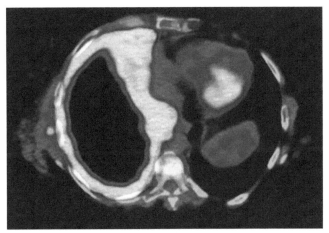

Figure S104-3 PET/CT fusion image reveals diffuse increased FDG uptake within the circumferential pleural thickening (same patient as in Figure S104-1). *Courtesy of Dr. Lucia Flors Blasco.*

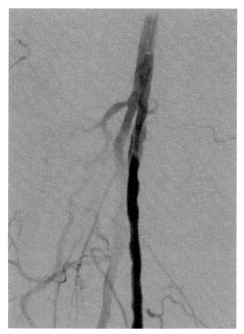

Figure S105-1 DSA image from RLE angiogram showing a flow-limiting dissection in the SFA just distal to its bifurcation from the profunda femoral artery. *Courtesy of Dr. Minhaj S. Khaja.*

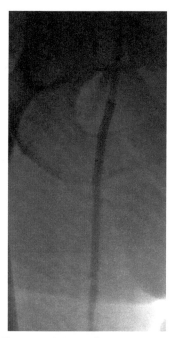

Figure S105-2 Fluoroscopic image from RLE angiogram after deployment of a stent across the lesion with no further dissection seen. *Courtesy of Dr. Minhaj S. Khaja.*

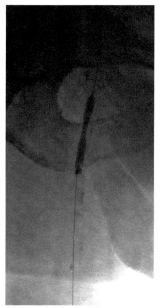

Figure S105-3 Native image of low-pressure, prolonged balloon inflation at the site of SFA dissection. *Courtesy of Dr. Minhaj S. Khaja.*

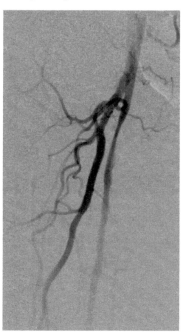

Figure S105-4 DSA image from RLE angiogram after balloon inflation showing continued stenosis of the proximal SFA necessitating stent placement. *Courtesy of Dr. Minhaj S. Khaja.*

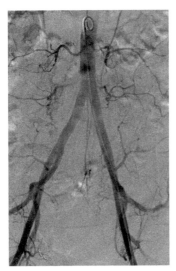

Figure S106-1 DSA image from abdominal aortogram revealing a highly tortuous artery coursing along the right side of the aorta, the ovarian artery (red arrow). *Courtesy of Dr. Wael E. Saad.*

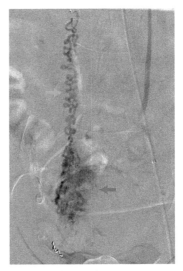

Figure S106-2 DSA image from selective ovarian angiogram confirming an enlarged right ovarian artery (blue arrow) with blush of the uterine fibroid (red arrow). *Courtesy of Dr. Wael E. Saad.*

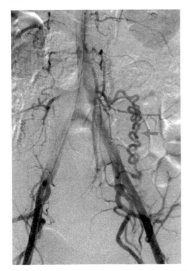

Figure S106-3 DSA image from an aortogram in a different patient reveals an enlarged left ovarian artery (red arrow).

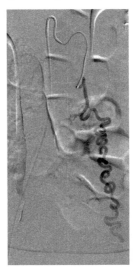

Figure S106-4 DSA image from selective left ovarian angiogram in the same patient as in Figure S106-3 confirms an enlarged left ovarian artery.

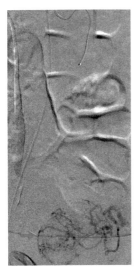

Figure S106-5 Late image from the selective left ovarian DSA demonstrates fibroid perfusion by the left ovarian artery (red arrow).

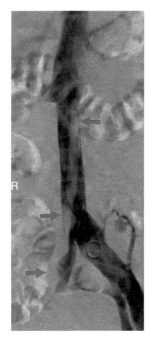

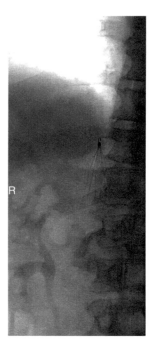

Figure S107-1 DSA image from cavogram demonstrates large, ovoid filling defect within the right iliac vein extending into the inferior vena cava (red arrows), consistent with a large free-floating acute thrombus.

Figure S107-2 Native image in the same patient confirming suprarenal placement of an IVC filter.

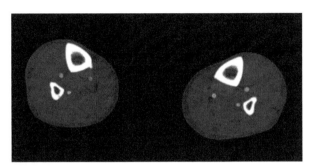

Figure S108-1 Axial image from CTA with runoff demonstrating highly calcified tibial vessels bilaterally. Endoluminal evaluation is limited due to overlying calcification. *Courtesy of Dr. Narasimham L. Dasika.*

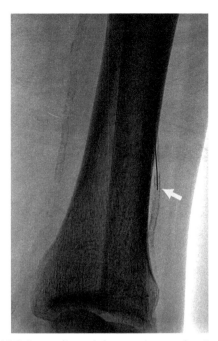

Figure S108-2 Spot radiograph from angiogram showing highly calcified posterior tibial artery (red arrow) and anterior tibial artery with wire in place (yellow arrow). *Courtesy of Dr. Narasimham L. Dasika.*

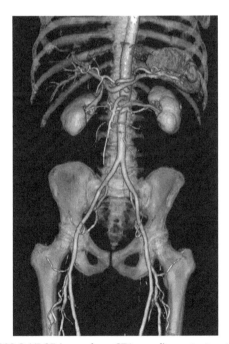

Figure S108-3 VR 3D image from CTA revealing patent aortoiliac and outflow vessels to the midthigh. Note that there is no significant atherosclerotic disease in the aorta, iliac arteries, or femoral arteries. *Courtesy of Dr. Narasimham L. Dasika.*

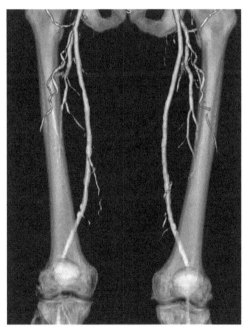

Figure S108-4 VR 3D image from CTA revealing patent femoropopliteal vessels to the knee. Note that there is no significant atherosclerotic disease in the imaged vessels. *Courtesy of Dr. Narasimham L. Dasika.*

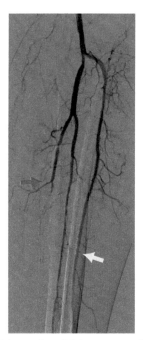

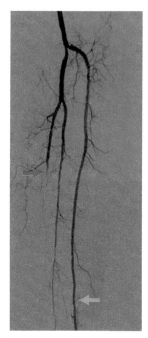

Figure S108-5 DSA image from left lower extremity angiogram prior to intervention confirming abrupt occlusion of the posterior tibial artery (red arrow), multifocal stenoses within the peroneal artery, and poor opacification of the anterior tibial artery (yellow arrow). *Courtesy of Dr. Narasimham L. Dasika.*

Figure S108-6 DSA image from left lower extremity angiogram after intervention revealing continued abrupt occlusion of the posterior tibial artery (red arrow), multifocal stenoses within the peroneal artery, and significantly improved inline flow through the anterior tibial artery (blue arrow). *Courtesy of Dr. Narasimham L. Dasika.*

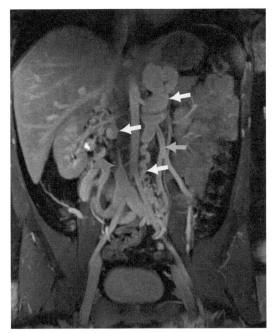

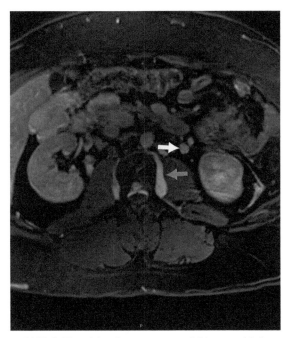

Figure S109-1 T1-weighted postcontrast coronal image from MR venogram demonstrating chronic IVC occlusion (red arrow), prominent retroperitoneal collateral veins (yellow arrows), and dilated gonadal vein (blue arrow). The distal portion of the IVC is patent and there is proximal tapering of the infrarenal segment. *Courtesy of Dr. Lucia Flors Blasco.*

Figure S109-2 T1-weighted postcontrast axial image with fat suppression demonstrating prominent lumbar venous plexus (red arrow) and left gonadal vein (yellow arrow). *Courtesy of Dr. Lucia Flors Blasco.*

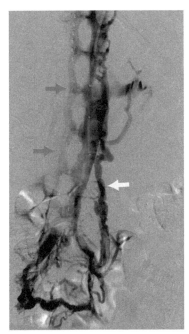

Figure S109-3 Delayed phase venogram image from a different patient demonstrating "stair-stepping" appearance of lumbar venous plexus (red arrows) as shown in Figure S109-2. Dilated gonadal vein noted as well (yellow arrow). *Courtesy of Dr. Minhaj S. Khaja.*

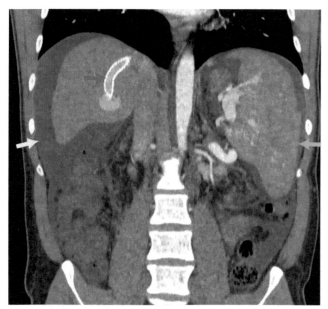

Figure S110-1 Coronal reconstruction from CECT demonstrates a patent TIPS (red arrow), ascites, (yellow arrow), and splenomegaly (blue arrow). *Courtesy of Dr. Minhaj S. Khaja.*

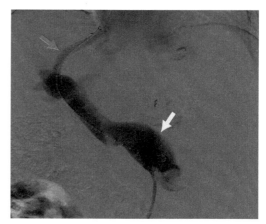

Figure S110-2 DSA image from portography confirming an enlarged splenic vein (yellow arrow) and patent TIPS (red arrow). *Courtesy of Dr. Minhaj S. Khaja.*

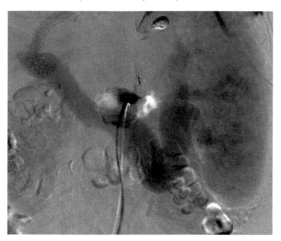

Figure S110-3 DSA image from indirect portogram (delayed phase of celiac angiogram) confirming an enlarged, tortuous splenic vein (red arrow) and splenomegaly. *Courtesy of Dr. Minhaj S. Khaja.*

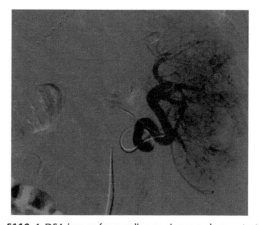

Figure S110-4 DSA image from celiac angiogram demonstrating a tortuous, splenic artery with splenomegaly, prior to embolization. *Courtesy of Dr. Minhaj S. Khaja.*

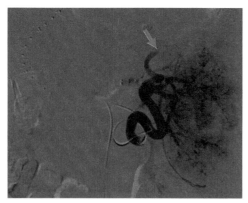

Figure S110-5 DSA image from celiac angiogram postembolization of an upper pole branch (red arrow). *Courtesy of Dr. Minhaj S. Khaja.*

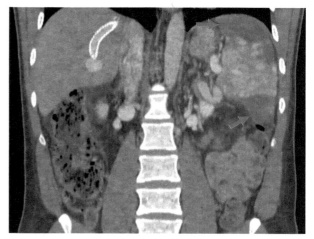

Figure S110-6 Coronal reconstruction from CECT 1 month postembolization revealing regions of infarction within the spleen (red arrows), a patent TIPS, and resolution of ascites. *Courtesy of Dr. Minhaj S. Khaja.*

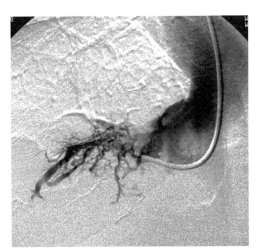

Figure S111-1 DSA image from venogram revealing a spider web-like appearance of the accessory right hepatic vein. *Courtesy of Dr. Daniel Brown.*

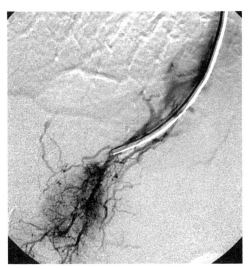

Figure S111-2 DSA image from venogram demonstrating a spider web-like appearance of the main right hepatic vein in the same patient. *Courtesy of Dr. Daniel Brown.*

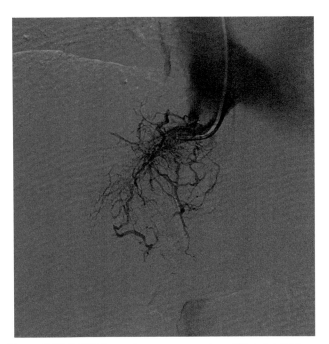

Figure S111-3 DSA image from venogram in a different patient revealing a similar spider-web-like appearance of the right hepatic vein. *Courtesy of Dr. Wael E. Saad.*

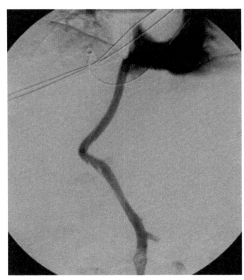

Figure S111-4 DSA image from portogram after TIPS placement in the patient seen in Figure S111-3 confirming a patent TIPS. *Courtesy of Dr. Wael E. Saad.*

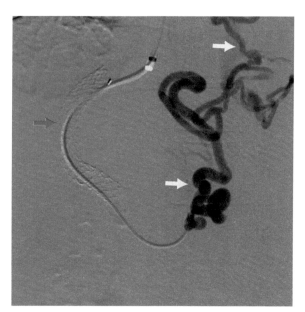

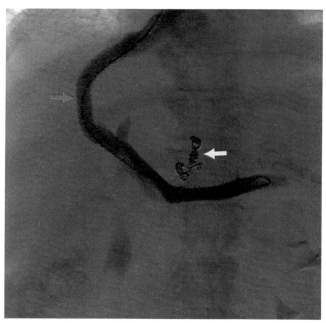

Figure S112-1 Selective DSA image of esophageal varices (yellow arrows) after the placement of a TIPS (red arrow) demonstrates multiple varices. The TIPS was widely patent (not shown). *Courtesy of Dr. Bill S. Majdalany.*

Figure S112-2 Native image from portogram confirming successful coil embolization (yellow arrow) of esophageal varices and a widely patent TIPS (red arrow). *Courtesy of Dr. Bill S. Majdalany.*

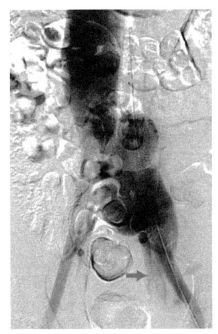

Figure S113-1 DSA image from pelvic aortogram revealing an aortocaval fisutala in conjunction to an aortic pseudoaneurysm. Note the left common iliac vein (red arrow) adjacent to the left common iliac artery (green arrow) as well as the IVC (blue arrow).

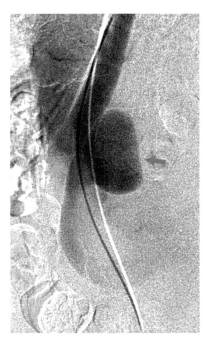

Figure S113-2 Oblique DSA image from pelvic aortogram demonstrating the aortic pseudoaneurysm (red arrow) and early IVC filling from fistulous tract (blue arrow).

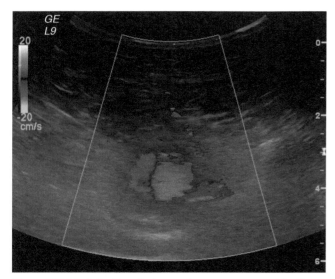

Figure S114-1 Color Doppler image demonstrates to and fro flow within the imaged structure. Given the history, this likely represents the access site pseduoaneurysm. *Courtesy of Dr. Minhaj S. Khaja.*

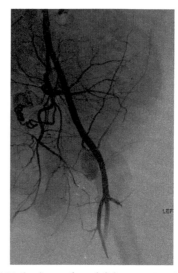

Figure S114-2 Native image from left lower extremity angiogram confirms a pseudoaneurysm (red arrow) extending from the proximal left common femoral artery. *Courtesy of Dr. Minhaj S. Khaja.*

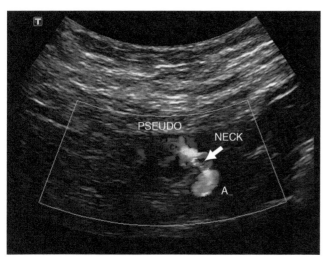

Figure S114-3 Color Doppler image shows the pseudoaneurysm, its neck (arrow), and originating artery. *Courtesy of Dr. Minhaj S. Khaja.*

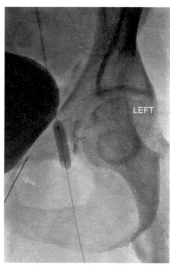

Figure S114-4 Native image from left lower extremity angiogram demonstrates an inflated balloon across the pseudoaneurysm neck (red arrow) and percutaneous access of the pseudoaneurysm (blue arrow) for thrombin injection. *Courtesy of Dr. Minhaj S. Khaja.*

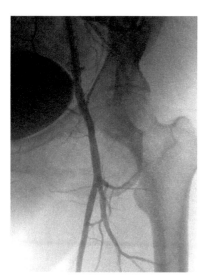

Figure S114-5 Native image from left lower extremity angiogram following balloon-occluded thrombin injection of pseudoaneurysm confirms lack of flow within the pseudoaneurysm. Completion angiogram to the foot did not show evidence of any complication (not shown). *Courtesy of Dr. Minhaj S. Khaja.*

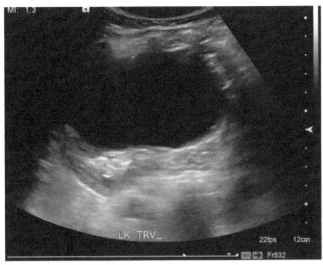

Figure S115-1 Transverse image from gray-scale ultrasound of the left kidney revealing a large, anechoic structure, found to be an isolated renal cyst. *Courtesy of Dr. Ranjith Vellody.*

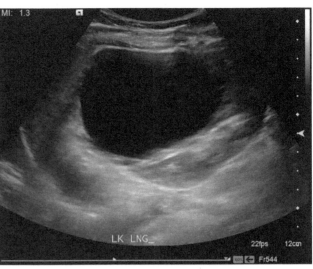

Figure S115-2 Sagittal image from gray-scale ultrasound of the left kidney confirming the isolated renal cyst. *Courtesy of Dr. Ranjith Vellody.*

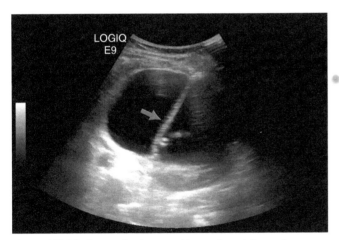

Figure S115-3 Gray-scale ultrasound image from intervention showing the tube (red arrow) within the renal cyst after placement. *Courtesy of Dr. Ranjith Vellody.*

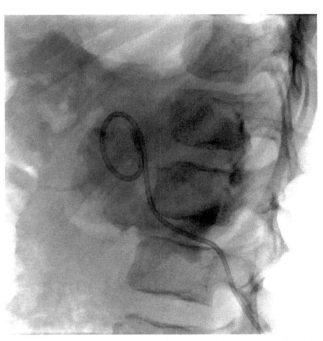

Figure S115-4 Fluoroscopic image from drain placement confirming its position. *Courtesy of Dr. Ranjith Vellody.*

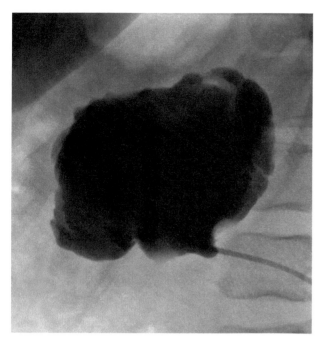

Figure S115-5 Fluoroscopic image from cyst sclerosis with contrast measuring the volume. This was followed by ethanol once the contrast was removed. *Courtesy of Dr. Ranjith Vellody.*

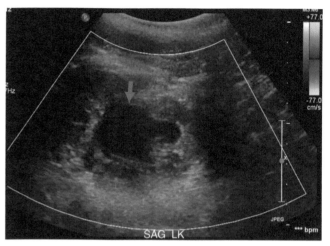

Figure S115-6 Color Doppler image of the left kidney 1 month following aspiration demonstrating a significantly smaller renal cyst (red arrow). *Courtesy of Dr. Ranjith Vellody.*

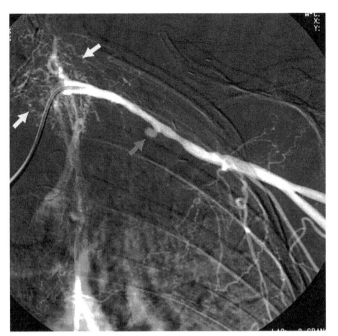

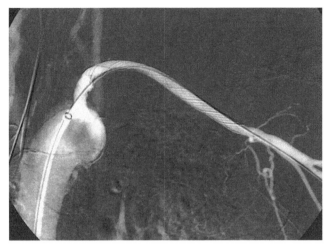

Figure S116-1 DSA image from left upper extremity angiogram revealing a small pseudoaneurysm arising from the left subclavian-axillary artery (red arrow). Also noted is hypervascularity along the base of the neck (yellow arrows), consistent with patient's metastatic disease.

Figure S116-2 DSA image following stent graft placement in the subclavian and axillary arteries with exclusion of the pseudoaneurysm.

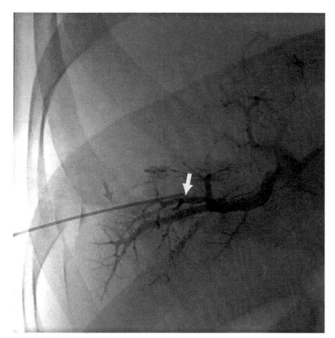

Figure S117-1 Fluoroscopic image from transhepatic portal vein access showing needle (red arrow) and portal vein access (yellow arrow). *Courtesy of Dr. Wael E. Saad.*

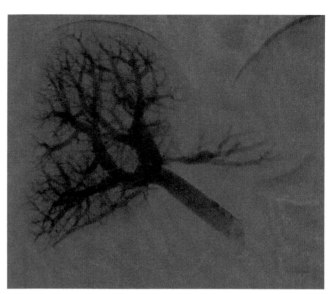

Figure S117-2 DSA image from portogram revealing the portal venous system and its distal radicals. Direct portal pressure was 5 mm Hg in this patient. *Courtesy of Dr. Wael E. Saad.*

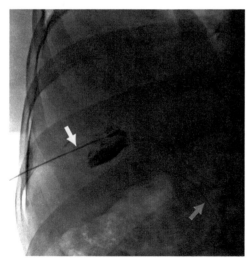

Figure S117-3 Fluoroscopic image after wire passage. The wire (red arrow) is seen conforming to the portal venous system. Needle also noted (yellow arrow). A small region of contrast noted with the parenchyma. *Courtesy of Dr. Wael E. Saad.*

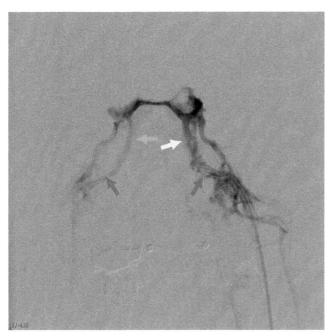

Figure S118-1 DSA image from venogram with catheters positioned in the bilateral inferior petrosal sinuses (red arrows). Contrast is injected into the left IPS (yellow arrow), fills the ipsilateral cavernous sinus and superior petrosal sinus, and refluxes into the contralateral IPS (blue arrow) and SPS. *Courtesy of Dr. J. Fritz Angle.*

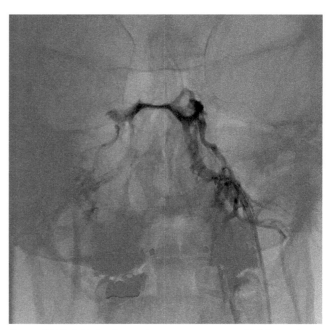

Figure S118-2 Native image from same venogram highlights the relative position of the sinuses to osseous landmarks. *Courtesy of Dr. J. Fritz Angle.*

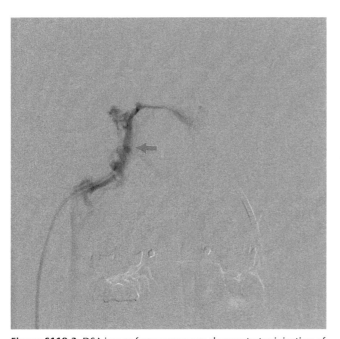

Figure S118-3 DSA image from venogram demonstrates injection of contrast into the right IPS (red arrow) with filling of the ipsilateral cavernous sinus. *Courtesy of Dr. J. Fritz Angle.*

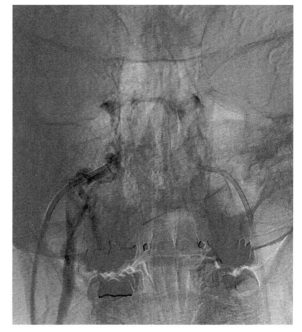

Figure S118-4 Native image from same venogram highlights the relative position of the sinuses to osseous landmarks. *Courtesy of Dr. J. Fritz Angle.*

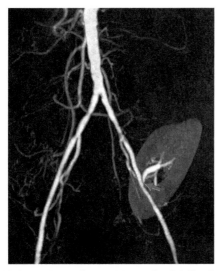

Figure S119-1 MIP image from MRA reveals a left iliac fossa renal transplant with a focal stenosis of the transplant renal artery at the site of anastomosis between the donor renal artery and the recipient left external iliac artery (red arrow). *Courtesy of Dr. Narasimham L. Dasika.*

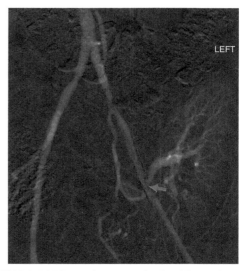

Figure S119-2 DSA image from nonselective CO_2 angiography confirms the stenosis of the transplant renal artery as seen on MRA (red arrow). *Courtesy of Dr. Narasimham L. Dasika.*

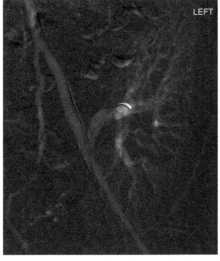

Figure S119-3 DSA image from selective CO_2 angiography redemonstrates the anastomotic stenosis. *Courtesy of Dr. Narasimham L. Dasika.*

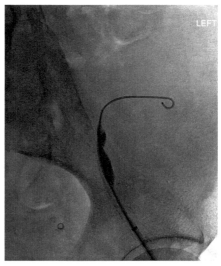

Figure S119-4 Intraprocedural fluoroscopic image reveals a "waist" on the balloon at the site of stenosis. *Courtesy of Dr. Narasimham L. Dasika.*

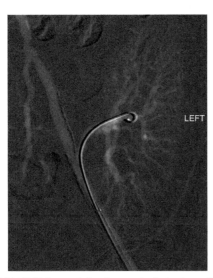

Figure S119-5 DSA image following angioplasty shows improved flow through the site of stenosis. *Courtesy of Dr. Narasimham L. Dasika.*

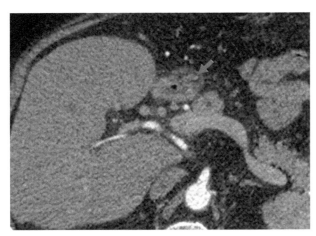

Figure S120-1 Axial image from CTA revealing a region of hyperdensity within the second portion of the duodenum (red arrow). *Courtesy of Dr. Minhaj S. Khaja.*

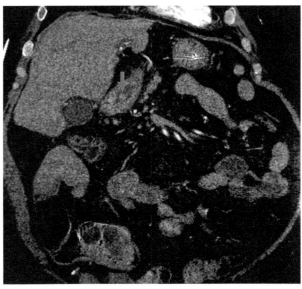

Figure S120-2 Coronal reconstruction from CTA demonstrating the same region of hyperdensity in the duodenum (red arrow). *Courtesy of Dr. Minhaj S. Khaja.*

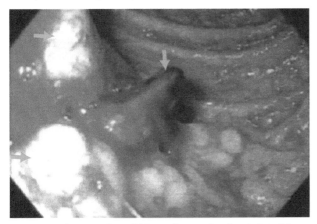

Figure S120-3 Image from EGD confirms a duodenal ulcer (blue arrows) with a visible vessel and active bleeding (green arrow). *Courtesy of Dr. Minhaj S. Khaja.*

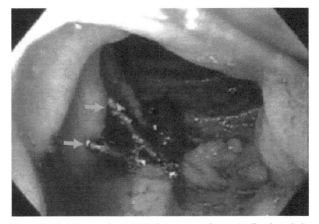

Figure S120-4 Image from EGD showing endoscopically placed clips at the site of bleeding (blue arrows), which may aid in directed embolization. *Courtesy of Dr. Minhaj S. Khaja.*

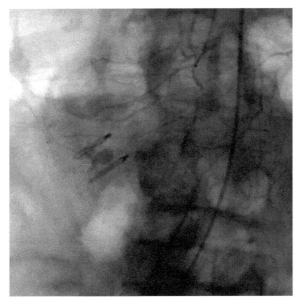

Figure S120-5 Native image from angiography highlighting the site of bleeding (red arrow), centered between the endoscopically placed clips, arising from branches of the pancreaticoduodenal arcade. *Courtesy of Dr. Minhaj S. Khaja.*

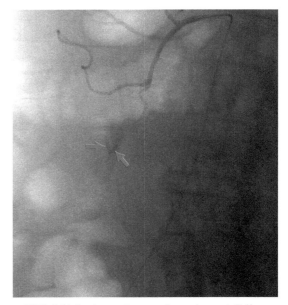

Figure S120-6 Native image from angiography post-Gelfoam embolization with no further evidence of bleeding adjacent to the clips (red arrows). *Courtesy of Dr. Minhaj S. Khaja.*

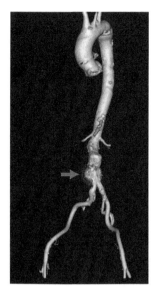

Figure S121-1 VR image from CTA revealing a multilobular infrarenal abdominal aortic aneurysm (red arrow). *Courtesy of Dr. John E. Rectenwald.*

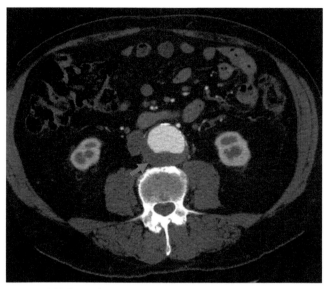

Figure S121-2 Axial image from CTA demonstrating the AAA with mural thrombus (red arrow). *Courtesy of Dr. John E. Rectenwald.*

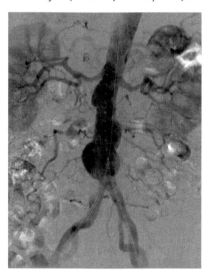

Figure S121-3 DSA image from aortogram confirming multilobular AAA. *Courtesy of Dr. John E. Rectenwald.*

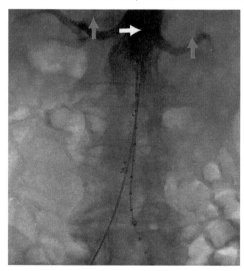

Figure S121-4 DSA image from aortogram showing the renal artery origins (red arrows). The main body of the stent graft is undeployed but in position (yellow arrow). *Courtesy of Dr. John E. Rectenwald.*

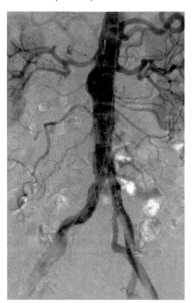

Figure S121-5 DSA image from aortogram postdeployment of main body and contralateral limb demonstrating exclusion of the aneurysm with no endoleak seen. *Courtesy of Dr. John E. Rectenwald.*

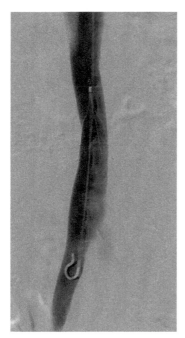

Figure S122-1 DSA image from inferior cavagram demonstrating a Gunther Tulip IVC filter in place. No thrombus is seen within the filter. *Courtesy of Dr. Minhaj S. Khaja.*

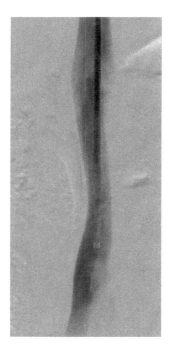

Figure S122-2 DSA image from inferior cavagram after retrieval of the IVC filter confirming there is no caval injury. *Courtesy of Dr. Minhaj S. Khaja.*

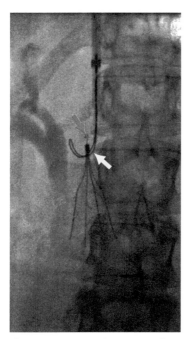

Figure S122-3 Fluoroscopic image from retrieval via right IJ access showing the snare (yellow arrow) just beyond the hook of the filter (red arrow). *Courtesy of Dr. Minhaj S. Khaja.*

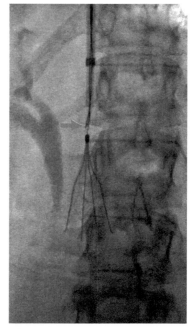

Figure S122-4 Fluoroscopic image from retrieval showing the snare tightly cinched around the hook of the filter (red arrow). *Courtesy of Dr. Minhaj S. Khaja.*

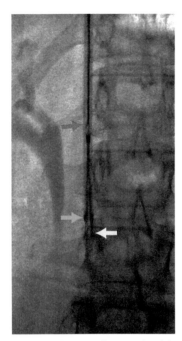

Figure S122-5 Fluoroscopic image from retrieval demonstrating retraction of the filter with snare around the hook (red arrow). The filter struts (red arrowhead) are just distal to the tip of the sheath (blue arrow). *Courtesy of Dr. Minhaj S. Khaja.*

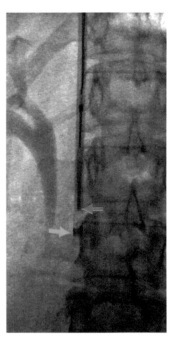

Figure S122-6 Fluoroscopic image from retrieval showing further retraction of the filter. The filter struts (red arrow) are now within the sheath (blue arrow). *Courtesy of Dr. Minhaj S. Khaja.*

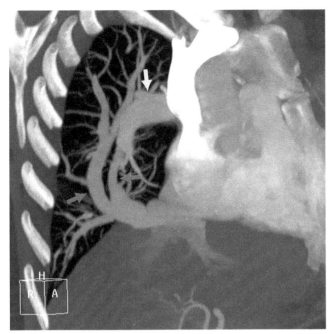

Figure S123-1 MIP oblique image from CT pulmonary angiogram (CTPA) revealing two right lower lobe pulmonary veins (red arrows) coming together and draining into the most cephalad portion of the IVC. The right pulmonary artery is also noted (yellow arrow). This configuration is consistent with infracardiac PAPVR. *Courtesy of Dr. Wael E. Saad.*

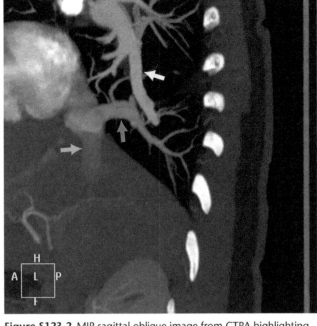

Figure S123-2 MIP sagittal oblique image from CTPA highlighting the anomalous pulmonary vein (red arrow) as it drains into the IVC (blue arrow). Again noted is the adjacent pulmonary artery (yellow arrow). *Courtesy of Dr. Wael E. Saad.*

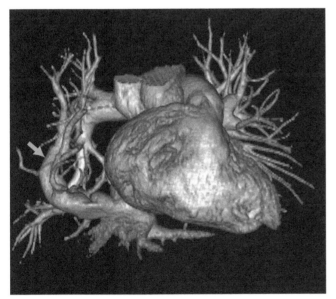

Figure S123-3 3D VR image from the same patient as in Figures S123-1 and S123-2 showing the anomalous pulmonary vein (blue arrow) drain into the IVC. *Courtesy of Dr. Wael E. Saad.*

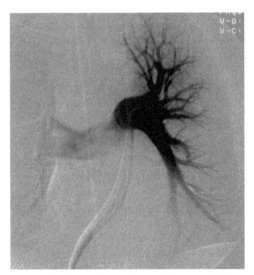

Figure S123-4 DSA image from early arterial phase of left pulmonary angiogram in a different patient, which is unremarkable. *Courtesy of Dr. Wael E. Saad.*

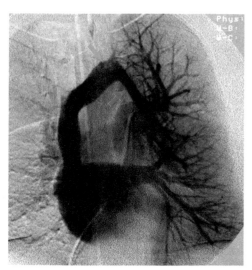

Figure S123-5 DSA image from late venous phase of pulmonary angiogram revealing an anomalous pulmonary vein (red arrow) draining into the left brachiocephalic vein (blue arrow). This configuration is consistent with supracardiac PAPVR. *Courtesy of Dr. Wael E. Saad.*

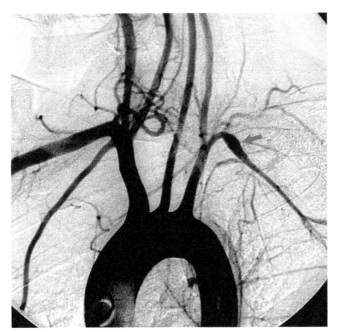

Figure S124-1 DSA image from thoracic aortogram revealing smooth narrowing of the left subclavian artery (blue arrow). Also noted is a mildly dilated proximal subclavian artery (red arrow). *Courtesy of Dr. Daniel Brown.*

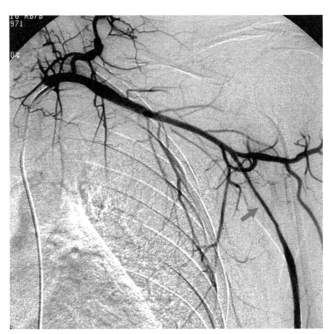

Figure S124-2 DSA image from left upper extremity angiogram demonstrating a smooth, elongated stenosis of the left axillary artery (red arrow). *Courtesy of Dr. Daniel Brown.*

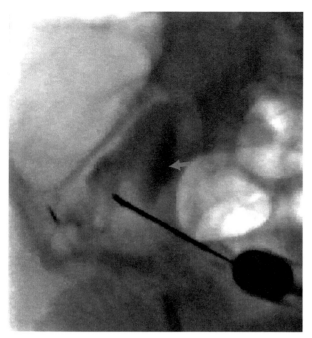

Figure S125-1 Intraprocedure fluoroscopic image showing percutaneous access of the cecum. Contrast is injected to confirm access (red arrow). *Courtesy of Dr. Ranjith Vellody.*

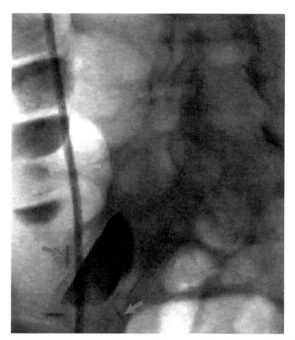

Figure S125-2 Fluoroscopic image demonstrating elongated Chait Trapdoor catheter with stiffener (blue arrow). Note the retention sutures affixing the cecum to the abdominal wall (red arrows). *Courtesy of Dr. Ranjith Vellody.*

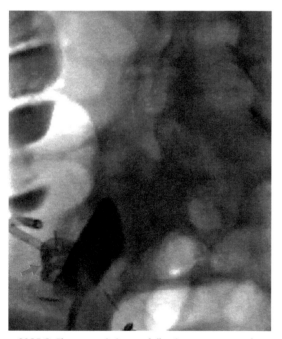

Figure S125-3 Fluoroscopic image following cecostomy placement illustrating coiled Chait Trapdoor catheter in the cecum (red arrow). *Courtesy of Dr. Ranjith Vellody.*

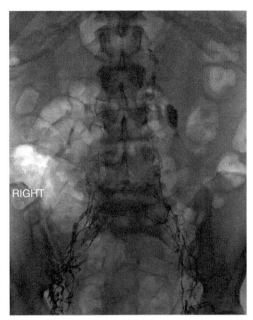

Figure S126-1 Radiograph of the pelvis during lymphangiogram demonstrating appropriate pelvic drainage. This drainage will provide the roadmap for cannulation of the cisterna chyli. *Courtesy of Dr. Bill S. Majdalany.*

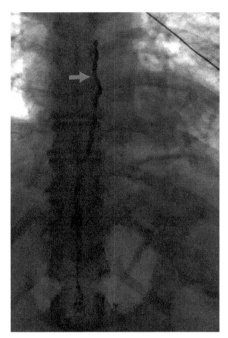

Figure S126-2 Fluoroscopic image of the chest showing coiling (red arrow) of the thoracic duct with residual contrast material opacifying the distal lymphatic drainage. *Courtesy of Dr. Bill S. Majdalany.*

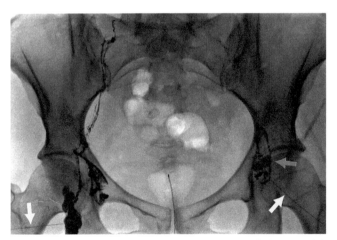

Figure S126-3 Pelvic radiograph during slow, controlled intranodal injection of lipiodol. Access needles (yellow arrows) and lymph nodes (red arrows) are shown. *Courtesy of Dr. Bill S. Majdalany.*

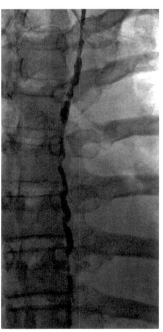

Figure S126-4 Fluoroscopic image of the chest revealing the opacified thoracic duct. *Courtesy of Dr. Bill S. Majdalany.*

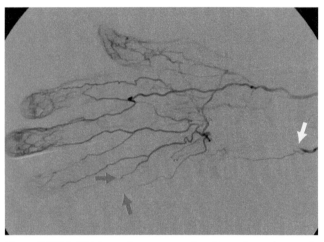

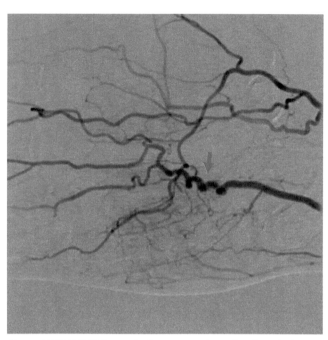

Figure S127-1 DSA image from upper extremity angiography reveals the absence of the ulnar artery at the wrist (yellow arrow). Digital artery occlusion is present in the fifth digit (red arrows).

Figure S127-2 DSA image in the same patient after thrombolysis demonstrates the classic corkscrew appearance of the ulnar artery at the site of repeated trauma to the vessel (red arrow).

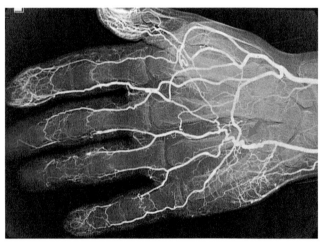

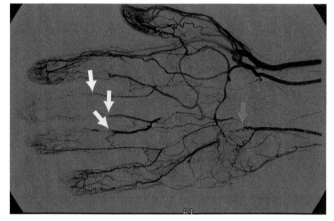

Figure S127-3 DSA image of the hand in a different patient shows the similar corkscrew pattern of the ulnar artery (red arrow). *Courtesy of Dr. Narasimham L. Dasika.*

Figure S127-4 DSA image of the hand in another different patient shows the similar corkscrew pattern of the ulnar artery (red arrow) with downstream occlusions in the third and fourth digits (yellow arrows). *Courtesy of Dr. Narasimham L. Dasika.*

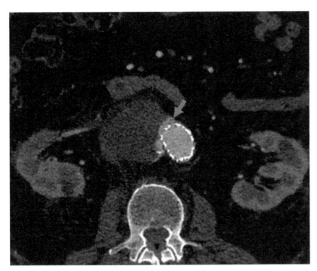

Figure S128-1 Axial image from CTA reveals extraluminal contrast, within the aneurysm sac at the rostral extent of the stent graft (red arrow). The aneurysm sac is mostly thrombosed. *Courtesy of Dr. Alan H. Matsumoto.*

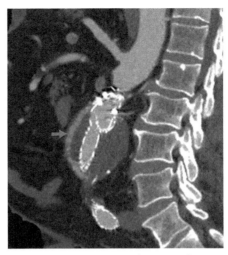

Figure S128-2 Sagittal reconstruction from CTA shows extraluminal contrast along the anterior margin of the aneurysm sac (red arrow). *Courtesy of Dr. Alan H. Matsumoto.*

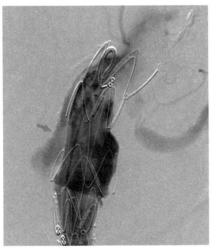

Figure S128-3 DSA image from aortogram in a different patient confirming a type IA endoleak (red arrow). *Courtesy of Dr. Alan H. Matsumoto.*

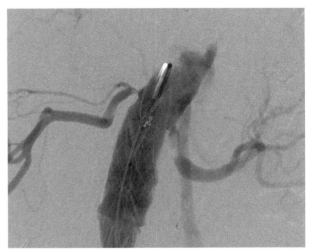

Figure S128-4 DSA image from aortogram after endoleak exclusion with a balloon-expandable stent at the rostral end of the stent graft. *Courtesy of Dr. Alan H. Matsumoto.*

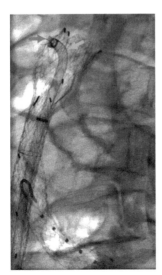

Figure S128-5 Fluoroscopic image from endoleak repair in a different patient demonstrating fixation of the endograft to the aorta using helical anchors (Aptus Endosystems, Sunnyvale, California). The anchor (red arrow) is shown being placed by the deployment guide (blue arrow). *Courtesy of Dr. John E. Rectenwald.*

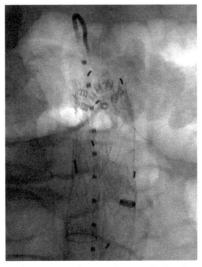

Figure S128-6 Fluoroscopic image after repair showing eight helical anchors placed circumferentially at the proximal seal zone of the endograft. *Courtesy of Dr. John E. Rectenwald.*

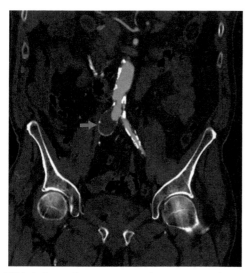

Figure S129-1 Coronal reconstruction from CTA reveals a calcified abdominal aorta with a completely occluded and aneurysmal right common iliac artery (red arrow). *Courtesy of Dr. Luke R. Wilkins.*

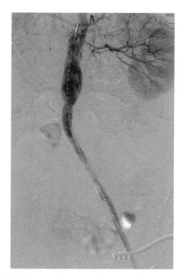

Figure S129-2 DSA image from aortogram demonstrates placement of an aorto-uniiliac graft with nonopacification of the right common iliac artery. *Courtesy of Dr. Luke R. Wilkins.*

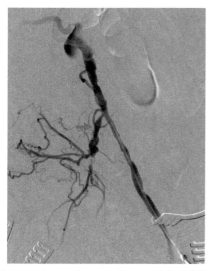

Figure S129-3 DSA image from angiogram of the left iliac arteries demonstrates a patent left internal iliac artery with ectatic region (red arrow). *Courtesy of Dr. Luke R. Wilkins.*

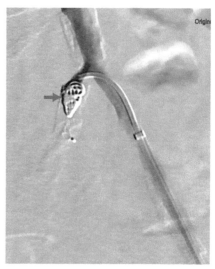

Figure S129-4 DSA image from repeat angiogram following catheter guided placement of embolization coils into the left internal iliac artery (red arrow). *Courtesy of Dr. Luke R. Wilkins.*

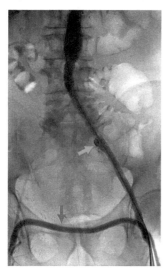

Figure S129-5 Native image from angiogram of the abdominal aorta demonstrates placement of an aorto-uniiliac endograft, coil embolization of the ipsilateral internal iliac artery (blue arrow), and placement of a femorofemoral bypass graft (red arrow). *Courtesy of Dr. Luke R. Wilkins.*

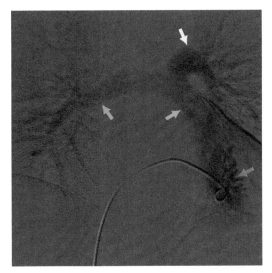

Figure S130-1 DSA image from pulmonary angiogram delineating the right ventricle (red arrow), main pulmonary artery (blue arrow), and the main left (yellow arrow) and right (green arrow) pulmonary arteries. *Courtesy of Dr. Wael E. Saad.*

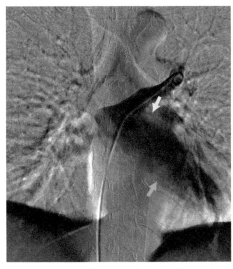

Figure S130-2 DSA image demonstrating the left superior pulmonary vein (red arrow), left atrium (yellow arrow), and left ventricle (blue arrow). *Courtesy of Dr. Wael E. Saad.*

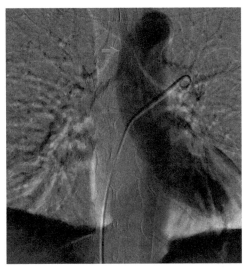

Figure S130-3 DSA image later in the injection showing the thoracic aorta (red arrow). *Courtesy of Dr. Wael E. Saad.*

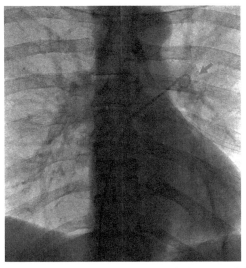

Figure S130-4 Fluoroscopic image showing the location of the catheter, projecting directly over the left pulmonary artery (red arrow). Its true location was found to be in the superior pulmonary vein as seen in Figure S130-2. *Courtesy of Dr. Wael E. Saad.*

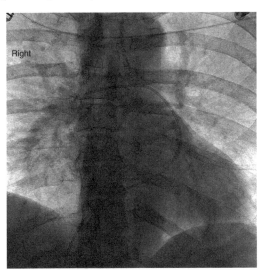

Figure S130-5 Fluoroscopic image showing the expected location of the right pulmonary artery. Subsequent images demonstrated normal right pulmonary arterial anatomy (not shown). *Courtesy of Dr. Wael E. Saad.*

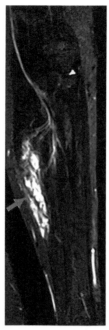

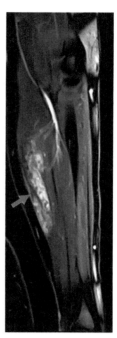

Figure S131-1 Sagittal T2-weighted image with fat-saturation of the upper extremity reveals a lobulated, septated mass with fairly homogeneous high-intensity signal in the soft tissues of the ventral left forearm (red arrow). *Courtesy of Dr. Auh Whan Park.*

Figure S131-2 Sagittal contrast-enhanced T1-weighted image demonstrates the same venous channels in the left forearm (red arrow). *Courtesy of Dr. Auh Whan Park.*

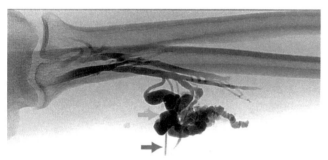

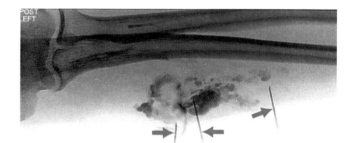

Figure S131-3 Intraprocedural fluoroscopic image confirming the extensive soft tissue venous malformation (blue arrow). A direct needle access is noted (red arrow). *Courtesy of Dr. Auh Whan Park.*

Figure S131-4 Fluoroscopic image after sclerotherapy shows stagnant contrast within the lesion. Multiple needles are noted (red arrows). *Courtesy of Dr. Auh Whan Park.*

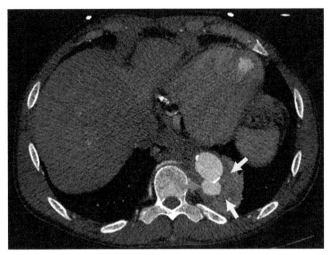

Figure S132-1 Axial image from CTA revealing an aortic pseudoaneurysm located on the posterior wall of the thoracic aorta (red arrow) with adjacent fluid (yellow arrows). *Courtesy of Dr. David M. Williams.*

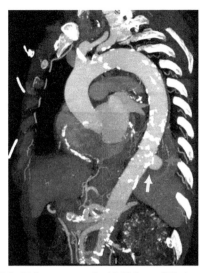

Figure S132-2 Oblique parasagittal MIP from CTA demonstrating the pseudoaneurysm (red arrow) which is surrounded by fluid (yellow arrow). *Courtesy of Dr. David M. Williams.*

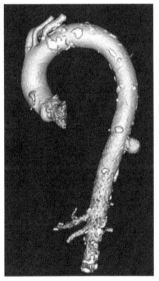

Figure S132-3 3D reconstruction of the thoracic aorta demonstrating the pseudoaneurysm arising from the posterior wall. There is a lack of calcification surrounding the pseudoaneurysm. *Courtesy of Dr. David M. Williams.*

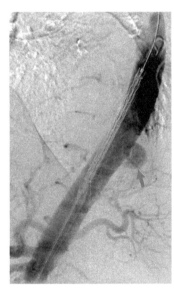

Figure S132-4 DSA image from thoracic aortogram showing the pseudoaneurysm (red arrow) with undeployed stent graft in place (blue arrow). *Courtesy of Dr. David M. Williams.*

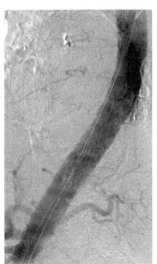

Figure S132-5 DSA image after the deployment of the stent graft confirming exclusion of the pseudoaneurysm. *Courtesy of Dr. David M. Williams.*

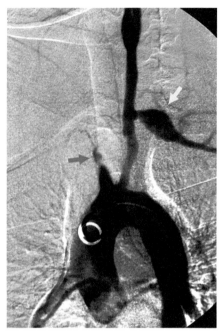

Figure S133-1 DSA image from thoracic aortogram reveals a focal narrowing near the ostium of the brachiocephalic artery (red arrow). There is also evidence of prior bypass from the left common carotid artery (yellow arrow).

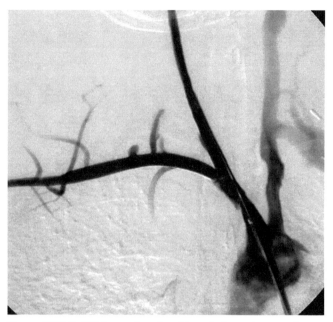

Figure S133-2 DSA image from brachiocephalic angiogram after stent placement shows patency of the brachiocephalic, right common carotid, and right subclavian arteries, respectively.

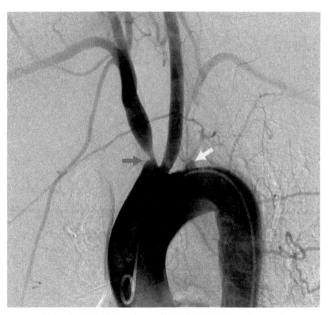

Figure S133-3 DSA image from thoracic aortogram in a different patient demonstrates significant narrowing at the ostium of the brachiocephalic (red arrow) and subclavian (yellow arrow) arteries, respectively. Note that the patient has a common origin of the brachiocephalic artery and left common carotid artery as well.

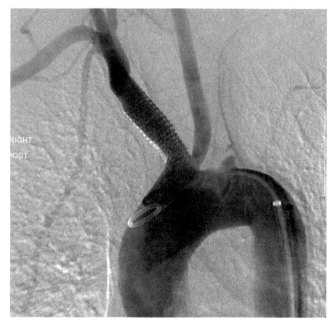

Figure S133-4 DSA image from aortogram following brachiocephalic artery stent placement with widely patent stent. The left subclavian artery was not treated at this time.

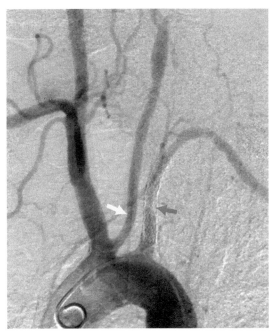

Figure S134-1 DSA image from thoracic aortography revealing stenosis within the left subclavian artery stent (red arrow). Additionally noted is a common origin of the left common carotid and brachiocephalic arteries (yellow arrow). *Courtesy of Dr. Wael E. Saad.*

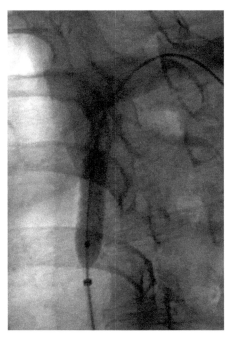

Figure S134-2 Intraprocedural fluoroscopic image showing balloon angioplasty of the lesion. *Courtesy of Dr. Wael E. Saad.*

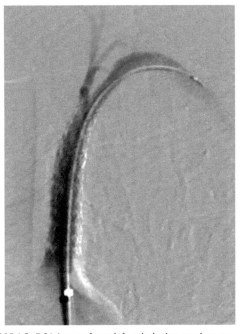

Figure S134-3 DSA image from left subclavian angiogram demonstrating a widely patent stent after angioplasty. *Courtesy of Dr. Wael E. Saad.*

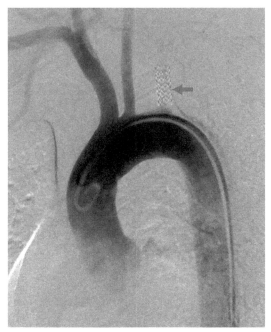

Figure S134-4 DSA image from thoracic aortography in a different patient illustrating occlusion of the left subclavian artery stent (red arrow). *Courtesy of Dr. Wael E. Saad.*

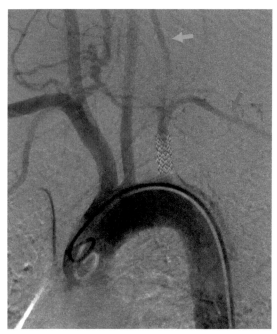

Figure S134-5 DSA image later in the aortogram revealing retrograde filling of the left subclavian artery (red arrow) via the left vertebral artery (blue arrow). *Courtesy of Dr. Wael E. Saad.*

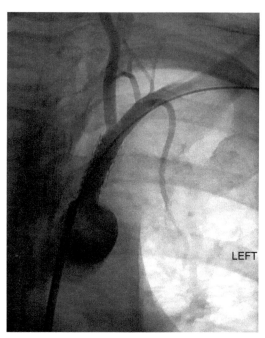

Figure S134-6 Native image from left subclavian angiogram following angioplasty showing a patent left subclavian artery stent. *Courtesy of Dr. Wael E. Saad.*

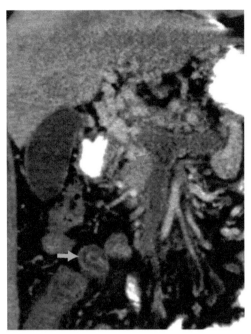

Figure S135-1 Coronal reconstruction from CECT reveals thrombosis of the portomesenteric veins (red arrow) with edema of the small bowel (blue arrow). *Courtesy of Dr. Wael E. Saad.*

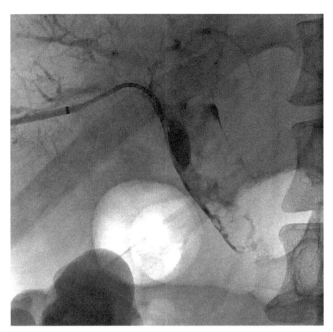

Figure S135-2 Native image from transhepatic portogram confirming extensive clot within the portal veins. *Courtesy of Dr. Wael E. Saad.*

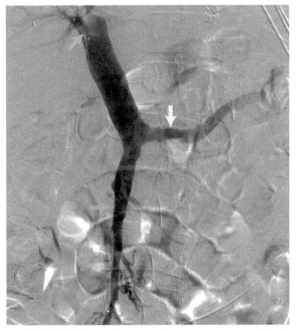

Figure S135-3 DSA image from transhepatic portogram following thrombolysis illustrates a significant improvement in patency of the main portal vein (red arrow), SMV (green arrow), and splenic vein (yellow arrow) with some residual clot at the portal vein bifurcation (blue arrow). *Courtesy of Dr. Wael E. Saad.*

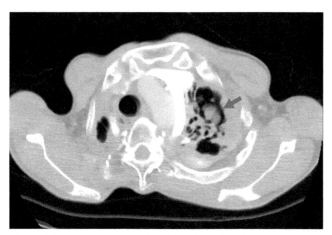

Figure S136-1 Pretreatment CT of the chest showing extensive bronchiectasis in the left upper lobe with pleural thickening and an anterior cavitation with internal solid mass (arrow) representing a mycetoma.

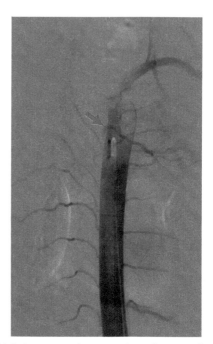

Figure S136-2 Aortogram demonstrating a hypertrophied, tortuous left bronchial artery (arrow).

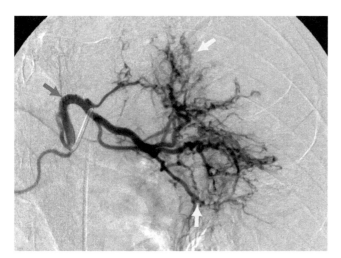

Figure S136-3 Selective bronchial arteriography redemonstrating the enlarged left bronchial artery (red arrow) with corkscrew appearance of the distal branches (yellow arrows).

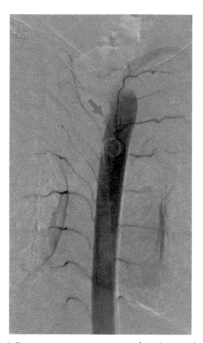

Figure S136-4 Posttreatment aortogram showing occlusion of the left bronchial artery (arrow demarcating origin).

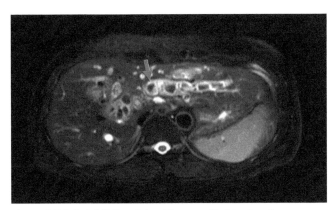

Figure S137-1 Axial T2-weighted image with fat saturation demonstrates a dilated bile duct with low-intensity filling defects consistent with stones (red arrow). *Courtesy of Dr. Narasimham L. Dasika.*

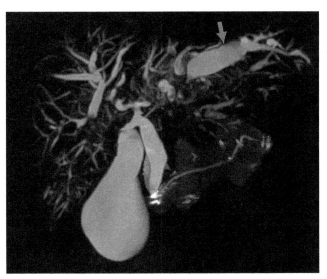

Figure S137-2 3D MIP from an MRCP shows a dilated left biliary system (red arrow) with nonvisualization of the central ducts due to obstructing stones. *Courtesy of Dr. Narasimham L. Dasika.*

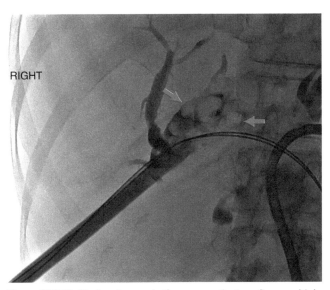

Figure S137-3 Cholangiogram in the same patient confirms multiple lucent filling defects within the biliary tree (red arrows). Again, the right biliary system is not well visualized. *Courtesy of Dr. Narasimham L. Dasika.*

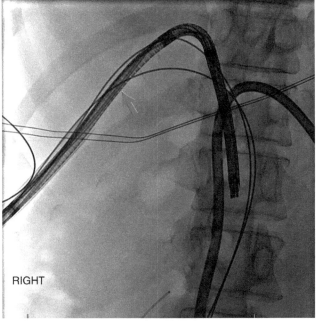

Figure S137-4 Fluoroscopic image demonstrates insertion of a choledochoscope (red arrow) into the biliary tree for removal of stones. *Courtesy of Dr. Narasimham L. Dasika.*

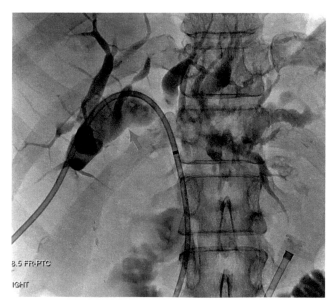

Figure S137-5 Cholangiogram 1 month after stone removal shows persistent biliary ductal dilation, but previously seen stones on the right are not present (red arrow). *Courtesy of Dr. Narasimham L. Dasika.*

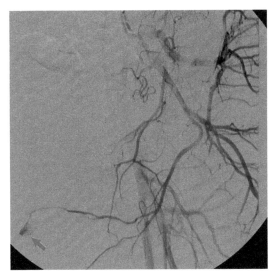

Figure S138-1 Oblique DSA image from left internal iliac artery angiogram revealing an early blush in the corpus cavernosum (red arrow). *Courtesy of Dr. Narasimham L. Dasika.*

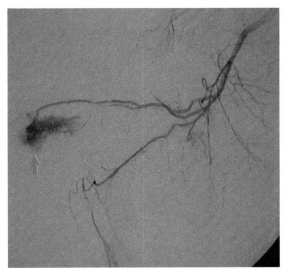

Figure S138-2 DSA image from selective angiogram of left internal pudendal artery confirming extensive blush in the corpus cavernosum (red arrow), primarily extending from the dorsal penile artery. *Courtesy of Dr. Narasimham L. Dasika.*

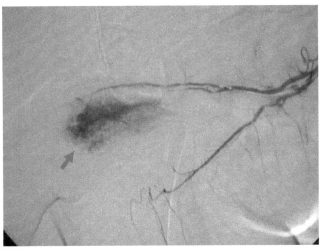

Figure S138-3 DSA image from selective proper penile artery injection redemonstrating the arterial-cavernosal shunt prior to embolization (red arrow). *Courtesy of Dr. Narasimham L. Dasika.*

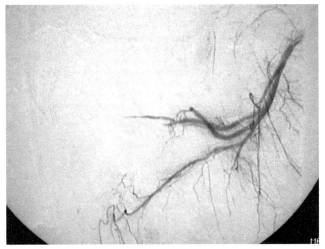

Figure S138-4 DSA image from selective left internal pudendal artery injection following embolization highlighting cessation of flow through the previously seen shunt. *Courtesy of Dr. Narasimham L. Dasika.*

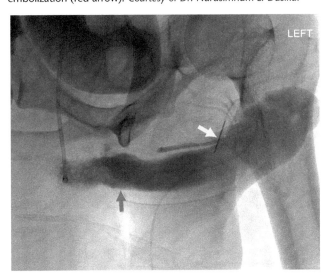

Figure S138-5 Native oblique image from direct contrast injection (yellow arrow) of the corpus cavernosum in a different patient revealing pooling of contrast within the corpus cavernosum (red arrow) suggesting low-flow priapism. *Courtesy of Dr. Narasimham L. Dasika.*

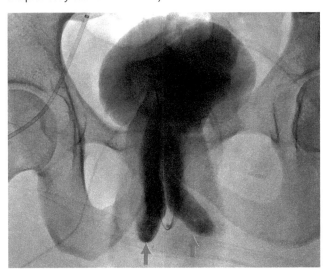

Figure S138-6 Native frontal image from direct contrast injection of the corpus cavernosum in the same patient as in Figure S138-5 highlighting pooling of contrast within the corpora cavernosa (red arrows) suggesting low-flow priapism. *Courtesy of Dr. Narasimham L. Dasika.*

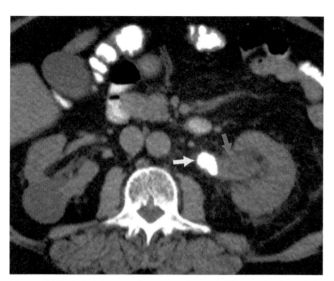

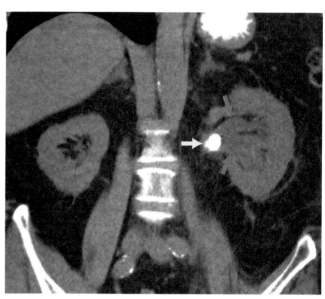

Figure S139-1 Axial image from unenhanced CT reveals a large left ureteropelvic junction (UPJ) calculus (yellow arrow) with dilation of the renal collecting system (red arrow).

Figure S139-2 Coronal reconstruction from CT shows large UPJ stone (yellow arrow) with dilated renal collecting system (red arrows).

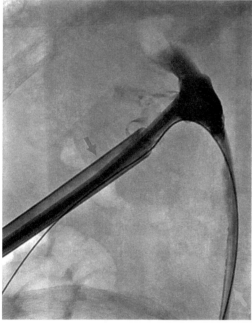

Figure S139-3 Intraoperative radiograph from percutaneous nephrolithotomy procedure demonstrates a large sheath (red arrow) in place with a wire in the ureter (blue arrow).

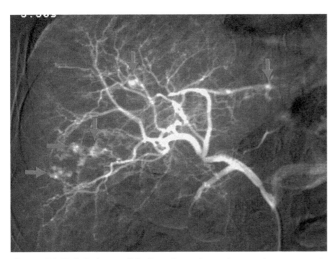

Figure S140-1 Early arterial-phase hepatic angiogram image reveals multiple foci of dense, discrete, nodular contrast opacification, scattered throughout the hepatic parenchyma (red arrows).

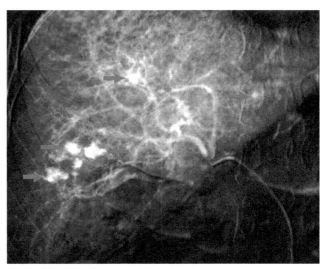

Figure S140-2 Late arterial/hepatic parenchymal-phase angiogram image demonstrates progressive centripetal contrast fill-in of the aforementioned lesions (red arrows).

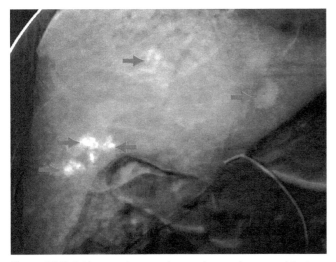

Figure S140-3 Venous-phase angiogram image shows persistent contrast opacification of lesions (red arrows).

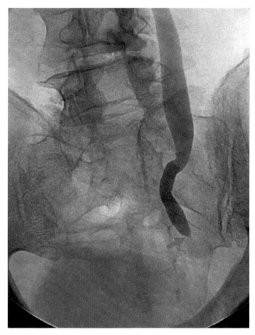

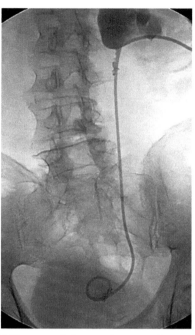

Figure S141-1 Fluoroscopic image from antegrade pyelogram reveals a tight stricture of the left ureter at the ureterovesical junction (red arrow), with consequent hydroureter. No filling defect is outlined.

Figure S141-2 Fluoroscopic image after stent placement shows that the stricture was successfully crossed, nephroureteral stent was placed, and the stent is function properly (contrast within the bladder).

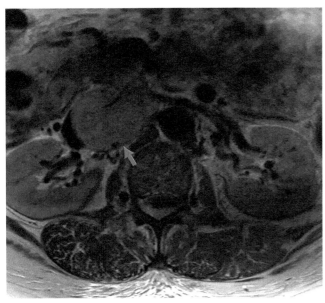

Figure S142-1 Axial T2-weighted MR image reveals a heterogeneous, iso- to hyperintense within and compressing the IVC (red arrow). *Courtesy of Dr. Wael E. Saad.*

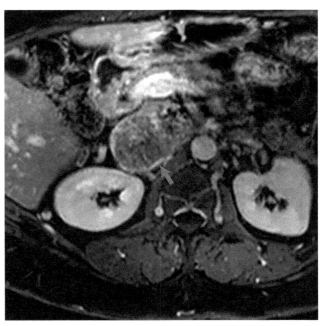

Figure S142-2 Axial contrast-enhanced T1-weighted MR image with fat-saturation demonstrates a heterogeneously enhancing mass within and compressing the IVC (red arrow). There was no mass seen within the kidneys (not shown). *Courtesy of Dr. Wael E. Saad.*

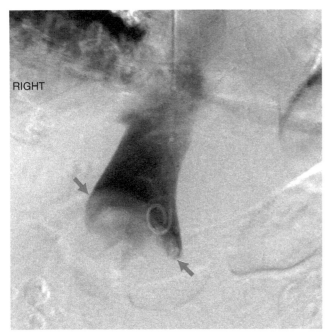

RIGHT

Figure S142-3 DSA image from cavagram confirms a large, lobulated filling defect within the IVC (red arrows). *Courtesy of Dr. Wael E. Saad.*

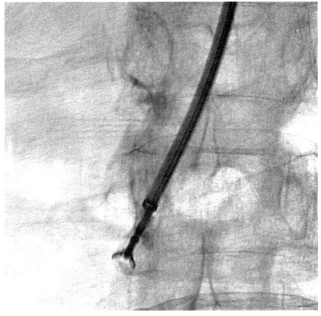

Figure S142-4 Intraprocedural fluoroscopic image shows the opening of biopsy forceps for an endovascular biopsy. *Courtesy of Dr. Wael E. Saad.*

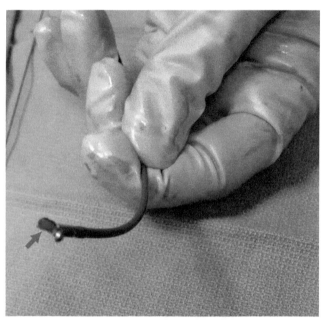

Figure S142-5 Photograph of biopsy forceps confirms tissue within the forceps (blue arrow). Pathology confirmed leiomyosarcoma of the IVC. *Courtesy of Dr. Wael E. Saad.*

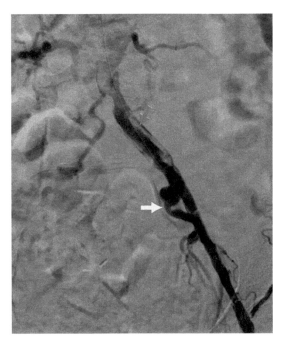

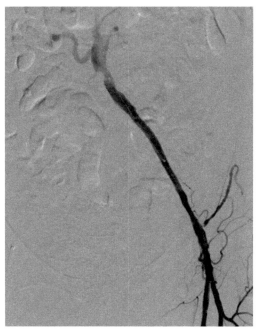

Figure S143-1 DSA image from left lower extremity angiogram reveals a linear defect in the left common iliac artery with differential enhancement on either side, compatible with a dissection, with likely concomitant thrombus (red arrow). The internal iliac artery appears to fill from the true lumen (yellow arrow).

Figure S143-2 DSA image from left lower extremity angiogram following angioplasty and stenting, demonstrating normal LCIA caliber. Note that the left internal iliac artery is no longer visible, suggesting it has been excluded by the treatment. Collateral perfusion via the right internal iliac artery (not shown) should ensure the patient does not experience significant symptoms as a result.

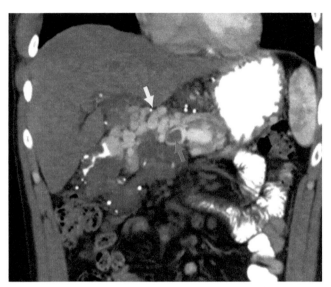

Figure S144-1 Coronal reconstruction from CECT revealing numerous venous collaterals in the porta hepatis seen during the portal venous phase (yellow arrow). Also noted is a thrombus in the main portal vein (red arrow). *Courtesy of Dr. Wael E. Saad.*

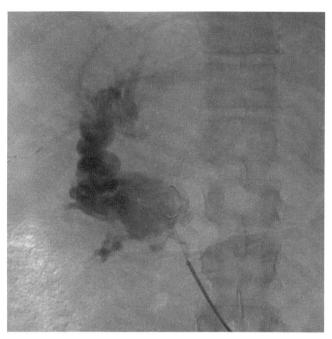

Figure S144-2 Native image from portogram via surgical cutdown and direct SMV access confirms serpiginous collateral veins in the porta hepatis. *Courtesy of Dr. Wael E. Saad.*

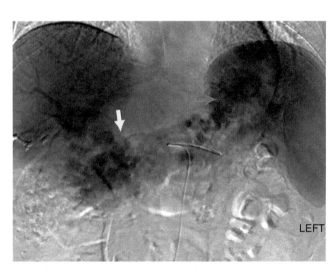

Figure S144-3 Portal venous phase DSA image from splenic angiogram in the same patient shows tortuous collateral veins in the porta hepatis (yellow arrow) and the splenic hilum (red arrow). *Courtesy of Dr. Wael E. Saad.*

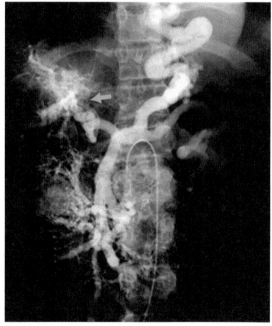

Figure S144-4 Portal venous phase image from angiogram in a different patient reveals cavernous transformation of the portal vein (blue arrowhead) with a severely dilated gastroesophageal varix (red arrow). *Courtesy of Dr. Wael E. Saad.*

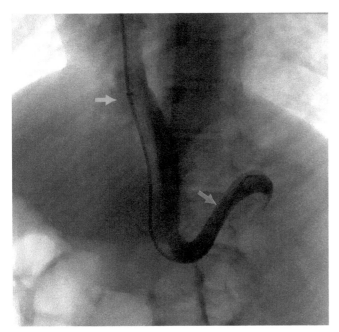

Figure S145-1 Native image from splenic venography via transjugular access revealing splenic vein (red arrow) drainage into the IVC (blue arrow) without evidence of a portal vein. *Courtesy of Dr. Ranjith Vellody.*

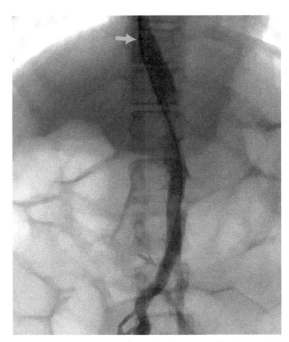

Figure S145-2 Native image from SMV venography via transjugular access showing SMV (red arrow) drainage into the IVC (blue arrow) without evidence of a portal vein. *Courtesy of Dr. Ranjith Vellody.*

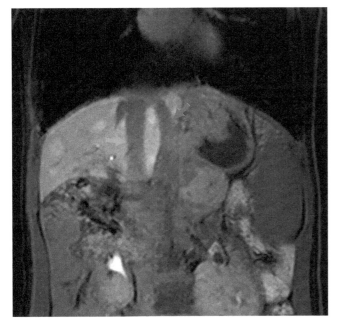

Figure S145-3 Coronal image from contrast-enhanced MRI showing the IVC (blue arrow) and common drainage pathway of SMV and splenic vein (red arrow). *Courtesy of Dr. Ranjith Vellody.*

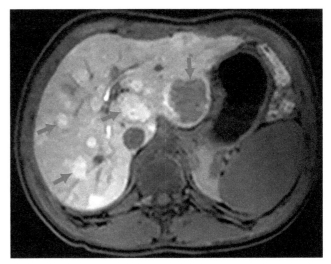

Figure S145-4 Axial image from contrast-enhanced MRI demonstrating multiple hepatic tumors (red arrows). *Courtesy of Dr. Ranjith Vellody.*

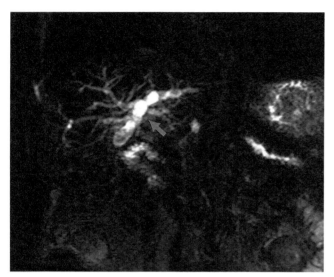

Figure S146-1 Coronal MRCP image reveals moderate, diffuse intrahepatic biliary dilatation to the level of the biliary-enteric anastomosis (red arrow) with abrupt termination at this location, compatible with biliary-enteric anastomotic stricture.

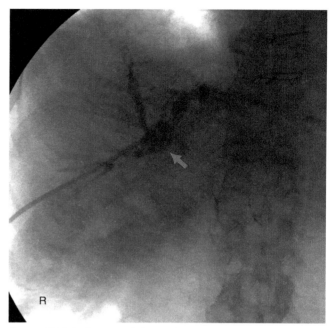

Figure S146-2 Fluoroscopic image from cholangiogram demonstrates moderate diffuse intrahepatic biliary dilatation with abrupt termination of contrast at the level of the hepaticojejunostomy (red arrow). No evidence of contrast leak seen.

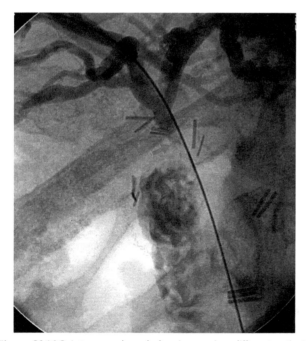

Figure S146-3 Intraprocedure cholangiogram in a different patient shows an anastomotic stricture (red arrow). *Courtesy of Dr. Daniel Brown.*

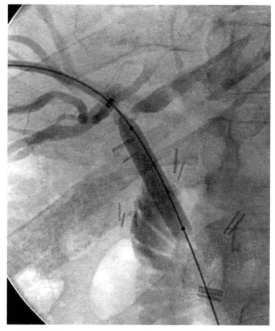

Figure S146-4 Fluoroscopic image from cholangiogram with balloon dilatation of the anastomotic stricture in the same patient as in Figure S146-3. *Courtesy of Dr. Daniel Brown.*

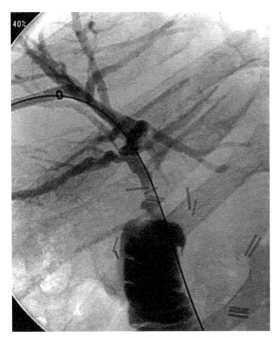

Figure S146-5 Intraprocedure cholangiography in the same patient as in Figure S146-3 shows improved luminal size and flow through the site of prior stricture (red arrow). *Courtesy of Dr. Daniel Brown.*

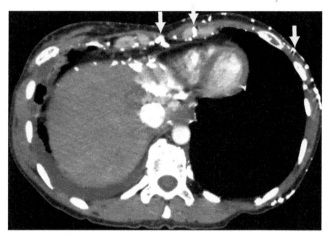

Figure S147-1 Axial image from CECT (base of the heart level) reveals hyperenhancement within numerous chest wall/abdominal wall collaterals (yellow arrows) and of the left lobe of the liver (red arrow). *Courtesy of Dr. Wael E. Saad.*

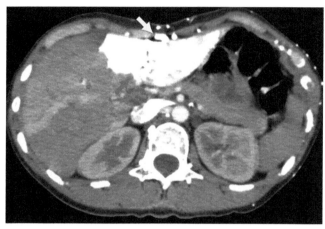

Figure S147-2 Axial image from CECT (midrenal level) demonstrates hyperenhancement of the left lobe of the liver (red arrow) and recanalized paraumbilical vein (yellow arrow). *Courtesy of Dr. Wael E. Saad.*

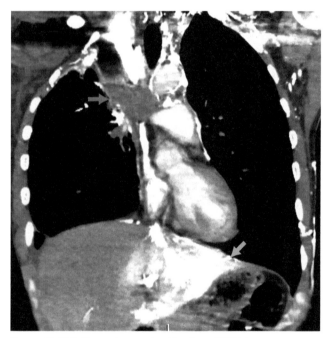

Figure S147-3 Coronal reconstruction from CECT shows a mass compressing the SVC (blue arrow) with hyperenhancement of left lobe of the liver (red arrow). *Courtesy of Dr. Wael E. Saad.*

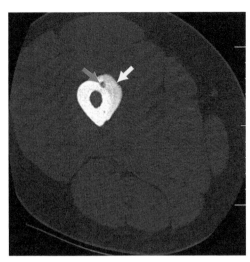

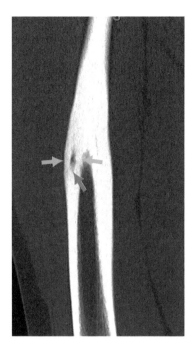

Figure S148-1 Axial image from unenhanced CT revealing a region of hypodensity within the cortex of the femur (red arrow) with surrounding sclerosis (yellow arrow) consistent with osteoid osteoma lesion. *Courtesy of Dr. Ranjith Vellody.*

Figure S148-2 Coronal reconstruction from CT demonstrating the same region of hypodensity within the cortex of the femur (red arrow) with surrounding sclerosis (blue arrows) consistent with osteoid osteoma lesion. *Courtesy of Dr. Ranjith Vellody.*

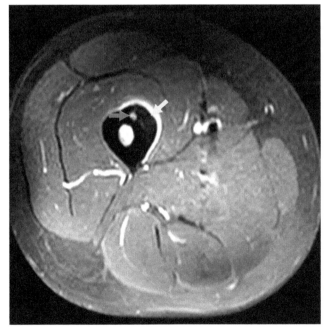

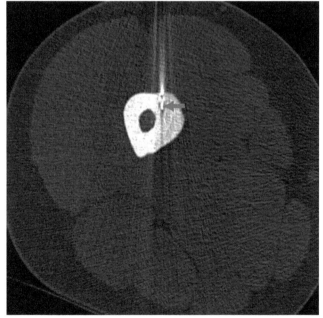

Figure S148-3 Axial T1-weighted image from contrast-enhanced MR confirming nidus (red arrow) with mildly enhancing adjacent sclerosis (yellow arrow). *Courtesy of Dr. Ranjith Vellody.*

Figure S148-4 Axial image from CT-guided RF ablation with RF probe within the lesion (red arrow). *Courtesy of Dr. Ranjith Vellody.*

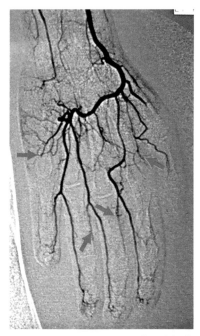

Figure S149-1 DSA image from angiography of the hand revealing several areas of stenotic or occluded digital arteries (red arrows).

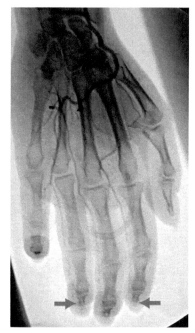

Figure S149-2 Native image from angiography of the hand demonstrating bony resorption of the distal phalanges in the same patient (red arrows).

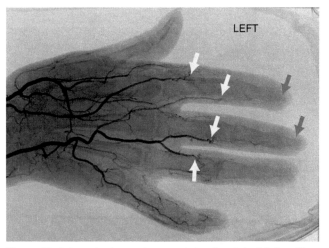

Figure S149-3 Native image from angiography of the left hand in a different patient showing several areas of stenotic or occluded digital arteries (yellow arrows) and acro-osteolysis (red arrows). *Courtesy of Dr. Narasimham L. Dasika.*

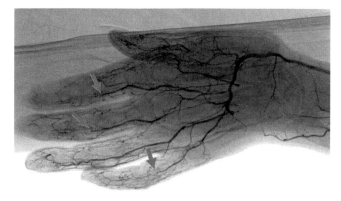

Figure S149-4 Native image from angiography of the right hand in the same patient as in Figure S149-3 confirming bilateral appearance of several stenotic or occluded digital arteries (red arrows). *Courtesy of Dr. Narasimham L. Dasika.*

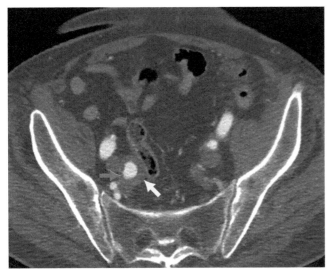

Figure S150-1 Axial image from CTA reveals a right internal iliac artery aneurysm (red arrow) with adjacent mural thrombus (yellow arrow).

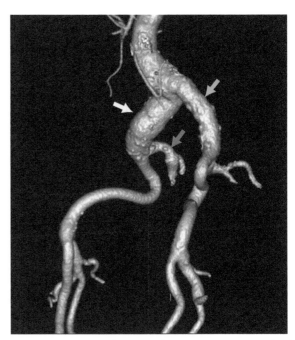

Figure S150-2 VR image from CTA demonstrates aneurysmal right common iliac (yellow arrow), right internal iliac (red arrow), and left common iliac (blue arrow) arteries.

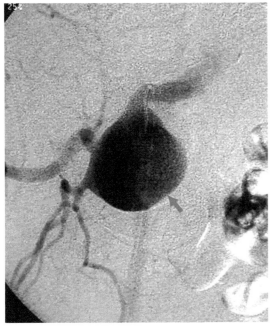

Figure S150-3 DSA image from pelvic angiogram in a different patient demonstrates focal fusiform dilation of the right internal iliac artery (red arrow), consistent with aneurysm. Also noted are branch vessels (blue arrows).

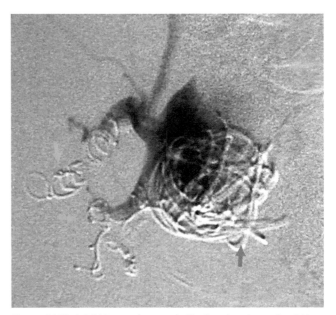

Figure S150-4 DSA image from embolization showing coils within the main aneurysm (red arrow), but also within the branch vessels (blue arrows).

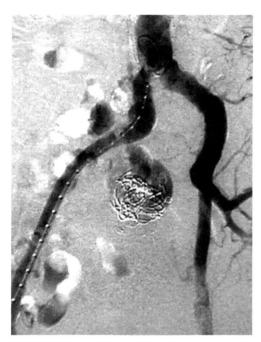

Figure S150-5 DSA image from pelvic angiogram postembolization with a marker pigtail catheter, being used to measure the vessel for stent graft placement across the origin.

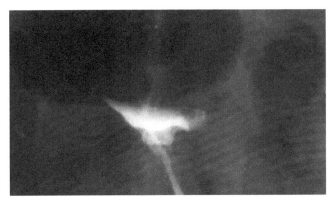

Figure S151-1 Fluoroscopic image from nonselective hysterosalpingogram reveals proximal fallopian tube occlusion, bilaterally. *Courtesy of Dr. David Hovsepian.*

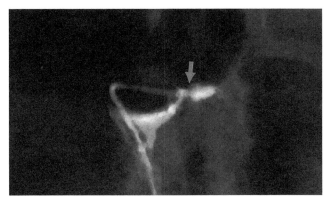

Figure S151-2 Intraprocedural image demonstrates catheterization of the left fallopian tube orifice (red arrow). *Courtesy of Dr. David Hovsepian.*

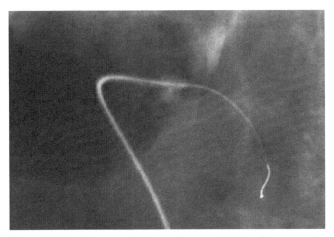

Figure S151-3 Fluoroscopic image shows guidewire advancement beyond the occlusion. *Courtesy of Dr. David Hovsepian.*

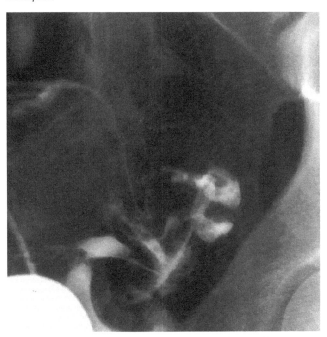

Figure S151-4 Intraprocedural image from completion salpingogram confirms spill of contrast into the peritoneal cavity after recanalization. *Courtesy of Dr. David Hovsepian.*

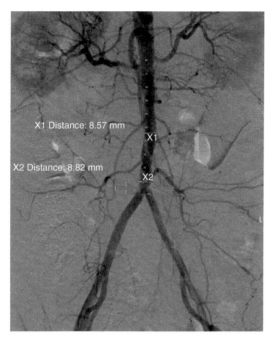

X1 Distance: 8.57 mm

X1

X2 Distance: 8.82 mm

X2

Figure S152-1 DSA image from aortogram reveals significant narrowing of the distal aorta (red arrows) that extends into the bilateral common iliac arteries. *Courtesy of Dr. Alan H. Matsumoto.*

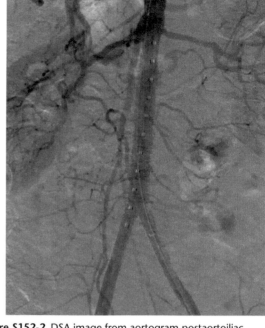

Figure S152-2 DSA image from aortogram postaortoiliac reconstruction demonstrates improved aortoiliac flow and patency of the recently placed stents. *Courtesy of Dr. Alan H. Matsumoto.*

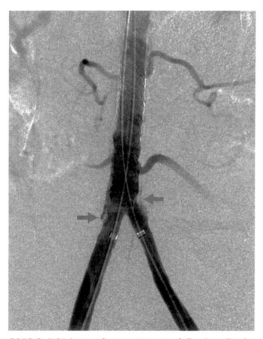

Figure S152-3 DSA image from aortogram following distal aortic stenting shows atheromatous plaque at the common iliac artery origins (red arrows). *Courtesy of Dr. Alan H. Matsumoto.*

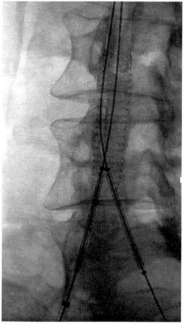

Figure S152-4 Intraoperative radiograph demonstrating kissing iliac stents in place prior to deployment. *Courtesy of Dr. Alan H. Matsumoto.*

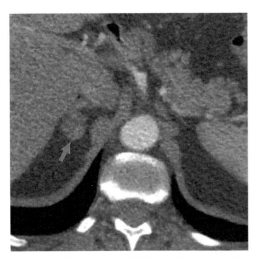

Figure S153-1 Axial image from CECT revealing a mass in the right adrenal gland (red arrow), which may represent an adrenal adenoma. *Courtesy of Dr. Kyung J. Cho.*

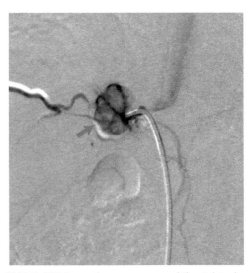

Figure S153-2 DSA image from venogram of the right adrenal vein demonstrating a vascularized mass in the adrenal gland consistent with a right adrenal adenoma (red arrow). *Courtesy of Dr. Kyung J. Cho.*

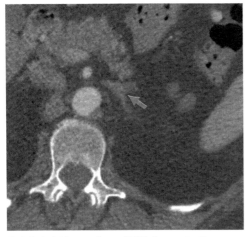

Figure S153-3 Axial image from CECT demonstrating a normal left adrenal gland (red arrow). *Courtesy of Dr. Kyung J. Cho.*

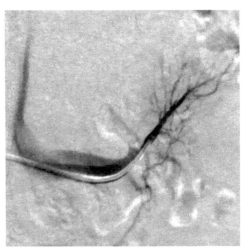

Figure S153-4 DSA image from venogram of the left adrenal vein demonstrating a normal left adrenal gland. *Courtesy of Dr. Kyung J. Cho.*

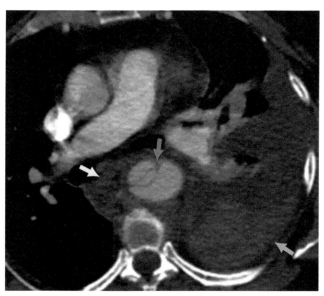

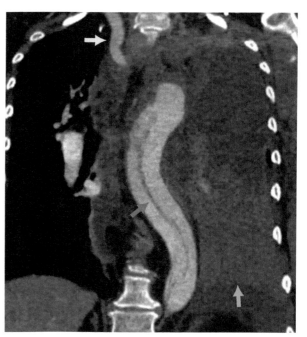

Figure S154-1 Axial CTA image reveals dissection flap within the descending thoracic aorta (red arrow) with left-sided hemothorax (blue arrow) and mediastinal hematoma (yellow arrow), consistent with rupture. *Courtesy of David M. Wiliams.*

Figure S154-2 Coronal reconstruction highlights the dissection flap (red arrow) and large left-sided hemothorax (blue arrow). Additionally noted is partial visualization of an aberrant right subclavian artery (yellow arrow). *Courtesy of David M. Wiliams.*

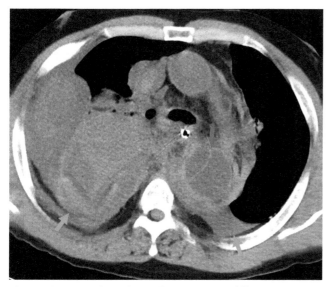

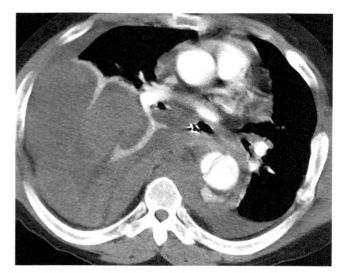

Figure S154-3 Axial-unenhanced CT image in a different patient demonstrates a dissection flap in the descending thoracic aorta (red arrow) with bilateral hemothorax (blue arrows). *Courtesy of Dr. Kyung Cho.*

Figure S154-4 Axial CTA image in the same patient as in Figure S154-3 confirms the findings of aortic dissection with rupture as above. *Courtesy of Dr. Kyung Cho.*

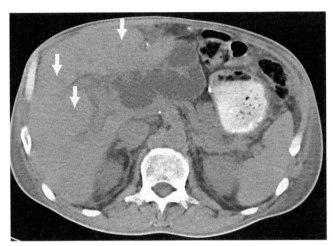

Figure S155-1 Axial image from unenhanced CT showing dilated bilateral biliary ducts (yellow arrows) and severely dilated loop of bowel coursing transversely in the midabdomen (red arrow).

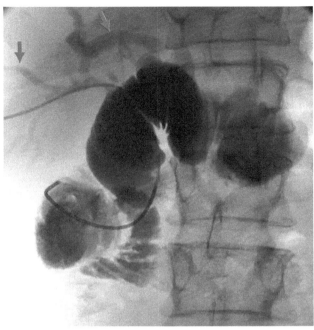

Figure S155-2 Fluoroscopic image of the abdomen confirming a percutaneously placed drainage catheter in the dilated afferent loop with the distal tip at the most proximal portion of the loop. Dilated biliary ducts can also be seen (red arrows).

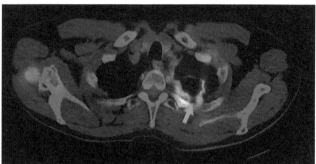

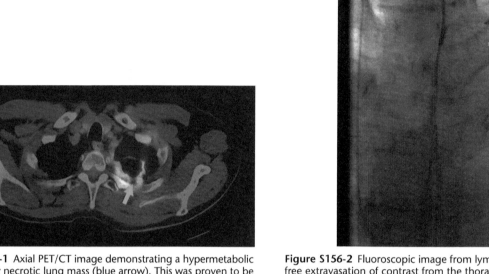

Figure S156-1 Axial PET/CT image demonstrating a hypermetabolic and centrally necrotic lung mass (blue arrow). This was proven to be nonsmall cell lung cancer for which the patient underwent a left thoracotomy and left upper lobe resection with chest wall reconstruction. *Courtesy of Dr. Bill S. Majdalany.*

Figure S156-2 Fluoroscopic image from lymphangiogram revealing free extravasation of contrast from the thoracic duct into the left pleural space and base of the neck (red arrows), diagnostic for a chylothorax. *Courtesy of Dr. Bill S. Majdalany.*

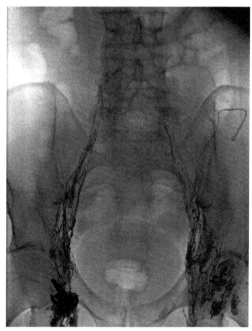

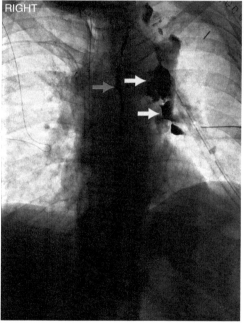

Figure S156-3 Fluoroscopic image from lymphangiogram demonstrating bilateral inguinal nodes (targets of injection) with multiple lymphatic vessels extending along the bilateral pelvis prior to opacifying the cisterna chyli and, subsequently, the thoracic duct. *Courtesy of Dr. Bill S. Majdalany.*

Figure S156-4 Fluoroscopic image of the chest following TDE. Lipiodol is seen within lymph nodes (yellow arrows). Also noted are coils within the thoracic duct (red arrow). *Courtesy of Dr. Bill S. Majdalany.*

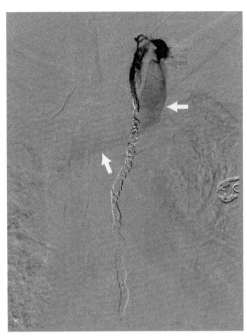

Figure S156-5 DSA image from lymphangiogram in a different patient after TDE delineating the thoracic duct emptying into the venous angle (red arrow) and flow within the left brachiocephalic vein (yellow arrows). *Courtesy of Dr. Bill S. Majdalany.*

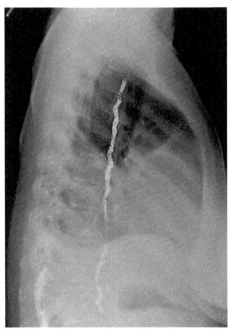

Figure S156-6 Lateral chest radiograph showing numerous coils within the thoracic duct in the same patient as in Figure S156-5. *Courtesy of Dr. Bill S. Majdalany.*

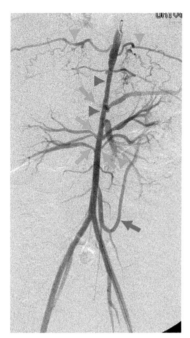

Figure S157-1 AP DSA image from early phase of abdominal aortogram reveals diffuse aortic narrowing with suprarenal aortic coarctation (red arrowheads). Also noted are dilated intercostal arteries (blue arrowheads), dilated IMA (red arrow), and stenoses of the multiple renal arteries (blue arrows). There is poor filling of the hepatic artery (green arrow) and SMA (green arrowhead). *Courtesy of Dr. Narasimham L. Dasika.*

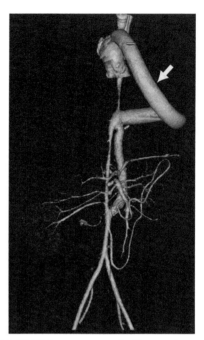

Figure S157-2 3D VR image postsurgical bypass demonstrates extensive bypass graft from ascending aorta to infrarenal aorta (yellow arrow). *Courtesy of Dr. Narasimham L. Dasika.*

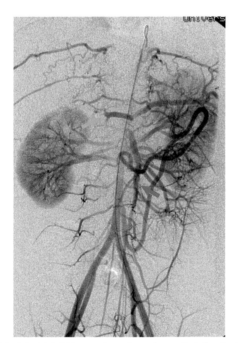

Figure S157-3 AP DSA image from late phase of abdominal aortogram shows no flow within the hepatic artery past the GDA (blue arrow) but improved delayed flow within the SMA (red arrow) from the IMA. *Courtesy of Dr. Narasimham L. Dasika.*

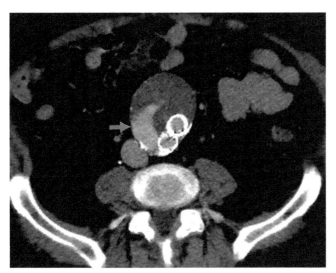

Figure S158-1 Late arterial phase axial image from CTA reveals contrast within the aneurysm sac in a patient s/p EVAR (red arrow). *Courtesy of Dr. Minhaj S. Khaja.*

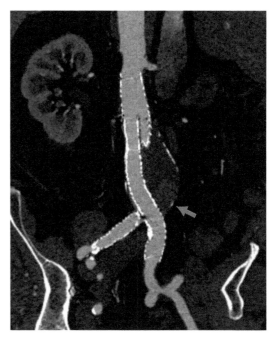

Figure S158-2 Curved MPR image from CTA shows extraluminal contrast along the right iliac limb, but not at its distal seal zone (red arrow). *Courtesy of Dr. Minhaj S. Khaja.*

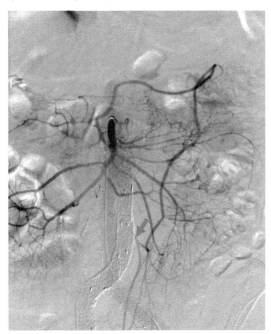

Figure S158-3 DSA image from SMA angiography shows filling of the IMA via the arc of Riolan (red arrow). *Courtesy of Dr. Minhaj S. Khaja.*

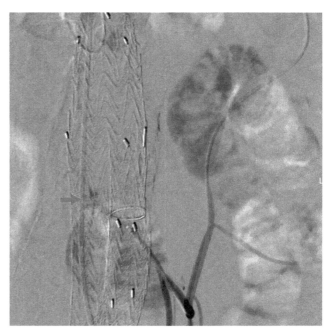

Figure S158-4 DSA image from IMA angiogram via SMA collateral pathway (Arc of Riolan) confirms contrast blush within the aneurysm sac (red arrow). *Courtesy of Dr. Minhaj S. Khaja.*

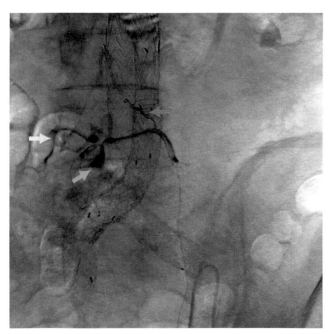

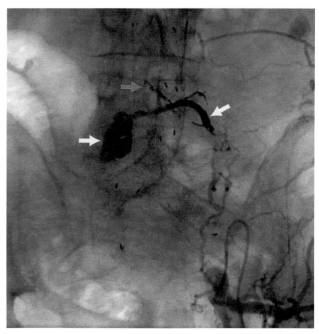

Figure S158-5 Native image from lumbar angiogram via iliolumbar collateral pathway reveals filling of contrast within the aneurysm sac (blue arrow) and outflow of contrast through the contralateral lumbar artery (yellow arrow). Also noted are coils within the IMA ostium (red arrow). *Courtesy of Dr. Minhaj S. Khaja.*

Figure S158-6 Native image from iliolumbar angiogram following embolization of the endoleak with ethylene vinyl alcohol copolymer (yellow arrows) and coils (red arrow) confirms occlusion of collateral vessels and no filling of the aneurysm sac. *Courtesy of Dr. Minhaj S. Khaja.*

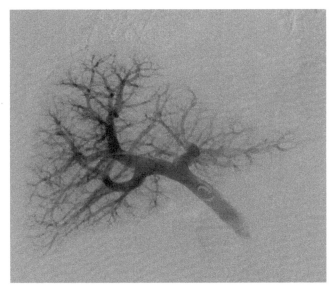

Figure S159-1 DSA image from portogram via transhepatic access reveals a patent right and left portal system, prior to embolization. *Courtesy of Dr. Wael E. Saad.*

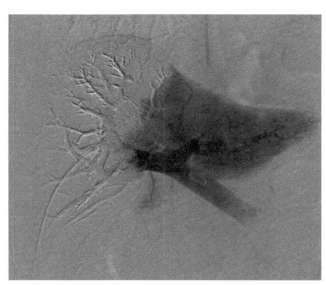

Figure S159-2 DSA image from portogram after right portal vein embolization demonstrates occluded right portal vein branches with cast formation from *n*-BCA glue. *Courtesy of Dr. Wael E. Saad.*

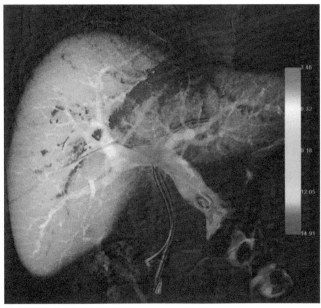

Figure S159-3 Color-coded, quantitative DSA image s/p iFlow (Siemens AG) processing demonstrating high-intensity perfusion within portal venous system. Flow of blood within the hepatic veins is coded as low intensity, shown in blue. *Courtesy of Dr. Wael E. Saad.*

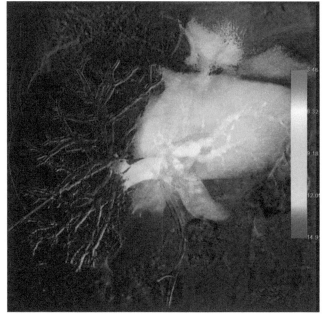

Figure S159-4 Color-coded, quantitative DSA image after right portal vein embolization s/p iFlow (Siemens AG) processing demonstrating high-intensity perfusion within the left portal venous system. The embolized right hepatic lobe appears low-intensity blue. *Courtesy of Dr. Wael E. Saad.*

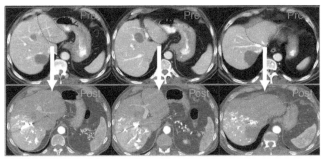

Figure S159-5 CECT images pre and postembolization demonstrating hypertrophy of the left hepatic lobe function liver remnant after right portal vein embolization. *Courtesy of Dr. Wael E. Saad.*

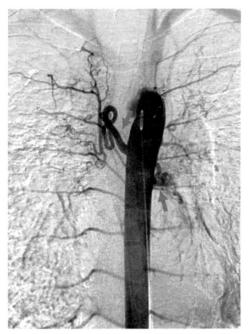

Figure S160-1 DSA image from descending thoracic aortogram demonstrates enlarged bronchial arteries (red arrows), right greater than left, and hypervascularity in a patient with hemoptysis.

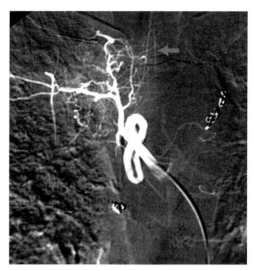

Figure S160-2 DSA image from a selective right bronchial arteriogram shows a tortuous bronchial artery. Importantly, a spinal artery is seen to arise from the proximal aspect of the right bronchial artery (red arrow). The vessel takes a characteristic hairpin turn before entering the vertebral canal to supply the spinal cord.

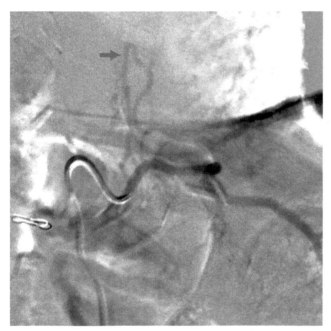

Figure S160-3 DSA image of a selective left intercostal angiogram in a different patient reveals a segmental medullary artery in classic hairpin configuration (red arrow) arising from the intercostal artery.

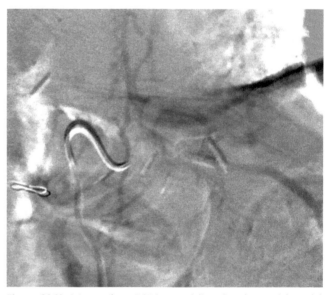

Figure S160-4 Later-phase DSA image delineating the cranial-caudal extent of the vessel from the single level injection.

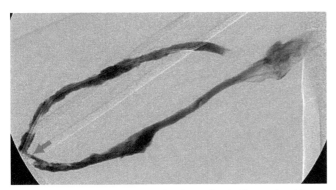

Figure S161-1 DSA image from fistulography (midprocedure) in a patient who presented with a thrombosed graft shows stenosis at the apex of the graft (red arrow) with multiple filling defects representing thrombus.

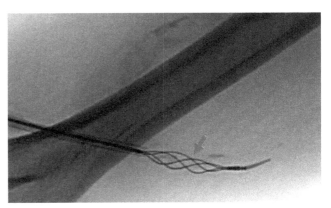

Figure S161-2 Native image from declot procedure showing a mechanical thrombectomy device within the graft (red arrow).

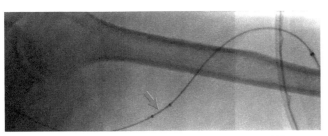

Figure S161-3 Native image from declot procedure in a different patient showing a rheolytic thrombectomy device within a fistula (red arrow).

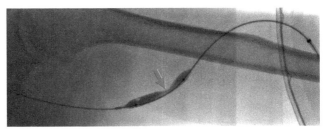

Figure S161-4 Native image from declot procedure in the same patient as in Figure S161-3 demonstrating a balloon with "waist" at the site of stenosis (red arrow).

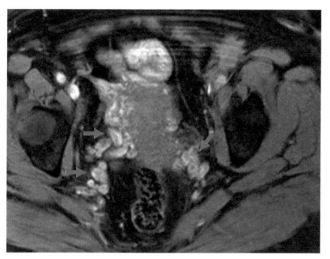

Figure S162-1 Axial T1-weighted fat-saturated postcontrast image reveals bilateral serpiginous parauterine vessels (red arrows).

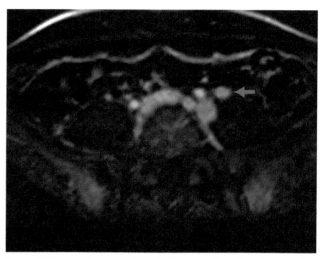

Figure S162-2 Axial image from MRV shows the dilated, patent left ovarian vein (red arrow).

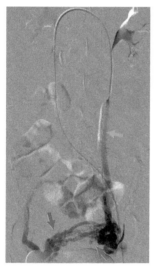

Figure S162-3 Digital subtraction venography (DSV) image confirms a dilated left ovarian vein (blue arrow) with cross-pelvic collaterals (red arrows).

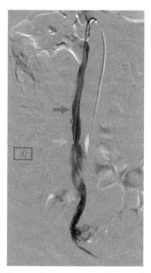

Figure S162-4 DSV image from venography confirms retrograde flow into an enlarged right ovarian vein (red arrow). Two distinct venous channels are present, branching near the tip of the catheter (blue arrow) and traveling distally to the congested vessels in the pelvis.

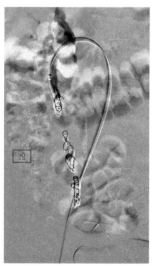

Figure S162-5 DSV image of the right gonadal vein postcoil embolization of both venous channels does not show any passage of contrast distally or any collateral draining veins.

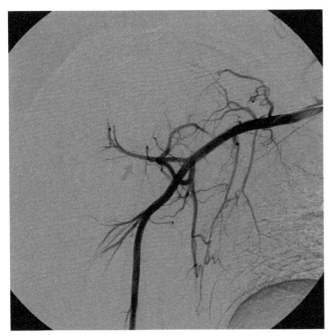

Figure S163-1 DSA image from right upper extremity angiogram with shoulder in a neutral position showing patent posterior humeral circumflex artery (red arrow).

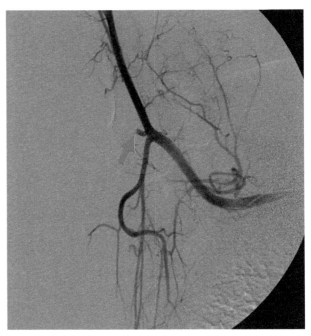

Figure S163-2 DSA image from angiogram while arm is in abduction and external rotation revealing complete occlusion and absence of flow beyond the proximal posterior humeral circumflex artery (red arrow).

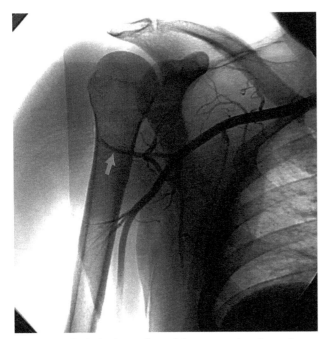

Figure S163-3 Native image from right upper extremity angiogram with shoulder in a neutral position showing patent posterior humeral circumflex artery (red arrow).

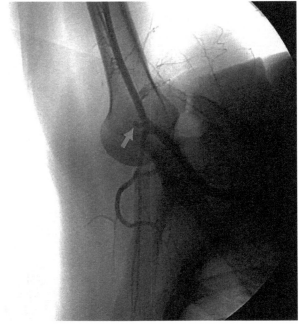

Figure S163-4 Native image from angiogram while arm is in abduction and external rotation revealing complete occlusion and absence of flow beyond the proximal posterior humeral circumflex artery (red arrow).

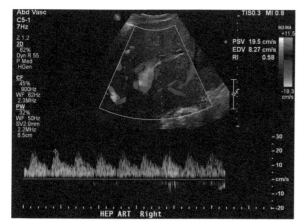

Figure S164-1 Color Doppler image from liver ultrasound demonstrates arterial resistive index of 0.58 within the right hepatic artery in a patient with graft dysfunction. *Courtesy of Dr. Wael E. Saad.*

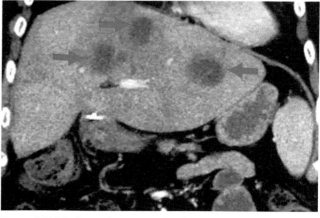

Figure S164-2 Coronal reconstruction from CT in the same patient reveals regions of hypodensity within the liver (red arrows) compatible with ischemic necrosis and biloma formation. *Courtesy of Dr. Wael E. Saad.*

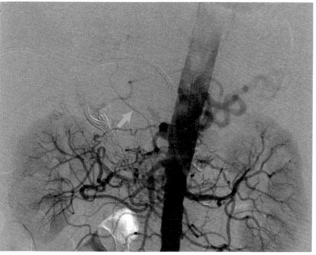

Figure S164-3 DSA image from early phase of aortogram reveals occlusion of the hepatic artery (red arrow) with numerous collaterals including a retroportal artery (blue arrow). *Courtesy of Dr. Wael E. Saad.*

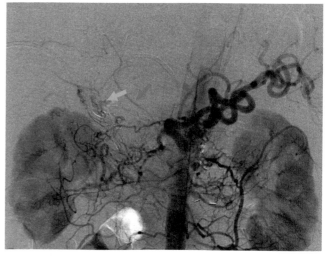

Figure S164-4 DSA image from midphase of aortogram illustrates omental arterial branches (blue arrow) and the retroportal artery (red arrow). *Courtesy of Dr. Wael E. Saad.*

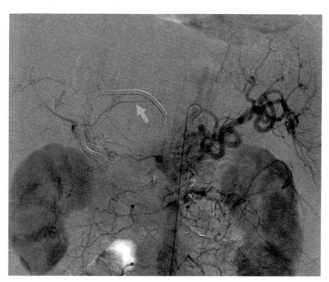

Figure S164-5 DSA image from late-phase of aortogram shows reconstitution of the left (blue arrow) and right (red arrow) hepatic arteries by the omental and retroportal branches seen earlier. *Courtesy of Dr. Wael E. Saad.*

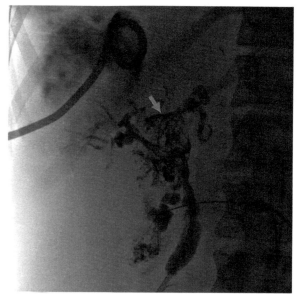

Figure S164-6 Radiograph from cholangiogram in a different patient reveals biliary necrosis with casts (red arrow). This appearance has been described as "shaggy biliary necrosis" (editor's term). *Courtesy of Dr. Wael E. Saad.*

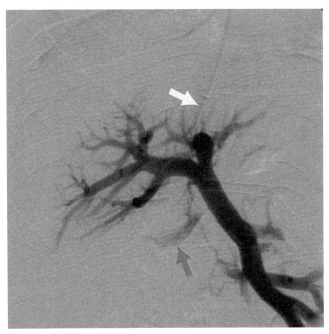

Figure S165-1 DSA image from portogram during TIPS placement revealing extravasation from the portal vein along the caudal margin of the liver (red arrow). Transjugular TIPS access noted (yellow arrow). *Courtesy of Dr. Wael E. Saad.*

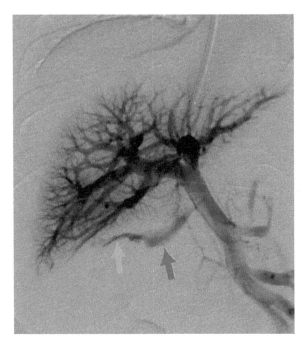

Figure S165-2 Late-phase DSA image from portogram during TIPS placement confirming extension (blue arrow) of extravasation (red arrow) along the caudal margin of the liver. *Courtesy of Dr. Wael E. Saad.*

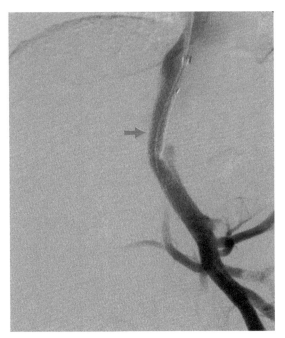

Figure S165-3 DSA image from portogram following TIPS placement (red arrow) showing patency of the TIPS without evidence of extravasation from portal venous injury. *Courtesy of Dr. Wael E. Saad.*

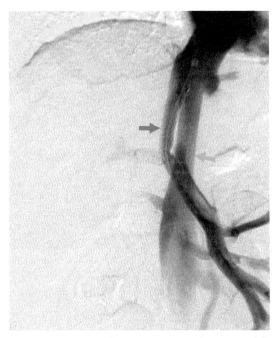

Figure S165-4 DSA image from portogram and cavagram following TIPS placement (red arrow) showing patency of the TIPS and its placement in relation to the IVC (blue arrow). *Courtesy of Dr. Wael E. Saad.*

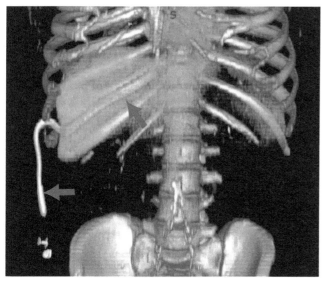

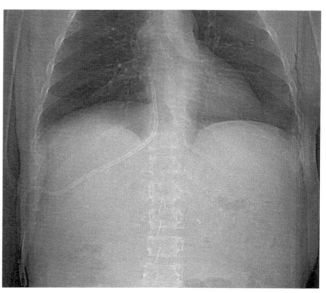

Figure S166-1 3D reconstruction from CT abdomen demonstrating a transhepatic central venous catheter (red arrows) traversing the liver and terminating in the right atrium.

Figure S166-2 Scout images from CT in the same patient as above showing the course of the transhepatic central venous catheter.

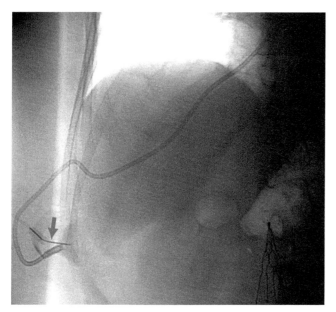

Figure S166-3 Fluoroscopic image in a different patient illustrating a transhepatic central venous catheter with a needle accessing the subcutaneous port (red arrow).

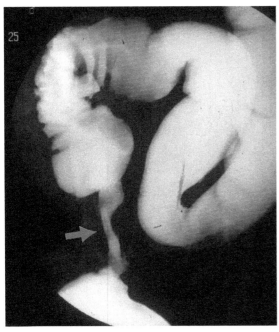

Figure S167-1 AP fluoroscopic image from barium enema revealing a region of stricture at the rectosigmoid junction consistent with colorectal cancer (red arrow). *Courtesy of Dr. Narasimham L. Dasika.*

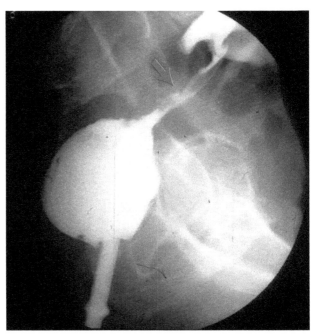

Figure S167-2 Lateral fluoroscopic image from barium enema redemonstrating a region of stricture at the rectosigmoid junction consistent with colorectal cancer (red arrow). *Courtesy of Dr. Narasimham L. Dasika.*

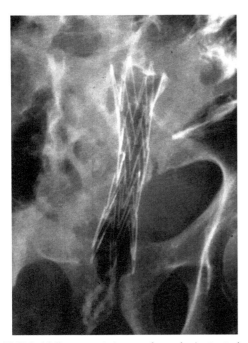

Figure S167-3 AP fluoroscopic image after colonic stent placement confirming its position. *Courtesy of Dr. Narasimham L. Dasika.*

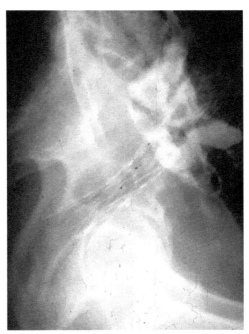

Figure S167-4 Lateral fluoroscopic image after colonic stent placement confirming its position. *Courtesy of Dr. Narasimham L. Dasika.*

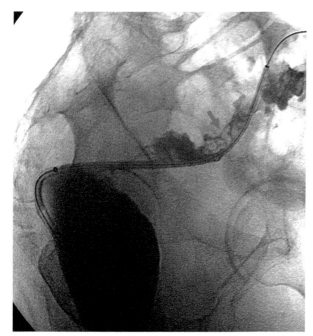

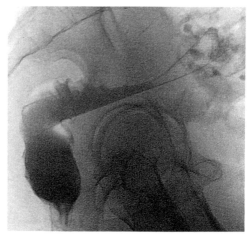

Figure S167-5 Lateral fluoroscopic image from enema in a different patient showing Wallstent across the obstruction prior to deployment and expansion. Contrast highlights the colon proximal to the obstruction with poor transit across the long segment of obstruction (red arrow). *Courtesy of Dr. James R. Duncan.*

Figure S167-6 Lateral fluoroscopic image after Wallstent placement confirming flow of contrast and alleviation of obstruction. *Courtesy of Dr. James R. Duncan.*

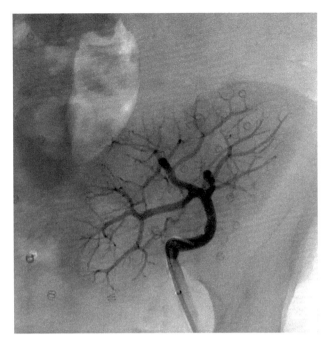

Figure S168-1 Native image from transplant renal angiogram showing perfusion throughout the kidney. *Courtesy of Dr. Minhaj S. Khaja.*

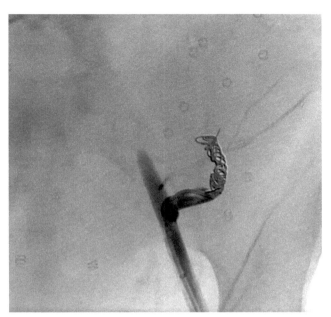

Figure S168-2 Native image from angiogram confirming embolization/ablation of the transplant renal artery with absolute alcohol and coils. *Courtesy of Dr. Minhaj S. Khaja.*

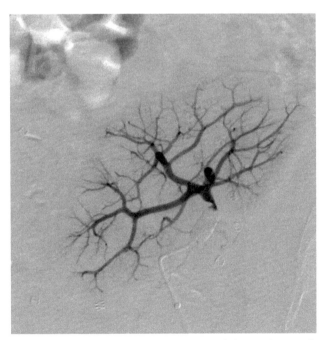

Figure S168-3 DSA image from balloon-occluded transplant renal angiogram delineating the arterial anatomy. This is performed to confirm the volume of inflation of the balloon to avoid reflux of alcohol and to calculate the volume of alcohol required to fill the distal arterial branches. *Courtesy of Dr. Minhaj S. Khaja.*

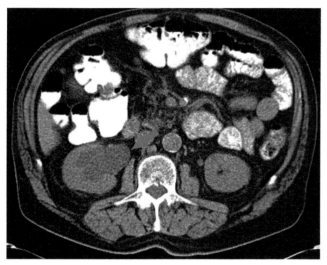

Figure S169-1 Axial noncontrast CT image reveals right-sided hydronephrosis (red arrow).

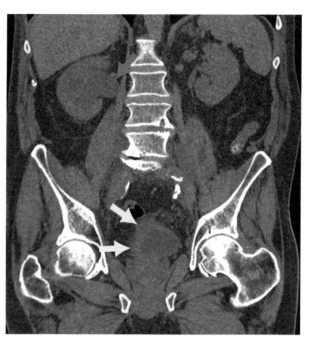

Figure S169-2 Coronal reconstruction demonstrates right-sided hydronephrosis (red arrow). Lateral bladder wall thickening is partially visualized at the expected location of ureteral insertion (yellow arrows). Patient was ultimately diagnosed with transitional cell carcinoma with ureteral obstruction at the UVJ.

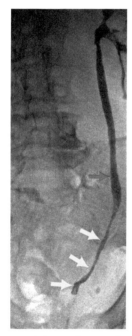

Figure S169-3 Fluoroscopic image from pyelography confirms ureteral dilatation (red arrow). Ureteral stricture is evident distally at the UVJ from the patient's known bladder wall carcinoma (yellow arrows).

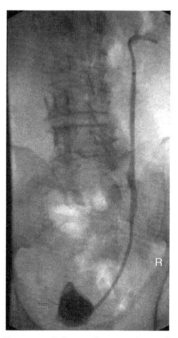

Figure S169-4 Fluoroscopic image from pyelography postnephroureteral catheter placement. Focal stricture at the UVJ is traversed with contrast noted distally in the bladder (red arrow).

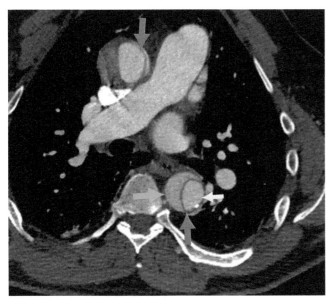

Figure S170-1 Axial image from CTA of the chest revealing a type A aortic dissection with flap (red arrows) involving the ascending and descending thoracic aorta. True (yellow arrow) and false (blue arrow) lumens are also seen clearly in the descending thoracic aorta. *Courtesy of Dr. David M. Williams.*

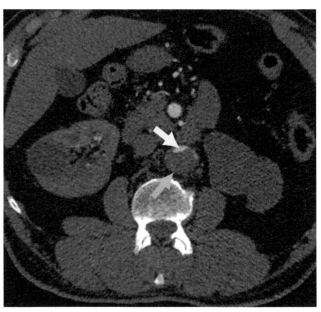

Figure S170-2 Axial image from CTA in the infrarenal aorta demonstrates severe compression of the true lumen (yellow arrow) by the enlarged, partially false lumen (blue arrow). *Courtesy of Dr. David M. Williams.*

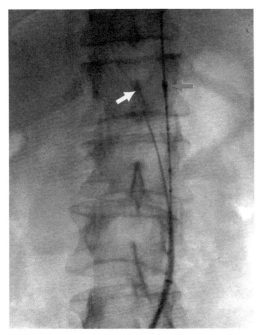

Figure S170-3 Intraoperative radiograph from aortic fenestration procedure shows intravascular ultrasound (IVUS) probe in the true lumen (red arrow) with wire in the false lumen (yellow arrow) following fenestration. *Courtesy of Dr. David M. Williams.*

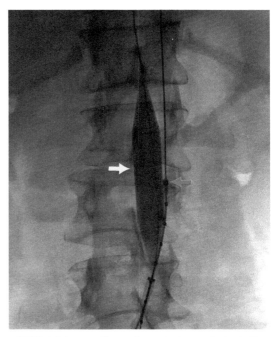

Figure S170-4 Intraoperative radiograph demonstrates balloon aortoplasty (yellow arrow) across the newly created fenestration. IVUS probe again noted within the true lumen (red arrow). *Courtesy of Dr. David M. Williams.*

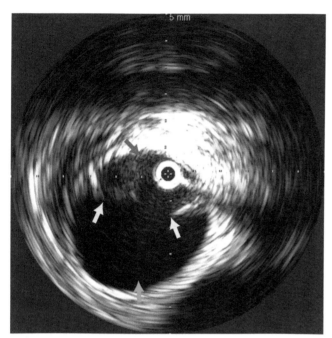

Figure S170-5 IVUS image after balloon fenestration highlights the true lumen (red arrow), false lumen (blue arrow), and fenestration site (between yellow arrows). *Courtesy of Dr. David M. Williams.*

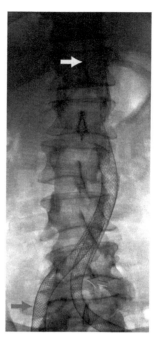

Figure S170-6 Intraoperative radiograph following stenting illustrates suprarenal (yellow arrow) as well as infrarenal aortoiliac stents (red arrows). *Courtesy of Dr. David M. Williams.*

Note: Page numbers followed by e indicate online material.

INDEX OF TERMS

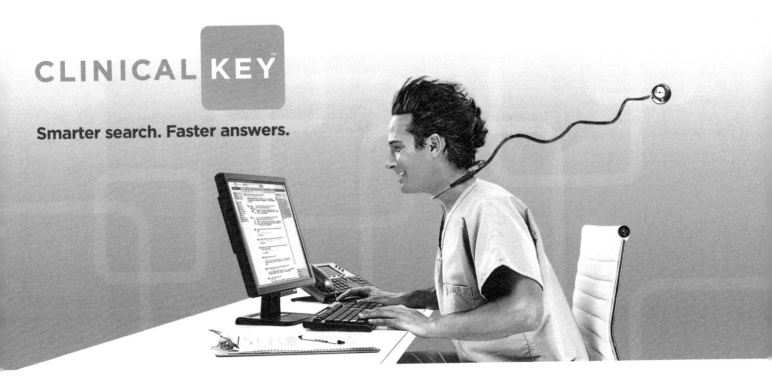

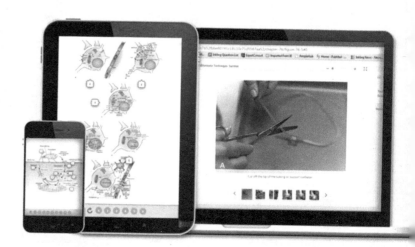

Any screen.
Any time.
Anywhere.

Activate the eBook version
of this title at no additional charge.

Expert Consult eBooks give you the power to browse and find content,
view enhanced images, share notes and highlights—both online and offline.

Unlock your eBook today.

1. Visit **expertconsult.inkling.com/redeem**
2. Scratch off your code
3. Type code into "Enter Code" box
4. Click "Redeem"
5. Log in or Sign up
6. Go to "My Library"

It's that easy!

Scan this QR code to redeem your
eBook through your mobile device:

Place Peel Off
Sticker Here

For technical assistance:
email expertconsult.help@elsevier.com
call 1-800-401-9962 (inside the US)
call +1-314-447-8200 (outside the US)

ELSEVIER